GUIDE TO NUTRITIONAL SUPPLEMENTS

GUIDE TO NUTRITIONAL SUPPLEMENTS

Editor
BENJAMIN CABALLERO

Elsevier Ltd., The Boulevard, Langford Lane, Kidlington, Oxford, OX5 1GB, UK

© 2009 Elsevier Ltd.

The following articles are US Government works in the
public domain and not subject to copyright:

CAROTENOIDS/Chemistry, Sources and Physiology

VEGETARIAN DIETS

Material in this work originally appeared in the *Encyclopedia of Human Nutrition, Second Edition,*
edited by Benjamin Caballero, Lindsay Allen and Andrew Prentice (Elsevier, Ltd 2005).

Library of Congress Control Number: 2009929980

A catalogue record for this book is available from the British Library

ISBN 978-0-12-375109-6

This book is printed on acid-free paper
Printed and bound in the EU

EDITORIAL ADVISORY BOARD

PREFACE

The use of dietary supplements continues to increase worldwide. In the US, sales of dietary supplement is reaching $30 billion per year, but their use transcend cultural barriers, and dietary supplement products now can be found virtually anywhere in the world.

One reason for the widespread use of dietary supplements is the increasing concern in the general population about diet-related chronic diseases, such as diabetes, arthritis, and cardiovascular diseases. In addition, limited access to preventive health care (particularly in the US) may encourage people to self-medicate, as a means to reduce any perceived risk of disease. Claims on the curative properties of dietary supplements abound, many times based on individual testimonials or unsubstantiated data. Still, most health practitioners are likely to confront the decision of whether to recommend (or to allow) a nutritional supplement, based on their own experience and on the best scientific evidence available.

This compilation of articles from the acclaimed EHN focuses on nutritional supplements[1]. These include the traditional, well-known substances such as vitamins and major minerals, present in most diets consumed by humans. They also include other food constituents such as certain fatty acids and amino acids, fiber, carotenoids, and other compounds. Some of these may not have a defined nutritional role, but do affect health by their involvement in specific physiological functions. In addition, several chapters describe key biological mechanisms related to dietary supplement effects, such as cellular antioxidant activity.

We trust that the scientific information provided in this compilation will assist the health care professional and the educated consumer in making reasonable choices when dealing with the sometimes limited evidence on supplements' effects. We also hope that this book will provide a scientific basis for assessing the validity of claims and indications of the ever increasing number of supplements that are coming into the market.

Benjamin Caballero
Johns Hopkins University, Maryland USA

---

[1] The other group of supplements would include botanicals, extracts from animal tissues, and other compounds not commonly present in human diets.

CONTRIBUTORS

L H Allen
University of California at Davis,
Davis, CA, USA

J J B Anderson
University of North Carolina,
Chapel Hill, NC, USA

L J Appel
Johns Hopkins University,
Baltimore, MD, USA

M J Arnaud
Nestle S.A.,
Vevey, Switzerland

A Ariño
University of Zaragoza,
Zaragoza, Spain

G E Bartley
Agricultural Research Service,
Albany, CA, USA

C J Bates
MRC Human Nutrition Research,
Cambridge, UK

J A Beltrán
University of Zaragoza,
Zaragoza, Spain

D A Bender
University College London,
London, UK

I F F Benzie
The Hong Kong Polytechnic University,
Hong Kong, China

A Cassidy
School of Medicine, University of East Anglia,
Norwich, UK

L Cobiac
CSIRO Health Sciences and Nutrition,
Adelaide, SA, Australia

C H C Dejong
University Hospital Maastricht,
Maastricht, The Netherlands

M L Dreyfuss
Johns Hopkins Bloomberg School of Public Health,
Baltimore, MD, USA

J Dwyer
Tufts University,
Boston, MA, USA

C A Edwards
University of Glasgow,
Glasgow, UK

J L Ensunsa
University of California at Davis,
Davis, CA, USA

C Feillet-Coudray
National Institute for Agricultural Research,
Clermont-Ferrand, France

H C Freake
University of Connecticut,
Storrs, CT, USA

L Galland
Applied Nutrition Inc.,
New York, NY, USA

M Gueimonde
University of Turku,
Turku, Finland

Z L Harris
Johns Hopkins Hospital and School of Medicine,
Baltimore, MD, USA

A Herrera
University of Zaragoza,
Zaragoza, Spain

B S Hetzel
Women's and Children's Hospital,
North Adelaide, SA, Australia

J M Hodgson
University of Western Australia, Perth, WA, Australia

M F Holick
Boston University Medical Center,
Boston, MA, USA

C Hotz
National Institute of Public Health,
Morelos, Mexico

R Houston
Emory University, Atlanta,
GA, USA

B K Ishida
Agricultural Research Service,
Albany, CA, USA

W P T James
International Association for the Study of Obesity
International Obesity Task Force Offices,
London, UK

S A Jebb
MRC Human Nutrition Research,
Cambridge, UK

I T Johnson
Institute of Food Research,
Norwich, UK

C L Keen
University of California at Davis,
Davis, CA, USA

J E Kerstetter
University of Connecticut,
Storrs, CT, USA

M Kiely
University College Cork,
Cork, Ireland

P Kirk
University of Ulster,
Coleraine, UK

R D W Klemm
Johns Hopkins University,
Baltimore, MD, USA

D Kritchevsky
Wistar Institute,
Philadelphia, PA, USA

R Lang
University of Teeside,
Middlesbrough, UK

A Laurentin
Universidad Central de Venezuela,
Caracas, Venezuela

A R Leeds
King's College London,
London, UK

B Lönnerdal
University of California at Davis,
Davis, CA, USA

Y C Luiking
University Hospital Maastricht,
Maastricht, The Netherlands

R J Maughan
Loughborough University,
Loughborough, UK

S S McDonald
Raleigh, NC, USA

J McPartlin
Trinity College,
Dublin, Ireland

R P Mensink
Maastricht University,
Maastricht, The Netherlands

A R Michell
St Bartholomew's Hospital,
London, UK

D M Mock
University of Arkansas for Medical Sciences,
Little Rock, AR, USA

T A Mori
University of Western Australia, Perth, WA, Australia

P A Morrissey
University College Cork,
Cork, Ireland

J L Napoli
University of California,
Berkeley, CA, USA

F Nielsen
Grand Forks Human Nutrition Research Center,
Grand Forks, ND, USA

S S Percival
University of Florida,
Gainesville, FL, USA

M F Picciano
National Institutes of Health,
Bethesda, MD, USA

S Pin
Johns Hopkins Hospital and School of Medicine,
Baltimore, MD, USA

Y Rayssiguier
National Institute for Agricultural Research,
Clermont-Ferrand, France

P Roncalés
University of Zaragoza,
Zaragoza, Spain

A C Ross
The Pennsylvania State University,
University Park, PA, USA

M J Sadler
MJSR Associates,
Ashford, UK

S Salminen
University of Turku,
Turku, Finland

C P Sánchez-Castillo
National Institute of Medical Sciences and Nutrition,
Salvador Zubirán, Tlalpan, Mexico

K J Schulze
Johns Hopkins Bloomberg School of Public Health,
Baltimore, MD, USA

J Shedlock
Johns Hopkins Hospital and School of Medicine,
Baltimore, MD, USA

R Shrimpton
Institute of Child Health,
London, UK

A P Simopoulos
The Center for Genetics, Nutrition and Health,
Washington, DC, USA

P B Soeters
University Hospital Maastricht,
Maastricht, The Netherlands

K Srinath Reddy
All India Institute of Medical Sciences,
New Delhi, India

S Stanner
British Nutrition Foundation,
London, UK

J J Strain
University of Ulster,
Coleraine, UK

C L Stylianopoulos
Johns Hopkins University,
Baltimore, MD, USA

S A Tanumihardjo
University of Wisconsin-Madison,
Madison, WI, USA

E H M Temme
University of Leuven,
Leuven, Belgium

D I Thurnham
University of Ulster,
Coleraine, UK

D L Topping
CSIRO Health Sciences and Nutrition,
Adelaide, SA, Australia

M G Traber
Oregon State University,
Corvallis, OR, USA

M C G van de Poll
University Hospital Maastricht,
Maastricht, The Netherlands

M L Wahlqvist
Monash University,
Victoria, VIC, Australia

P A Watkins
Kennedy Krieger Institute and Johns Hopkins University
School of Medicine,
Baltimore, MD, USA

K P West Jr
Johns Hopkins University,
Baltimore, MD, USA

H Wiseman
King's College London,
London, UK

X Xu
Johns Hopkins Hospital and School of Medicine,
Baltimore, MD, USA

Z Yang
University of Wisconsin-Madison,
Madison, WI, USA

S H Zeisel
University of North Carolina at Chapel Hill,
Chapel Hill, NC, USA

X Zhu
University of North Carolina at Chapel Hill,
Chapel Hill, NC, USA

S Zidenberg-Cherr
University of California at Davis,
Davis, CA, USA

CONTENTS

AMINO ACIDS

Specific Functions

M C G van de Poll, Y C Luiking, C H C Dejong and P B Soeters, University Hospital Maastricht, Maastricht, The Netherlands

Introduction

Apart from being the building blocks of proteins, many amino acids are indispensable for certain vital functions or have specific functions of their own. They can function as neurotransmitters, as precursors for neurotransmitters and other important metabolites, including crucial oligo- and polypeptides, as a stimulus for hormonal release, and in inter-organ nitrogen transport and nitrogen excretion. Consequently, manipulation of free amino acid levels by dietary or topical supplementation may support and modulate these specific functions.

Amino Acid Flux, Concentration, and Function

Many amino acids have specific functions or support specific functions by serving as precursors or substrates for reactions in which vital end products are produced. The availability of amino acids to serve these purposes is determined by the rate at which they are released into the plasma and other pools in which these reactions take place, as well as by the rate of disappearance through excretion, protein synthesis, or conversion to other amino acids. The rate of this release, referred to as amino acid flux, is determined by the breakdown of (dietary) proteins or the conversion from other amino acids. Increased demand for one or more amino acids generally leads to an increased flux of the required amino acids across specific organs. Since it is the flux of an amino acid that determines its availability for metabolic processes, the flux is far more important for maintenance of specific functions than the plasma concentration. In fact it is striking that fluxes of some amino acids can double without significantly affecting plasma levels despite the fact that the plasma pool may be quantitatively negligible compared to the flux per hour. Plasma amino acid concentrations must therefore be subject to strong regulatory mechanisms. Increased demand and utilization of a specific amino acid may lead to decreased plasma and tissue concentrations, which may act as a signal to increase flux. Thus, a low plasma concentration in itself does not necessarily imply that the supply of the amino acid in question is inadequate, but it may indicate that there is increased turnover of the amino acid and that deficiencies may result when dietary or endogenous supply is inadequate. Other factors determining amino acid concentration are induction of enzymes and stimulation or blocking of specific amino acid transporters affecting the exchange and distribution of amino acids between different compartments. The regulation of plasma and tissue concentrations of specific amino acids may also be executed by the fact that release of the amino acid by an organ (e.g., muscle) and the uptake of that amino acid by another organ (e.g., liver) are subject to a highly integrated network including the action of cytokines and other hormones.

By repeated conversion of one amino acid to another, metabolic pathways arise by which (part of) the carbon backbone of a single amino acid can pass through a succession of different amino acids. Because of this interconvertibility, groups of amino acids rather than one specific amino acid contribute to specific functions. Apart from the rate at which these amino acids interconvert, the rate at which they gain access to the tissue where the specific end products exert their functions is also an important determinant of deficiencies of amino acids.

Amino acid Deficiencies and Supplementation

In many diseases and during undernutrition diminished turnover of amino acids can occur. These deficiencies may concern specific amino acids in certain diseases or a more generalized amino acid deficiency. The resulting functional deficits can contribute to the symptoms, severity, and progress of the disease. In some instances these deficits can be counteracted by simple supplementation of the deficient amino acids. Amino acid supplementation is also applied to enhance turnover and improve amino acid function in nondeficient patients. However, amino acid supplementation in nondeficient states does not necessarily lead to an increased function since the organism utilizes what is programed by regulating hormones and cytokines. An additional factor to consider is that metabolic processes can be subject to counter-regulatory feedback mechanisms. Some important metabolic processes served by a specific amino acid require only a marginal part of the total flux of that amino acid. The question may be raised whether true shortages may arise in such pathways, and supplemented amino acids may be disposed of in pathways other than those serving to improve a specific function.

Assessment of Amino Acid Function

The effectiveness of amino acid supplementation, particularly with respect to clinical effectiveness, can be assessed at four levels. First, the intervention should lead to an increased local or systemic concentration of the amino acid in question. The conversion of amino acids in (interorgan) metabolic pathways can lead to an increase in the levels of amino acids other than the one supplemented, increasing or mediating its functionality. Alternatively, supplementation of one amino acid may decrease the uptake of other amino acids because they compete for a common transporter. Second, the metabolic process for which the supplemented amino acid forms the substrate should be stimulated or upregulated by this increased amino acid availability. Third, this enhanced metabolic activity must lead to physiological changes. Fourth, these changes must be clinically effective in a desirable fashion.

Table 1 Specific functions of amino acids and their intermediate products

Amino acid	Intermediate products	Function	Supplementation efficacy
Alanine	Pyruvate	Gluconeogenesis Nitrogen transport	Data too limited
Arginine	Nitric oxide	Vasodilation Immunomodulation Neurotransmission	Positive effects of arginine-containing immunonutrition on morbidity in surgical and trauma patients suggested; further research required
	Urea	Ammonia detoxification	
	Creatine	Muscle constituent/fuel	
	Agmatine	Cell signaling Ornithine precursor	
Citrulline	Arginine production		
Ornithine	Polyamines	Cell differentiation	Improves healing of burns (ornithine α-ketoglutarate)
		Proline precursor	
Proline	Hydroxyproline	Hepatocyte DNA, protein synthesis Collagen synthesis	
Asparagine		Aspartic acid precursor	(Asparaginase-induced asparagine depletion is therapeutic in leukemia)
Aspartic acid	Oxaloacetate, fumarate	Gluconeogenesis	
Methionine		Cysteine precursor	
	Creatine	(*see* arginine)	
Cysteine (Cystine)	Glutathione	Antioxidant	Improves antioxidant status in undernutrition, inflammatory diseases
	Taurine	Bile acid conjugation, neuronal cell development, regulation of membrane potential, calcium transport, antioxidant	Reduces contrast-induced nephropathy in renal failure Mucolysis, symptom reduction in COPD Hepatoprotective in acetaminophen intoxication
Glutamic acid	Glutamine α-ketoglutarate Glutathione γ-aminobutyric acid	Ammonia disposal Gluconeogenesis Antioxidant Inhibition CNS Excitation CNS (NMDA receptor)	

Glutamine	Ammonia	Inter-organ nitrogen transport	Reduces infectious morbidity in trauma patients, burn patients, and surgical patients
		Renal HCO_3^- production	
	Purines, pyrimidines	RNA synthesis, DNA synthesis	
		Glutamic acid precursor	
Glycine		Inhibition CNS (glycine receptor)	Adjuvant to antipsychotics, probably reduces negative symptoms of schizophrenia
		Excitation CNS (NMDA receptor)	
	Glutathione	Antioxidant	
	Creatine	(*see* arginine)	
		Serine precursor	
Serine	D-serine	Excitation CNS (NMDA receptor)	Adjuvant to antipsychotics, probably reduces negative symptoms of schizophrenia
		Glycine precursor	
		Cysteine precursor	
Threonine	Glycine	Brain development	
	Serine		
Histidine	Histamine	Immunomodulation	
		Gastric acid secretion	
Lysine	Carnitine	Mitochondrial oxidation of long-chain fatty acids	Reduces chronic stress-induced anxiety
	Glutamate		
Branched chain amino acids			
Isoleucine	α-keto-β-methylvaleric acid		Upper gastrointestinal hemorrhage
Leucine	α-ketoisocaproic acid	Important in regulation of energy and protein metabolism	Improve protein malnutrition and restore amino acid and neurotransmitter balance in hepatic failure and hepatic encephalopathy (supplemented BCAA)
		Substrate for glutamine synthesis	
Valine	α-ketoisovaleric acid		
Aromatic amino acids			
Phenylalanine		Tyrosine precursor	
Tyrosine	L-dopa	Dopamine synthesis	Possible slight improvement of cognitive functions after physical or mental exhaustion. Metabolites are powerful pharmacotherapeutic drugs
	Dopamine	Movement, affect on pleasure, motivation	
	Noradrenaline, adrenaline	Activation of sympathetic nervous system (fight-or-flight response)	
	Tri-iodothyronine, thyroxine	Regulation of basal metabolic rate	
Tryptophan	Kynureninic acid	CNS inhibition	No scientific evidence for beneficial effects of supplementation
	Quinolinic acid	CNS excitation	
	Serotonin	Mood regulation	
		Sleep regulation	
		Intestinal motility	
	Melatonin	Regulation of circadian rhythms	

Different fonts indicate: nonessential amino acids, **essential amino acids**, and *conditionally essential amino acids*.

Alanine

Alanine and glutamine are the principal amino acid substrates for hepatic gluconeogenesis and ureagenesis. Alanine is produced in peripheral tissues in transamination processes with glutamate, branched chain amino acids, and other amino acids; following its release in the systemic circulation, alanine is predominantly taken up by the liver and to a lesser extent by the kidney. Here, alanine can be deaminated to yield pyruvate and an amino group, which can be used for transamination processes, ureagenesis, or can be excreted in urine. Thus, the alanine released from peripheral tissues may be converted to glucose in the liver or kidney and eventually become a substrate for peripheral (mainly muscular) glycolysis. This so-called glucose-alanine cycle may be especially relevant during metabolic stress and critical illness when the endogenous alanine release from peripheral tissues is increased. Simultaneously, alanine serves as a nitrogen carrier in this manner. Alanine is often used as the second amino acid in glutamine dipeptides that are applied to increase solubility and stability of glutamine in nutritional solutions.

Supplementation

No clinical benefits have been ascribed to supplementation with alanine, although it has never been considered whether the beneficial effects of the dipeptide alanine-glutamine, which are generally ascribed to glutamine, may also be due to alanine. In this context, it should be realized, however, that alanine itself constitutes the strongest drive for hepatic ureagenesis (leading to breakdown of alanine).

Arginine, Citrulline, Ornithine, and Proline (Figure 1)

Arginine is a nitrogen-rich amino acid because it contains three nitrogen atoms and is the precursor for nitric oxide (NO). The conversion to NO is catalyzed by the enzyme nitric oxide synthase (NOS), and results in coproduction of the amino acid citrulline. Depending on its site of release, NO exerts several functions including stimulation of the pituitary gland, vasodilation, neurotransmission, and immune modulation. Arginine is also a precursor for urea synthesis in the urea cycle, which has an important function in the detoxification of ammonia and excretion of waste nitrogen from the body. A full urea cycle is only present in the liver, but the arginase enzyme that converts arginine to urea and ornithine is to a limited extent also found in other tissues and cells, such as brain, kidney, small intestine, and red blood cells. Ornithine is utilized for the formation of proline, polyamines (putrescine, spermine, and spermidine), glutamic acid, and glutamine. Arginine is involved in collagen formation, tissue repair, and wound healing via proline, which is hydroxylated to form hydroxyproline. This role in wound healing may additionally be mediated by stimulation of collagen synthesis by NO, although this claim is still under investigation. It is currently thought that arginine availability is regulated by the balance between NOS and arginase enzyme activity, which subsequently determines substrate availability for NO and ornithine production. Proline also stimulates hepatocyte DNA and protein synthesis. Polyamines are potent inducers of cell differentiation.

In addition to synthesis of NO, urea, and ornithine, arginine is used for synthesis of creatine, which is an important constituent of skeletal muscle and neurons and acts as an energy source for these tissues. Furthermore, arginine may be catabolyzed to agmatine, which acts as a cell-signaling molecule. Arginine not only acts as an intermediate in the synthesis of functional products, but also is a potent stimulus for the release of several hormones, such as insulin, glucagon, somatostatin, and growth hormone, illustrating its pharmacological characteristics.

Arginine can be synthesized by the body from citrulline. However, since virtually all arginine produced in the liver is trapped within the urea cycle, the kidney is the only arginine-synthesizing organ that significantly contributes to the total body pool of free arginine. Diminished renal arginine synthesis has been found in patients with renal failure and in highly catabolic conditions, like sepsis, burn injury, or trauma (which may be related to concomitant renal failure). In these situations arginine may be considered a conditionally essential amino acid and it has been suggested that arginine supplementation can become useful in these situations.

Citrulline is formed from glutamine, glutamic acid, and proline in the intestine. Plasma citrulline concentration reflects intestinal metabolic function and has recently been introduced as a potential marker for (reduced) enterocyte mass.

Supplementation

Based on its pluripotent functions, arginine has been widely used in supplemental nutrition for surgical patients, patients with burns, and patients with sepsis and cancer in order to modify the inflammatory response, to enhance organ perfusion, and to stimulate wound healing. However, the benefits of arginine supplementation in these conditions are not uniformly proven and accepted. Moreover, arginine is never given alone but is

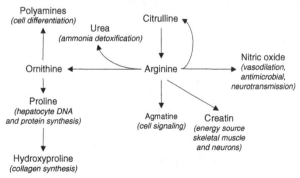

Figure 1 Specific functions of arginine metabolism.

always provided in a mixture of amino acids and other nutrients. The use of NO donors that have vasodilatory actions is an established therapeutic modality in coronary artery disease and for erectile dysfunction. Given this fact it remains worthwhile to clarify the need for arginine supplementation as the natural substrate for NO synthesis in other conditions.

Using citrulline as an arginine-delivering substrate has been suggested, but has not been applied clinically. Ornithine is supplied as part of the ornithine-α-ketoglutarate molecule (see glutamine). Creatine is widely used by professional and recreational athletes as a nutritional supplement, although the ascribed performance-enhancing effects have not been proven.

Asparagine and Aspartic Acid

Asparagine can be converted by asparaginase to ammonia and aspartic acid, which is the precursor of the citrate cycle intermediates oxaloacetate and fumarate; this reaction is reversible. In fasting humans asparagine and aspartic acid are utilized as precursors for *de novo* synthesis of glutamine and alanine in muscle.

Supplementation

The claim that asparagine or aspartic acid supplementation improves endurance has not been confirmed in human studies. Asparaginase, which degrades asparagine, is widely used in the treatment of pediatric leukemia since the resulting asparagine depletion leads to apoptosis of leukemic cells.

Cysteine, Cystine, Methionine, and Taurine (Figure 2)

Methionine is converted to cysteine and its dipeptide cystine. In addition methionine is a precursor for creatine (see arginine). The potential for formation of disulfide bonds between its thiol (-SH) groups makes protein-bound cysteine important in the folding and structural assembly of proteins. Reduced cysteine thiol groups are found in protein (albumin), free cysteine, and in the principal intracellular antioxidant tripeptide glutathione (see glycine, glutamic acid) for which free cysteine is the synthesis rate-limiting constituent. Through the formation of disulfides (e.g., cystine, cysteinyl-glutathione, glutathione disulfide, mercaptalbumin) thiol-

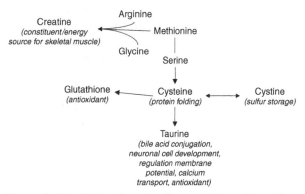

Figure 2 Specific functions of sulfur-containing amino acids.

containing molecules can scavenge oxygen-derived free radicals. The ratio between oxidized and reduced thiol groups reflects the cellular redox state. Owing to its small pool size cysteine deficiencies rapidly occur during malnutrition.

Cysteine is also the precursor for taurine, which is abundant in all mammalian cells, particularly in neuronal cells and lymphocytes, but is not a true amino acid and is not incorporated in proteins. Taurine is involved in the conjugation of bile acids and may act as an antioxidant. Moreover, taurine is an osmolyte by virtue of the fact that through its transporter its intracellular concentrations are between 50 and 100-fold higher than in the extracellular compartment. This gradient contributes to the maintenance of the cellular hydration state. Similarly, it has been proposed that taurine is involved in stabilization of cell membrane potential and regulation of Ca^{2+} transport through several calcium-ion channels. Based upon these characteristics it has been suggested that taurine is involved in the control of cardiac muscle cell contraction, which has led to the addition of taurine to commercially available energy drinks. Its high level in lymphocytes suggests an important role in immunological resistance to infections. Taurine plays an important part in the development and maintenance of neuronal and especially retinal cells.

Supplementation

Although methionine is the only sulfur-containing essential amino acid, it has not been considered as part of supplementation regimes. Since cysteine easily oxidizes to cystine, which has a poor solubility, it is generally supplemented in the form of *n*-acetylcysteine (NAC). Both directly and indirectly, as a precursor for glutathione, NAC has attracted attention as a potentially protective agent against oxidative injury in numerous conditions including endurance exercise, ischemia reperfusion injury, adult respiratory distress syndrome (ARDS), and cystic fibrosis. In addition, NAC has mucolytic properties in chronic obstructive pulmonary disease (COPD) patients by reducing disulfide bonds of polymers in mucus, blocking their reactivity. Currently, only robust evidence exists for the usefulness of NAC supplementation in the protection against nephropathy, induced by administration of iodine-containing contrast agents for radiological imaging in patients with chronic renal failure, in the reduction of the number of exacerbations and disability in COPD patients, and in the treatment of liver injury induced by acetaminophen intoxication. On the other hand it has been suggested that glutathione depletion by buthionine sulfoximine administration potentiates the effect of radiotherapy by increasing the susceptibility of tumor cells to radiation-induced oxidative injury.

In a few studies it has been demonstrated that taurine supplementation improves retinal development in premature babies receiving parenteral nutrition. Human data on the efficacy of taurine supplementation in so-called energy drinks are very limited. In the absence of taurine supplementation in children taurine concentrations drop, suggesting its conditional indispensability also in the postneonatal period. This has led to the addition of taurine to standard feeding formulas for infants and growing children.

Glutamine, Glutamic acid, and Ornithine α-Ketoglutarate (Figure 3)

Glutamine is the most abundant amino acid in plasma and in tissue. In glutamine-consuming cells it is readily converted by the enzyme glutaminase to form ammonia and glutamic acid, which is the primary intermediate in almost all routes of glutamine degradation. In the presence of ammonia this process can occur in reverse, catalyzed by the enzyme glutamine synthetase. In contrast to glutamic acid, glutamine can easily pass through the cellular membrane, thus exporting waste nitrogen out of the cell and serving as an inter-organ nitrogen carrier. In the kidney glutamine donates NH_3, which is the acceptor for protons released from carbonic acid, to form NH_4^+ and thus facilitates the formation of HCO_3^-, which is essential in plasma pH regulation.

Following conversion to glutamic acid and subsequently α-ketoglutarate, glutamine may supplement intermediates of the citrate cycle. In this manner glutamine serves as the preferred fuel for rapidly dividing cells of, for example, the immune system cells and intestinal mucosa. In the brain glutamic acid is the most abundant excitatory neurotransmitter and the precursor for gamma-aminobutyric acid, which is an important inhibitory neurotransmitter. Glutamine is a direct precursor for purine and pyrimidine and therefore is involved in RNA and DNA synthesis and cell proliferation. In addition it is a constituent of the tripeptide glutathione, which is the principal intracellular antioxidant in eukaryotes (see also sections on cysteine and glycine).

Supplementation

Of all the compounds discussed above glutamine is the most extensively applied in clinical and experimental amino acid supplementation, often in the form of the more soluble and stable dipeptides alanyl- and glycyl-glutamine. Glutamic acid and α-ketoglutarate are less ideally suited for use in feeding formulas because of poor inward transport of glutamic acid and poor solubility and stability of α-ketoglutarate. Moreover, glutamic acid has been related to the 'Chinese restaurant syndrome,' characterized by light-headiness and nausea after consumption of Chinese food containing glutamic acid for flavor improvement. However, scientific evidence is weak. Numerous experimental and clinical studies have suggested that glutamine supplementation has positive effects on immune function, intestinal mucosal integrity, nitrogen balance, and glutathione concentration in a wide variety of conditions. Nevertheless, the true benefit of glutamine supplementation is difficult to quantify in clinical practice. Its benefit has especially been claimed in the critically ill and surgical patients in whom clinical outcome is multifactorial. Recent meta-analyses support the view that glutamine supplementation is safe and may reduce infectious morbidity and hospital stay in surgical patients. A

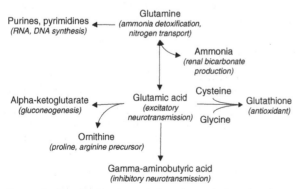

Figure 3 Specific functions of glutamine and glutamine degradation products.

positive effect of glutamine supplementation on morbidity and mortality in critical illness, trauma patients, and burn patients has been demonstrated in a few well-designed clinical trials. However, due to the paucity of such trials reliable meta-analyses are not possible in these latter patient categories. It has been demonstrated in some small clinical series that supplementation with ornithine α-ketoglutarate may improve wound healing in burn patients, benefiting from the combined actions of both α-ketoglutarate and ornithine (see sections on arginine and ornithine).

Glycine, Serine, and Threonine

Threonine is an essential amino acid, which can be converted to glycine in the liver and subsequently to serine. Glycine is a constituent of glutathione (see also sections on cysteine and glutamic acid) and is a versatile neurotransmitter in the central nervous system. Through the glycine receptor it has a direct inhibitory neurotransmitter function but it is also a ligand for the glycine site at the N-methyl-D-aspartate (NMDA) glutamic acid receptor. Activation of this glycine site is needed for NMDA activation, which makes glycine a mediator in the excitatory neurotransmitter effects of glutamic acid. Besides a role in the central nervous system, glycine is also thought to possess anti-inflammatory properties, but to date these properties have only been demonstrated in the test tube. Furthermore, glycine can react with arginine and methionine to form creatine (see section on arginine). Finally, glycine, like taurine, is a conjugate for bile acids.

Glycine is convertible to serine in a reversible reaction, which can be converted to its stereoisomeric form D-serine; this is also a ligand for the glycine site at the NMDA receptor. Furthermore, serine is an intermediate in the pathway from methionine to cysteine and a precursor for pyrimidines and purines and as such is involved in cell proliferation. It is also a precursor for gluconeogenesis, albeit of lesser importance than glutamine and alanine.

Supplementation

Based upon their excitatory effects on the central nervous system both glycine and D-serine have been implicated in the treatment of schizophrenia. As adjuvant therapy to standard psychopharmacological treatment they may reduce the negative symptoms of the disease.

High doses of threonine in adults have been used as tentative therapy for spastic syndromes, a therapy that probably acts through increased glycine formation. A negative effect of excessive threonine, which is abundant in bovine infant formula nutrition, has been considered in experimental studies on brain development, and it has been suggested that this happens through its conversion to glycine and serine, or through competition of amino acid transport across the blood–brain barrier.

Histidine

Histidine is the precursor for histamine, which is important for the immune system by mediating growth and functionality of immune cells. Excessive release of histamine from mast cells induces the clinical signs of allergy (dilation of capillaries and larger blood vessels, increased capillary permeability and swelling, itching, and anaphylactic shock). These phenomena are effected via the H_1 receptor, which is found in smooth muscle cells of the vascular wall and bronchi, among others. Furthermore, histamine acts as a neurotransmitter and mediates gastric acid production. The latter occurs via the H_2 receptor found in gastric mucosa. There is no literature available on the potential relationship between histidine availability and histamine production and action.

Supplementation

H_1 receptor antagonists are applied in the treatment of allergy and H_2 receptor antagonists have been shown to be very effective in the inhibition of gastric acid secretion and have greatly improved the treatment of individuals with peptic ulcer disease and acid reflux esophagitis. Histamine is present in abundance in many dietary sources; no beneficial effects of supplementation of either histidine or histamine are known.

Branched Chain Amino Acids (Isoleucine, Leucine, Valine)

Branched chain amino acids (BCAAs) are essential amino acids, which together compose approximately a third of the daily amino acid requirement in humans. BCAAs, and especially leucine, play an important role in the regulation of energy and protein metabolism. BCAAs are primarily oxidized in skeletal muscle and not in the liver. BCAAs donate their amino groups to furnish glutamic acid in muscle in transamination reactions yielding the α-ketoacids α-ketoisocaproic acid, α-keto-β-methylvaleric acid, and α-ketoisovaleric acid. These transamination products of BCAAs can enter the citrate cycle and contribute to ATP production by aerobic substrate oxidation, which is important during the change from rest to exercise. After consumption of protein-containing meals, a large part of the BCAA passes through the liver and is taken up by muscle where it primarily contributes to protein synthesis and the synthesis of glutamine, which accounts for about 70% of the amino acid release from muscle. The importance of the essential branched chain amino acids for protein synthesis is strikingly exemplified by the negative nitrogen balance and catabolism that follows upper gastrointestinal bleeding caused by ingestion of large amounts of hemoglobin (which lacks isoleucine). Leucine has been suggested to regulate the turnover of protein in muscle cells by inhibiting protein degradation and enhancing protein synthesis. This has led to a worldwide interest in the possible use of BCAAs in general, and leucine in particular, for metabolic support.

In liver failure the plasma concentrations of the aromatic amino acids (AAAs) tyrosine, phenylalanine, and tryptophan increase, probably because they are predominantly broken down in the liver, whereas the plasma levels of BCAAs decrease while they are degraded in excess in muscle as a consequence of hepatic failure-induced catabolism. As AAAs and BCAAs are all neutral amino acids and share a common transporter across the blood–brain barrier (system L carrier), changes in their plasma ratio are reflected in the brain, subsequently disrupting the neurotransmitter profile of the catecholamines and indoleamines (see sections on tyrosine and tryptophan). It has been hypothesized that this disturbance contributes to the multifactorial pathogenesis of hepatic encephalopathy. In line with this hypothesis it has been suggested that normalization of the amino acid pattern by supplementing extra BCAAs counteracts hepatic encephalopathy.

Supplementation

Specialized formulas that are widely used for hepatic failure and hepatic encephalopathy are based on a high content of BCAAs to improve protein malnutrition and restore the amino acid and neurotransmitter balance. Although BCAA-enriched formulas have been proven to improve neurological status in comatose liver patients it is not certain that this is achieved by the addition of BCAAs specifically, because of a lack of adequate control groups.

Since BCAAs compete with tryptophan for uptake by the brain, they have (in line with the ascribed benefits in hepatic encephalopathy) been applied as competitive antagonists for tryptophan transport, reducing tryptophan-induced cognitive impairment (see also section on tryptophan).

Isoleucine, which is absent in the hemoglobin molecule, can be supplemented to patients with upper gastrointestinal bleeding to restore the balance of amino acids that are taken up by the splanchnic organs. This has been demonstrated to improve mainly protein synthesis in liver and muscle in small observational studies. Prospective randomized clinical trials are, however, still lacking.

Lysine

Lysine is an essential amino acid that is mainly provided by meat products and is therefore limited in diets where wheat is the primary protein source. Lysine is also the first rate-limiting amino acid in milk-fed newborns for growth and protein synthesis. Lysine is catabolized to glutamate and acetyl-CoA and is also the precursor for the synthesis of carnitine, which is needed for mitochondrial oxidation of long-chain fatty acids.

Supplementation

Lysine supplementation in patients with renal failure is contraindicated, as the amino acid shows some degree of nephrotoxicity.

Phenylalanine and Tyrosine

Phenylalanine is hydroxylated to tyrosine by the enzyme phenylalanine hydroxylase. The inborn disease phenylketonuria is characterized by a deficiency of this enzyme.

Tyrosine is the precursor for dihydroxyphenylalanine (dopa), which can successively be converted to the catecholamines dopamine, noradrenaline (norepinephrine) and adrenaline (epinephrine). Although only a small proportion of tyrosine is used in this pathway, this metabolic route is extremely relevant. Dopamine is an important neurotransmitter in different parts of the brain and is involved in movement and affects pleasure and motivation. Disruption of dopamine neurons in the basal ganglia is the cause of Parkinson's disease. Noradrenaline and ardrenaline are the most important neurotransmitters in the sympathetic nervous system. The sympathetic nervous system becomes activated during different forms of emotional and physical arousal, and results in the induction of phenomena such as increased blood pressure and heart rate, increased alertness, and decreased intestinal motility (fight-or-flight response). Besides acting as a precursor for catecholamines, tyrosine can be iodinated and as such is the precursor for the thyroid hormones triiodothyronine and thyroxine. These hormones are important regulators of general whole body rate of metabolic activity.

Supplementation

The processes described in the paragraph above quantitatively contribute only marginally to total tyrosine turnover and the limited data on tyrosine supplementation in phenylketonuria suggest that tyrosine deficiency is not causal in the development of cognitive dysfunction in the disease. In two studies tyrosine supplementation has been found to modestly increase mental status and cognitive performance following exhausting efforts such as prolonged wakefulness and intensive military training. In contrast, tyrosine derivatives (L-dopa, noradrenaline, adrenaline) have strong pharmacological properties. L-dopa is the direct precursor of dopamine synthesis and has been found to have strong beneficial effects in Parkinson's disease. The fact that administration of tyrosine as the physiological precursor of catecholamines has no or minor effects on catecholamine-induced sympathetic activity, whereas the effects of the catecholamines or more direct precursors is very strong, suggests that tyrosine hydroxylation to L-dopa is not limited by substrate availability.

Tryptophan

Functional end products of the essential amino acid tryptophan arise mainly through two distinctive pathways. The major pathway is degradation of tryptophan by oxidation, which fuels the kynurenine pathway (See 02011). The second and quantitatively minor pathway is hydroxylation of tryptophan and its subsequent decarboxylation to the indoleamine 5-hydroxytryptamine (serotonin) and subsequently melatonin. The metabolites of the kynurenine pathway, indicated as kynurenines, include quinolic acid and kynurenic acid. Quinolinic acid is an agonist of the NMDA receptor (see also section on glutamic acid), while kynurenic acid is a nonselective NMDA-receptor antagonist with a high affinity for the glycine site of the NMDA receptor (see also section on

glycine), and as such is a blocker of amino acid-modulated excitation of the central nervous system. Imbalance between kynurenic acid and quinolinic acid can lead to excitotoxic neuronal cell death and is believed to play a role in the development of several neurological diseases such as Huntington's chorea and epilepsy. In addition, an immunomodulatory role is suggested for several metabolites of the kynurenine pathway.

Serotonin is synthesized in the central nervous system and is involved in the regulation of mood and sleep. In addition it is found in high quantities in neurons in the gastrointestinal tract where it is involved in regulation of gut motility. Tryptophan competes with BCAAs for transport across the blood–brain barrier and the ratio between tryptophan and BCAAs therefore determines the uptake of both (groups of) amino acids by the brain (see section on BCAAs). Since albumin has a strong tryptophan-binding capacity, the plasma albumin concentration is inversely related to the plasma concentration of free tryptophan and as such influences the BCAA to tryptophan ratio and hence the brain uptake of both BCAAs and tryptophan. It has been suggested that increased plasma AAAs (tyrosine, phenylalanine, and tryptophan) levels in patients with liver failure are caused by the inability of the liver to degrade these amino acids. The resulting change in the ratio between AAA and BCAA plasma levels has been implied in the pathogenesis of hepatic encephalopathy since this may cause marked disturbances in transport of both AAAs and BCAAs across the blood–brain barrier, leading to disturbed release of indoleamines and catecholamines in the brain (see also section on BCAAs). High tryptophan concentrations have been associated with chronic fatigue disorders and hepatic encephalopathy while low tryptophan plasma concentrations have been implicated in the etiology of mood disorders, cognitive impairment, and functional bowel disorders. Melatonin, which is produced in the degradation pathway of serotonin during the dark period of the light-dark cycle, is an important mediator of circadian rhythms.

Supplementation

Inhibition of serotonin reuptake from the neuronal synapse and the subsequent increase in its functionality is one of the mainstays of the pharmacological treatment of depression. Like many amino acids, tryptophan is commercially available as a nutritional supplement or as a so-called smart drug, claiming to reduce symptoms of depression, anxiety, obsessive-compulsive disorders, insomnia, fibromyalgia, alcohol withdrawal, and migraine. However, no convincing clinical data are available to support these claims. In contrast tryptophan depletion induced by ingestion of a tryptophan-deficient amino acid mixture, is widely used in experimental psychiatry to study the biological background of various psychiatric disorders.

Further Reading

Cynober LA (ed.) (2004) *Metabolic and Therapeutic Aspects of Amino Acids in Clinical Nutrition*, 2nd edn. Boca Raton: CRC Press.

Fürst P and Young V (2000) *Proteins, Peptides and Amino Acids in Enteral Nutrition*. Nestlé Nutrition Workshop Series Clinical & Performance Program. vol. 3. Vevey: Nestec Ltd Nestec and Basel: Karger.

Guyton AC and Hall JE (1996) *Textbook of Medical Physiology*, 9th edn. Philadelphia: W.B. Saunders.

Labadarios D and Pichard C (2002) *Clinical Nutrition: early Intention*. Nestlé Nutrition Workshop Series Clinical & Performance Program. vol. 7. Vevey: Nestec Ltd Nestec and Basel: Karger.

Newsholme P, Procopio J, Lima MMR, Ptihon-Curi TC, and Curi R (2003) Glutamine and glutamate – their central role in cell metabolism and function. *Cell Biochemistry and Function* **21**: 1–9.

Wu G and Morris SM (1998) Arginine metabolism: nitric oxide and beyond. *Biochemical Journal* **336**: 1–17.

Young V, Bier DM, Cynober L, Hayashi Y, and Kadowaki M (eds.) (2003) The third Workshop on the Assessment of adequate Intake of Dietary Amino Acids. *J Nutr Supplement* **134**: 1553S–1672S.

ANEMIA

Iron-Deficiency Anemia

K J Schulze and M L Dreyfuss, Johns Hopkins Bloomberg School of Public Health, Baltimore, MD, USA

Anemia is defined by abnormally low circulating hemoglobin concentrations. A variety of etiologies exist for anemia, including dietary deficiencies of folate or vitamin B_{12} (pernicious or macrocytic anemia), infections and inflammatory states (anemia of chronic disease), and conditions that result in insufficient production of red blood cells (aplastic anemia) or excessive destruction of red blood cells (hemolytic anemia). However, worldwide, the most prevalent form of anemia is that of iron deficiency, which causes anemia characterized by hypochromic and normo- or microcytic red blood cells. Iron deficiency anemia remains a health problem in both the developed and the developing world. This article discusses the metabolism of iron; the assessment of iron deficiency; iron requirements across the life span; and the consequences, prevention, and treatment of iron deficiency and iron deficiency anemia.

Iron Metabolism

The adult body contains 2.5–5 g of iron, approximately two-thirds of which is present in hemoglobin. Other essential iron-containing systems include muscle myoglobin (3%) and a variety of iron-containing enzymes (5–15%), including cytochromes. In addition to the role of iron in oxygen transfer via hemoglobin and myoglobin, iron is involved in energy metabolism and also affects neural myelination and neurotransmitter metabolism. Iron stores vary considerably but may represent up to 30% of body iron, and iron that circulates with transferrin represents less than 1% of body iron. Men have a higher concentration of iron per kilogram body weight than women because they have larger erythrocyte mass and iron stores.

More than 90% of body iron is conserved through the recycling of iron through the reticuloendothelial system (**Figure 1**). Iron is transported through the body by the protein transferrin, which carries up to two iron atoms. The distribution of iron to body tissues is mediated by transferrin receptors (TfRs), which are upregulated in the face of increased tissue demand for iron. The transferrin/TfR complex is internalized via cell invagination, iron is released into the cell cytosol, and transferrin is recycled back to the cell surface.

In hematopoietic cells, iron is used to produce hemoglobin through its combination with zinc protoporphyrin to form heme. Therefore, protoporphyrin accumulates relative to hemoglobin in red blood cells during iron deficiency. Mature red blood cells circulate in the body for approximately 120 days before being destroyed. Macrophage cells

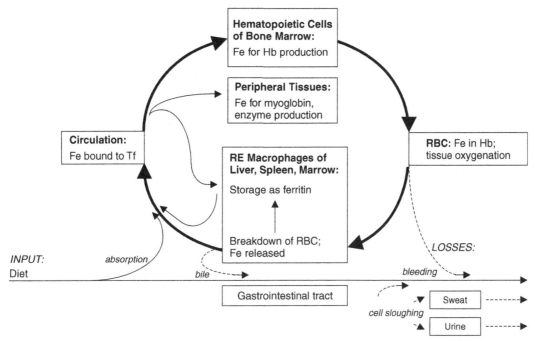

Figure 1 Iron metabolism and balance: inputs, losses, and recycling of iron through the reticuloendothelial system. Fe, iron; Tf, transferrin; Hb, hemoglobin; RBC, red blood cell; RE, reticuloendothelial.

of the liver and spleen phagocytize senescent red blood cells and the iron released in this process is recycled back to the circulation or, when iron is readily available, incorporated with ferritin or hemosiderin for storage. A typical ferritin molecule may contain 2000 iron atoms. Hemosiderin is a less soluble variant of ferritin that may contain even greater amounts of iron.

The production of transferrin receptors and ferritin is regulated by iron response proteins (IRPs) that 'sense' intracellular iron concentrations and interact with iron response elements (IREs) of protein mRNA. When cellular iron concentrations are low, the IRP–IRE interaction works to prevent translation of mRNA to ferritin or to stabilize mRNA to enhance the translation of transferrin receptors. Identifying other proteins regulated through the IRP–IRE interaction is an area of particular interest. Although body iron is highly conserved, daily basal losses of iron of ∼1 mg/day do occur even in healthy individuals. These basal losses occur primarily through the gastrointestinal tract (in bile, sloughing of ferritin-containing enterocytes, and via blood loss), and sweat and urine are additional minor sources of iron loss (**Figure 1**). Iron losses are not strictly regulated; rather, iron balance is achieved through the regulation of dietary iron absorption.

Dietary Iron Absorption

The efficiency of iron absorption depends on both the bioavailability of dietary iron and iron status. Typically, 5–20% of the iron present in a mixed diet is absorbed. Dietary iron exists in two forms, heme and non-heme. Heme iron is derived from animal source food and is more bioavailable than non-heme iron, with approximately 20–30% of heme iron absorbed via endocytosis of the entire heme molecule. Iron is then released into the enterocyte by a heme oxidase.

Non-heme iron exists in plant products and its bioavailability is compromised by the concurrent ingestion of tannins, phytates, soy, and other plant constituents, that decrease its solubility in the intestinal lumen. Bioavailability of non-heme iron is increased by concurrent ingestion of ascorbic acid and meat products. Non-heme iron is reduced from the ferric to the ferrous form in the intestinal lumen and transported into enterocytes via the divalent metal transporter (DMT-1). Once inside the enterocyte, iron from heme and non-heme sources is similarly transported through the cell and across the basolateral membrane by the ferroportin transporter in conjunction with the ferroxidase hephaestin after which it can be taken up by transferrin into the circulation. The regulation of iron across the basolateral membrane of the enterocyte is considered the most important aspect of iron absorption.

The absorption efficiency of non-heme iron in particular is also inversely related to iron status. The factor responsible for communicating body iron status to the enterocyte to allow for the up- or downregulation of iron absorption remained elusive until recently, when the hormone hepcidin was identified. Hepcidin declines during iron deficiency, and its decline is associated with an increased production of the DMT-1 and ferroportin transporters in a rat model, although its exact mode of action is unknown. Hepcidin may also regulate iron absorption and retention or release of iron from body stores during conditions of enhanced erythropoiesis and inflammation.

Iron Requirements

Iron requirements depend on iron losses and growth demands for iron across life stages. To maintain iron balance or achieve positive iron balance, therefore, the amount of iron absorbed from the diet must equal or exceed the basal losses plus any additional demands for iron attributable to physiologic state (e.g., growth, menstruation, and pregnancy) and/or pathological iron losses (e.g., excess bleeding). When iron balance is negative, iron deficiency will occur following the depletion of the body's iron reserves. Thus, ensuring an adequate supply of dietary iron is of paramount importance. The risk of iron deficiency and iron deficiency anemia varies across the life cycle as iron demand and/or the likelihood of consuming adequate dietary iron changes.

Basal Iron Loss

Because basal iron losses are due to cell exfoliation, these losses are relative to interior body surfaces, totaling an estimated 14 µg/kg body weight/day, and are approximately 0.8 mg/day for nonmenstruating women and 1.0 mg/day for men. Basal losses in infants and children have not been directly determined and are estimated from data available on adult men. Basal losses are reduced in people with iron deficiency and increased in people with iron overload. The absorbed iron requirement for adult men and nonmenstruating women is based on these obligate iron losses.

Infancy and Childhood

The iron content of a newborn infant is approximately 75 mg/kg body weight, and much of this iron is found in hemoglobin. The body iron of the newborn is derived from maternal–fetal iron transfer, 80% of which occurs during the third trimester of pregnancy. Preterm infants, with less opportunity to

establish iron stores, have a substantially reduced endowment of body iron at birth than term infants.

During the first 2 months of life, there is a physiologic shift of body iron from hemoglobin to iron stores. For the first 6 months of life, the iron requirement of a term infant is satisfied by storage iron and breast milk iron, which is present in low concentrations but is highly bioavailable (50–100%) to the infant. However, by 6 months of age in term infants, and even earlier in preterm infants, iron intake and body stores become insufficient to meet the demands for growth (expanding erythrocyte mass and growth of body tissues), such that negative iron balance will ensue at this time without the introduction of iron supplements or iron-rich weaning foods.

A full-term infant almost doubles its body iron content and triples its body weight in the first year of life. Although growth continues through childhood, the rate of growth declines following the first year of life. Similarly, the requirement for iron expressed per kilogram body weight declines through childhood from a high of 0.10 mg/kg in the first 6 months to 0.03 mg/kg/d by 7–10 years of age until increasing again during the adolescent growth spurt. Throughout the period of growth, the iron concentration of the diet of infants and children must be greater than that of an adult man in order to achieve iron balance.

Adolescence

Adolescents have very high iron requirements, and the iron demand of individual children during periods of rapid growth is highly variable and may exceed mean estimated requirements. Boys going through puberty experience a large increase in erythrocyte mass and hemoglobin concentration. The growth spurt in adolescent girls usually occurs in early adolescence before menarche, but growth continues postmenarche at a slower rate. The addition of menstrual iron loss to the iron demand for growth leads to particularly high iron requirements for postmenarchal adolescent girls.

Menstruation

Although the quantity of menstrual blood loss is fairly constant across time for an individual, it varies considerably from woman to woman. The mean menstrual iron loss is 0.56 mg/day when averaged over a monthly cycle. However, menstrual blood losses are highly skewed so that a small proportion of women have heavy losses. In 10% of women, menstrual iron loss exceeds 1.47 mg/day and in 5% it exceeds 2.04 mg/day. Therefore, the daily iron requirement for menstruating women is set quite high to cover the iron needs of most of the population. Menstrual blood loss is decreased by oral contraceptives but increased by intrauterine devices. However, recent progesterone-releasing versions of the device lead to decreased menstrual blood loss or amenorrhea.

Pregnancy and Lactation

The body's iron needs during pregnancy are very high despite the cessation of menstruation during this period. Demand for iron comes primarily from the expansion of the red blood cell mass (450 mg), the fetus (270 mg), the placenta and cord (90 mg), and blood loss at parturition (150 mg). However, the requirement for iron is not spread evenly over the course of pregnancy, as depicted in **Figure 2**, with iron requirements actually reduced in the first trimester because menstrual blood loss is absent and fetal demand for iron is negligible. Iron requirements increase dramatically through the second and third trimesters to support expansion of maternal red blood cell mass and fetal growth. The maternal red cell mass expands approximately 35% in the second and third trimesters to meet increased maternal oxygen needs. When iron deficiency is present, the expansion of the red cell mass is compromised, resulting in anemia. Furthermore, an expansion of the plasma fluid that is proportionately greater than that of the red cell mass results in a physiologic anemia attributable to hemodilution.

To attempt to meet iron requirements during pregnancy, iron absorption becomes more efficient in the second and third trimesters. Iron absorption nearly doubles in the second trimester and can increase up to four times in the third trimester. Despite this dramatic increase in iron absorption, it

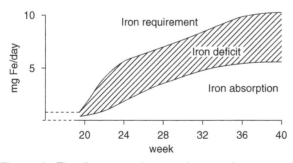

Figure 2 The discrepancy between iron requirements and availability of iron from dietary absorption in pregnant women beyond 20 weeks of gestation. The resulting iron deficit is maintained as pregnancy progresses into the second and third trimesters. (Reproduced with permission from the Food and Agriculture Organization of the United Nations (2001) Iron. In *Human Vitamin and Mineral Requirements: Report of a Joint FAO/WHO Expert Consultation, Bangkok, Thailand*, pp. 195–221. Rome: FAO.)

is virtually impossible for pregnant women to acquire sufficient iron through diet alone because of the concurrent increase in iron requirements during the latter half of pregnancy (**Figure 2**).

There is also an iron cost of lactation to women of approximately 0.3 mg/day as iron is lost in breastmilk. However, this is compensated by the absence of menstrual iron losses and the gain in iron stores achieved when much of the iron previously invested in expansion of the red cell mass is recovered postpartum.

Pathological Losses

Conditions that cause excessive bleeding additionally compromise iron status. Approximately 1 mg of iron is lost in each 1 ml of packed red blood cells. Excessive losses of blood may occur from the gastrointestinal tract, urinary tract, and lung in a variety of clinical pathologies, including ulcers, malignancies, inflammatory bowel disease, hemorrhoids, hemoglobinuria, and idiopathic pulmonary hemosiderosis. In developing countries, parasitic infestation with hookworm and schistosomiasis can contribute substantially to gastrointestinal blood loss and iron deficiency.

Recommended Nutrient Intakes for Iron

Recommended intakes of dietary iron are based on the requirement for absorbed iron and assumptions about the bioavailability of iron in the diet. They are meant to cover the iron needs of nearly the entire population group. Thus, the amount of dietary iron necessary to meet an iron requirement depends in large part on the bioavailability of iron in the diet (**Figure 3**). Americans consume approximately 15 mg of iron daily from a diet that is considered moderately to highly bioavailable (10–15%) due to the meat and ascorbic acid content. Studies in European countries suggest that iron intake averages 10 mg/day, representing a decline in dietary iron. Although estimates of total iron intake in developing countries are not substantially lower than that, iron is often consumed in plant-based diets that inhibit its absorption and contain few animal products to counterbalance that effect, such that the bioavailability of iron is closer to 5%. Thus, **Figure 3** demonstrates the total amount of dietary iron that would be necessary to meet the iron requirements of various population groups based on its bioavailability. Where intakes are sufficient and bioavailability adequate, dietary iron can meet the iron needs of adolescent boys and adult men and also lactating and postmenopausal women. However, regardless

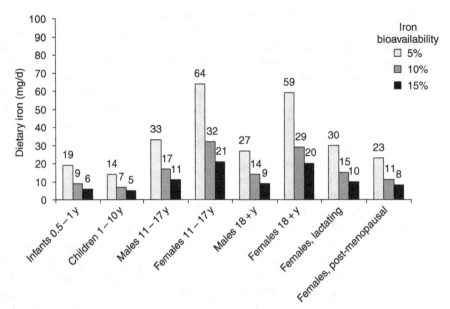

Figure 3 The Recommended Nutrient Intake (RNI) for iron given different levels of bioavailability of iron in the diet: 5%, low; 10%, moderate; and 15%, high. The RNI is based on the amount of iron necessary to meet requirements of 95% of the population for each age/sex group. Because typical iron intakes range from 10 to 15 mg/day, iron requirements are nearly impossible to meet on low-bioavailability diets. (Data from the Food and Agriculture Organization of the United Nations (2001) Iron. In *Human Vitamin and Mineral Requirements: Report of a Joint FAO/WHO Expert Consultation, Bangkok, Thailand*, pp. 195–221. Rome: FAO.)

of bioavailability, iron requirements are not met by many adolescent girls and adult menstruating women who have above average menstrual blood loss. Few if any population groups can achieve iron intakes sufficient to meet iron requirements when bioavailability of iron is poor.

Dietary recommendations for infants are based on the iron content and bioavailability of human milk. The iron in infant formula is much less bioavailable (10%) than that of human milk and is thus present in greater concentrations than that of human milk. Infants who are not breast-fed should consume iron-fortified formula. Complementary foods offered after 6 months of age can potentially meet iron needs if they have a high content of meat and ascorbic acid. This is rarely the case in developing or developed countries, and fortified infant cereals and iron drops are often introduced at this time in developed countries. In developing countries where diets are poor in bioavailable iron, iron-fortified weaning foods are not commonly consumed, and iron supplements are rarely given to infants and children.

Pregnant women rarely have sufficient iron stores and consume diets adequate to maintain positive iron balance, particularly in the latter half of pregnancy, as previously discussed. They cannot meet their iron requirements through diet alone even in developed countries, where high iron content diets with high bioavailability are common.

Supplementation is universally recommended for pregnant women, as discussed later.

Indicators of Iron Deficiency and Anemia

Indicators of iron deficiency can be used to distinguish the degree of iron deficiency that exists across the spectrum from the depletion of body iron stores to frank anemia (**Table 1**). Indicator cutoffs vary by age, sex, race, and physiologic state (e.g., pregnancy), so using a proper reference is important when interpreting indicators of iron deficiency.

Serum ferritin is directly related to liver iron stores—a gold standard for iron deficiency that is infrequently used due to the invasive nature of the test. Different sources place the cutoff for serum ferritin concentrations indicative of depleted stores at 12 or 15 μg/l. Once iron stores are exhausted, serum ferritin is not useful for determining the extent of iron deficiency. Serum ferritin is also useful for diagnosing iron excess. A major limitation of serum ferritin is the fact that it acts as an acute phase reactant and therefore is mildly to substantially elevated in the presence of inflammation or infection, complicating its interpretation when such conditions exist.

Transferrin saturation is measured as the ratio between total serum iron (which declines during iron deficiency) and total iron binding capacity (which increases during iron deficiency). Typically,

Table 1 Indicators for assessing the progression of iron deficiency from depletion of iron stores to iron deficiency anemia

Stage of iron deficiency	Consequence	Indicator
Depletion	Decline in storage iron	↓ Serum ferritin
Deficiency	Decreased circulating iron	↓ Serum iron ↑ Total iron binding capacity ↓ Transferrin saturation
	Insufficient tissue iron	↑ Transferrin receptor
	Impaired heme synthesis	↑ Protoporphyrin/heme
Depletion	Impaired red blood cell production	↓ Hemoglobin ↓ Hematocrit ↓ Red blood cell indices

transferrin is approximately 30% saturated, and low transferrin saturation (< 16%) is indicative of iron deficiency. Transferrin saturation concentrations higher than 60% are indicative of iron overload associated with hereditary hemochromatosis. The use of transferrin saturation to distinguish iron deficiency is limited because of marked diurnal variation and its lack of sensitivity as an indicator.

Elevated circulating TfRs are a sensitive indicator of the tissue demand for iron. Circulating TfR is not affected by inflammation, a limitation of other indicators of iron status. Furthermore, expressing TfR as a ratio with ferritin appears to distinguish with a great deal of sensitivity iron deficiency anemia from anemia of chronic disease, making this combined measure potentially very useful in settings in which these conditions coexist.

Elevated erythrocyte zinc protoporphyrin indicates iron-deficient erythropoiesis. Protoporphyrin concentrations may also be elevated by inflammation and lead exposure.

Finally, although hemoglobin concentrations or percentage hematocrit are not specific for iron deficiency, these measures are used most frequently as a proxy for iron deficiency in field settings because of their technical ease. Anemia is defined as a hemoglobin concentration of less than 110 g/l for those 6 months to 5 years old and for pregnant women, 115 g/l for those 5–11 years old, 120 g/l for nonpregnant females older than 11 years and for males 12–15 years old, or 130 g/l for males older than 15 years of age. Other measures of red blood cell

characteristics include total red blood cell counts, mean corpuscular volume, and mean hemoglobin volume.

The choice of indicators and the strategy for assessment will depend on technical feasibility and whether a screening or survey approach is warranted. When more than 5% of a population is anemic, iron deficiency is considered a public health problem, and population-based surveys may be useful for assessing and monitoring the prevalence of iron deficiency. When anemia is less prevalent, screening for iron deficiency in high-risk groups or symptomatic individuals is a more efficient approach. Hemoglobin alone would be insufficient to diagnose iron deficiency in an individual, but hemoglobin distributions can offer clues as to the extent to which anemia is attributable to iron deficiency in a population. Preferred indicators, such as transferrin and/or ferritin, may not be feasible due to blood collection requirements, cost, or technical difficulty in a population survey, but they may be indispensable for characterizing iron status of a population subgroup or individual.

Prevalence of Iron Deficiency and Iron Deficiency Anemia

Although iron deficiency anemia is considered the most prevalent nutritional deficiency globally, accurate prevalence estimates are difficult to obtain. Worldwide, prevalence estimates for iron deficiency anemia have ranged from 500 million to approximately 2 billion people affected. However, most global prevalence estimates are based on anemia surveys, which will overestimate the amount of anemia attributable to iron deficiency but underestimate the prevalence of less severe iron deficiency. There is clearly a disparity in anemia prevalence between the developing and developed world, with ~50% of children and nonpregnant women in the developing world considered anemic compared with ~10% in the developed world. The prevalence of anemia increases during pregnancy, with ~20% of US women anemic during pregnancy and estimates of anemia prevalence in some developing countries exceeding 60%.

Data from the US NHANES III (1988–1994) survey, which used a variety of indicators of iron status, showed that 9% of US toddlers were iron deficient and 3% had iron deficiency anemia. Eleven percent of adolescent females and women of reproductive age were iron deficient, and 3–5% of these women had iron deficiency anemia. Iron deficiency in the developed world is more common among low-income minorities.

Consequences of Iron Deficiency and Iron Deficiency Anemia

Iron deficiency anemia has been implicated in adverse pregnancy outcomes, maternal and infant mortality, cognitive dysfunction and developmental delays in infants and children, and compromised physical capacity in children and adults. However, data to support causal relationships with some of these outcomes is limited, and the extent to which outcomes are associated with iron deficiency specifically or more generally with anemia regardless of the etiology is the subject of debate.

A variety of observational studies demonstrate an association of maternal hemoglobin concentrations during pregnancy with birth weight, the likelihood of low birth weight and preterm birth, and perinatal mortality, such that adverse pregnancy outcomes are associated in a 'U-shaped' manner with the lowest and highest maternal hemoglobin concentrations. Anemia during pregnancy may not be specific to iron deficiency, and randomized trials utilizing a strict placebo to firmly establish a causal link between iron status per se and adverse pregnancy outcomes are rare because of ethical concerns about denying women iron supplements during pregnancy. However, two randomized trials, one conducted in a developed country and the other in a developing country, have shown a positive impact of iron supplementation during pregnancy on birth weight. In the developed country study, control women with evidence of compromised iron stores were offered iron supplements at 28 weeks of gestation after 8 weeks of randomized iron supplementation. In the developing country study, the control group received supplemental vitamin A and the intervention group received folic acid in addition to iron.

Mortality among pregnant women and infants and children also increases with severe anemia. However, most data showing this relationship are observational and clinic based. Anemia in such circumstances is unlikely to be attributable to iron deficiency alone; furthermore, the degree to which mild to moderate anemia influences mortality outcomes is not well established.

Iron deficiency and iron deficiency anemia have been associated with impaired cognitive development and functioning. These effects of iron deficiency may be mediated in part by the deprivation of functional iron in brain tissue, and the impact of iron deprivation may vary depending on its timing in relation to critical stages of brain development. Iron interventions in anemic school-age children generally result in improved school performance. The results of iron interventions in infants and preschool-age children are less clear, perhaps in part because cognition is more difficult to measure in this age group.

Studies have shown a negative impact of iron deficiency anemia on work productivity among adult male and female workers in settings requiring both strenuous labor (rubber plantation) and less intensive efforts (factory work). The impact of iron deficiency anemia on performance may be mediated by a reduction in the oxygen-carrying capacity of blood associated with low hemoglobin concentration and by a reduction in muscle tissue oxidative capacity related to reductions in myoglobin and effects on iron-containing proteins involved in cellular respiration.

Interventions: Prevention and Treatment of Iron Deficiency Anemia

Supplementation

Iron supplementation is the most common intervention used to prevent and treat iron deficiency anemia. Global guidelines established by the International Nutritional Anemia Consultative Group, the World Health Organization, and UNICEF identify pregnant women and children 6–24 months of age as the priority target groups for iron supplementation because these populations are at the highest risk of iron deficiency and most likely to benefit from its control. However, recommendations are given for other target groups, such as children, adolescents, and women of reproductive age, who may also benefit from iron supplementation for the prevention of iron deficiency. The recommendations are given in **Table 2**. Recommended dose and/or duration of supplementation are increased for populations where the prevalence of anemia is 40% or higher. The recommended treatment for severe anemia (Hb < 70 g/l) is to double prophylactic doses for 3 months and then to continue the preventive supplementation regimen.

Ferrous sulfate is the most common form of iron used in iron tablets, but fumarate and gluconate are also sometimes used. A liquid formulation is available for infants, but it is not used often in anemia control programs in developing countries because of the expense compared to tablets. Crushed tablets can be given to infants and young children as an alternative, but this has not been very successful programmatically.

Efforts to improve the iron status of populations worldwide through supplementation have met with mixed success. Given the frequency with which iron tablets must be taken to be effective, a lack of

Table 2 Guidelines for iron supplementation to prevent iron deficiency anemia

Target group	Dose	Duration
Pregnant women	60 mg iron + 400 μg folic acid daily	6 months in pregnancy[a,b]
Children 6–24 months (normal birth weight)	12.5 mg iron[c] + 50 μg folic acid daily	6–12 months of age[d]
Children 6–24 months (low birth weight)	12.5 mg iron + 50 μg folic acid daily	2–24 months of age
Children 2–5 years	20–30 mg iron[c] daily	
Children 6–11 years	30–60 mg iron daily	
Adolescents and adults	60 mg iron daily[e]	

[a]If 6-months' duration cannot be achieved during pregnancy, continue to supplement during the postpartum period for 6 months or increase the dose to 120 mg iron daily during pregnancy.
[b]Continue for 3 months postpartum where the prevalence of pregnancy anemia is ≥ 40%.
[c]Iron dosage based on 2 mg iron/kg body weight/day.
[d]Continue until 24 months of age where the prevalence of anemia is ≥ 40%.
[e]For adolescent girls and women of reproductive age, 400 μg folic acid should be included with iron supplementation.
Adapted with permission from Stoltzfus RJ and Dreyfuss ML (1998) *Guidelines for the Use of Iron Supplements to Prevent and Treat Iron Deficiency Anemia.* Washington, DC: International Nutritional Anemia Consultative Group.

efficacy of iron supplementation in research studies and programs has often been attributed to poor compliance and the presence of side effects such as nausea and constipation. Ensuring compliance in some settings also requires extensive logistical support. Although in developing countries the maximum coverage of iron supplementation programs for pregnant women is higher than 50%, other high-risk groups are less frequently targeted for iron supplementation.

Comparative trials have demonstrated that both weekly and daily iron supplementation regimens significantly increase indicators of iron status and anemia, but that daily supplements are more efficacious at reducing the prevalence of iron deficiency and anemia, particularly among pregnant women and young children who have high iron demands. Therefore, daily iron supplements continue to be the recommended choice for pregnant women and young children because there is often a high prevalence of iron deficiency anemia in these populations. Weekly supplementation in school-age children and adolescents holds promise for anemia prevention programs because it reduces side effects, improves compliance, and lowers costs. Further assessment of the relative effectiveness of the two approaches is needed to determine which is more effective in the context of programs.

Fortification

Iron fortification of food is the addition of supplemental iron to a mass-produced food vehicle consumed by target populations at risk of iron deficiency anemia. Among anemia control strategies, iron fortification has the greatest potential to improve the iron status of populations. However, its success has been limited by technical challenges

of the fortification process: (i) the identification of a suitable iron compound that does not alter the taste or appearance of the food vehicle but is adequately absorbed and (ii) the inhibitory effect of phytic acid and other dietary components that limit iron absorption. Water-soluble iron compounds, such as ferrous sulfate, are readily absorbed but cause rancidity of fats and color changes in some potential food vehicles (e.g., cereal flours). In contrast, elemental iron compounds do not cause these sensory changes but are poorly absorbed and are unlikely to benefit iron status. Research on iron compounds and iron absorption enhancers that addresses these problems has yielded some promising alternatives. Encapsulated iron compounds prevent some of the sensory changes that occur in fortified food vehicles. The addition of ascorbic acid enhances iron absorption from fortified foods, and NaFe–EDTA provides highly absorbable iron in the presence of phytic acid.

Many iron-fortified products have been tested for the compatibility of the fortificant with the food vehicle and for the bioavailability of the fortified iron, but few efficacy or effectiveness trials have been done. Iron-fortified fish sauce, sugar, infant formula, and infant cereal have been shown to improve iron status. In contrast, attempts to fortify cereal flours with iron have met with little success because they contain high levels of phytic acid and the characteristics of these foods require the use of poorly bioavailable iron compounds.

In the developed world, iron fortification has resulted in decreased rates of iron deficiency and anemia during the past few decades. Some debate remains, however, about the potential for the acquisition of excess iron, which has been associated with increased chronic disease risk in some studies. In Europe, Finland and Denmark have recently discontinued food fortification programs because of concerns of iron overload. Individuals with hereditary hemochromatosis, ~5/1000 individuals in populations of European descent, are at particular risk of iron overload.

Control of Parasitic Infections

Because geohelminths such as hookworm also contribute to iron deficiency, programs that increase iron intakes but do not address this major source of iron loss are unlikely to be effective at improving iron status. Other infections and inflammation also cause anemia, as does malaria, and the safety of iron supplementation during infection or malaria has been debated. Where malaria and iron deficiency coexist, the current view is that iron supplementation is sufficiently beneficial to support its use. Ideally, however, where multiple etiologies of anemia coexist, these etiologies need to be recognized and simultaneously addressed.

Other Micronutrients

Other nutrients and their deficiencies that can impact iron status, utilization, or anemia include vitamin A, folate, vitamin B_{12}, riboflavin, and ascorbic acid (vitamin C). Improving iron status can also increase the utilization of iodine and vitamin A from supplements. On the other hand, it is increasingly recognized that simultaneous provision of iron and zinc in supplements may decrease the benefit of one or both of these nutrients. These complex micronutrient interactions and their implications for nutritional interventions are incompletely understood but have significant implications for population-based supplementation strategies.

Summary

Iron deficiency anemia exists throughout the world, and pregnant women and infants 6–24 months old are at highest risk because of their high iron requirements. Women of reproductive age, school-age children, and adolescents are also high-risk groups that may require attention in anemia control programs. Although numerous indicators exist to characterize the progression of iron deficiency to anemia, difficulties remain with their use and interpretation, particularly in the face of other causes of anemia. Despite the proven efficacy of iron supplementation

and fortification to improve iron status, there are few examples of effective anemia prevention programs. More innovative programmatic approaches that aim to improve iron status, such as geohelminth control or prevention of other micronutrient deficiencies, deserve more attention. Challenges remain in preventing and controlling iron deficiency anemia worldwide.

See also: **Folic Acid**.

Further Reading

ACC/SCN (2001) Preventing and treating anaemia. In: Allen LH and Gillespie SR (eds.) *What Works? A Review of the Efficacy and Effectiveness of Nutrition Interventions*. Geneva: ACC/SCN in collaboration with the Asian Development Bank, Manila.

Anonymous (2001) Supplement II: Iron deficiency anemia: Reexamining the nature and magnitude of the public health problem. *Journal of Nutrition* 131: 563S–703S.

Anonymous (2002) Supplement: Forging effective strategies to combat iron deficiency. *Journal of Nutrition* 132: 789S–882S.

Bothwell TH, Charlton RW, Cook JD, and Finch CA (1979) *Iron Metabolism in Man*. Oxford: Blackwell Scientific.

Cook JD, Skikne BS, and Baynes RD (1994) Iron deficiency: The global perspective. *Advances in Experimental Medicine and Biology* 356: 219–228.

Eisenstein RS and Ross KL (2003) Novel roles for iron regulatory proteins in the adaptive response to iron deficiency. *Journal of Nutrition* 133: 1510S–1516S.

Fairbanks VP (1999) Iron in medicine and nutrition. In: Shils M, Olson JA, Shike M, and Ross AC (eds.) *Modern Nutrition in Health and Disease*, 9th edn, pp. 193–221. Philadelphia: Lippincott Williams & Wilkins.

Food and Agriculture Organization of the United Nations (2001) Iron. In: . *Human Vitamin and Mineral Requirements: Report of a Joint FAO/WHO Expert Consultation, Bangkok, Thailand*, pp. 195–221. Rome: FAO.

Frazer DM and Anderson GJ (2003) The orchestration of body iron intake: How and where do enterocytes receive their cues? *Blood Cells, Molecules, and Diseases* 30(3): 288–297.

Koury MJ and Ponka P (2004) New insights into erythropoiesis: The roles of folate, vitamin B_{12}, and iron. *Annual Review of Nutrition* 24: 105–131.

Leong W-I and Lonnerdal B (2004) Hepcidin, the recently identified peptide that appears to regulate iron absorption. *Journal of Nutrition* 134: 1–4.

Roy CN and Enns CA (2000) Iron homeostasis: New tales from the crypt. *Blood* 96(13): 4020–4027.

Stoltzfus RJ and Dreyfuss ML (1998) *Guidelines for the Use of Iron Supplements to Prevent and Treat Iron Deficiency Anemia*. Washington, DC: International Nutritional Anemia Consultative Group.

World Health Organization (2001) *Iron Deficiency Anaemia Assessment, Prevention and Control: A Guide for Programme Managers*. Geneva: WHO.

ANTIOXIDANTS

Contents
Diet and Antioxidant Defense
Intervention Studies
Observational Studies

Diet and Antioxidant Defense

I F F Benzie, The Hong Kong Polytechnic University, Hong Kong SAR, China
J J Strain, University of Ulster, Coleraine, UK

Introduction

Oxygen is an essential 'nutrient' for most organisms. Paradoxically, however, oxygen damages key biological sites. This has led to oxygen being referred to as a double-edged sword. The beneficial side of oxygen is that it permits energy-efficient catabolism of fuel by acting as the ultimate electron acceptor within mitochondria. During aerobic respiration, an oxygen atom accepts two electrons, forming (with hydrogen) harmless water. The less friendly side of oxygen is the unavoidable and continuous production of partially reduced oxygen intermediates within the body. These 'free radicals' (reactive oxygen species; ROS) are more reactive than ground-state oxygen and cause oxidative changes to carbohydrate, DNA, lipid, and protein. Such changes can affect the structures and functions of macromolecules, organelles, cells, and biological systems. This induces oxidant stress if allowed to proceed unopposed.

The human body is generally well equipped with an array of 'antioxidative' strategies to protect against the damaging effects of ROS. Our endogenous antioxidants are inadequate, however, as we are unable to synthesize at least two important antioxidant compounds, vitamin C and vitamin E. Ingestion of these, and perhaps other, antioxidants is needed to augment our defenses and prevent or minimize oxidative damage. In this article, the causes and consequences of oxidant stress and the types and action of antioxidants will be described, the source and role of dietary antioxidants will be discussed, and current evidence relating to dietary antioxidants and human health will be briefly reviewed.

Oxidant Stress

Oxidant, or oxidative, stress is a pro-oxidant shift in the oxidant–antioxidant balance caused by a relative or absolute deficiency of antioxidants (**Figure 1**). A pro-oxidant shift promotes damaging oxidative changes to important cellular constituents, and this may, in turn, lead to cellular dysfunction and, ultimately, to aging, disability, and disease.

Molecular oxygen is relatively unreactive in its ground state. However, molecular oxygen can be reduced in several ways within the body to produce more reactive species (**Table 1**). These species include radical and nonradical forms of oxygen, some of which contain nitrogen or chlorine. A 'free radical' is capable of independent existence and has a single (unpaired) electron in an orbital. Electrons stabilize as pairs with opposing spins within an orbital. An unpaired electron seeks a partner for stability, and this increases the reactivity of the radical. A partner electron can be obtained by removing ('abstracting') an electron from another species or co-reactant. The result of this interaction may be either quenching by reduction (electron addition) of the radical with the production of a new radical by oxidation (electron loss) of the reductive ('antioxidant') co-reactant or quenching of two radicals if the co-reactant is also a radical (one quenched by reduction (electron addition) and one by oxidation (electron removal)).

Free radicals produced *in vivo* include superoxide, the hydroxyl radical, nitric oxide, oxygen-centered organic radicals such as peroxyl and alkoxyl radicals, and sulfur-centered thiyl radicals. Other oxygen-containing reactive species that are not radicals are also formed. These include hydrogen peroxide, peroxynitrite, and hypochlorous acid. While these are not radical species, they are actually or potentially damaging oxidants. The collective term ROS is often used to describe both radical and nonradical species.

What Causes Oxidant Stress?

Oxidant stress is caused by the damaging action of ROS. There are two main routes of production of ROS in the body: one is deliberate and useful; the

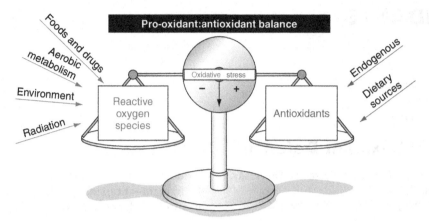

Figure 1 Antioxidant defenses balance reactive oxygen species load and oppose oxidant stress.

other is accidental but unavoidable (**Figure 2**). Deliberate production of ROS is seen, for example, during the respiratory burst of activated phagocytic white cells (macrophages, neutrophils, and monocytes). Activated phagocytes produce large amounts of superoxide and hypochlorous acid for microbial killing. The ROS nitric oxide is produced constitutively and inducibly, is a powerful vasodilator, and is vital for the maintenance of normal blood pressure. Nitric oxide also decreases platelet aggregability, decreasing the likelihood of the blood clotting within the circulation. Hydrogen peroxide is produced enzymatically from superoxide by the action of the superoxide dismutases (SODs) and is recognized increasingly as playing a central role in cell signalling and gene activation. Nonetheless, while some ROS are physiologically useful, they are damaging if they accumulate in excess as a result of, for example, acute or chronic inflammation or ischaemia.

Accidental, but unavoidable, production of ROS occurs during the passage of electrons along the mitochondrial electron transport chain. Leakage of electrons from the chain leads to the single-electron reduction of oxygen, with the consequent formation of superoxide. This can be regarded as a normal, but undesirable, by-product of aerobic metabolism. Around 1–3% of electrons entering the respiratory chain are estimated to end up in superoxide, and this results in a large daily ROS load *in vivo*. If anything increases oxygen use, such as exercise, then more ROS will be formed, and oxidant stress may increase owing to a pro-oxidant shift. Significant amounts of ROS are also produced during the metabolism of drugs and pollutants by the mixed-function cytochrome P-450 oxidase (phase I) detoxifying system and as a consequence of the transformation of xanthine dehydrogenase to its truncated oxidase form, which occurs as a result of ischemia. This causes a flood of superoxide to be formed when

Table 1 Reactive oxygen species found *in vivo* in general order of reactivity (from lowest to highest)

Name of species	Sign/ formula	Radical (R) or nonradical (NR)	Comment
Molecular oxygen	O_2	R	Biradical, with two unpaired electrons; these are in parallel spins, and this limits reactivity
Nitric oxide	$NO^{\cdot}$	R	Important to maintain normal vasomotor tone
Superoxide	$O_2^{\cdot-}$	R	Single electron reduction product of O_2; large amounts produced *in vivo*
Peroxyl	$ROO^{\cdot}$	R	R is often a carbon of an unsaturated fatty acid
Singlet oxygen	$^1\Delta_g O_2$ $^1\Sigma_g^+ O_2$	NR	'Energized' nonradical forms of molecular oxygen; one unpaired electron is transferred to the same orbital as the other unpaired electron
Hydrogen peroxide	H_2O_2	NR	Small, uncharged, freely diffusible ROS formed by dismutation of superoxide
Hydroperoxyl	$HOO^{\cdot}$	R	Protonated, more reactive form of superoxide; formed at sites of low pH
Alkoxyl	$RO^{\cdot}$	R	R is carbon in a carbon-centered radical formed by peroxidation of unsaturated fatty acid
Hypochlorous	$HOCl$	NR	Formed in activated phagocytes to aid in microbial killing
Peroxynitrite	$HNOO^-$	NR	Highly reactive product of nitric oxide and superoxide
Hydroxyl	$^{\cdot}OH$	R	Fiercely, indiscriminately reactive radical

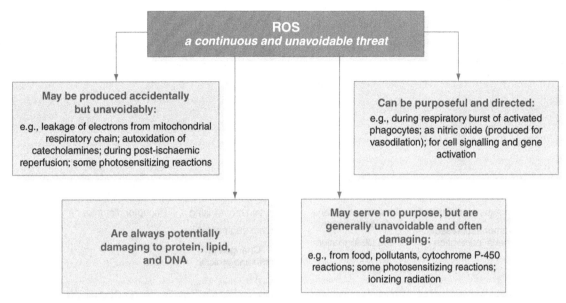

Figure 2 Sources of reactive oxygen species found *in vivo*.

the oxygen supply is restored. In addition, if free iron is present (as may happen in iron overload, acute intravascular hemolysis, or cell injury), there is a risk of a cycle of ROS production via iron-catalyzed 'autoxidation' of various constituents in biological fluids, including ascorbic acid, catecholamines, dopamine, hemoglobin, flavins, and thiol compounds such as cysteine or homocysteine. Preformed reactive species in food further contribute to the oxidant load of the body, and ROS are also produced by pathological processes and agents such as chronic inflammation, infection, ionizing radiation, and cigarette smoke. Breathing oxygen-enriched air results in enhanced production of ROS within the lungs, and various toxins and drugs, such as aflatoxin, acetaminophen, carbon tetrachloride, chloroform, and ethanol, produce reactive radical species during their metabolism or detoxification and excretion by the liver or kidneys. Clearly, all body tissues are exposed to ROS on a regular or even constant basis. However, sites of particularly high ROS loads within the human body include the mitochondria, the eyes, the skin, areas of cell damage, inflammation, and post-ischemic reperfusion, the liver, the lungs (especially if oxygen-enriched air is breathed), and the brain.

What does Oxidant Stress Cause?

A sudden and large increase in ROS load can overwhelm local antioxidant defenses and induce severe oxidant stress, with cell damage, cell death, and subsequent organ failure. However, less dramatic chronic oxidant stress may lead to depletion of defenses and accumulation of damage and ultimately cause physiological dysfunction and pathological change resulting in disability and disease. This is because oxidant stress causes oxidative changes to DNA, lipid, and protein. These changes lead in turn to DNA breaks, mutagenesis, changed phenotypic expression, membrane disruption, mitochondrial dysfunction, adenosine triphosphate depletion, intracellular accumulation of non-degradable oxidized proteins, increased atherogenicity of low-density lipoproteins, and crosslinking of proteins with subsequent loss of function of specialized protein structures, for example, enzymes, receptors, and the crystallins of the ocular lens. In addition, the aldehydic degradation products of oxidized polyunsaturated fatty acids (PUFAs) are carcinogenic and cytotoxic. Increased oxidant stress can also trigger apoptosis, or programed cell death, through a changed redox balance, damage to membrane ion-transport channels, and increased intracellular calcium levels (**Figure 3**).

Oxidant stress, through its effects on key biological sites and structures, is implicated in chronic noncommunicable diseases such as coronary heart disease, cancer, cataract, dementia, and stroke (**Figure 4**). Oxidant stress is also thought to be a key player in the aging process itself. A cause-and-effect relationship between oxidant stress and aging

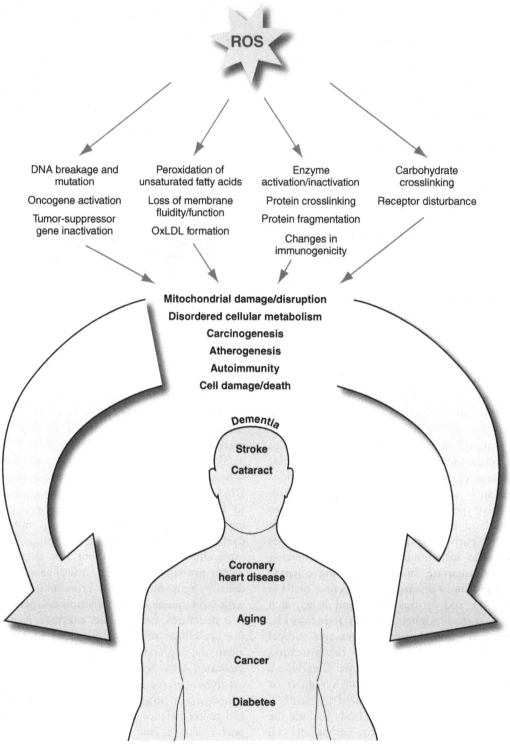

Figure 3 Possible involvement of reactive oxygen species (ROS) in ageing and chronic degenerative disease. OxLDL, oxidized low density lipoprotein.

and disease has not been confirmed, however, and it is very unlikely that oxidant stress is the sole cause of aging and chronic degenerative disease. Nonetheless, there is evidence that oxidant stress contributes substantially to age-related physiological decline and pathological changes. Consequently, if it

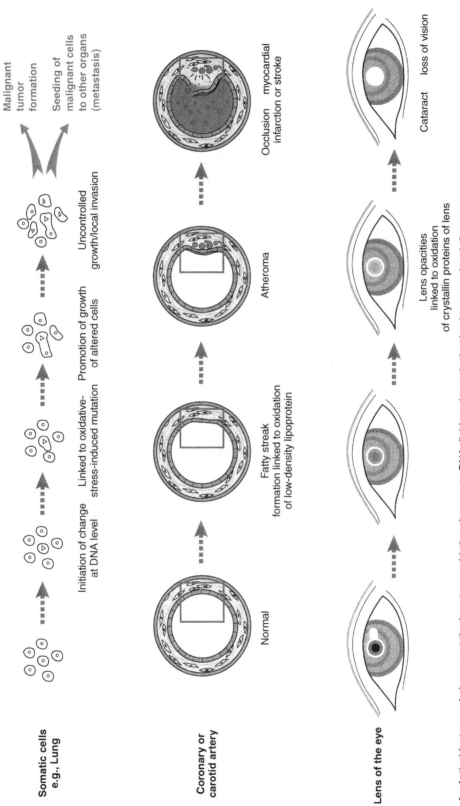

Somatic cells e.g., Lung

Initiation of change at DNA level

Linked to oxidative-stress-induced mutation

Promotion of growth of altered cells

Uncontrolled growth/local invasion

Malignant tumor formation

Seeding of malignant cells to other organs (metastasis)

Coronary or carotid artery

Normal

Fatty streak formation linked to oxidation of low-density lipoprotein

Atheroma

Occlusion myocardial infarction or stroke

Lens of the eye

Lens opacities linked to oxidation of crystallin proteins of lens

Cataract loss of vision

Figure 4 Antioxidants may help prevent the long-term oxidative changes to DNA, lipid, and protein that lead to age-related disease.

is accepted that oxidant stress is associated with aging and degenerative disease, then opposing oxidant stress by increasing antioxidant defense offers a potentially effective means of delaying the deleterious effects of aging, decreasing the risk of chronic disease, and achieving functional longevity. For this reason, there has been great interest in recent years in the source, action, and potential health benefits of dietary antioxidants.

Antioxidant Defense

An antioxidant can be described in simple terms as anything that can delay or prevent oxidation of a susceptible substrate. Our antioxidant system is complex, however, and consists of various intracellular and extracellular, endogenous and exogenous, and aqueous and lipid-soluble components that act in concert to prevent ROS formation (preventative antioxidants), destroy or inactivate ROS that are formed (scavenging and enzymatic antioxidants), and terminate chains of ROS-initiated peroxidation of biological substrates (chain-breaking antioxidants). In addition, metals and minerals (such as selenium, copper, and zinc) that are key components of antioxidant enzymes are often referred to as antioxidants.

There are many biological and dietary constituents that show 'antioxidant' properties *in vitro*. For an antioxidant to have a physiological role, however, certain criteria must be met.

1. The antioxidant must be able to react with ROS found at the site(s) in the body where the putative antioxidant is found.
2. Upon interacting with a ROS, the putative antioxidant must not be transformed into a more reactive species than the original ROS.
3. The antioxidant must be found in sufficient quantity at the site of its presumed action *in vivo* for it to make an appreciable contribution to defense at that site: if its concentration is very low, there must be some way of continuously recycling or resupplying the putative antioxidant.

Antioxidants Found Within the Human Body

The structures of the human body are exposed continuously to a variety of ROS. Humans have evolved an effective antioxidant system to defend against these damaging agents. Different sites of the body contain different antioxidants or contain the same

antioxidants but in different amounts. Differences are likely to reflect the different requirements and characteristics of these sites.

Human plasma and other biological fluids are generally rich in scavenging and chain-breaking antioxidants, including vitamin C (ascorbic acid) and 'vitamin E.' Vitamin E is the name given to a group of eight lipid-soluble tocopherols and tocotrienols. In the human diet, γ-tocopherol is the main form of vitamin E, but the predominant form in human plasma is α-tocopherol. Bilirubin, uric acid, glutathione, flavonoids, and carotenoids also have antioxidant activity and are found in cells and/or plasma. Scavenging and chain-breaking antioxidants found *in vivo* are derived overall from both endogenous and exogenous sources. Cells contain, in addition, antioxidant enzymes, the SODs, glutathione peroxidase, and catalase. The transition metals iron and copper, which can degrade preexisting peroxides and form highly reactive ROS, are kept out of the peroxidation equation by being tightly bound to, or incorporated within, specific proteins such as transferrin and ferritin (for iron) and caeruloplasmin (for copper). These proteins are regarded as preventive antioxidants. Caeruloplasmin ferroxidase activity is also important for the non-ROS-producing route of ferrous (Fe(II)) to ferric (Fe(III)) oxidation and for incorporating released iron into ferritin for 'safe' iron storage. Haptoglobin (which binds released hemoglobin), hemopexin (which binds released hem), and albumin (which binds transition-metal ions and localizes or absorbs their oxidative effects) can also be regarded as antioxidants in that they protect against metal-ion-catalyzed redox reactions that may produce ROS. An overview of the major types of antioxidants within the body and their interactions is given in **Table 2** and **Figure 5**.

Table 2 Types of antioxidants

Physical barriers *prevent* ROS generation or ROS access to important biological sites; e.g., UV filters, cell membranes

Chemical traps or sinks 'absorb' energy and electrons and *quench* ROS; e.g., carotenoids, anthocyanidins

Catalytic systems *neutralize or divert* ROS, e.g., the antioxidant enzymes superoxide dismutase, catalase, and glutathione peroxidase

Binding and redox inactivation of metal ions *prevent generation* of ROS by inhibiting the Haber–Weiss reaction; e.g., ferritin, caeruloplasmin, catechins

Sacrificial and chain-breaking antioxidants *scavenge and destroy* ROS; e.g., ascorbic acid (vitamin C), tocopherols (vitamin E), uric acid, glutathione, flavonoids

---

ROS, reactive oxygen species.

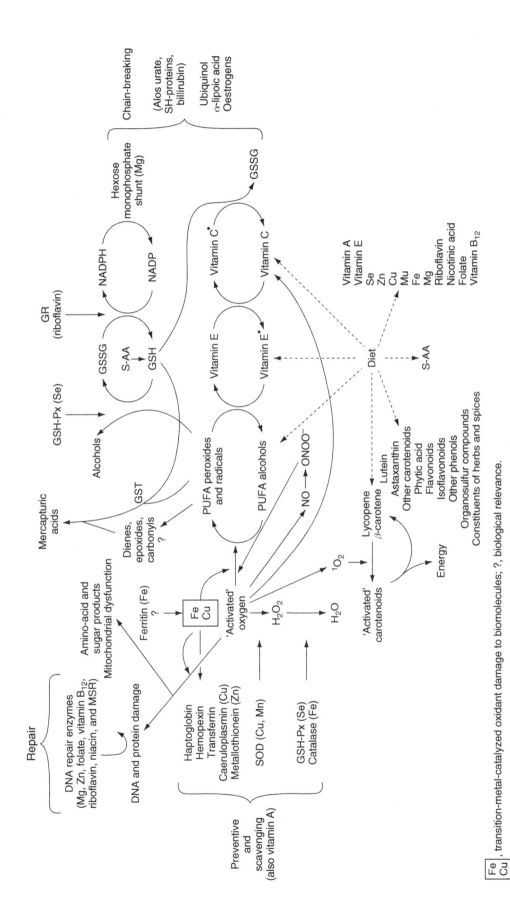

Figure 5 The integrated antioxidant defense system comprises both endogenous and dietary-derived antioxidants. GR, glutathione reductase (EC1.6.4.2); GSH, reduced glutathione; GSH-Px, glutathione peroxidase (EC1.11.1.9); GSSG, oxidized glutathione; GST, glutathione-S-transferase (EC 2.5.1.18); MSR, methionine sulfoxide reductase (EC1.8.4.5); NADPH and, NADP, are, respectively, the reduced and oxidized forms of the co-factor nicotinamide adenine dinucleotide phosphate; PUFA, polyunsaturated fatty acid; S-AA, sulfur amino-acids; SH, sulfhydryl; SOD, superoxide dismutase (EC1.15.1.1).

Dietary Antioxidants

The human endogenous antioxidant system is impressive but incomplete. Regular and adequate dietary intakes of (largely) plant-based antioxidants, most notably vitamin C, vitamin E, and folic acid, are needed. Fresh fruits and vegetables are rich in antioxidants (**Figure 6**), and epidemiological evidence of protection by diets rich in fruits and vegetables is strong. To decrease the risk of cancer of various sites, five or more servings per day of fruits and vegetables are recommended. However, it is not known whether it is one, some, or all antioxidant(s) that are the key protective agents in these foods. Furthermore, it may be that antioxidants are simple co-travellers with other, as yet unidentified, components of antioxidant-rich foods. Perhaps antioxidants are not 'magic bullets' but rather 'magic markers' of protective elements. Nonetheless, the US recommended daily intakes (RDIs) for vitamin C and vitamin E were increased in 2000 in recognition of the strong evidence that regular high intakes of these antioxidant vitamins are associated with a decreased risk of chronic disease and with lower all-cause mortality.

To date, research on dietary antioxidant micronutrients has concentrated mainly on vitamin C and vitamin E. This is likely to be because humans have an undoubted requirement for these antioxidants, which we cannot synthesize and must obtain in regular adequate amounts from food. However, there are a plethora of other dietary antioxidants. Some or all of the thousands of carotenoids, flavonoids, and phenolics found in plant-based foods, herbs, and beverages, such as teas and wines, may also be important for human health, although there are currently no RDIs for these. Furthermore, while there are recommended intakes for vitamin C, vitamin E, and folic acid, these vary among countries, and there is currently no agreement as regards the 'optimal' intake for health. In addition, there is growing evidence that other dietary constituents with antioxidant properties, such as quercetin and catechins (found in teas, wines, apples, and onions), lycopene, lutein, and zeaxanthin (found in tomatoes, spinach, and herbs) contribute to human health. Zinc (found especially in lamb, leafy and root vegetables, and shellfish) and selenium (found especially in beef, cereals, nuts, and fish) are incorporated into the antioxidant enzymes SOD and glutathione peroxidase, and the elements are therefore sometimes referred to as antioxidants.

The levels of ascorbic acid, α-tocopherol, folic acid, carotenoids, and flavonoids within the body are maintained by dietary intake. While the role and importance of dietary antioxidants are currently unclear, antioxidant defense can be modulated by increasing or decreasing the intake of foods containing these antioxidants. There are a number of reasons for recommending dietary changes in preference to supplementation for achieving increased antioxidant status, as follows.

1. It is not clear which antioxidants confer protection.
2. The hierarchy of protection may vary depending on body conditions.
3. A cooperative mix of antioxidants is likely to be more effective than an increased intake of one antioxidant.

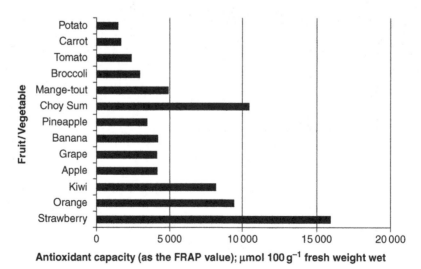

Antioxidant capacity (as the FRAP value); µmol 100 g⁻¹ fresh weight wet

Figure 6 Antioxidant capacity varies among different fruits and vegetables. FRAP, Ferric Reducing/Anti-oxidant Power.

4. Antioxidants, including vitamin A, β-carotene, vitamin C, selenium, and copper, can be harmful in large doses or under certain circumstances.
5. Antioxidant status is likely to be affected by the overall composition of the diet, e.g., the fatty-acid and phytochemical mix.
6. The iron status of the body, environmental conditions, and lifestyle undoubtedly affect antioxidant demand.

Antioxidant defense, therefore, is likely to be optimized through a balanced intake of a variety of antioxidants from natural sources rather than by pharmacological doses of one or a few antioxidants.

Dietary Recommendations for Increased Antioxidant Defense

Dietary recommendations that would result in increased antioxidant defense are not inconsistent with accepted recommendations for healthy eating. The recommendation to increase the consumption of plant-based foods and beverages is one that is widely perceived as health promoting, and the consistent and strong epidemiological links between high fruit and vegetable intake and the greater life expectancy seen in various groups worldwide whose diet is high in plant-based foods indicate that more emphasis should be given to this particular dietary recommendation. Vitamin C, vitamin E, various carotenoids, flavonoids, isoflavonoids, phenolic acids, organosulfur compounds, folic acid, copper, zinc, and selenium are all important for antioxidant defense, and these are found in plant-based foods and beverages such as fruits, vegetables, nuts, seeds, teas, herbs, and wines. Dietary strategies for health promotion should be directed towards optimizing the consumption of these items.

It is recommended generally that at least five servings of fruits and vegetables are eaten each day. This recommendation is based on a wealth of epidemiological evidence that, overall, indicates that 30–40% of all cancers can be prevented by diet. However, it is estimated that most individuals in developed countries eat less than half this amount of fruits and vegetables, and intake by people in developing nations is often very low. Furthermore, the antioxidant contents (both of individual antioxidants and in total) of foods vary widely among different food items and even within the same food item, depending on storage, processing, and cooking method. In addition, the issues of bioavailability and distribution must be considered, and it is of interest to see where dietary antioxidants accumulate (**Table 3**). Vitamin C is absorbed well at low doses and is concentrated in nucleated cells and in the eyes, but relative absorption within the gastrointestinal tract decreases as dose ingested increases. Of the eight isomers of 'vitamin E,' α-tocopherol and γ-tocopherol are distributed around the body and are found in various sites, including skin and adipose tissue. Vitamin E protects lipid systems, such as membranes and lipoproteins. While α-tocopherol is

Table 3 Dietary antioxidants: source, bioavailability, and concentrations in human plasma

	Dietary source	Bioavailability	Concentration	Comment
Ascorbic acid (vitamin C)	Fruits and vegetables, particularly strawberries, citrus, kiwi, Brussels sprouts, and cauliflower	100% at low doses (< 100 mg) decreasing to $< 15\%$ at > 10 g	25–80 μmol l^{-1}	Unstable at neutral pH, concentrated in cells and the eye
'Vitamin E' (in humans mainly α-tocopherol)	Green leafy vegetables, e.g., spinach, nuts, seeds, especially wheatgerm, vegetable oils, especially sunflower	10–95%, but limited hepatic uptake of absorbed tocopherol	15–40 μmol l^{-1} (depending on vitamin supply and lipid levels)	Major tocopherol in diet is γ form, but α form is preferentially taken up by human liver
Carotenoids (hundreds)	Orange/red fruits and vegetables (carrot, tomato, apricot, melon, yam), green leafy vegetables	Unclear, dose and form dependent, probably $< 15\%$	Very low (< 1 μmol l^{-1})	Lutein and zeaxanthin are concentrated in macula region of the eye
Flavonoids (enormous range of different types)	Berries, apples, onions, tea, red wine, some herbs (parsley, thyme), citrus fruits, grapes, cherries	Most poorly absorbed, quercetin absorption 20–50%, catechins $< 2\%$, dependent on form and dose	No data for most, likely < 3 μmol l^{-1} in total	Quercetin and catechins may be most relevant to humans health as intake is relatively high, there is some absorption, possible gastrointestinal-tract protection by unabsorbed flavonoids

by far the predominant form in human lipophilic structures, there is limited information on the bioavailabilities and roles of the other isomers. Gastrointestinal absorption of catechins (a type of flavonoid found in high quantity in tea) is very low, and, although it has been shown that plasma antioxidant capacity increases after ingesting catechin-rich green tea, catechins appear to be excreted via the urine fairly rapidly. Some are likely to be taken up by membranes and cells, although this is not clear, but most of the flavonoids ingested are likely to remain within the gastrointestinal tract. However, this does not necessarily mean that they have no role to play in antioxidant defense, as the unabsorbed antioxidants may provide local defense to the gut lining (**Figure 7**).

With regard to plasma and intracellular distributions of dietary antioxidants, if it is confirmed that increasing defense by dietary means is desirable, frequent small doses of antioxidant-rich food may be the most effective way to achieve this. Furthermore, ingestion of those foods with the highest antioxidant contents may be the most cost-effective strategy. For example, it has been estimated that around 100 mg of ascorbic acid (meeting the recently revised US RDI for vitamin C) is supplied by one orange, a few strawberries, one kiwi fruit, two slices of pineapple, or a handful of raw cauliflower or uncooked spinach leaves. Interestingly, apples, bananas, pears, and plums, which are probably the most commonly consumed fruits in Western countries, are very low in vitamin C. However, these, and other, fruits contain a significant amount of antioxidant power, which is conferred by a variety of other scavenging and chain-breaking antioxidants (**Figure 6**).

Dietary Antioxidants and Human Health

Plants produce a very impressive array of antioxidant compounds, including carotenoids, flavonoids, cinnamic acids, benzoic acids, folic acid, ascorbic acid, tocopherols, and tocotrienols, and plant-based foods are our major source of dietary antioxidants. Antioxidant compounds are concentrated in the oxidation-prone sites of the plant, such as the oxygen-producing chloroplast and the PUFA-rich seeds and oils. Plants make antioxidants to protect their own structures from oxidant stress, and plants increase antioxidant synthesis at times of additional need and when environmental conditions are particularly harsh.

Humans also can upregulate the synthesis of endogenous antioxidants, but this facility is very limited. For example, production of the antioxidant

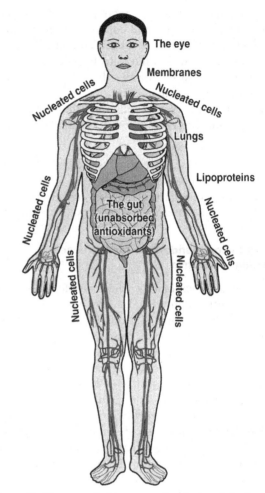

Figure 7 Dietary antioxidants are absorbed and distributed to various sites within the human body.

enzyme SOD is increased with regular exercise, presumably as an adaptation to the increased ROS load resulting from higher oxygen use. However, an increase in other endogenous antioxidants, such as bilirubin and uric acid, is associated with disease, not with improved health. Increasing the antioxidant status of the body by purposefully increasing the production of these antioxidants, therefore, is not a realistic strategy. However, the concept that increased antioxidant intake leads to increased antioxidant defense, conferring increased protection against oxidant stress and, thereby, decreasing the risk of disease, is a simple and attractive one. Antioxidant defense can be modulated by varying the dietary intake of foods rich in natural antioxidants. It has been shown that following ingestion of an antioxidant-rich food, drink, or herb the antioxidant status of the plasma does indeed increase. The question remains, however, as to whether increasing the antioxidant defense of the body by dietary means, while achievable, is a desirable strategy to promote human health and well-being.

There are many age-related disorders that, in theory at least, may be prevented or delayed by increased antioxidant defense. These disorders include arthritis, cancer, coronary heart disease, cataract, dementia, hypertension, macular degeneration, the metabolic complications of diabetes mellitus, and stroke. The rationale for prevention of disease by antioxidants is based on the following facts.

1. Epidemiological evidence shows that a high intake of antioxidant-rich foods, and in some cases antioxidant supplements, is associated with a lower risk of these diseases.
2. Experimental evidence shows that oxidation of cells and structures (such as low-density lipoprotein, DNA, membranes, proteins, and mitochondria) is increased in individuals suffering from these disorders.
3. Experimental evidence shows that antioxidants protect protein, lipid, and DNA from oxidative damage.
4. Experimental evidence shows that biomarkers of oxidative damage to key structures are ameliorated by an increased intake of dietary antioxidants.

However, the following cautionary statements must be noted.

1. While there is a large body of observational evidence supporting a protective effect of dietary antioxidants, it has been suggested that the importance of this has been overstated, and recent studies are less supportive.
2. While phenomenological evidence is strong that oxidative damage does occur in aging and in chronic degenerative diseases, cause-and-effect relationships have not been confirmed.
3. While experimental evidence is quite strong, studies have generally been performed *in vitro* using very high concentrations of antioxidants, making their physiological relevance unclear.
4. Evidence from intervention trials is of variable quality and conflicting; animal studies have shown positive results but have often used very high does of antioxidants, and the relevance to human health is unclear; large human intervention trials completed to date, such as the α-Tocopherol β-Carotene Cancer Prevention Study, Gruppo Italiano per Io Studio Delia Sopravivenza nell'Infarto Miocardico, the Heart Protection Study, the Heart Outcomes Prevention Evaluation, and the Primary Prevention Project, have been largely disappointing in that they have not shown the expected benefits. These studies are summarized in **Table 4**.

Overall, observational data are supportive of beneficial effects of diets rich in antioxidants (**Figure 8**), and intervention trials have often used high-risk groups or individuals with established disease (**Table 4**). In addition, intervention trials have generally used antioxidant supplements (usually vitamin C or vitamin E) rather than antioxidant mixtures or antioxidant-rich foods. Therefore, while observational data support a role for antioxidant-rich food in health promotion, whether or not it is the antioxidants in the food that are responsible for the benefit remains to be confirmed.

Summary and Concluding Remarks

Our diet contains a multitude of antioxidants that we cannot synthesize, and most are plant-based. The available evidence supports a role for antioxidant-rich foods in the promotion of health, although it is not yet clear how many antioxidants and how much of each are needed to achieve an optimal status of antioxidant defense and minimize disease risk. Nor is it clear whether the benefit is of a threshold type or whether it continues to increase with the amount of antioxidant ingested. It is also not yet known whether those dietary antioxidants for which there is no absolute known requirement play a significant role in human antioxidant defense and health or whether they are merely coincidental co-travellers with other, as yet unknown, antioxidant or nonantioxidant dietary constituents that have beneficial effects. A reasonable recommendation is to eat a variety of antioxidant-rich foods on a regular basis. This is likely to be beneficial and is not associated with any harmful effects. However, further study is needed before firm conclusions can be drawn regarding the long-term health benefits of increasing antioxidant defense per se, whether through food or supplements. The challenge in nutritional and biomedical science remains to develop tools that will allow the measurement of biomarkers of functional and nutritional status and to clarify human requirements for dietary antioxidants, the goal being the design of nutritional strategies to promote health and functional longevity.

Table 4 Summary of completed large antioxidant intervention trials

Name and aim of study	Subjects	Supplementation	Results/comments	Reference
The α-tocopherol β-carotene cancer prevention study (ATBC); primary prevention	29 133 high-risk subjects (male smokers, 50–69 years old; average of 20 cigarettes day^{-1} smoked for 36 years)	50 mg day^{-1} of α-tocopherol (synthetic) or 20 mg day^{-1} of β-carotene, or placebo, for 5–8 years (median follow-up 6.1 years)	Supplementation with α-tocopherol had no effect on lung-cancer incidence; no evidence of interaction between α-tocopherol and β-carotene; significant increase in fatal coronary events in men with history of heart disease, and 18% increase in lung-cancer incidence in β-carotene supplemented men; follow-up showed significant (32%) decrease in risk of prostate cancer and nonsignificant (8%) decrease in fatal coronary heart disease in α-tocopherol supplemented subjects	The Alpha-tocopherol, Beta-carotene Cancer Prevention Study Group (1994) *Journal of the National Cancer Institute* 88: 1560–1570 Pryor WA (2000) *Free Radical Biology and Medicine* 28: 141–164
The Cambridge Heart Antioxidant Study (CHAOS); secondary prevention	2002 high-risk subjects (angiographically proven cardiovascular disease)	d-α-tocopherol 400 IU or 800 IU per day (median follow-up 510 days; results on different doses combined into one treatment group)	Significant decrease (77%) in non-fatal MI in treatment group; slight nonsignificant (18%) increase in fatal cardiovascular events in treatment group, but most (21/27) in noncompliant subjects	Stephens NG *et al.* (1996) *Lancet* 347: 781–786
Gruppo Italiano per lo Studio Delia Sopravvivenza nell'Infarto Miocardico (GISSI); secondary prevention	11 324 survivors of MI within previous 3 months of enrollment	α-tocopherol (synthetic) 300 mg day^{-1} or omega 3 fatty acids (0.9 g day^{-1}) or both or neither for 3.5 years; subjects continued on normal medication (50% on statins)	Nonsignificant decrease (11%) in primary endpoints (death, nonfatal MI, and stroke) with vitamin E; high dropout rate (25%); open label study	Marchioli R (1999) *Lancet* 354: 447–455
Primary Prevention Project (PPP)	4495 subjects with ≥ 1 major cardiovascular risk factor	α-tocopherol (synthetic) 300 mg day^{-1} or aspirin 100 mg day^{-1} or both or neither, follow-up average of 3.6 years	Vitamin E had no significant effect on any primary endpoint (cardiovascular death, MI, or stroke)	Primary Prevention Project (2001) *Lancet* 357: 89–95
The Heart Outcomes Prevention Evaluation Study (HOPE); secondary prevention	9541 subjects (2545 women, 6996 men) aged ≥ 55 years, high-risk (cardiovascular disease or diabetes and ≥ 1 other CVD risk factor)	400 IU day^{-1} vitamin E (from 'natural sources') or Ramipril (angiotensin converting enzyme inhibitor) or both or neither; follow-up for 4–6 years	No significant effect of vitamin E on any primary endpoint (MI, stroke, or cardiovascular death)	The Heart Outcomes Prevention Evaluation Study Investigators (2000) *New England Journal of Medicine* 342: 154–160
Heart Protection Study	20 536 subjects, high-risk (diabetes, peripheral vascular disease or coronary heart disease)	Daily antioxidant cocktail (600 IU dl-α-tocopherol, 250 mg vitamin C, 20 mg β-carotene) or placebo for 5 years	No significant differences in hemorrhagic stroke or all-cause mortality between treatment and placebo groups	The Heart Protection Study Collaborative Group (2002) *Lancet* 360: 23–32

MI, myocardial infarction; CVD, cardiovascular disease.

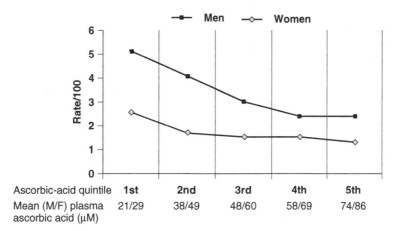

Figure 8 Age-adjusted rates of all-cause mortality by sex-specific ascorbic-acid quintiles in 8860 British men (squares) and 10 636 British women (diamonds).

Acknowledgments

The authors thank The Hong Kong Polytechnic University and The University of Ulster for financially supporting this work.

See also: **Antioxidants**: Observational Studies; Intervention Studies. **Ascorbic Acid**: Physiology, Dietary Sources and Requirements. **Carotenoids**: Chemistry, Sources and Physiology; Epidemiology of Health Effects. **Copper. Folic Acid. Riboflavin. Selenium. Vitamin E**: Physiology and Health Effects. **Zinc**: Physiology.

Further Reading

Ames BN and Wakimoto P (2002) Are vitamin and mineral deficiencies a major cancer risk? *Nature Reviews* 2: 694–704.

Asplund K (2002) Antioxidant vitamins in the prevention of cardiovascular disease: a systematic review. *Journal of Internal Medicine* 251: 372–392.

Benzie IFF (2003) Evolution of dietary antioxidants. *Journal of Comparative Biochemistry and Physiology* 136: 113–126.

Block G, Norkus E, Hudes M, Mandel S, and Helzlsouer K (2001) Which plasma antioxidants are most related to fruit and vegetable consumption? *American Journal of Epidemiology* 154: 1113–1118.

Chisholm GM and Steinberg D (2000) The oxidative modification hypothesis of atherogenesis: an overview. *Free Radical Biology and Medicine* 28: 1815–1826.

Clarkson PM and Thompson HS (2000) Antioxidants: what role do they play in physical activity and health? *American Journal of Clinical Nutrition* 72(Supplement 2): 637S–646S.

Cooke MS, Evans MD, Mistry N, and Lunec J (2002) Role of dietary antioxidants in the prevention of *in vivo* oxidative DNA damage. *Nutrition Research Reviews* 15: 19–41.

Halliwell B and Gutteridge JMC (1999) *Free Radicals in Biology and Medicine*, 3rd edn. Oxford: Clarendon Press.

Khaw KT, Bingham S, Welch A *et al.* (2001) Relation between plasma ascorbic acid and mortality in men and women in EPIC-Norfolk prospective study: a prospective population study. *Lancet* 357: 657–663.

Levine M, Wang Y, Padayatty SJ, and Morrow J (2001) A new recommended dietary allowance of vitamin C for healthy young women. *Proceedings of the National Academy of Science USA* 98: 9842–9846.

Lindsay DG and Clifford MN (eds.) (2000) Critical reviews produced within the EU Concerted Action 'Nutritional Enhancement of Plant-Based Food in European Trade' (NEODIET). *Journal of the Science of Food Agriculture* 80: 793–1137.

McCall MR and Frei B (1999) Can antioxidant vitamins materially reduce oxidative damage in humans? *Free Radical Biology and Medicine* 26: 1034–1053.

Polidori MC, Stahl W, Eichler O, Niestrol I, and Sies H (2001) Profiles of antioxidants in human plasma. *Free Radical Biology and Medicine* 30: 456–462.

Pryor WA (2000) Vitamin E and heart disease: basic science to clinical intervention trials. *Free Radical Biology and Medicine* 28: 141–164.

Szeto YT, Tomlinson B, and Benzie IFF (2002) Total antioxidant and ascorbic acid content of fresh fruits and vegetables: implications for dietary planning and food preservation. *British Journal of Nutrition* 87: 55–59.

World Cancer Research Fund and the American Institute for Cancer Research (1997) *Food, Nutrition and the Prevention of Cancer: A Global Perspective*. Washington, DC: American Institute for Cancer Research.

Intervention Studies

S Stanner, British Nutrition Foundation, London, UK

A predominantly plant-based diet reduces the risk of developing several chronic diseases, including cancer and cardiovascular disease (CVD) coronary heart disease and stroke. It is often assumed that antioxidants, including vitamin C, vitamin E, the carotenoids (e.g., β-carotene, lycopene, and lutein), selenium, and the flavonoids (e.g., quercetin, kaempferol, myricetin, luteolin, and apigenin), contribute to this protection by interfering passively with oxidative damage to DNA, lipids, and proteins. This hypothesis is supported by numerous *in vitro* studies in animals and humans. A large number of descriptive, case–control, and cohort studies have also demonstrated an inverse association between high intakes and/or plasma levels of antioxidants and risk of CVD and cancer at numerous sites, as well as other conditions associated with oxidative damage, such as age-related macular degeneration, cataracts, and chronic obstructive pulmonary disease (COPD).

These findings provided a strong incentive for the initiation of intervention studies to investigate whether a lack of dietary antioxidants is causally related to chronic disease risk and if providing antioxidant supplements confers benefits for the prevention and treatment of these conditions. This article summarizes the findings of the largest primary and secondary trials published to date and considers their implications for future research and current dietary advice.

Cardiovascular Disease

Of all the diseases in which excess oxidative stress has been implicated, CVD has the strongest supporting evidence. Oxidation of low-density lipoprotein (LDL) cholesterol appears to be a key step in the development of atherosclerosis, a known risk factor in the development of CVD. Small studies have demonstrated reductions in LDL oxidation (mostly *in vitro*) following supplementation with dietary antioxidants (particularly vitamin E, which is primarily carried in LDL-cholesterol), suggesting that they may provide protection against the development of heart disease. A number of large intervention trials using disease outcomes (rather than biomarkers such as LDL oxidation) have also been conducted to try to demonstrate a protective effect of vitamin E, β-carotene, and, to a lesser extent, vitamin C supplements on cardiovascular disease. Most have been carried out in high-risk groups (e.g., smokers) or those with established heart disease (i.e., people with angina or who have already suffered a heart attack).

Primary Prevention

The results of most primary prevention trials have not been encouraging (**Table 1**). For example, in the Finnish Alpha-Tocopherol Beta-Carotene Cancer Prevention (ATBC) study, approximately 30 000

male smokers received vitamin E (50 mg/day of α-tocopherol), β-carotene (20 mg/day), both, or an inactive substance (placebo) for approximately 6 years. There was no reduction in risk of major coronary events with any of the treatments despite a 50% increase in blood vitamin E concentrations and a 17-fold increase in β-carotene levels. Moreover, with vitamin E supplementation, there was an unexpected increase in risk of death from hemorrhagic stroke and a small but significant increase in mortality from all causes with β-carotene supplementation (RR, 1.08; 95% confidence interval (CI), 1–16). An increase in CVD deaths was also observed in the Beta-Carotene and Retinol Efficacy Trial (CARET), which tested the effects of combined treatment with β-carotene (30 mg/day) and retinyl palmitate (25 000 IU/day) in 18 000 men and women with a history of cigarette smoking or occupational exposure to asbestos compared to the placebo group (RR, 1.26; 95% CI, 0.99–1.61).

Secondary Prevention

The most positive results from secondary prevention trials came from the Cambridge Heart Antioxidant Study (CHAOS), a controlled trial on 2002 heart disease patients with angiographically proven coronary atherosclerosis randomly assigned to receive a high dose of vitamin E (400 or 800 IU/day) or placebo (**Table 2**). Those receiving the supplements were 77% less likely to suffer from nonfatal heart disease over the $1\frac{1}{2}$-year trial period than those who did not receive vitamin E (RR, 0.23; 95% CI, 0.11–0.47), although there was no reduction in CVD deaths. However, other large secondary prevention trials with longer follow-up have been less encouraging. For example, in a further analysis of the ATBC study, the β-carotene supplementation was associated with an increased risk of coronary heart disease (CHD) deaths among men who had a previous heart attack and were thus at high risk of subsequent coronary events. There were significantly more deaths from fatal CHD in the β-carotene group (RR, 1.75; 95% CI, 1.16–2.64) and in the combined β-carotene and vitamin E group compared to the placebo group (RR, 1.58; 95% CI, 1.05–2.40). The Heart Outcomes Prevention Evaluation Study (HOPE) observed no benefit from vitamin E supplementation (400 IU/day) on CVD or all-cause mortality. The Heart Protection Study in the United Kingdom examined the effect of 5 years of supplementation with a cocktail of antioxidant vitamins (600 mg vitamin E, 250 mg vitamin C, and 20 mg β-carotene) alone or in combination with the lipid-lowering drug Simvastatin or placebo in more than

Table 1 Summary of large intervention trials (> 1000 subjects) investigating the role of antioxidants and CVD in primary prevention

Trial	Characteristics of subjects	Sex	Length of follow-up (years)	Treatment	Effect of antioxidant supplementation
ATBC	29 133 smokers, Finland	Male	6	50 mg α-tocopherol and/or 20 mg β-carotene	No significant effect on fatal or nonfatal-CHD or total strokes with either supplement. Increase in deaths from hemorrhagic stroke in vitamin E group. Increase in hemorrhagic stroke (+62%) and total mortality (+8%) in β-carotene group
CARET	14 254 smokers, 4 060 asbestos workers, United States	Male and Female	4	30 mg β-carotene and 25 000 IU retinol	Increase in deaths from CVD (+26%) (terminated early)
LCPS	29 584 poorly nourished, China	Male and Female	5	15 mg β-carotene, 30 mg α-tocopherol, and 50 μg selenium	Small decline in total mortality (+9%). Reduction in deaths from stroke in men (−55%) but not women
PHS	22 071 physicians, United States	Male	12	50 mg β-carotene and/or aspirin (alternate days)	No effect on fatal or nonfatal myocardial infarction or stroke
PPP	4 495 with one or more CVD risk factors, Italy	Male and Female	$3\frac{1}{2}$	Low-dose aspirin and/or 300 mg α-tocopherol	No effect on CVD deaths or events (but inadequate power due to premature interruption of trial)
SCPS	1720 with recent nonmelanoma skin cancer, Australia	Male and Female	8	50 mg β-carotene	No effect on CVD mortality
VACP II	1 204 former asbestos workers, Australia	Male and Female	5	30 mg β-carotene or 25 000 IU retinol (no placebo group)	No effect of β-carotene on CHD deaths
WHS	39 876, United States	Female	2	50 mg β-carotene (alternate days)	No effect on fatal or nonfatal CVD

ATBC, Alpha Tocopherol Beta Carotene Prevention Study; CARET, Beta Carotene and Retinol Efficacy Trial; LCPS, Linxian Cancer Prevention Study; PHS, Physicians Health Study; PPP, Primary Prevention Project; SCPS, Skin Cancer Prevention Study; VACP, Vitamin A and Cancer Prevention; WHS, Women's Health Study; CHD, Coronary Heart Disease; CVD, Cardiovascular disease.

20 000 adults with CHD, other occlusive arterial disease, or diabetes mellitus. Although blood levels of antioxidant vitamins were substantially increased, no significant reduction in the 5-year mortality from vascular disease or any other major outcome was noted. In the Italian GISSI-Prevenzione Trial dietary fish oils reduced the risk of fatal or nonfatal CVD in men and women who had recently suffered from a heart attack but vitamin E supplementation (300 mg daily for $3\frac{1}{2}$ years) did not provide any benefit. In these three trials, no significant adverse effects of vitamin E were observed.

Systematic reviews and meta-analyses of the clinical trials to date have therefore concluded that despite evidence from observational studies, people with a high occurrence of CVD often have low intakes or plasma levels of antioxidant nutrients. Supplementation with any single antioxidant nutrient or combination of nutrients has not demonstrated any benefit for the treatment or prevention of CVD.

Cancer

The oxidative hypothesis of carcinogenesis asserts that carcinogens generate reactive oxygen species that damage RNA and DNA in cells, predisposing these cells to malignant changes and enhanced cancer risk. Most, but not all, damage is corrected by internal surveillance and repair systems involving dietary antioxidants, as well as endogenous antioxidant mechanisms. Antioxidants are therefore

Table 2 Summary of large intervention trials (>1000 subjects) investigating the role of antioxidants and CVD in secondary prevention[a]

Trial	Characteristics of subjects	Sex	Length of follow-up (years)	Treatment	Effect of antioxidant supplementation
ATBC	1862 smokers with previous MI, Finland	Male	$5\frac{1}{2}$	50 mg α-tocopherol and/ or 20 mg β-carotene	No effect on total coronary events (fatal and nonfatal)
					Increase in deaths from fatal CHD in β-carotene (+75%) and combined β-carotene/vitamin E group (+58%) vs placebo
	1795 heavy smokers with previous angina, Finland				No effect on symptoms or progression of angina or on total coronary events
CHAOS	2002 patients with coronary atherosclerosis, United Kingdom	Male and Female	$1\frac{1}{2}$	300 or 800 IU α-tocopherol	Reduction in nonfatal MI (−77%) but no effect on CVD mortality
GISSI	11324 patients with recent MI, Italy			300 mg α-tocopherol and/or 1 g n-3 PUFA	No benefit from vitamin E
HOPE	9541 known CVD or diabetes, Canada	Male and Female	4–6	400 IU α-tocopherol and/or ACE inhibitor	No effect on MI, stroke, or CVD death
HPS	20536 with known vascular disease or at high risk, United Kingdom	Male and Female	≥5	20 mg β-carotene, 600 mg α-tocopherol, and 250 mg vitamin C	No effect on fatal or nonfatal MI or stroke

[a]Secondary prevention is defined as including patients with known or documented vascular disease.
ACE, angiotensin converting enzyme; ATBC, Alpha Tocopherol Beta Carotene Prevention Study; CHAOS, Cambridge Heart Antioxidant Study; GISSI, GISSI Prevenzione Trial; HOPE, Heart Outcomes Prevention Evaluation Study; HPS, Heart Protection Study; CHD, Coronary Heart Disease; CVD, cardiovascular disease; MI, myocardial infarction; PUFA, polyunsatutated fatty acids.

proposed to prevent cell damage by neutralizing free radicals and oxidants, thus preventing subsequent development of cancer.

β-Carotene

Many of the randomized controlled trials (RCTs) investigating a protective role for antioxidant nutrients in cancer prevention (**Table 3**) have focused on β-carotene. A study in Linxian, China, of a rural population with poor nutritional status found that supplementation with a combination of β-carotene, selenium, and vitamin E for 5 years provided a 21% reduction in stomach cancer mortality and a 13% reduction in all cancer deaths. Although interesting, the population studied was likely to have very low intakes of a number of micronutrients and this study does not contribute to knowledge about the effects of individual antioxidants or offer any insight into their effects on populations with good nutritional status.

The findings of a number of large double-blind RCTs in well-fed subjects using high-dose β-

carotene supplements (either alone or in combination with other agents) have generally been unsupportive of any protective effect, although most have only focused on high-risk groups (e.g., smokers, asbestos workers, and older age groups). In the ATBC Cancer Prevention Trial, in which 29 000 male smokers were randomly assigned to receive β-carotene and/or α-tocopherol or placebo each day, β-carotene showed no protective effect on the incidence of any type of cancer after approximately 6 years. In fact, concern was raised following the publication of the findings of this trial because those randomized to receive this vitamin had an 18% higher risk of lung cancer (RR, 1.18; 95% CI, 3–36) as well as an 8% higher total mortality than nonrecipients. Subgroup analyses suggested that the adverse effect of β-carotene on lung cancer risk was restricted to heavy smokers and that the risk appeared to be transient, being lost at follow-up 4–6 years after cessation of supplementation.

The CARET was also terminated early because of similar findings; subjects receiving a combination of supplements (30 mg β-carotene and vitamin A daily)

Table 3 Summary of large intervention trials (> 1000 subjects) investigating the role of antioxidants and cancer in primary prevention

Trial	Characteristics of subjects	Sex	Length of follow-up (years)	Treatment	Effect of antioxidant supplementation
ATBC	29 133 smokers, Finland	Male	5–8	50 mg α-tocopherol and/or 20 mg β-carotene	18% increase in lung cancer in β-carotene group (no effect in vitamin E group) 34% reduction in incidence of prostate cancer in vitamin E group No effect of either vitamin on colorectal, pancreatic, or urinary tract cancer
CARET	14 254 smokers, 4060 asbestos workers, United States	Male and Female	4	30 mg β-carotene and 25 000 IU retinol	Lung cancer increased by 28%
HPS	20 536 at high CVD risk, United Kingdom	Male and Female	≥ 5	20 mg β-carotene, 600 mg α-tocopherol, and 250 mg vitamin C	No effect on cancer incidence or mortality
LCPS	29 584 poorly nourished, China	Male and Female	5	15 mg β-carotene, 30 mg α-tocopherol, and 50 μg selenium	Cancer deaths declined by 13% Stomach cancer declined by 21%
NSCPT	1621 (73% without skin cancer at baseline), Australia	Male and Female	$4\frac{1}{2}$	30 mg β-carotene with or without sunscreen application	No effect on basal cell or squamous cell carcinoma
PHS	22 071 physicians, United States	Male	12	50 mg β-carotene and/or aspirin (alternate days)	No effect on incidence of malignant neoplasms or nonmelanoma skin cancer
VACP II	1204 former asbestos workers, Australia	Male and Female	5	30 mg β-carotene or 25 000 IU retinol (no placebo group)	No effect of β-carotene on cancer mortality
WHS	39 876, United States	Female	2	50 mg β-carotene (alternate days)	No effect on cancer incidence

ATBC, Alpha Tocopherol Beta Carotene Prevention Study; CARET, Beta Carotene and Retinol Efficacy Trial; HPS, Heart Protection Study; LCPS, Linxian Cancer Prevention Study; NSCPT, Nambour Skin Cancer Prevention Trial; PHS, Physicians Health Study; VACP, Vitamin A and Cancer Prevention; WHS, Women's Health Study; CVD, Cardio Vascular disease.

experienced a 28% increased risk of lung cancer incidence compared with the placebo group (RR, 1.28; 95% CI, 1.04–1.57). Subgroup analyses also suggested that the effect was found in current, but not former, smokers. In contrast, in the Physicians Health Study, supplementation of male physicians with 50 mg β-carotene on alternate days had no effect on cancer incidence (men who were smokers did not experience any benefit or harm). The Heart Protection Study also demonstrated no effect on 5-year cancer incidence or mortality from supplementation with 20 mg β-carotene in combination with vitamins E and C in individuals at high risk of CVD, despite increases in blood concentrations of these nutrients (plasma β-carotene concentrations increased 4-fold). They did not, however, find any harmful effects from these vitamins.

A number of trials have attempted to investigate the effect of β-carotene supplementation on nonmelanoma skin cancer, the most common forms of which are basal cell and squamous cell carcinomas (these types of cells are both found in the top layer of the skin). However, none have shown any significant effect on skin cancer prevention. For example, the Physicians Health Study found no effect after 12 years of β-carotene supplementation on the development of a first nonmelanoma skin cancer. The Nambour Skin Cancer Prevention Trial of 1621 men and women followed for nearly 5 years (most of whom had no history of skin cancer at baseline) showed that those supplemented with 30 mg β-carotene did not experience any reduction in risk of basal cell or squamous cell carcinoma or the occurrence of solar keratoses (precancerous skin growths that are a strong determinant of squamous cell carcinoma). A 5-year trial of 1805 men and women with recent nonmelanoma skin cancer (the Skin Cancer Prevention Study) also found that supplementation with 50 mg of β-carotene gave no protection against either type of skin cancer, although this may have been because these cancers have a long latency period of approximately 12 years (**Table 4**).

Together, these trials suggest that β-carotene supplements offer no protection against cancer at any site and, among smokers, may actually increase the risk of lung cancer. Investigators have sought to explain these findings by proposing that components of cigarette smoke may promote oxidation of β-carotene in the lungs, causing it to exert a prooxidant (rather than antioxidant) effect and act as a tumor promoter.

Vitamin C

There are no published RCTs of vitamin C alone in primary prevention, but data from the small number of trials of vitamin C in combination with other nutrients have not provided any support for a role for high-dose vitamin C supplementation in cancer prevention (**Table 3**). The Linxian trial found no significant effect of supplementing Chinese men and women with 120 mg vitamin C and 30 µg molybdenum daily for 5 years on the risk of cancers of the oesophagus or stomach. The Polyp Prevention Study, a trial of 864 patients with previous adenoma, found no effect of either β-carotene or a combination of vitamins E and C (1000 mg) on the incidence of subsequent colorectal adenomas. The Heart Protection Study also found no beneficial effects of supplementation with these three vitamins on cancer mortality. However, trials have generally

been carried out on those with diets containing sufficient amounts of vitamin C and there is a need for further studies in people with low intakes.

Vitamin E

The ATBC trial showed no significant effect of α-tocopherol supplementation (50 mg/day) on risk of lung, pancreatic, colorectal, or urinary tract cancers among heavy smokers (**Table 3**). However, in a post hoc subgroup analysis a 34% reduction in the risk of prostate cancer was seen in men who received this supplement. Although interesting, prostate cancer was not a primary endpoint of this study, and no other studies have supported a preventative effect of vitamin E for prostate cancer. The Heart Protection Study found no effect of vitamin E in combination with vitamin C and β-carotene on cancer incidence or mortality. Two smaller, short-term intervention studies found no effect of α-tocopherol supplementation on mammary dysplasia or benign breast disease. Several trials have also been unable to demonstrate a protective effect of vitamin E supplementation on the risk or recurrence of colorectal adenomatous polyps.

Selenium

A few trials have suggested that selenium supplementation may have a protective effect on liver cancer in high-risk groups living in low-selenium areas. The provision of selenium-fortified salt to a town in Qidong, China, with high rates of primary liver cancer, reduced the incidence of this cancer by 35% compared with towns that did not receive this intervention (**Table 3**). Trials have also demonstrated the incidence of liver cancer to be

Table 4 Summary of large intervention trials (>1000 subjects) investigating the role of antioxidants and cancer in secondary prevention[a]

Trial	Characteristics of subjects	Sex	Length of follow-up (years)	Treatment	Effect of antioxidant supplementation
NPCT	1312 with history of basal or squamous cell carcinoma, United States	Male and Female	$4\frac{1}{2}$	200 µg selenium	No effect on incidence of skin cancer
					Reduce cancer mortality (50%), cancer incidence (37%), prostate cancer (63%), colorectal cancer (58%), and lung cancer (46%)
SCPS	1805 with recent nonmelanoma skin cancer, United States	Male and Female	5	50 mg β-carotene	No effect on occurrence of new nonmelanoma skin cancer

[a]Secondary prevention defined as subjects with documented cancer including nonmelanoma skin cancer (although some of the primary prevention trials did not exclude those with nonmelanoma skin cancer at baseline).
NPCT, Nutritional Prevention of Cancer Trial; SCPS: Skin Cancer Prevention Study.

significantly reduced in subjects with hepatitis B and among members of families with a history of liver cancer receiving a daily supplement of 200 μg of selenium for 4 and 2 years, respectively.

The Nutritional Prevention of Cancer Trial in the United States also supported a possible protective role of selenium (**Table 4**): 1312 patients (mostly men) with a previous history of skin cancer were supplemented with either placebo or 200 μg selenium per day for $4\frac{1}{2}$ years and those receiving selenium demonstrated significant reductions in the risk of cancer incidence (37%) and mortality (50%). Although selenium was not found to have a protective effect against recurrent skin cancer, the selenium-treated group had substantial reductions in the incidence of lung, colorectal, and prostate cancers of 46, 58, and 63%, respectively. Further analysis showed the protective effect on prostate cancer to be confined to those with lower baseline prostate-specific antigen and plasma selenium levels. Although these data need confirmation, they suggest that adequate selenium intake may be important for cancer prevention.

Other Diseases Associated with Oxidative Damage

Type 2 Diabetes

Type 2 diabetes is associated with elevated oxidative stress (especially lipid peroxidation) and declines in antioxidant defense. This is thought to be due in part to elevated blood glucose levels (hyperglycemia), but severe oxidative stress may also precede and accelerate the development of type 2 diabetes and then of diabetic complications (CVD and microvascular complications such as retinopathy, neuropathy, and nephropathy).

Small-scale human trials have shown administration of high doses of vitamin E to reduce oxidative stress and improve some CVD risk factors, such as blood glycated hemoglobin, insulin, and triglyceride levels, in people with diabetes. Such trials have also indicated benefit from vitamin E in improving endothelial function, retinal blood flow, and renal dysfunction. However, the findings of large clinical trials investigating the role of individual or a combination of antioxidant nutrients in reducing the risk of CVD and microvascular complications in people with diabetes have generally been disappointing. For example, the Heart Outcomes Prevention Evaluation Trial investigated the effects of vitamin E and the drug Ramipril in patients at high risk for CVD events and included a large number of middle-aged and elderly people with diabetes (more than 3600).

An average of $4\frac{1}{2}$ years of supplementation with 400 IU of vitamin E per day was found to exert no beneficial or harmful effect on CVD outcomes or on nephropathy. The Primary Prevention Project trial found no effect of vitamin E (300 mg/day) supplementation for 3 or 4 years in diabetic subjects, and the Heart Protection Study, which included a number of people with diabetes, also reported no benefit of a combination of antioxidant vitamins on mortality or incidence of vascular disease.

Chronic Obstructive Pulmonary Disease (COPD)

The generation of oxygen free radicals by activated inflammatory cells produces many of the pathophysiological changes associated with COPD. Common examples of COPD are asthma and bronchitis, each of which affects large numbers of children and adults. Antioxidant nutrients have therefore been suggested to play a role in the prevention and treatment of these conditions. A number of studies have demonstrated a beneficial effect of fruit and vegetable intake on lung function. For example, regular consumption of fresh fruit rich in vitamin C (citrus fruits and kiwi) has been found to have a beneficial effect on reducing wheezing and coughs in children.

Vitamin C is the major antioxidant present in extracellular fluid lining the lung, and intake in the general population has been inversely correlated with the incidence of asthma, bronchitis, and wheezing and with pulmonary problems. Although some trials have shown high-dose supplementation (1–2 g/day) to improve symptoms of asthma in adults and protect against airway responsiveness to viral infections, allergens, and irritants, this effect has been attributed to the antihistaminic action of the vitamin rather than to any antioxidant effect. The results of these trials have also been inconsistent, and a Cochrane review of eight RCTs concluded that there is insufficient evidence to recommend a specific role for the vitamin in the treatment of asthma. However, a need for further trials to address the question of the effectiveness of vitamin C in asthmatic children was highlighted.

Other dietary antioxidants have been positively associated with lung function in cohort studies but the findings of clinical trials have been mixed. In a study of 158 children with moderate to severe asthma, supplementation with vitamin E (50 mg/day) and vitamin C (250 mg/day) led to some improvement in lung function following ozone exposure. However, the much larger ATBC trial found no benefit from supplementation with α-tocopherol (50 mg/day) and β-carotene (20 mg/day) on symptoms of COPD, despite the fact that those with high dietary intakes and blood levels of these vitamins at baseline had a lower prevalence of chronic bronchitis and dyspnea. A small trial investigating the effects of selenium supplementation in asthmatics found that those receiving the supplements experienced a significant increase in glutathione peroxidase levels and reported improvement in their asthma symptoms. However, this improvement could not be validated by significant changes in the separate clinical parameters of lung function and airway hyperresponsiveness. Therefore, there is little evidence to support the role of other nutrients in COPD treatment.

Macular Degeneration and Cataracts

The eye is at particular risk of oxidative damage due to high oxygen concentrations, large amounts of oxidizable fatty acids in the retina, and exposure to ultraviolet rays. In Western countries, age-related macular degeneration (AMD) is the leading cause of blindness among older people. Cataracts are also widespread among the elderly and occur when the lens is unable to function properly due to the formation of opacities within the lens. These develop when proteins in the eye are damaged by photooxidation; these damaged proteins build up, clump, and precipitate. It has been proposed that antioxidants may prevent cellular damage in the eye by reacting with free radicals produced during the process of light absorption.

The results of intervention trials in this area have also been mixed. The Age-Related Eye Disease Study in the United States investigating the effects of combined antioxidant vitamins C (500 mg), E (400 IU), and β-carotene (15 mg) with and without 80 mg zinc daily for 6 years showed some protective effect (a reduction in risk of approximately 25%) on the progression of moderately advanced AMD but no benefit on the incidence or progression or early AMD or cataracts. The Lutein Antioxidant Supplementation Trial, a 12-month study of 90 patients with AMD, found significant improvements in visual function with 10 mg/day lutein (one of the major carotenoids found in the pigment of a normal retina) alone or in combination with a number of other antioxidant nutrients. The Roche European Cataract Trial, providing a combined daily supplement of β-carotene, vitamin C, and vitamin E among adults with early signs of age-related cataract, showed a small deceleration in the progression of cataract after 3 years.

However, the Linxian trial found no influence of vitamin supplementation on risk of cataract; the ATBC trial found no reduction in the prevalence of cataracts with vitamin E, β-carotene, or both among male smokers; and the Health Physicians Study of more than 22 000 men showed no benefit from 12 years of supplementation with β-carotene (50 mg on alternate days) on cataract incidence. In fact, current smokers at the beginning of this trial who received the supplement experienced an increased risk of cataract (by approximately 25%) compared to the placebo group. The Vitamin E, Cataract and Age-Related Maculopathy Trial also reported no effect of supplementation with vitamin E for 4 years (500 IU/day) on the incidence or progression of cataracts or AMD.

Possible Explanations for the Disagreement between the Findings of Observational Studies and Clinical Trials

Various explanations have been given for the different findings of observational studies and intervention trials. Clearly, nonrandomized studies are unable to exclude the possibility that antioxidants are simply acting as a surrogate measure of a healthy diet or lifestyle and that the protective effect of certain dietary patterns, which has been presumed to be associated with dietary antioxidants, may in fact be due to other compounds in plant foods, substitution of these foods for others, or a reflection of other health behaviors common to people who have a high fruit and vegetable intake. However, although intervention studies provide a more rigorous source of evidence than observational studies, they are not without weaknesses from a nutritional perspective and the trials have been criticized for a number of reasons:

- The nature of the supplements used: It has been suggested that the synthetic forms used in most trials may have different biological activity or potency from natural forms of these vitamins, although trials using the natural forms have not found different clinical effects. The type of isomer used has also been questioned (e.g., β-carotene versus other carotenoids such as lycopene or lutein or α-tocopherol versus γ-tocopherol). Trials have not investigated other potentially beneficial antioxidants in foods, such as flavonoids and lycopenes.
- The use of high doses of one or two antioxidants: Mechanistic and epidemiological data suggest that antioxidants act not only individually but also cooperatively and in some cases synergistically. Single supplements may interfere with the uptake, transport, distribution, and metabolism of other antioxidant nutrients. An optimal effect would

therefore be expected to be seen with a combination of nutrients at levels similar to those contained in the diet (corresponding to higher levels of intake associated with reduced risk in the observational studies). The findings of clinical trials testing the effect of a cocktail of antioxidant nutrients at low doses are awaited, but the Heart Protection Study did not demonstrate a protective effect of multiple antioxidants and a small RCT of 160 patients with coronary disease, using a combination of antioxidant nutrients (800 IU α-tocopherol, 1000 mg vitamin C, 25 mg β-carotene, and 100 μg selenium twice daily) for 3 years, showed no benefit for secondary prevention of vascular disease.

- Insufficient duration of treatment and follow-up: Most of the intervention trials published to date (except the Physicians Health Study, which found no effect despite 12 years of follow-up) had durations of treatment and follow-up lasting only approximately 4–6 years. Diseases such as cancer and CVD develop over a long period of time and trials may have been too short to demonstrate any benefit.

- The use of high-risk groups: Many of the supplementation trials have not been undertaken on normal 'healthy' individuals but on those with preexisting oxidative stress, either through smoking or through preexisting disease, among whom increasing antioxidant intake may not have been able to repair the oxidative damage process sufficiently to affect cancer or CVD risk.

- Lack of information about the impact of genetic variability: Unknown genetic factors (interacting with nutrition) may explain some of the lack of effect in intervention studies. A greater understanding of the impact of factors such as genotype, age, and ill health on the interactions between antioxidants and reactive oxygen species would be helpful in designing future trials.

The Supplementation en Vitamines et Minéraux AntioXydants Study (SU.VI.MAX) has taken account of many of these issues in its design. This is a randomized, placebo-controlled trial testing the efficacy of supplementation among more than 12 000 healthy men and women over an 8-year period with a cocktail of antioxidant vitamins (120 mg vitamin C, 30 mg vitamin E, and 6 mg β-carotene) and minerals (100 μg selenium and 20 mg zinc) at doses achievable by diet (approximately one to three times the daily recommended

dietary allowances) on premature death from CVD and cancer. Early reports suggest that this regime has not demonstrated an effect on CVD risk but has led to a 31% decrease in cancer incidence and a 37% reduction in total mortality among men but not women. This may reflect higher dietary intakes of these nutrients among the women in the trial compared to men, but publication of these results is still awaited. However, this is a good illustration of the type of nutritional approach that may be needed in the future.

Conclusion

Although there is a substantial body of evidence that diets rich in plant foods (particularly fruit and vegetables) convey health benefits, as do high plasma levels of several antioxidant nutrients found in these foods, a causal link between lack of antioxidants and disease occurrence or between antioxidant administration and disease prevention remains to be established. There is a lack of understanding of the mechanisms underpinning the apparent protective effect of plant foods and, as yet, no clear picture of which components are effective and hence no way of predicting whether all or just some plant foods are important in this respect.

If future trials do demonstrate a reduction in chronic disease risk with antioxidant supplementation, this cannot be definitively attributed to the antioxidant effect of these nutrients because other biological functions may also play a role. For example, in addition to retarding LDL oxidation, vitamin E may help to protect against CVD via its action on platelet aggregation and adhesion or by inhibition of the proliferation of smooth muscle cells. Furthermore, although vitamin C, vitamin E, and selenium have been shown to decrease the concentration of some of the biomarkers associated with oxidative stress, the relationship between many of these biomarkers and chronic disease remains to be elucidated.

The intervention studies highlight the lack of information on the safety of sustained intakes of moderate to high doses of micronutrient supplements and long-term harm cannot be ruled out, particularly in smokers. Further evidence is required regarding the efficacy, safety, and appropriate dosage of antioxidants in relation to chronic disease.

Currently, the most prudent public health advice continues to be to consume a variety of plant foods.

See also: **Antioxidants**: Diet and Antioxidant Defense; Observational Studies. **Ascorbic Acid**: Physiology, Dietary Sources and Requirements. **Carotenoids**: Chemistry, Sources and Physiology; Epidemiology of Health Effects. **Coronary Heart Disease**: Lipid Theory. **Selenium**. **Vitamin E**: Metabolism and Requirements; Physiology and Health Effects.

Further Reading

Asplund K (2002) Antioxidant vitamins in the prevention of cardiovascular disease: A systematic review. *Journal of Internal Medicine* **251**: 372–392.

British Nutrition Foundation (2001) *Briefing Paper: Selenium and Health*. London: British Nutrition Foundation.

British Nutrition Foundation (2003). *Plants: Diet and Health. A Report of the British Nutrition Foundation Task Force*. Goldberg G (ed.) Oxford: Blackwell Science.

Clarke R and Armitage J (2002) Antioxidant vitamins and risk of cardiovascular disease. Review of large-scale randomised trials. *Cardiovascular Drugs and Therapy* **16**: 411–415.

Evans J (2002) Antioxidant vitamin and mineral supplements for age-related macular degeneration. *Cochrane Database Systematic Review* **2**: CD000254.

Lawlor DA, Davey Smith G, Kundu D *et al.* (2004) Those confounded vitamins: What can we learn from the differences between observational versus randomised trial evidence? *Lancet* **363**: 1724–1727.

Lee I (1999) Antioxidant vitamins in the prevention of cancer. *Proceedings of the Association of American Physicians* **111**: 10–15.

Mares JA (2004) High-dose antioxidant supplementation and cataract risk. *Nutrition Review* **62**: 28–32.

Morris C and Carson S (2003) Routine vitamin supplementation to prevent cardiovascular disease: A summary of the evidence for the US Preventive Services Task Force. *Annals of Internal Medicine* **139**: 56–70.

National Academy of Sciences Food and Nutrition Board (2000) *Dietary Reference Intakes for Vitamin C, Vitamin E, Selenium and Carotenoids*. Washington, DC: National Academy Press.

Ram F, Rowe B, and Kaur B (2004) Vitamin C supplementation for asthma. *Cochrane Database Systematic Review* **3**: CD000993.

Stanner SA, Hughes J, Kelly CNM *et al.* (2004) A review of the epidemiological evidence for the 'antioxidant hypothesis'. *Public Health Nutrition* **7**: 407–422.

Vivekananthan D, Penn MS, Sapp SK *et al.* (2003) Use of antioxidant vitamins for the prevention of cardiovascular disease: Meta-analysis of randomised trials. *Lancet* **361**: 2017–2023.

Observational Studies

I F F Benzie, The Hong Kong Polytechnic University, Hong Kong, China

Introduction

The study of temporal and geographical variation in disease prevalence in association with differences in environment, diet, and lifestyle helps identify possible factors that may modulate the risk of disease within and across populations. As such, observational epidemiology is a powerful, albeit blunt, tool that serves to inform and guide experimental studies and intervention trials. In the case of dietary antioxidants and chronic age-related disease, there is a logical biochemical rationale for the protective effect of antioxidants, and there is strong, and consistent observational evidence supportive of this. The way in which dietary antioxidants are believed to act is described in a separate chapter. In this chapter, observational evidence relating to dietary antioxidants and the risk of disease states is discussed.

Epidemiology: Setting the Scene

The risk of developing a disease can be increased by exposure to a disease-promoting factor or decreased by a protective factor. In terms of antioxidants, high risk is generally assumed to be associated with low intakes, plasma levels, or tissue concentrations of antioxidants. Epidemiological studies often express results in terms of the relative risk (RR) of mortality or disease. The RR is generally given as the mean and 95% confidence interval (CI). In general, an RR of 0.80 indicates an average reduction in risk of 20%; however, RR values must be interpreted with caution and the CI must be considered. If the CI spans 1.0, the RR is not statistically significant, regardless of its magnitude.

Different approaches are used in observational epidemiology. Cross-cultural studies compare standardized mortality rates (from all causes or from a specific disease) or disease prevalence and the factor of interest ('exposure variable') in different populations within or between countries. These can be regarded as 'snapshot' observational surveys. Case–control studies compare the factor of interest in people who have a disease (the cases) with that in those who do not (the controls). Prospective trials are longitudinal studies of apparently disease-free subjects whose health is monitored over years or decades; the exposure variable of interest is compared, retrospectively, between those who develop the disease of interest and those who do not.

The Observational View of Dietary Antioxidants

Cancer and cardiovascular disease (CVD) are the two leading causes of death worldwide, diabetes mellitus is reaching epidemic proportions, and dementia and maculopathy are largely untreatable irreversible disorders that are increasingly common in our aging population. The prevalence and standardized mortality rates of these diseases vary considerably between and within populations. Mortality from CVD varies more than 10-fold amongst different populations, and incidences of specific cancers vary 20-fold or more across the globe. This enormous variation highlights the multiple factors at play in the etiology of chronic age-related diseases. These factors include smoking habit, socioeconomic status, exposure to infectious agents, cholesterol levels, certain genetic factors, and diet. Dietary factors have long been known to play an important role in determining disease risk. Indeed, 30–40% of overall cancer risk is reported to be diet-related, and there is a wealth of compelling observational evidence that a lower risk of cancer, CVD, diabetes, and other chronic age-related disorders is associated with diets that are rich in antioxidants.

In terms of dietary antioxidants, the major research focus to date has been on the water-soluble vitamin C (ascorbic acid) and the lipophilic vitamin E. 'Vitamin E' is a group of eight lipid-soluble tocopherols and tocotrienols; however, the most widely studied form to date is α-tocopherol because it is the most abundant form in human plasma. Neither vitamin C nor vitamin E can be synthesized by humans, so they must be obtained in the diet, most coming from plant-based foods and oils. Deficiency of either of these vitamins is rare and can be prevented by the daily intake of a few milligrams of each. However, an adequate intake to prevent simple deficiency is unlikely to be sufficient for optimal health. Based on observational findings and experimental evidence that vitamin C and vitamin E protect key biological sites from oxidative damage *in vitro*, it has been suggested that there is a threshold of intake or plasma concentration for these antioxidants that confers minimum disease risk and promotes optimal health. The strength of the data supporting the health benefits of increased intakes of these vitamins was acknowledged in the US Food and Nutrition Board recommendation in 2000 to increase the daily intake of vitamin C to $75\,mg\,day^{-1}$ for women and $90\,mg\,day^{-1}$ for men and to increase that of vitamin E to $15\,mg\,day^{-1}$ for both men and women. However, whether these new recommended intakes are 'optimal' is a contentious issue.

Supplementation trials with vitamin C or vitamin E have not to date shown the expected health benefits. The reasons for this mismatch between observational and supplementation data are not yet known, but some suggested reasons are outlined in **Table 1**. Nonetheless, despite the apparent lack of effect in supplementation trials, the variety and strength of observational findings, backed by a solid body of *in vitro* biochemical data, keep dietary antioxidants in the research spotlight, and in recent years attention has focused on the influence of 'non-nutrient' dietary antioxidants, such as polyphenolic compounds, in addition to the effects of vitamin C and vitamin E. The current evidence for vitamin C, vitamin E, and non-nutrient dietary antioxidants in relation to the major causes of morbidity and mortality in developed countries is discussed briefly below.

Vitamin C

Low plasma ascorbic-acid concentrations have been reported to be strongly predictive of mortality, particularly in men. Results of a prospective trial in the UK (EPIC-Norfolk Prospective Study), in which 19 496 men and women aged 45–79 years were followed for 4 years, showed that men and women in the highest quintile of plasma ascorbic-acid concentration in samples collected within 1 year of

Table 1 Possible reasons for the conflict in results between observational epidemiological and supplementation trials

- Antioxidants are likely to work in cooperation with each other; more of one may increase the need for another
- The action of an antioxidant within a heterogeneous food matrix may be different from that in pure supplemental form
- A high intake of antioxidants may help to promote health when taken regularly over decades but may have little discernable effect over a few months or years
- A high intake of antioxidants may slow or even prevent some of the deleterious age-related changes that lead to chronic disease, but antioxidants are unlikely to reverse established pathological changes
- Benefits of increased antioxidant intake may be seen only in those with marginal or depleted antioxidant status at baseline
- The effect of antioxidant supplementation may be seen only in subgroups of the study population, e.g., in those individuals with certain single-nucleotide polymorphisms
- The key players may not be the most widely studied antioxidants; for example, γ-tocopherol, rather than α-tocopherol, may play an important role in modulation of cancer risk but has been little studied to date
- Antioxidants can act as pro-oxidants under certain conditions, and the net effect of a dietary antioxidant may well depend on dose and conditions at its site of action
- Antioxidant action per se may not be the key mechanism of action of protection; for example, immunomodulatory, anti-inflammatory, anti-proliferative, and pro-apoptotic effects of dietary agents (antioxidants or otherwise) may be more relevant to overall effects in terms of disease risk

entry into the study had significantly ($p < 0.0001$) lower all-cause mortality than those in the lowest quintile. Highest-quintile concentrations of plasma ascorbic acid (mean $\pm$ standard deviation) were $72.6 \pm 11.5 \, \mu mol \, l^{-1}$ for men and $85.1 \pm 13.7 \, \mu mol \, l^{-1}$ for women; lowest quintiles were $20.8 \pm 7.1 \, \mu mol \, l^{-1}$ and $30.3 \pm 10.1 \, \mu mol \, l^{-1}$, respectively, for men and women. In men and women in the highest quintile, RRs (CI) for all-cause mortality were, respectively, 0.48 (0.33–0.70) and 0.50 (0.32–0.81), relative to those in the lowest quintile. Mortality from ischemic heart disease was also significantly ($p < 0.001$) lower in the highest quintiles: for men the RR (CI) was 0.32 (0.15–0.75), and for women it was 0.07 (0.01–0.67). The relationship held for CVD and cancer in men ($p < 0.001$), but no significant difference in cancer mortality was seen in women, and CVD rates in women were affected less than those in men. The mean ascorbic-acid level in each quintile in women was around $10 \, \mu mol \, l^{-1}$ higher than that in men. Interestingly, the relationship between ascorbic-acid concentration and mortality was continuous throughout the range of plasma ascorbic-acid concentrations found. It was estimated that a $20 \, \mu mol \, l^{-1}$ increase in plasma ascorbic acid (achievable by one or two additional servings of fruit and vegetables each day) was associated with a 20% decrease in all-cause mortality, independent of age, blood pressure, cholesterol, smoking habit, and diabetes. Interestingly, also, mortality was not associated with supplement use, indicating that dietary sources of vitamin C are crucial.

In the Third National Health and Nutrition Examination Survey (NHANES III) in the USA, the plasma ascorbic-acid concentrations of 7658 men and women were not found to be independently associated with a history of cardiovascular disease in participants who reported no alcohol consumption; however, in 3497 participants who consumed alcohol a significantly lower prevalence of pre-existing angina was found in those with high plasma ascorbic acid ($> 56 \, \mu mol \, l^{-1}$) than in those with 'low to marginal' levels ($< 22 \, \mu mol \, l^{-1}$). No significant association was seen between plasma ascorbic acid and previous myocardial infarction or stroke in this cross-sectional survey. In the NHANES II prospective study, a 43% decrease in mortality was associated with higher plasma ascorbic-acid levels in more than 3000 men followed for up to 16 years. Plasma ascorbic-acid levels in the highest and lowest quartiles in this study were more than $73 \, \mu mol \, l^{-1}$ and less than $28.4 \, \mu mol \, l^{-1}$, respectively. The corresponding values in women were again higher, at more than $85 \, \mu mol \, l^{-1}$ and less than $39.7 \, \mu mol \, l^{-1}$,

respectively, and no significant relationship between plasma ascorbic-acid levels and mortality was seen in women.

The Kuopio IHD (ischemic heart disease) Risk Factor Study followed 1605 men for 5 years and reported an RR (CI) of 0.11 (0.04–0.30) for acute myocardial infarction in those men with higher plasma ascorbic-acid concentrations. The Medical Research Council Trial of Assessment and Management of Older People in the Community, a prospective trial in the UK of 1214 elderly subjects followed for a median of 4.4 years, showed that those in the highest quintile of plasma ascorbic-acid level ($> 66 \, \mu mol \, l^{-1}$) at entry had less than half the risk of dying in the follow-up period compared with those in the lowest quintile (plasma ascorbic-acid level of $< 17 \, \mu mol \, l^{-1}$). Data on men and women were not analyzed separately, but there were fewer men (27%) in the highest quintile of ascorbic-acid level. No relationship was seen between mortality and plasma levels or intake of β-carotene or lipid-standardized α-tocopherol. Interestingly, while the relationship between mortality and the concentration of plasma ascorbic acid was strong, there was no significant association between mortality and estimated dietary intake of vitamin C. This may reflect the difficulty in obtaining accurate dietary information, but it also suggests that different individuals may well need different intakes to achieve certain plasma levels of ascorbic acid.

There have been many case–control and cohort studies performed in Europe and the USA and published in the past 15 years, and some data from Asia have been gathered. In most case–control studies no significant relationship has been demonstrated between intake and/or plasma ascorbic-acid levels and the risk of cardiovascular events; however, the combination of findings from individual studies is revealing. In a detailed analysis of 11 cohort studies comparing high and low intakes of ascorbic acid in 50 000 subjects overall, with 2148 CVD events during follow-up, a Peto's Odds Ratio (95% CI) of 0.89 (0.79–0.99) for CVD was calculated, indicating a modest reduction in risk associated with a high intake of vitamin C. In an analysis of five cohort studies comparing high and low plasma ascorbic-acid levels, involving 13 018 subjects overall with 543 CVD events during follow-up, a Peto's Odds Ratio for CVD of 0.58 (0.47–0.72) was calculated. This was interpreted as showing high plasma ascorbic-acid levels to be a powerful predictor of freedom from CVD during follow-up.

The relationship between antioxidant-rich diets and protection from cancer is strong and clear; however, the influences of individual antioxidants are difficult to isolate. Cancer risk increases as total calorie intake increases, and this confounds prospective and retrospective dietary studies. Cancer causes many biochemical changes, and cancer treatment is harsh, and this confounds the results of studies comparing antioxidant levels in plasma in cases and controls unless the samples were collected and analysed before cancer developed (which may be a considerable time before diagnosis). Currently, the evidence for a cancer-opposing effect of high intakes or plasma concentrations of ascorbic acid is conflicting. To date, the strongest evidence of a role for vitamin C in lowering cancer risk is in relation to cancer of the stomach, with a low intake of vitamin C being associated with a two-to-three-fold increase in the risk of stomach cancer. A Spanish study showed a 69% lower risk of stomach cancer in those in the highest quintile of vitamin C intake, and low levels of ascorbic acid in gastric juice are found in patients with chronic atrophic gastritis or *Helicobacter pylori* infection, both of which are associated with a greatly increased risk of gastric cancer. Whether the decrease in ascorbic acid is directly related to the development of gastric cancer is not known, but it is known that ascorbic acid inactivates carcinogenic nitrosamines within the stomach. There is also evidence of a decreased risk of cancer of the mouth, pharynx, pancreas, lung, cervix, and breast in association with increased vitamin C intake, though not all studies find this. It has been estimated that if the diets of postmenopausal women were enriched with vitamin C, a 16% decrease in breast cancer in these women would result. No significant association was reported between vitamin C intake and the incidence of ovarian cancer in 16 years of follow-up of 80 326 women in the Nurses' Health Study. A study of 100 children with brain tumours showed a three-fold increase in risk in those children whose mothers had a low intake of vitamin C during pregnancy, suggesting that the dietary intake of vitamin C by pregnant women may help to determine the future cancer risk in their children. In a prospective study of 19 496 British men and women aged 45–79 years and followed for 4 years (the EPIC (European Prospective Investigation into Cancer and Nutrition) study), the RR (CI) of mortality from cancer for a $20\,\mu mol\,l^{-1}$ increase in plasma ascorbic acid was 0.85 (0.74–0.99). In men there was a strong and continuous decrease in cancer risk with increasing plasma ascorbic-acid concentrations, with an RR (CI) in the highest quintile relative to the lowest quintile of 0.47 (0.27–0.88); i.e., the average risk in those with the highest plasma ascorbic-acid concentrations was less than half that of those in the

lowest quintile. In women the decrease in RR did not reach statistical significance. The NHANES II study reported that men in the lowest quartile of ascorbic-acid level had a 62% higher risk of death from cancer during 12 years of follow-up than those in the highest quartile. However, this relationship was not seen in women. Of possible relevance here is the common finding in these studies that men, in general, had lower ascorbic-acid levels than women.

Vitamin C is concentrated in ocular tissues and fluids, particularly in the anterior aspect (cornea and lens). A case–control study in Spain reported a 64% reduction in the risk of cataract ($p < 0.0001$) in those with a plasma ascorbic-acid concentration of more than $49\,\mu mol\,l^{-1}$; however, no significant association with the dietary intake of vitamin C was seen. In a case–control study in the Netherlands, the prevalence of age-related maculopathy was reported to be twice as high in those with low antioxidant intake (from fruits and vegetables); however the data on vitamin C intake or plasma levels and maculopathy are conflicting. Lipid-soluble antioxidants, especially zeaxanthin and lutein (dietary-derived carotenoids that are highly concentrated in the lipid-rich fovea), may be more relevant in this condition than water-soluble vitamin C.

High plasma concentrations of ascorbic acid are reportedly associated with better memory performance, and lower plasma and cerebrospinal-fluid concentrations of ascorbic acid were found in patients with Alzheimer's disease than in non-demented controls. Individuals who took vitamin C supplements were reported to have a lower prevalence of Alzheimer's disease on follow-up after 4.3 years. However, not all studies have shown a significant association between vitamin C intake or plasma levels and cognitive decline or dementia.

Vitamin E

An extensive review noted that the data in relation to a connection between vitamin E and CVD risk are strong and convincing. In a large cross-cultural European (WHO/MONICA) observational study, a strong inverse relationship ($r^2 = 0.60$, $p < 0.005$) was found between plasma concentrations of lipid-standardized vitamin E and mortality from coronary heart disease (CHD) across 16 populations. In a detailed analysis, this relationship was found to be stronger than that between mortality and plasma cholesterol, smoking, and diastolic blood pressure combined ($r^2 = 0.44$, $p < 0.02$). In a case–control study in Scotland, patients with previously undiagnosed angina pectoris were found to have lower levels of plasma lipid-standardized vitamin E than controls. After adjustment for classical CHD risk factors, men in the highest quintile of lipid-standardized vitamin E level had an almost three-fold decrease in risk. Confusingly, some studies have reported a higher CVD risk in individuals with increased plasma total vitamin E, but these results are probably driven by elevated blood lipids. Vitamin E is carried in the lipoproteins, and it is important to lipid standardize plasma concentrations of this, and other, lipophilic antioxidants.

The Nurses' Health Study (women) and the Health Professionals Study (men) were initiated in the USA in 1980 and 1986, respectively, and recruited almost 200 000 subjects. It was found that women at the high end of vitamin E intake from diet alone had a small and non-significant decrease in CVD risk; however, those women in the highest quintile of vitamin E intake (more than 100 IU day^{-1}) had an RR (CI) for CVD of 0.54 (0.36–0.82). It should be noted that an intake of 100 IU day^{-1} of vitamin E is achievable only by using supplements: intake from food alone is unlikely be more than 15 IU day^{-1}. In this study, protection against CVD was seen only in those women who had taken vitamin E supplements for at least 2 years. In the Health Professionals Follow-up Study the findings were very similar. Supplemental, but not dietary, intake of vitamin E (more than 100 IU day^{-1}) in men was associated with a significant decrease in CVD risk, averaging over 30%, but again the effect was seen only if supplements had been taken for at least 2 years. A separate study in the USA of more than 11 000 elderly subjects showed that the use of vitamin E supplements was associated with a significant decrease in the risk of heart disease (RR (CI) of 0.53 (0.34–0.84)). The results also showed a significant decrease in all-cause mortality in users of vitamin E supplements and suggested that long-term use was beneficial. A study in Finland of more than 5000 men and women showed an average of 40% lower CVD risk in the highest versus the lowest tertile of vitamin E intake. Interestingly, most (97%) of subjects in this study did not take supplements, indicating that the protective effect was due to higher intake from food. An inverse association between dietary vitamin E intake and heart disease was also seen in The Women's Iowa Health Study, which involved almost 35 000 postmenopausal women. In this study, an RR (CI) of 0.38 (0.18–0.80) for CVD mortality was seen in women in the highest quintile relative to those in the lowest quintile of vitamin E intake from food alone. However, the Medical Research Council Trial of Assessment and Management of Older People in the Community (UK) found no relation between either dietary intake of vitamin E or plasma concentration of lipid-standardized α-tocopherol and all-cause mortality or death from CVD in 1214 elderly participants followed for a median of 4.4 years.

Cancer is caused by mutations in key genes. Anything that protects DNA will, in theory, help to prevent cancer-causing mutations. Lipid peroxide degradation products are reported to be carcinogenic, and vitamin E opposes lipid peroxidation, possibly conferring indirect protection against cancer. Furthermore, by interacting with reactive species elsewhere in the cell, vitamin E may spare other antioxidants, thereby also indirectly protecting DNA. Vitamin E reportedly protects against cancer of the upper digestive tract, skin cancer, including melanoma, and lung cancer. Follow-up analysis of the placebo group of the Finnish ATBC (Alpha Tocopherol Beta Carotene) study (incidentally, a study that showed no protection against lung cancer in a high-risk group supplemented with α-tocopherol and/or β-carotene) showed that there was a 36% higher incidence of lung cancer in those in the lowest quartile than in those in the highest quartile of diet-derived vitamin E. Vitamin E from dietary sources, but not supplements, has been reported to confer modest protection against breast cancer; however, as with vitamin C, no association was seen between vitamin E intake and the risk of ovarian cancer in the Nurses' Health Study follow-up.

Colorectal cancer is the second and third most common cancer in men and women, respectively. Dietary influences on the risk of colorectal cancer are currently unclear, and, based on recent findings of large prospective trials, it has been suggested that the influence of antioxidant-rich foods has been overstated. Nonetheless, there is evidence that vitamin E may be protective. In a case–control study in the USA of almost 1000 cases of rectal cancer, the risk was reported to be modestly decreased in women with a high vitamin E intake, but not in men. In a meta-analysis of five prospective nested case–control studies, there was a marginal decrease in the incidence of colorectal cancer in those in the highest quartile of plasma α-tocopherol, although no significant inverse association was seen in any of the studies individually. In the Iowa Women's Health Study, women with the highest risk of colon cancer were those with the lowest intake of vitamin E, although the relationship was significant only in women aged 55–59 years.

In addition to its antioxidant properties, vitamin E is reported to have immune-boosting and anti-inflammatory effects and to inhibit cell division, all of which may help explain the reported relationship between low intake or plasma concentrations of vitamin E and increased risk of various cancers. Currently, there is much interest in vitamin E in association with selenium in relation to the prevention of prostate, lung, and colon cancer. Indeed, the combination of vitamin E with other antioxidant micronutrients may be much more important than vitamin E alone. Furthermore, the different members of the vitamin E family may play cooperative or complementary roles in modulating the risk of disease. In terms of cancer prevention, γ-tocopherol is attracting much interest. Dietary intake of this form of vitamin E can be up to three times higher than that of α-tocopherol. Corn, canola, palm, soya bean, and peanut oils contain more γ-tocopherol than α-tocopherol. Despite a higher intake, however, our plasma levels of γ-tocopherol are only around 10% of those of α-tocopherol, owing to preferential placement of the α-form into very low-density lipoproteins. Interestingly, higher tissue levels of α-tocopherol are reportedly found in animals fed both α-tocopherol and γ-tocopherol than in animals fed α-tocopherol alone, suggesting that intake of both forms may enhance the enrichment of tissues. Furthermore, the lower reaches of the gastrointestinal tract may contain high levels of γ-tocopherol, and this may help to destroy fecal mutagens. None of the epidemiological studies to date have estimated the dietary intake of γ-tocopherol, but the few studies that have measured plasma levels of γ-tocopherol show interesting results. In a nested case–control study of 6000 Japanese men, there was a statistically significant inverse relationship between the risk of cancer of the upper digestive tract and plasma levels of γ-tocopherol but not α-tocopherol. In a nested case–control study in the USA, a statistically significant protective effect against prostate cancer was found only when both plasma α-tocopherol and γ-tocopherol levels were high, with a five-fold decrease in prostate cancer in those in the highest quintile relative to those in the lowest quintile. Some of the putative effect of γ-tocopherol may be mediated through its antioxidant properties; however, γ-tocopherol has other properties relevant to cancer prevention, including effects on oncogenes and tumor suppressor genes and on cell cycle events, that the α-form does not have or demonstrates to a lesser extent. It is of interest that most vitamin E supplementation trials to date have used α-tocopherol. It may be that intake of both isomers is needed for optimal tissue uptake and effect. Furthermore, in view of the ability of α-tocopherol to displace bound γ-tocopherol, supplementation with the α-form alone may be counterproductive, in that it may deplete tissues of γ-tocopherol. Further studies are needed in this area.

The brain is rich in unsaturated fatty acids, and there is a reasonable rationale for the protection of lipid-rich neurones by vitamin E. Plasma and cerebrospinal α-tocopherol concentrations were found to be low in patients with Alzheimer's disease in some but not all studies. Cognitive function is reported to be directly correlated with plasma α-tocopherol levels. A high intake of vitamin E is associated with a decreased risk of the subsequent development of Alzheimer's disease, and an 8 month delay in significant worsening of Alzheimer's disease was reported in association with increased intakes of vitamin E. In the NHANES III study, better memory performance in elderly participants was reportedly found in those with higher plasma α-tocopherol levels. Based on data such as these, vitamin E (2000 IU day^{-1}) is currently being studied in relation to its possible ability to delay the onset of Alzheimer's disease in people with mild cognitive impairment.

'Non-Nutrient' Antioxidants

Plant-based foods contain a multitude of antioxidants other than vitamin C and vitamin E. The two major classes of these other dietary-derived antioxidants are the carotenoids and the polyphenolic flavonoids. There are hundreds of different carotenoids and thousands of flavonoids, and these compounds give fruits, vegetables, teas, and herbs their wonderful colors in shades of red, orange, yellow, and purple. These compounds are synthesized exclusively in plants and have no known function in human metabolism. No deficiency state for either class of compounds has been identified in humans. Consequently, there is no recommended daily intake or agreed requirement for any of these compounds, and they are regarded as 'non-nutrients.' Nonetheless, there is evidence that diets rich in carotenoids and flavonoids are beneficial to health. For example, in a study of 1299 elderly people in the USA, those with diets rich in carotenoid-containing fruits and vegetables were found to have a significantly decreased rate of CVD and fatal myocardial infarction: the RRs (CI) when the highest and lowest quartiles of intake were compared were 0.54 (0.34–0.86) for fatal CVD and 0.25 (0.09–0.67) for fatal myocardial infarction.

The carotenoid lycopene has been reported to lower the risk of prostate cancer, but the evidence for a relationship between carotenoid intake and the risk of other cancers is conflicting. Increased intake of lutein and zeaxanthin may help to delay or prevent age-related maculopathy, because these carotenoids are concentrated in the macula and are likely to be very important in local protection of the lipid-rich retina. To date, however, epidemiological findings point to health benefits of foods containing carotenoids, and the influence, if any, of individual carotenoids remains to be established.

The same is true for the polyphenolic flavonoids, anthocyanins, and various other plant-based non-nutrient antioxidants in the diet. Many of these have antioxidant powers far higher than those of vitamin C and vitamin E when tested in *in vitro* systems. Dietary intake can be similar to that of vitamin C (100 mg day^{-1} or higher), but, as their bioavailability is low, plasma levels of individual flavonoids and other phenolic antioxidants are very low or undetectable. The major dietary polyphenolic compounds are quercetin, kaempferol, myricitin, and the catechins. These flavonoids are found in onions, apples, kale, broccoli, Brussels sprouts, teas, grapes, and wine. Moderate wine intake, especially of red wine (which is very rich in polyphenolic antioxidants), is associated with a significant decrease in the risk of CHD. Tea consumption, especially a high intake of green tea, is associated with a lower risk of CVD and cancer. However, which of the myriad compounds contribute to the reported health benefits is not yet clear. It may be many; it may be none. It must be remembered that association does not prove causality. Equally, the lack of significant effects of supplementation trials in healthy subject does not mean that there is no effect. As outlined in **Table 1**, and further delineated in **Table 2**, observational studies have several limitations, and there are various reasons why a conflict may exist between what we observe and the outcome of supplementation trials.

Summary and Research Needs

Strong evidence from a variety of sources indicates that a high intake of vitamin C or something very closely associated with it in the diet is protective against cancer and CVD, the major causes of disability and death in our aging communities. Indeed, it may be that plasma ascorbic-acid concentration can predict overall mortality risk. This interesting concept remains to be confirmed. The evidence for the benefits of a high intake of vitamin E is also strong, but research is needed into which member(s) of the vitamin E family are most important. The evidence for the benefits of carotenoids and flavonoids stems largely from observational studies that show a decreased risk of disease in association with a high intake of foods or beverages rich in these non-nutrient antioxidants rather than the agents themselves. However, individuals who take these foods in large quantities are often more health conscious, take fewer total calories, do not smoke, exercise more, and eat less red meat and saturated fat. The relationship between diet and health is clear, but diet is

Table 2 Limitations of observational epidemiological studies of diet and disease

- Cross-cultural study has no power if rates of disease and/or population means of the exposure variable of interest do not vary significantly between the populations being compared
- Behavioral, genetic, and geographical, rather than dietary, variation may account for differences detected
- A 'snapshot' view of recent dietary habits or current status may not be representative of those in earlier or later life, and differences during these periods will confound and confuse the results
- In case–control studies, the disease process itself, drug treatment, or post-diagnosis changes in diet or lifestyle may cause or mask changes in the exposure variable
- Subclinical or undetected disease may be present in controls, decreasing contrast with cases
- Retrospective dietary recall may be unreliable, food tables may be out of date or incomplete, and analysis methods may be inaccurate
- In nested case–control studies, long-term follow-up is needed and may rely on a distant 'snapshot' measure of the exposure variable as a representative index of past and future levels
- Instability or inaccurate measurement of the exposure variable will lead to bias in the results
- Assessment methods and 'high' or 'low' thresholds may vary in different areas supplying data
- If protection is maximal above a 'threshold' level of the exposure variable, then no effect will be detectable if levels in most of the study population are below or above the threshold
- Prospective studies are very expensive, requiring a very large study group and years or decades of follow-up
- Prospective trials generally have disease or death as the measured outcome; this means that the participants in the trial cannot benefit from its findings

complex and dynamic, the underlying mechanisms of chronic diseases are uncertain, and the influence of individual dietary antioxidants is difficult to discern within the heterogeneous framework of the human diet and lifestyle. Antioxidants do appear to play a role in protecting key biological sites, but further study is needed to establish which, how, and where and to establish the doses needed to achieve optimal effect. To date there is no evidence that high intakes of antioxidants in the diet are harmful. It is not yet known, however, whether intake above a threshold level brings additional benefit or whether the benefit of increased intake is limited to those with initially poor or marginal antioxidant status. Furthermore, antioxidants are likely to act within a coordinated system, and more of one may require more of others for beneficial effects to be achieved. Achieving 'target thresholds' of several antioxidants may be critical to achieving the optimal effect of each, and threshold plasma concentrations of $50\,\mu mol\,l^{-1}$ and $30\,\mu mol\,l^{-1}$ for vitamin C and vitamin E, respectively, with a ratio of more than 1.3, have been proposed for minimizing the risk of CHD.

To establish cause and effect and to make firm recommendations about the type and dose of antioxidants needed to achieve optimal health requires much in the way of further study. Of particular interest and value in such study is the growing field of orthomolecular nutrition, in which advances in genomics and proteomics are used to determine gene–nutrient interaction and the influence of diet on epigenetic phenomena. Such molecular-based studies, guided by epidemiological data and incorporated into future supplementation trials, will help answer the questions about the mechanisms of action and which, if any, antioxidants are important, how much, and for whom. However, while many questions relating to dietary antioxidants and health remain unanswered, to understand how to obtain a mixture of antioxidants and promote health we need look only at the macro level of food rather than at the micro level of specific constituents or molecular level of response. Fruits, vegetables, teas, herbs, wines, juices, and some types of chocolate are rich in antioxidants. It is known that diets rich in a variety of such foods are beneficial to health. The results of molecular-based experimental studies will determine whether these two truths are linked in a cause-and-effect relationship.

Acknowledgments

The author thanks The Hong Kong Polytechnic University and The World Cancer Research Fund International for financially supporting this work.

See also: **Antioxidants**: Diet and Antioxidant Defense.

Further Reading

Ames BN and Wakimoto P (2002) Are vitamin and mineral deficiencies a major cancer risk? *Nature Reviews* 2: 694–704.

Asplund K (2002) Antioxidant vitamins in the prevention of cardiovascular disease: a systematic review. *Journal of Internal Medicine* 251: 372–392.

Benzie IFF (2003) Evolution of dietary antioxidants. *Journal of Comparative Biochemistry and Physiology* 136A: 113–126.

Block G, Norkus E, Hudes M, Mandel S, and Helzlsouer K (2001) Which plasma antioxidants are most related to fruit and vegetable consumption? *American Journal of Epidemiology* 154: 1113–1118.

Brigelius-Flohé R, Kelly FJ, Salonen JT *et al.* (2002) The European perspective on vitamin E: current knowledge and future research. *American Journal of Clinical Nutrition* 76: 703–716.

Clarkson PM and Thompson HS (2000) Antioxidants: what role do they play in physical activity and health? *American Journal of Clinical Nutrition* 72: 637S–646S.

Duthie GG, Gardner PT, and Kyle JAM (2003) Plant polyphenols: are they the new magic bullet? *Proceedings of the Nutrition Society* 62: 599–603.

Gey KF (1998) Vitamins E plus C and interacting co-nutrients required for optimal health: a critical and constructive review of epidemiology and supplementation data regarding cardiovascular disease and cancer. *Biofactors* 7: 113–175.

Grundman M and Delaney P (2002) Antioxidant strategies for Alzheimer's disease. *Proceedings of the Nutrition Society* 61: 191–202.

Khaw KT, Bingham S, Welch A *et al.* (2001) Relation between plasma ascorbic acid and mortality in men and women in EPIC-Norfolk prospective study: a prospective population study. *Lancet* 357: 657–663.

Lindsay DG and Clifford MN (eds.) (2000) Critical reviews within the EU Concerted Action 'Nutritional enhancement of plant-based food in European trade' ('NEODIET'). *Journal of the Science of Food and Agriculture* 80: 793–1137.

McCall MR and Frei B (1999) Can antioxidant vitamins materially reduce oxidative damage in humans? *Free Radical Biology and Medicine* 26: 1034–1053.

Mensink RP and Plat J (2002) Post-genomic opportunities for understanding nutrition: the nutritionist's perspective. *Proceedings of the Nutrition Society* 61: 404–463.

Padayatty SJ, Katz A, Wang Y *et al.* (2003) Vitamin C as an antioxidant: evaluation of its role in disease prevention. *Journal of the American College of Nutrition* 22: 18–35.

Pryor WA (2000) Vitamin E and heart disease: basic science to clinical intervention trials. *Free Radical Biology and Medicine* 28: 141–164.

World Cancer Research Fund and the American Institute for Cancer Research (1997) *Food, Nutrition and the Prevention of Cancer: A Global Perspective.* Washington DC: American Institute for Cancer Research.

ASCORBIC ACID

Physiology, Dietary Sources and Requirements

D A Bender, University College London, London, UK

Ascorbic acid is a vitamin (vitamin C) for only a limited number of species: man and the other primates, bats, the guinea pig, and a number of birds and fishes.

In other species ascorbic acid is not a vitamin, but is an intermediate in glucuronic acid catabolism, and its rate of synthesis bears no relation to physiological requirements for ascorbate. Species for which ascorbate is a vitamin lack the enzyme gulonolactone oxidase (EC 1.11.3.8) and have an alternative pathway for glucuronic acid metabolism.

Ascorbic acid functions as a relatively nonspecific, radical-trapping antioxidant and also reduces the tocopheroxyl radical formed by oxidation of vitamin E. It has a specific metabolic function as the redox coenzyme for dopamine β-hydroxylase and peptidyl glycine hydroxylase, and it is required to maintain the iron of 2-oxoglutarate-dependent hydroxylases in the reduced state.

Absorption, Transport, and Storage

In species for which ascorbate is not a vitamin, intestinal absorption is passive, while in human beings and guinea pigs there is sodium-dependent active transport of the vitamin at the brush border membrane, with a sodium-independent mechanism at the basolateral membrane. Dehydroascorbate is absorbed passively in the intestinal mucosa and is reduced to ascorbate before transport across the basolateral membrane.

At intakes up to about 100 mg per day, 80–95% of dietary ascorbate is absorbed, falling from 50% of a 1 g dose to 25% of a 6 g and 16% of a 12 g dose. Unabsorbed ascorbate is a substrate for intestinal bacterial metabolism.

Ascorbate and dehydroascorbate circulate in the bloodstream both in free solution and bound to albumin. About 5% of plasma vitamin C is normally in the form of dehydroascorbate. Ascorbate enters cells by sodium-dependent active transport; dehydroascorbate is transported by the insulin-dependent glucose transporter and is accumulated intracellularly by reduction to ascorbate. In poorly controlled diabetes mellitus, tissue uptake of dehydroascorbate is impaired because of competition by glucose, and there may be functional deficiency of vitamin C despite an apparently adequate intake.

About 70% of blood-borne ascorbate is in plasma and erythrocytes (which do not concentrate the vitamin from plasma). The remainder is in white cells, which have a marked ability to concentrate ascorbate; mononuclear leukocytes achieve 80-fold concentration, platelets 40-fold, and granulocytes 25-fold, compared with the plasma concentration.

There is no specific storage organ for ascorbate; apart from leukocytes (which account for 10% of total blood ascorbate), the only tissues showing a significant concentration of the vitamin are the adrenal and pituitary glands. Although the concentration of ascorbate in muscle is relatively low, skeletal muscle contains much of the body pool of 5–8.5 mmol (900–1500 mg) of ascorbate.

Metabolism and Excretion

As shown in **Figure 1**, oxidation of ascorbic acid proceeds by a one-electron process, forming monodehydroascorbate, which disproportionates to ascorbate and dehydroascorbate. Most tissues also contain monodehydroascorbate reductase (EC 1.6.5.4), a flavoprotein that reduces the radical back to ascorbate. Dehydroascorbate is reduced to ascorbate by dehydroascorbate reductase (EC 1.8.5.1), a glutathione-dependent enzyme; little is oxidized to diketogulonic acid in human beings.

Both ascorbate and dehydroascorbate are filtered at the glomerulus, then reabsorbed by facilitated diffusion. When glomerular filtration exceeds the capacity of the transport systems, at a plasma concentration of ascorbate above about 85 µmol/l, the vitamin is excreted in the urine in amounts proportional to intake.

It has been reported that approximately 25% of the dietary intake of ascorbate is excreted as oxalate; this would account for about 40% of the total urinary excretion of oxalate. However, there is no known metabolic pathway for the synthesis of oxalate from ascorbate, and it is likely that all or most of the oxalate found in urine after loading doses of ascorbate is formed nonenzymically, after the urine has been collected. Even in people at risk of forming oxalate renal stones it is unlikely that normal or

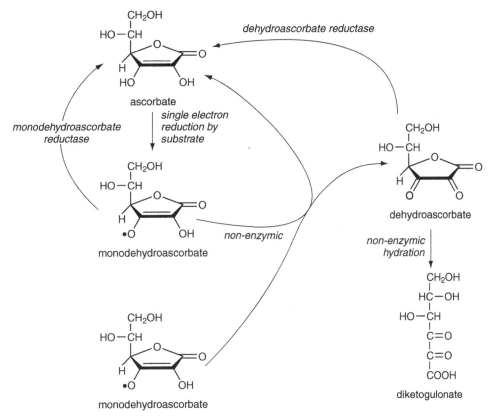

Figure 1 The metabolism of ascorbate. Monodehydroascorbate reductase, EC 1.6.5.4; dehydroascorbate reductase, EC 1.8.5.1.

high intakes of ascorbate pose any additional hazard.

Metabolic Functions of Ascorbic Acid

Ascorbic acid has specific and well-defined roles in two classes of enzymes: copper-containing hydroxylases and the 2-oxoglutarate-linked, iron-containing hydroxylases. It also increases the activity of a number of other enzymes *in vitro*—a nonspecific reducing action rather than reflecting a metabolic function of the vitamin. In addition, ascorbic acid has a number of less specific effects due to its action as a reducing agent and oxygen radical quencher. There is also evidence that ascorbate has a role in regulating the expression of connective tissue protein (and some other) genes; its mechanism of action is unknown.

Copper-Containing Hydroxylases

Dopamine β-hydroxylase (EC 1.14.17.1) is a copper-containing enzyme involved in the synthesis of the catecholamines noradrenaline and adrenaline from tyrosine in the adrenal medulla and central nervous system. The active enzyme contains Cu^+, which is oxidized to Cu^{2+} during the hydroxylation of the substrate; reduction back to Cu^+ specifically requires ascorbate, which is oxidized to monodehydroascorbate.

A number of peptide hormones have a terminal amide, and amidation is essential for biological activity. The amide group is derived from a glycine residue in the precursor peptide, by proteolysis to leave a carboxy terminal glycine. This is hydroxylated on the α-carbon; the hydroxyglycine decomposes nonenzymically to yield the amidated peptide and glyoxylate. This reaction is catalyzed by peptidyl glycine hydroxylase (peptidyl α-amidase, EC 1.14.17.3); like dopamine β-hydroxylase, it is a copper-containing enzyme, and it requires ascorbate as the electron donor.

2-Oxoglutarate-Linked, Iron-Containing Hydroxylases

A number of iron-containing hydroxylases (**Table 1**) share a common reaction mechanism, in which hydroxylation of the substrate is linked to decarboxylation of 2-oxoglutarate. Ascorbate is required for

Table 1 Vitamin C-dependent, 2-oxoglutarate-linked hydroxylases

Aspartate β-hydroxylase	EC 1.14.11.16
γ-Butyrobetaine hydroxylase	EC 1.14.11.1
p-Hydroxyphenylpyruvate hydroxylase	EC 1.14.11.27
Procollagen lysine hydroxylase	EC 1.14.11.4
Procollagen proline 3-hydroxylase	EC 1.14.11.7
Procollagen proline 4-hydroxylase	EC 1.14.11.2
Pyrimidine deoxynucleotide dioxygenase	EC 1.14.11.3
Thymidine dioxygenase	EC 1.14.11.10
Thymine dioxygenase	EC 1.14.11.6
Trimethyllysine hydroxylase	EC 1.14.11.8

the activity of all of these enzymes, but it does not function as either a stoichiometric substrate or a conventional coenzyme (which would not be consumed in the reaction).

Proline and lysine hydroxylases are required for the postsynthetic modification of collagen, and proline hydroxylase also for the postsynthetic modification of osteocalcin in bone and the Cl$_q$ component of complement. Aspartate β-hydroxylase is required for the postsynthetic modification of protein C, the vitamin K-dependent protease which hydrolyzes activated factor V in the blood-clotting cascade. Trimethyllysine and γ-butyrobetaine hydroxylases are required for the synthesis of carnitine.

The best studied of this class of enzymes is procollagen proline hydroxylase; it is assumed that the others follow essentially the same mechanism. As shown in **Figure 2**, the first step is binding of oxygen to the enzyme-bound iron, followed by attack on the 2-oxoglutarate substrate, resulting in decarboxylation to succinate, leaving a ferryl radical at the active site of the enzyme. This catalyzes the hydroxylation of proline, restoring the free iron to undergo further reaction with oxygen.

It has long been known that ascorbate is oxidized during the reaction, but not stoichiometrically with hydroxylation of proline and decarboxylation of 2-oxoglutarate. The purified enzyme is active in the absence of ascorbate, but after about 5–10 s (about 15–30 cycles of enzyme action) the rate of reaction falls. The loss of activity is due a side reaction of the highly reactive ferryl radical in which the iron is oxidized to Fe^{3+}, which is catalytically inactive—so-called uncoupled decarboxylation of 2-oxoglutarate. Activity is only restored by ascorbate, which reduces the iron back to Fe^{2+}.

The Role of Ascorbate in Iron Absorption

Inorganic dietary iron is absorbed as Fe^{2+} and not as Fe^{3+}; ascorbic acid in the intestinal lumen not only maintains iron in the reduced state but also chelates it, increasing absorption considerably. A dose of 25 mg of vitamin C taken together with a meal increases the absorption of iron

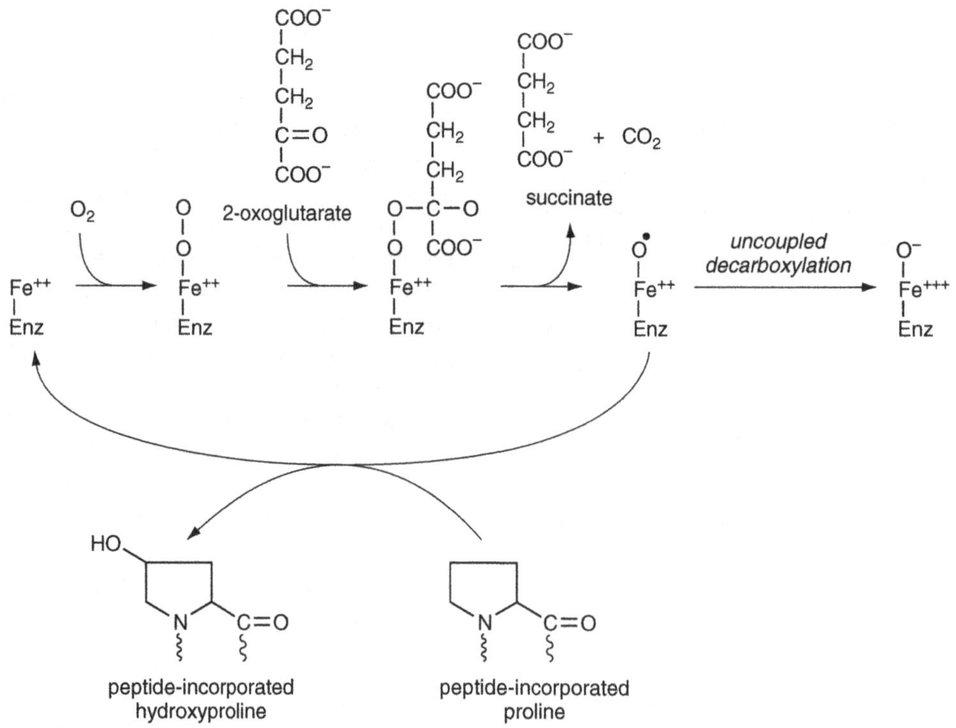

Figure 2 The reaction of procollagen proline hydroxylase.

approximately 65%, while a 1 g dose gives a 9-fold increase. This is an effect of ascorbic acid present together with the test meal; neither intravenous administration of vitamin C nor supplements several hours before the test meal affects iron absorption, although the ascorbate secreted in gastric juice should be effective. This is not a specific effect of ascorbate; a variety of other reducing agents including alcohol and fructose also enhance the absorption of inorganic iron.

Inhibition of Nitrosamine Formation

Oral bacteria can reduce nitrate to nitrite which, under the acidic conditions of the stomach, can react with amines in foods to form carcinogenic N-nitrosamines. In addition to dietary sources, a significant amount of nitrate is formed endogenously by the metabolism of nitric oxide—1 mg/kg body weight/day (about the same as the average dietary intake), increasing 20-fold in response to inflammation and immune stimulation, and nitrate is secreted in saliva.

Ascorbate reacts with nitrite forming NO, NO_2, and N_2, so preventing the formation of nitrosamines. In addition to ascorbate in foods, there is considerable secretion of ascorbate in the gastric juice, and inhibition of gastric secretion for treatment of gastric ulcers, as well as reducing vitamin B_{12} absorption, also inhibits this presumably protective gastric secretion of ascorbate.

However, while ascorbate can deplete nitrosating compounds under anaerobic conditions, the situation may be reversed in the presence of oxygen. Nitric oxide reacts with oxygen to form N_2O_3 and N_2O_4, both of which are nitrosating reagents, and can also react with ascorbate to form NO and monodehydroascorbate. It is thus possible for ascorbate to be depleted, with no significant effect on the total concentration of nitrosating species. It remains to be determined whether or not ascorbate has any significant effect in reducing the risk of nitrosamine formation and carcinogenesis.

Antioxidant and Prooxidant Actions of Ascorbate

Chemically, ascorbate is a potent reducing agent, both reducing hydrogen peroxide and also acting as a radical trapping antioxidant, reacting with superoxide and a proton to yield hydrogen peroxide or with the hydroxy radical to yield water. In each case the product is monodehydroascorbate, which, as shown in **Figure 1**, undergoes dismutation to ascorbate and dehydroascorbate. In studies of ascorbate depletion in men there is a significant increase in abnormalities of sperm

DNA, suggesting that vitamin C may have a general, nonspecific radical-trapping antioxidant function.

Ascorbate also acts to reduce the tocopheroxyl radical formed by oxidation of vitamin E in cell membranes and plasma lipoproteins. It thus has a vitamin E sparing antioxidant action, coupling lipophilic and hydrophilic antioxidant reactions.

The antioxidant efficiency of ascorbate is variable. From the chemistry involved, it would be expected that overall 2 mol of tocopheroxyl radical would be reduced per mole of ascorbate because of the reaction of 2 mol of monodehydroascorbate to yield ascorbate and dehydroascorbate. However, as the concentration of ascorbate increases, so the molar ratio decreases, and it is only at very low concentrations of ascorbate that it tends toward the theoretical ratio. This is because, as well as its antioxidant role, ascorbate can be a source of hydroxyl and superoxide radicals.

At high concentrations, ascorbate can reduce molecular oxygen to superoxide, being oxidized to monodehydroascorbate. Both Fe^{3+} and Cu^{2+} ions are reduced by ascorbate, again yielding monodehydroascorbate; the resultant Fe^{2+} and Cu^+ are reoxidized by reaction with hydrogen peroxide to yield hydroxide ions and hydroxyl radicals. Thus, as well as its antioxidant role, ascorbate has prooxidant action; the net result will depend on the relative rates of formation of superoxide and hydroxyl radicals by autooxidation and metal-catalyzed reactions of ascorbate, and the trapping of these radicals by ascorbate.

It seems likely that the prooxidant actions of ascorbate are of relatively little importance *in vivo*. Except in cases of iron overload there are almost no transition metal ions in free solution, they are all bound to proteins, and because the renal transport system is readily saturated, plasma and tissue concentrations of ascorbate are unlikely to rise to a sufficient extent to lead to significant radical formation.

Assessment of Vitamin C Status

The early method of assessing vitamin C nutritional status was by testing the extent of saturation of the body's reserves by giving a test dose of 500 mg (2.8 mmol) and measuring the amount excreted in the urine. In a subject with high status, more or less all of the test dose is recovered over a period of 5 or 6 h.

More sensitive assessment of status is achieved by measuring the concentration of the vitamin in whole blood, plasma, or leukocytes. Criteria of adequacy

Table 2 Plasma and leukocyte ascorbate concentrations as criteria of vitamin C nutritional status

		Deficient	*Marginal*	*Adequate*
Whole blood	m mol/l	< 17	17–28	28
	mg/l	< 3.0	3.0–5.0	> 5.0
Plasma	m mol/l	< 11	11–17	> 17
	mg/l	< 2.0	2.0–3.0	> 3.0
Leukocytes	p mol/10^6 cells	< 1.1	1.1–2.8	> 2.8
	μ g/10^6 cells	< 0.2	0.2–0.5	> 0.5

are shown in **Table 2**. The determination of ascorbate in whole blood is complicated by nonenzymic oxidation of the vitamin by hemoglobin, and most studies rely on plasma or leukocyte concentrations of ascorbate.

A problem arises in the interpretation of leukocyte ascorbate concentrations because of the different capacity of different classes of leukocytes to accumulate the vitamin. Granulocytes are saturated at a concentration of about 530 pmol/10^6 cells, while mononuclear leukocytes can accumulate 2.5 times more ascorbate. A considerable mythology has developed to the effect that vitamin C requirements are increased in response to infection, inflammation, and trauma, based on reduced leukocyte concentrations of ascorbate in these conditions. However, the fall in leukocyte ascorbate can be accounted for by an increase in the proportion of granulocytes in response to trauma and infection (and hence a fall in the proportion of mononuclear leukocytes). Total leukocyte ascorbate is not a useful index of vitamin C status without a differential white cell count.

There is increased formation of 8-hydroxyguanine (a marker of oxidative radical damage) in DNA during (short-term) vitamin C depletion, and the rate of removal of 8-hydroxyguanine from DNA by excision repair, and hence its urinary excretion, is affected by vitamin C status. This suggests that measurement of urinary excretion of 8-hydroxyguanine may provide a biomarker of optimum status, as a basis for estimating requirements.

Requirements

While the minimum requirement for ascorbate is firmly established, there are considerable differences between the reference intakes published by different national and international authorities. Depending on the chosen criteria of adequacy, and assumptions made in interpreting experimental results, it is possible to produce arguments in support of reference intakes ranging from 30 to 100 mg/day. Studies of intakes associated with reduced risks of cancer and cardiovascular disease suggest an average requirement of 90–100 mg/day and a reference intake of 120 mg/day.

Minimum Requirement

The minimum requirement for vitamin C was established in the 1940s in a depletion/repletion study, which showed that an intake of less than 10 mg per day was adequate to prevent the development of scurvy, or to cure the clinical signs. At this level of intake, wound healing is impaired, and optimum wound healing requires a mean intake of 20 mg per day. Allowing for individual variation, this gives reference intake of 30 mg/day, which was the UK figure until 1991 and the WHO/FAO figure until 2001.

Requirements Estimated from the Plasma and Leukocyte Concentrations of Ascorbate

The plasma concentration of ascorbate shows a sigmoidal relationship with intake. Below about 30 mg/day it is extremely low and does not reflect increasing intake to any significant extent. As the intake rises above 30 mg/day, so the plasma concentration begins to increase sharply, reaching a plateau of 70–85 μmol/l, at intakes between 70 and 100 mg/day, when the renal threshold is reached and the vitamin is excreted quantitatively with increasing intake.

The point at which the plasma concentration increases more or less linearly with increasing intake represents a state where reserves are adequate and ascorbate is available for transfer between tissues. This corresponds to an intake of 40 mg/day and is the basis of the UK, EU, and FAO figures. At this level of intake the total body pool is about 5.1 mmol (900 mg). It has been argued that setting requirements and reference intakes on the basis of the steep part of a sigmoidal curve is undesirable, and a more appropriate point would be the intake at which the plasma concentration reaches a plateau, at an intake of around 100–200 mg/day.

The US/Canadian reference intakes of 75 mg for women and 90 mg for men are based on studies of leukocyte saturation during depletion/repletion studies.

Requirements Estimated from Maintenance of the Body Pool of Ascorbate

An alternative approach to estimating requirements is to determine the fractional rate of catabolism of total body ascorbate; an appropriate intake would then be that required to replace losses and maintain the body pool.

Clinical signs of scurvy are seen when the total body pool of ascorbate is below 1.7 mmol (300 mg). The pool increases with intake, reaching a maximum of about 8.5 mmol (1500 mg) in adults—114 μmol (20 mg)/kg body weight. The basis for the 1989 US RDA of 60 mg was the observed mean fractional turnover rate of 3.2% of a body pool of 20 mg/kg body weight/day, with allowances for incomplete absorption of dietary ascorbate and individual variation.

It has been argued that a total body pool of 5.1 mmol (900 mg) is adequate; it is threefold higher than the minimum required to prevent scurvy, and there is no evidence that there are any health benefits from a body pool greater than 600 mg. The observed body pool of 8.5 mmol in depletion/repletion studies was found in subjects previously consuming a self-selected diet, with a relatively high intake of vitamin C, and therefore might not represent any index of requirement. Assuming a total body pool of 5.1 mmol and catabolism of 2.7%/day, allowing for efficiency of absorption and individual variation gives a reference intake of 40 mg/day.

Because the fractional turnover rate was determined during a depletion study, and the rate of ascorbate catabolism varies with intake, it has been suggested that this implies a rate of 3.6%/day before depletion. On this basis, and allowing for incomplete absorption and individual variation, various national authorities arrive at a recommended intake of 80 mg.

The rate of ascorbate catabolism is affected by intake, and the requirement to maintain the body pool cannot be estimated as an absolute value. A habitual low intake, with a consequent low rate of catabolism, will maintain the same body pool as a habitual higher intake with a higher rate of catabolism.

Dietary Sources and High Intakes

It is apparent from the list of rich sources of vitamin C in **Table 3** that the major determinant of vitamin C intake is the consumption of fruit and vegetables; deficiency is likely in people whose habitual intake of fruit and vegetables is very low. However, clinical

Table 3 Rich sources of vitamin C

	Portion (g)	mg/portion
Black currants	80	160
Oranges	250	125
Orange juice	200	100
Strawberries	100	60
Grapefruit	140	56
Melon	200	50
Green peppers	45	45
Sweet potato	150	38
Loganberries	85	34
Spinach	130	33
Red currants	80	32
White currants	80	32
Pineapple	125	31
Brussels sprouts	75	30
Mangoes	100	30
Satsumas	100	30
Tangerines	100	30
Turnips	120	30
Gooseberries	70	28
Potato chips	265	27
Broccoli	75	26
Swedes	120	24
Spring greens	75	23
Artichokes, globe	220	22
Potatoes	140	21
Avocados	130	20
Leeks	125	20
Lemons	25	20
Okra	80	20
Peas	75	20
Raspberries	80	20
Tomato juice	100	20
Plantain, green	85	17
Bilberries	80	16
Blackberries	80	16
Kidney	150	15
Tomatoes	75	15
Bananas	135	14
Cauliflower	65	13
Beans, broad	75	11
Cabbage	75	11
Nectarines	110	11
Parsnips	110	11
Rhubarb	100	10

signs of deficiency are rarely seen in developed countries. The range of intakes by healthy adults in Britain reflects fruit and vegetable consumption: the 2.5 percentile intake is 19 mg per day (men) and 14 mg per day (women), while the 97.5 percentile intake from foods (excluding supplements) is 170 mg per day (men) and 160 mg per day (women). Smokers may be at increased risk of deficiency; there is some evidence that the rate of ascorbate catabolism is 2-fold higher in smokers than in nonsmokers.

There is a school of thought that human requirements for vitamin C are considerably higher than those discussed above. The evidence is largely based on observation of the vitamin C intake of gorillas in captivity, assuming that this is the same as their intake in the wild (where they eat considerably less fruit than under zoo conditions), and then assuming that because they have this intake, it is their requirement—an unjustified assumption. Scaling this to human beings suggests a requirement of 1–2 g per day.

Intakes in excess of about 80–100 mg per day lead to a quantitative increase in urinary excretion of unmetabolized ascorbate, suggesting saturation of tissue reserves. It is difficult to justify a requirement in excess of tissue storage capacity.

A number of studies have reported low ascorbate status in patients with advanced cancer—perhaps an unsurprising finding in seriously ill patients. One study has suggested, on the basis of an uncontrolled open trial, that 10 g daily doses of vitamin C resulted in increased survival. Controlled studies have not demonstrated any beneficial effects of high-dose ascorbic acid in the treatment of advanced cancer.

High doses of ascorbate are popularly recommended for the prevention and treatment of the common cold. The evidence from controlled trials is unconvincing, and meta-analysis shows no evidence of a protective effect against the incidence of colds. There is, however, consistent evidence of a beneficial effect in reducing the severity and duration of symptoms. This may be due to the antioxidant actions of ascorbate against the oxidizing agents produced by, and released from, activated phagocytes, and hence a decreased inflammatory response.

Scorbutic guinea pigs develop hypercholesterolemia. While there is no evidence that high intakes of vitamin C result in increased cholesterol catabolism, there is evidence that monodehydroascorbate inhibits hydroxymethylglutaryl CoA reductase, resulting in reduced synthesis of cholesterol, and high intakes of ascorbate may have some hypocholesterolaemic action. There is limited evidence of benefits of high intakes of vitamin C in reducing the incidence of stroke, but inconsistent evidence with respect to coronary heart disease.

Regardless of whether or not high intakes of ascorbate have any beneficial effects, large numbers of people habitually take between 1 and 5 g per day of vitamin C supplements. There is little evidence of any significant toxicity from these high intakes. Once the plasma concentration of ascorbate reaches the renal threshold, it is excreted more or less quantitatively with increasing intake.

Because the rate of ascorbate catabolism increases with increasing intake, it has been suggested that abrupt cessation of high intakes of ascorbate may result in rebound scurvy because of 'metabolic conditioning' and a greatly increased rate of catabolism. While there have been a number of anecdotal reports, there is no evidence that this occurs.

See also: **Antioxidants**: Diet and Antioxidant Defense. **Vitamin E**: Physiology and Health Effects.

Further Reading

Basu TK and Schorah CI *Vitamin C in Health and Disease.* 1981 p. 160. London: Croom Helm.

Bender DA Ascorbic acid (vitamin C). In: *Nutritional Biochemistry of the Vitamins*, 2nd edn. 2003, pp. 357384. New York: Cambridge University Press.

Benzie IF Vitamin C: Prospective functional markers for defining optimal nutritional status. *Proceedings of the Nutrition Society* **58**: 1999469476.

Chatterjee IB Ascorbic acid metabolism. *World Review of Nutrition and Dietetics* **30**: 19786987.

England S and Seifter S The biochemical functions of ascorbic acid. *Annual Review of Nutrition* **6**: 1986365406.

Ginter E Marginal vitamin C deficiency, lipid metabolism and atherogenesis. *Advances in Lipid Research* **16**: 1978167220.

Rivers JM Safety of high-level vitamin C ingestion. *Annals of the New York Academy of Sciences* **498**: 1987445451.

Sato P and Udenfriend S Studies on vitamin C related to the genetic basis of scurvy. *Vitamins and Hormones* **36**: 19783352.

Sauberlich HE Pharmacology of vitamin C. *Annual Review of Nutrition* **14**: 1994371391.

Smirnoff N Ascorbic acid: Metabolism and functions of a multi-facetted molecule. *Current Opinion in Plant Biology* **3**: 2000229235.

BIOTIN

D M Mock, University of Arkansas for Medical
Sciences, Little Rock, AR, USA

Biotin is a water-soluble vitamin that is generally
classified in the B complex group. Biotin was discovered in nutritional experiments that demonstrated a factor in many foodstuffs capable of
curing the scaly dermatitis, hair loss, and neurologic
signs induced in rats fed dried egg white. Avidin, a
glycoprotein found in egg white, binds biotin very
specifically and tightly. From an evolutionary standpoint, avidin probably serves as a bacteriostat in egg
white; consistent with this hypothesis is the observation that avidin is resistant to a broad range of
bacterial proteases in both the free and biotin-
bound form. Because avidin is also resistant to pancreatic proteases, dietary avidin binds to dietary
biotin (and probably any biotin from intestinal
microbes) and prevents absorption, carrying the biotin through the gastrointestinal tract. Biotin is
synthesized by many intestinal microbes; however,
the contribution of microbial biotin to absorbed
biotin, if any, remains unknown. Cooking denatures
avidin, rendering this protein susceptible to digestion and unable to interfere with absorption of
biotin.

Absorption and Transport

Digestion of Protein-Bound Biotin

The content of free biotin and protein-bound biotin
in foods is variable, but the majority of biotin in
meats and cereals appears to be protein-bound via
an amide bond between biotin and lysine. Neither
the mechanisms of intestinal hydrolysis of protein-
bound biotin nor the determinants of bioavailability
have been clearly delineated. Because this bond is
not hydrolyzed by cellular proteases, release is likely
mediated by a specific biotin—amide hydrolase (biotinidase, EC 3.5.1.12). Biotinidase mRNA is present
in pancreas and, in lesser amounts, in intestinal

mucosa. Biotinidase is also present in many other
tissues, including heart, brain, liver, lung, skeletal
muscle, kidney, plasma, and placenta. Biotinidase
also likely plays a critical role in intracellular recycling of biotin by releasing biotin from intracellular
proteins such as carboxylases during protein
turnover.

Intestinal Absorption and Transport into Somatic Cells

At physiologic pH, the carboxylate group of biotin is
negatively charged. Thus, biotin is at least modestly
water-soluble and requires a transporter to cross cell
membranes such as enterocytes for intestinal absorption,
somatic cells for utilization, and renal tubule cells for
reclamation from the glomerular filtrate. In intact intestinal preparations such as loops and everted gut sacks,
biotin transport exhibits two components. One component is saturable at a k_m of approximately $10\,\mu M$ biotin;
the other is not saturable even at very large concentrations of biotin. This observation is consistent with passive diffusion. Absorption of biocytin, the biotinyl-lysine
product of intraluminal protein digestion, is inefficient
relative to biotin, suggesting that biotinidase releases
biotin from dietary protein. The transporter is present
in the intestinal brush border membrane. Transport is
highly structurally specific, temperature dependent, Na^+
coupled, and electroneutral. In the presence of a sodium
ion gradient, biotin transport occurs against a concentration gradient.

In rats, biotin transport is upregulated with
maturation and by biotin deficiency. Although carrier-mediated transport of biotin is most active in
the proximal small bowel of the rat, the absorption of
biotin from the proximal colon is still significant, supporting the potential nutritional significance of biotin
synthesized and released by enteric flora. Clinical studies have provided evidence that biotin is absorbed from
the human colon, but studies in swine indicate that
absorption of biotin from the hindgut is much less
efficient than from the upper intestine; furthermore,
biotin synthesized by enteric flora is probably not present at a location or in a form in which bacterial biotin
contributes importantly to absorbed biotin. Exit of

biotin from the enterocyte (i.e., transport across the basolateral membrane) is also carrier mediated. However, basolateral transport is independent of Na^+, electrogenic, and does not accumulate biotin against a concentration gradient.

Based on a study in which biotin was administered orally in pharmacologic amounts, the bioavailability of biotin is approximately 100%. Thus, the pharmacologic doses of biotin given to treat biotin-dependent inborn errors of metabolism are likely to be well absorbed. Moreover, the finding of high bioavailability of biotin at pharmacologic doses provides at least some basis for predicting that bioavailability will also be high at the physiologic doses at which the biotin transporter mediates uptake.

Studies of a variety of hepatic cell lines indicate that uptake of free biotin is similar to intestinal uptake; transport is mediated by a specialized carrier system that is Na^+ dependent, electroneutral, and structurally specific for a free carboxyl group. At large concentrations, transport is mediated by diffusion. Metabolic trapping (e.g., biotin bound covalently to intracellular proteins) is also important. After entering the hepatocyte, biotin diffuses into the mitochondria via a pH-dependent process.

Two biotin transporters have been described: a multivitamin transporter present in many tissues and a biotin transporter identified in human lymphocytes. In 1997, Prasad and coworkers discovered a Na^+-coupled, saturable, structurally specific transporter present in human placental choriocarcinoma cells that can transport pantothenic acid, lipoic acid, and biotin. This sodium-dependent multivitamin transporter has been named SMVT and is widely expressed in human tissues. Studies by Said and coworkers using RNA interference specific for SMVT provide strong evidence that biotin uptake by Caco-2 and HepG2 cells occurs via SMVT; thus, intestinal absorption and hepatic uptake are likely mediated by SMVT. The biotin transporter identified in lymphocytes is also Na^+ coupled, saturable, and structurally specific. Studies by Zempleni and coworkers provide evidence in favor of monocarboxylate transporter-1 as the lymphocyte biotin transporter.

A child with biotin dependence due to a defect in the lymphocyte biotin transporter has been reported. The SMVT gene sequence was normal. The investigators speculate that lymphocyte biotin transporter is expressed in other tissues and mediates some critical aspect of biotin homeostasis.

Ozand and collaborators described several patients in Saudi Arabia with biotin-responsive basal ganglia disease. Symptoms include confusion, lethargy, vomiting, seizures, dystonia, dysarthria, dysphagia, seventh nerve paralysis, quadriparesis, ataxia, hypertension, chorea,

and coma. A defect in the biotin transporter system across the blood–brain barrier was postulated. Additional work by Gusella and coworkers has suggested that SLC19A3 may be responsible for the reported defect.

The relationship of these putative biotin transporters to each other and their relative roles in intestinal absorption, transport into various organs, and renal reclamation remain to be elucidated.

Transport of Biotin from the Intestine to Peripheral Tissues

Biotin concentrations in plasma are small relative those of other water-soluble vitamins. Most biotin in plasma is free, dissolved in the aqueous phase of plasma. However, small amounts are reversibly bound and covalently bound to plasma protein (approximately 7 and 12%, respectively); binding to human serum albumin likely accounts for the reversible binding. Biotinidase has been proposed as a biotin binding protein or biotin carrier protein for the transport into cells. A biotin binding plasma glycoprotein has been observed in pregnant rats. Although the importance of protein binding in the transport of biotin from the intestine to the peripheral tissues is not clear, the immunoneutralization of this protein led to decreased transport of biotin to the fetus and early death of the embryo.

Transport of Biotin into the Central Nervous System

Biotin is transported across the blood–brain barrier. The transporter is saturable and structurally specific for the free carboxylate group on the valeric acid side chain. Transport into the neuron also appears to involve a specific transport system with subsequent trapping of biotin by covalent binding to brain proteins, presumably carboxylases.

Placental Transport of Biotin

Biotin concentrations are 3- to 17-fold greater in plasma from human fetuses compared to those in their mothers in the second trimester, consistent with active placental transport. The microvillus membrane of the placenta contains a saturable transport system for biotin that is Na^+ dependent and actively accumulates biotin within the placenta, consistent with SMVT.

Transport of Biotin into Human Milk

More than 95% of the biotin in human milk is free in the skim fraction. The concentration of biotin varies substantially in some women and exceeds the concentration in serum by one or two orders of magnitude, suggesting that there is a system for transport into milk. Metabolites account for more than half of the total biotin plus metabolites in early and transitional human milk. With postpartum maturation, the biotin concentration increases, but inactive metabolites still account for approximately one-third of the total biotin plus metabolites at 5 weeks postpartum. Studies have not detected a soluble biotin binding protein.

Metabolism and Urinary Excretion of Biotin and Metabolites

Biotin is a bicyclic compound (**Figure 1**). One of the rings contains an ureido group (—N—CO—N—). The tetrahydrothiophene ring contains sulfur and has a valeric acid side chain. A significant proportion of biotin undergoes catabolism before excretion (**Figure 1**). Two principal pathways of biotin catabolism have been identified in mammals. In the first pathway, the valeric acid side chain of biotin is degraded by β-oxidation. β-Oxidation of biotin leads to the formation of bisnorbiotin, tetranorbiotin, and related intermediates that are known to result from β-oxidation of fatty acids. The cellular site of this β-oxidation of biotin is uncertain. Spontaneous (nonenzymatic) decarboxylation of the unstable β-keto acids (β-keto-biotin and β-keto-bisnorbiotin) leads to formation of bisnorbiotin methylketone and tetranorbiotin methylketone; these catabolites appear in urine.

In the second pathway, the sulfur in the thiophane ring of biotin is oxidized, leading to the formation of biotin-L-sulfoxide, biotin-D-sulfoxide, and biotin sulfone. Sulfur oxidation may be catalyzed by a NADPH-dependent process in the smooth endoplasmic reticulum. Combined oxidation of the ring sulfur and β-oxidation of the side chain lead to metabolites such as bisnorbiotin sulfone. In mammals, degradation of the biotin ring to release carbon dioxide and urea is quantitatively minor. Biotin metabolism is accelerated in some individuals by anticonvulsants and during pregnancy, thereby increasing in urine the ratio of biotin metabolites to biotin.

Animal studies and studies using brush border membrane vesicles from human kidney cortex indicate that biotin is reclaimed from the glomerular filtrate against a concentration gradient by a saturable, Na^+-dependent, structurally specific system, but biocytin does not inhibit tubular reabsorption of biotin. Subsequent egress of biotin from the tubular cells occurs via a basolateral membrane transport system that is not dependent on Na^+. Studies of patients with biotinidase deficiency suggest that there may be a role for biotinidase in the renal handling of biotin.

On a molar basis, biotin accounts for approximately half of the total avidin-binding substances in human serum and urine (**Table 1**). Biocytin, bisnorbiotin, bisnorbiotin methylketone, biotin-D,L-sulfoxide, and biotin sulfone account for most of the balance.

Biliary Excretion of Biotin and Metabolites

Biliary excretion of biotin and metabolites is quantitatively negligible based on animal studies. When [^{14}C]biotin was injected intravenously into rats, biotin, bisnorbiotin, biotin-D,L-sulfoxide, and bisnorbiotin methylketone accounted for less than 2% of the administered ^{14}C, but urinary excretion accounted for 60%. Although the concentrations of biotin, bisnorbiotin, and biotin-D,L-sulfoxide were approximately 10-fold greater in bile than in serum of pigs, the bile-to-serum ratios of biotin and metabolites were more than 10-fold less than those of bilirubin, which is actively excreted in bile.

Metabolic Functions

In mammals, biotin serves as an essential cofactor for five carboxylases, each of which catalyses a critical step in intermediary metabolism. All five of the mammalian carboxylases catalyze the incorporation of bicarbonate as a carboxyl group into a substrate and employ a similar catalytic mechanism.

Biotin is attached to the apocarboxylase by a condensation reaction catalyzed by holocarboxylase synthetase (**Figure 1**). An amide bond is formed between the carboxyl group of the valeric acid side chain of biotin and the ε-amino group of a specific lysyl residue in the apocarboxylase; these regions contain sequences of amino acids that are highly conserved for the individual carboxylases both within and between species.

In the carboxylase reaction, the carboxyl moiety is first attached to biotin at the ureido nitrogen opposite the side chain; then the carboxyl group is transferred to the substrate. The reaction is driven by the hydrolysis of ATP to ADP and inorganic phosphate. Subsequent reactions in the pathways of the mammalian carboxylases release carbon dioxide from the product of the carboxylase reaction. Thus, these reaction sequences rearrange the substrates into more useful intermediates but do not violate the classic observation that mammalian metabolism does not result in the net fixation of carbon dioxide.

Regulation of intracellular mammalian carboxylase activity by biotin remains to be elucidated. However, the interaction of biotin synthesis and production of holoacetyl-CoA carboxylase in *Escherichia coli* has been extensively studied. In the bacterial

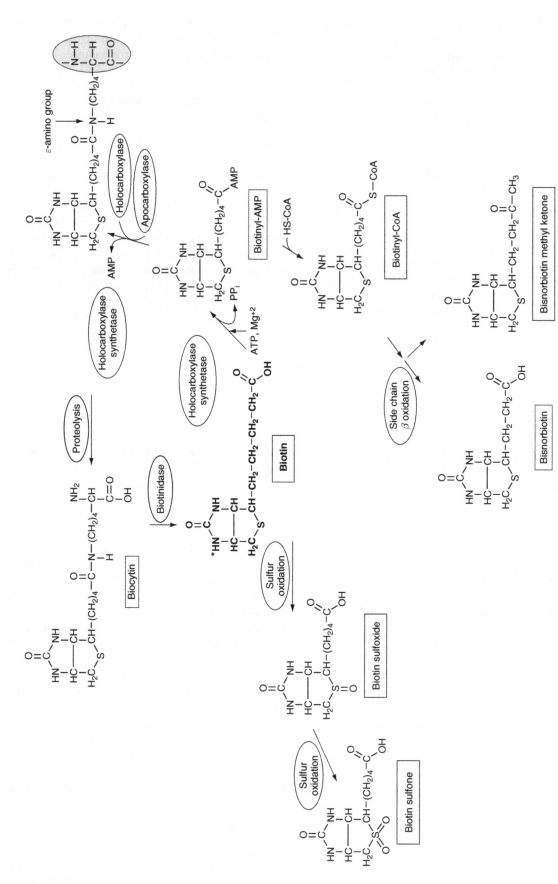

Figure 1 Biotin metabolism and degradation. Ovals denote enzymes or enzyme systems; rectangles denote biotin, intermediates, and metabolites. AMP, adenosine monophosphae; ATP, adenosine triphosphate; CoA, coenzyme A; PP$_i$, pyrophosphate; *, site of attachment of carboxyl moiety.

Table 1 Normal range for biotin and metabolites in human serum and urine[a]

Compound	Serum (pmol/l)	Urine (nmol/24 h)
Biotin	133–329	18–127
Bisnorbiotin	21–563	6–39
Biotin-D,L-sulfoxide	0–120	5–19
Bisnorbiotin methylketone	0–120	2–13
Biotin sulfone	ND	1–8
Biocytin	0–26	1–13
Total biotinyl compounds	294–1021[b]	46–128

[a]Normal ranges are reported ($n = 15$ for serum; $n = 16$ for urine, except biocytin, $n = 10$).
[b]Including unidentified biotin metabolites.
ND, not determined.

system, the apocarboxylase protein and biotin (as the intermediate biotinyl-AMP) act together to control the rate of biotin synthesis by direct interaction with promoter regions of the biotin operon, which in turn controls a cluster of genes that encode enzymes that catalyze the synthesis of biotin.

The five biotin-dependent mammalian carboxylases are acetyl-CoA carboxylase isoforms I and II (also known as α-ACC (EC 6.4.1.2) and β-ACC (EC 6.4.1.2)), pyruvate carboxylase (EC 6.4.1.1), methylcrotonyl-CoA carboxylase (EC 6.4.1.4), and propionyl-CoA carboxylase (EC 6.4.1.3). ACC catalyzes the incorporation of bicarbonate into acetyl-CoA to form malonyl-CoA (**Figure 2**). There are two isoforms of ACC. Isoform I is located in the cytosol and produces malonyl-CoA, which is rate limiting in fatty acid synthesis (elongation). Isoform II is located on the outer mitochondrial membrane and controls fatty acid oxidation in mitochondria through the inhibitory effect of malonyl-CoA on fatty acid transport

into mitochondria. An inactive mitochondrial form of ACC may serve as storage for biotin.

The three remaining carboxylases are mitochondrial. Pyruvate carboxylase (PC) catalyzes the incorporation of bicarbonate into pyruvate to form oxaloacetate, an intermediate in the Krebs tricarboxylic acid cycle (**Figure 2**). Thus, PC catalyzes an anaplerotic reaction. In gluconeogenic tissues (i.e., liver and kidney), the oxaloacetate can be converted to glucose. Deficiency of PC is probably the cause of the lactic acidemia, central nervous system lactic acidosis, and abnormalities in glucose regulation observed in biotin deficiency and biotinidase deficiency. β-Methylcrotonyl-CoA carboxylase (MCC) catalyzes an essential step in the degradation of the branched-chain amino acid leucine (**Figure 2**). Deficient activity of MCC leads to metabolism of 3-methylcrotonyl-CoA to 3-hydroxyisovaleric acid and 3-methylcrotonylglycine by an alternate pathway. Thus, increased urinary excretion of these abnormal metabolites reflects deficient activity of MCC.

Propionyl-CoA carboxylase (PCC) catalyzes the incorporation of bicarbonate into propionyl-CoA to form methylmalonyl-CoA; methylmalonyl-CoA undergoes isomerization to succinyl-CoA and enters the tricarboxylic acid cycle (**Figure 2**). In a manner analogous to MCC deficiency, deficiency of PCC leads to increased urinary excretion of 3-hydroxypropionic acid and 3-methylcitric acid.

In the normal turnover of cellular proteins, holocarboxylases are degraded to biocytin or biotin linked to an oligopeptide containing at most a few amino acid residues (**Figure 1**). Biotinidase releases biotin for recycling. Genetic deficiencies of holocarboxylase synthetase and biotinidase cause the two types of multiple carboxylase deficiency that were previously designated the neonatal and juvenile forms.

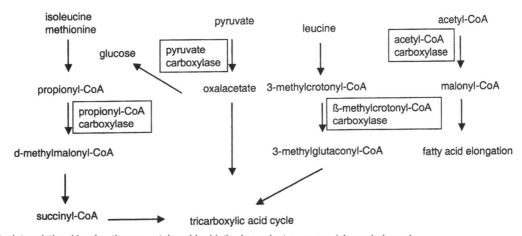

Figure 2 Interrelationship of pathways catalyzed by biotin-dependent enzymes (shown in boxes).

A Potential Role for Biotin in Gene Expression

In 1995, Hymes and Wolf discovered that biotinidase can act as a biotinyl-transferase; biocytin serves as the source of biotin, and histones are specifically biotinylated. Approximately 25% of total cellular biotinidase activity occurs in the nucleus. Zempleni and coworkers demonstrated that the abundance of biotinylated histones varies with the cell cycle, that biotinylated histones are increased approximately twofold compared to quiescent lymphocytes, and that histones are debiotinylated enzymatically in a process that is at least partially catalyzed by biotinidase. These observations suggest that biotin plays a role in regulating DNA transcription and regulation.

Although the mechanisms remain to be elucidated, biotin status has been shown to clearly effect gene expression. Cell culture studies suggest that cell proliferation generates an increased demand for biotin, perhaps mediated by increased synthesis of biotindependent carboxylases. Solozano-Vargas and coworkers reported that biotin deficiency reduces messenger RNA levels of holocarboxylase synthetase, α-ACC, and PCC and postulated that a cyclic GMP-dependent signaling pathway is involved in the pathogenesis.

Studies have been conducted on diabetic humans and rats that support an effect of biotin status on carbohydrate metabolism. Genes studied include glucokinase, phosphoenolpyruvate carboxykinase (PEPCK), and expression of the asialoglycoprotein receptor on the surface of hepatocytes. The effect of biotin status on PEPCK expression was particularly striking when diabetic rats were compared to nondiabetic rats. However, most studies have been performed on rats in which metabolic pathways have been perturbed prior to administration of biotin. Thus, the role of biotin in regulation of these genes during normal biotin status remains to be elucidated.

Hyperammonemia is a finding in biotin deficiency. Maeda and colleges have reported that ornithine transcarbamoylase (an enzyme in the urea cycle) is significantly reduced in biotin-deficient rats.

Assessment of Biotin Status

Measurement of Biotin

For measuring biotin at physiological concentrations (i.e., $100 \, \text{pmol} \, \text{l}^{-1}$ to $100 \, \text{nmol} \, \text{l}^{-1}$), a variety of assays have been proposed, and a limited number have been used to study biotin nutritional status. Most published studies of biotin nutritional status have used one of two basic types of biotin assays: bioassays (most studies) or avidin-binding assays (several recent studies).

Bioassays are generally sensitive enough to measure biotin in blood and urine. However, the bacterial bioassays (and perhaps the eukaryotic bioassays as well) suffer interference from unrelated substances and variable growth response to biotin analogues. Bioassays give conflicting results if biotin is bound to protein.

Avidin-binding assays generally measure the ability of biotin (i) to compete with radiolabeled biotin for binding to avidin (isotope dilution assays), (ii) to bind to avidin coupled to a reporter and thus prevent the avidin from binding to a biotin linked to solid phase, or (iii) to prevent inhibition of a biotinylated enzyme by avidin. Avidin-binding assays generally detect all avidin-binding substances, although the relative detectabilities of biotin and analogues vary between analogues and between assays, depending on how the assay is conducted. Chromatographic separation of biotin analogues with subsequent avidin-binding assay of the chromatographic fractions appears to be both sensitive and chemically specific.

Laboratory Findings of Biotin Deficiency

Although various indices have been used to assess biotin status, these have been validated in humans only twice during progressive biotin deficiency. In both studies, marginal biotin deficiency was induced in normal adults by feeding egg white. The urinary excretion of biotin declined dramatically with time on the egg-white diet, reaching frankly abnormal values in 17 of 21 subjects by day 20 of egg-white feeding. Bisnorbiotin excretion declined in parallel, providing evidence for regulated catabolism of biotin. In most subjects, urinary excretion of 3-hydroxyisovaleric acid increased steadily. By day 14 of egg-white feeding, 3-hydroxyisovaleric acid excretion was abnormally increased in 18 of 21 subjects, providing evidence that biotin depletion decreases the activity of MCC and alters leucine metabolism early in progressive biotin deficiency. Based on a study of only 5 subjects, 3-hydroxyisovaleric acid excretion in response to a leucine challenge may be even more sensitive than 3-hydroxyisovaleric acid excretion. Urinary excretions of 3-methylcrotonylglycine, 3-hydroxypropionic acid, and 3-methylcitric acid are not sensitive indicators of biotin deficiency compared to 3-hydroxyisovaleric acid excretion.

In a single study, plasma concentrations of free biotin decreased to abnormal values in only half of the subjects. This observation provides confirmation

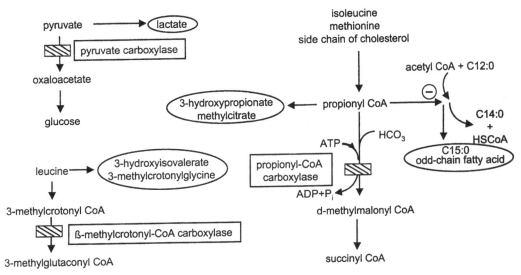

Figure 3 Organic acids and odd-chain fatty acids accumulate because biotin deficiency causes reduced activity of biotin-dependent enzymes. Hatched bars denote metabolic blocks at deficient carboxylases; ovals denote accumulation of products from alternative pathways.

of the impression that blood biotin concentration is not an early or sensitive indicator of marginal biotin deficiency.

Lymphocyte PCC activity is an early and sensitive indicator of marginal biotin deficiency. In 11 of 11 subjects, lymphocyte PCC activity decreased to abnormal values by day 28 of egg-white feeding and returned to normal in 8 of 11 within 3 weeks of resuming a general diet with or without biotin supplement.

Odd-chain fatty acid accumulation is also a marker of biotin deficiency. The accumulation of odd-chain fatty acid is thought to result from PCC deficiency (**Figure 3**); the accumulation of propionyl-CoA likely leads to the substitution of a propionyl-CoA moiety for acetyl-CoA in the ACC reaction and to the incorporation of a three- (rather than two-) carbon moiety during fatty acid elongation. However, in comparison to lymphocyte PCC activity and urinary excretion of 3-hydroxyisovaleric acid, odd-chain fatty acids accumulate in blood lipids more slowly during biotin deficiency and return to normal more gradually after biotin repletion.

Requirements and Allowances

Data providing an accurate estimate of the dietary and parenteral biotin requirements for infants, children, and adults are lacking. However, recommendations for biotin supplementation have been formulated for oral and parenteral intake for preterm infants, term infants, children, and adults (**Table 2**).

Dietary Sources, Deficiency, and High Intakes

Dietary Sources

There is no published evidence that biotin can be synthesized by mammals; thus, the higher animals must derive biotin from other sources. The ultimate source of biotin appears to be de novo synthesis by bacteria, primitive eukaryotic organisms such as yeast, moulds, and algae, and some plant species.

The great majority of measurements of biotin content of foods have used bioassays. Recent publications provide evidence that the values are likely to contain substantial errors. However, some worthwhile generalizations can be made. Biotin is widely distributed in natural foodstuffs, but the absolute content of even the richest sources is low compared to the content of most other water-soluble vitamins.

Table 2 Adequate intake of biotin

Life-stage group	Adequate intake (μg/day)
Infants (months)	
0–6	5
7–12	6
Children (years)	
1–3	8
4–8	12
Males and females (years)	
9–13	20
14–18	25
≥19	30
Pregnancy	30
Lactation	35

Table 3 Foods relatively rich in biotin

Food	ng biotin/g food	serving size (g)	μg biotin/serving
Chicken liver, cooked	1872.00	74	138.00
Beef liver, cooked	416.00	74	30.80
Egg, whole, cooked	214.00	47	10.00
Peanuts, roasted, salted	175.00	28	4.91
Egg, yolk, cooked	272.00	15	4.08
Salmon, pink, canned in water	59.00	63	3.69
Pork chop, cooked	45.00	80	3.57
Mushrooms, canned	21.60	120	2.59
Sunflower seeds, roasted, salted	78.00	31	2.42
Chili	5.20	441	2.29
Hot dog, chicken and pork, cooked	37.00	56	2.06
Egg, white, cooked	58.00	35	2.02
Banana pudding	10.20	170	1.73
Strawberries, fresh	15.00	111	1.67

Foods relatively rich in biotin are listed in **Table 3**. The average daily dietary biotin intake has been estimated to be approximately 35–70 μg.

Circumstances Leading to Deficiency

The fact that normal humans have a requirement for biotin has been clearly documented in two situations: prolonged consumption of raw egg white and parenteral nutrition without biotin supplementation in patients with short bowel syndrome and other causes of malabsorption. Based on lymphocyte carboxylase activities and plasma biotin levels, some children with severe protein–energy malnutrition are biotin deficient. Investigators have speculated that the effects of biotin deficiency may be responsible for part of the clinical syndrome of protein–energy malnutrition.

Biotin deficiency has also been reported or inferred in several other clinical circumstances, including long-term anticonvulsant therapy, Leiner's disease, sudden infant death syndrome, renal dialysis, gastrointestinal diseases, and alcoholism. Studies of biotin status during pregnancy and of biotin supplementation during pregnancy provide evidence that a marginal degree of biotin deficiency develops in at least one-third of women during normal pregnancy. Although the degree of biotin deficiency is not severe enough to produce overt manifestations of biotin deficiency, the deficiency is sufficiently severe to produce metabolic derangements. A similar marginal degree of biotin deficiency causes high rates of fetal malformations in some mammals. Moreover, data from a multivitamin supplementation study provide significant albeit indirect evidence that the marginal degree of biotin deficiency that occurs spontaneously in normal human gestation is teratogenic.

Clinical Findings of Frank Deficiency

The clinical findings of frank biotin deficiency in adults, older children, and infants are similar. Typically, the findings appear gradually after weeks to several years of egg-white feeding or parenteral nutrition. Thinning of hair and progression to loss of all hair, including eyebrows and lashes, has been reported. A scaly (seborrheic), red (eczematous) skin rash was present in the majority; in several, the rash was distributed around the eyes, nose, mouth, and perineal orifices. These cutaneous manifestations, in conjunction with an unusual distribution of facial fat, have been termed 'biotin deficiency facies.' Depression, lethargy, hallucinations, and paraesthesia of the extremities were prominent neurologic symptoms in the majority of adults. The most striking neurologic findings in infants were hypotonia, lethargy, and developmental delay.

The clinical response to administration of biotin has been dramatic in all well-documented cases of biotin deficiency. Healing of the rash was striking within a few weeks, and growth of healthy hair was generally present by 1 or 2 months. Hypotonia, lethargy, and depression generally resolved within 1 or 2 weeks, followed by accelerated mental and motor development in infants. Pharmacological doses of biotin (e.g., 1–10 mg) have been used to treat most patients.

High Intakes

Daily doses up to 200 mg orally and up to 20 mg intravenously have been given to treat biotin-responsive inborn errors of metabolism and acquired biotin deficiency. Toxicity has not been reported.

See also: **Microbiota of the Intestine**: Prebiotics.

Further Reading

Bender DA (1999) Optimum nutrition: Thiamin, biotin, and pantothenate. *Proceedings of the Nutritional Society* 58: 427–433.

Cronan JE Jr (2002) Interchangeable enzyme modules. Functional replacement of the essential linker of the biotinylated subunit of acetyl-CoA carboxylase with a linker from the lipoylated subunit of pyruvate dehydrogenase. *Journal of Biological Chemistry* 277: 22520–22527.

Flume MZ (2001) Final report on the safety assessment of biotin. *International Journal of Toxicology* 20(supplement 4): 1–12.

McCormick DB (2001) Bioorganic mechanisms important to coenzyme functions. In: Rucker RB, Suttie JW, McCormick DB, and Machlin LJ (eds.) *Handbook of Vitamins*, 3rd edn, pp. 199–212. New York: Marcel Dekker.

McMahon RJ (2002) Biotin in metabolism and molecular biology. *Annual Reviews in Nutrition* 22: 221–239.

Mock DM (1992) Biotin in human milk: When, where, and in what form? In: Picciano MF and Lonnerdal B (eds.) *Mechanisms Regulating Lactation and Infant Nutrient Utilization*. New York: John Wiley.

National Research Council, Food and Nutrition Board, and Institute of Medicine (1998) Dietary reference intakes for thiamin, riboflavin, niacin, vitamin B-6, folate, vitamin B-12, pantothenic acid, biotin, and choline. In *Recommended Dietary Allowances.*, pp. 374–389. Washington, DC. National Academy Press.

Pacheco-Alvarez D, Solorzano-Vargas RS, and Del Rio AL (2002) Biotin in metabolism and its relationship to human disease. *Archives of Medical Research* 33: 439–447.

Solbiati J, Chapman-Smith A, and Cronan JE Jr (2002) Stabilization of the biotinoyl domain of *Escherichia coli* acetyl-CoA carboxylase by interactions between the attached biotin and the protruding "thumb" structure. *Journal of Biological Chemistry* 277: 21604–21609.

Wolf B (2001) Disorders of biotin metabolism. In: Scriver CR, Beaudet AL, Sly WS, and Valle D (eds.) *The Metabolic and Molecular Basis of Inherited Disease*, vol. 3, pp. 3151–3177. New York: McGraw-Hill.

Zempleni J and Mock DM (2001) Biotin. In: Song WO and Beecher GR (eds.) *Modern Analytical Methodologies in Fat and Water-Soluble Vitamins*, pp. 459–466. Baltimore: John Wiley.

CAFFEINE

M J Arnaud, Nestle S.A., Vevey, Switzerland

During the period 1820–1827, three white crystalline substances called 'caffein' or 'coffein,' 'guaranin,' and 'thein' were isolated from green coffee beans, guarana, and tea, respectively. These substances were shown in 1838–1840 to be identical. Later, caffeine was also discovered in maté prepared from *Ilex paraguariensis* and kola nuts. Since then, caffeine has been shown to be a natural constituent of more than 60 plant species.

Two other related compounds, theophylline and theobromine, have also been isolated from tea and cocoa beans, respectively while a third, paraxanthine, was isolated from human urine (**Figure 1**). By the end of the nineteenth century, all of these methylated xanthines had been synthesized. Caffeine, both natural and synthetic, has been used as a flavoring agent in food and beverages and as an active component of a variety of over-the-counter pharmaceutical products and drugs. A regulation adopted by the European Commission requires the compulsory labeling 'high caffeine content' when soft drinks contain more than 150 mg caffeine per liter.

In addition to natural caffeine obtained by the industrial decaffeination process, caffeine can also be obtained by the methylation of theobromine and also by total chemical synthesis using dimethylcarbamide and malonic acid.

Chemistry

Caffeine (M_r 194.19) is also called, more systematically, 1,3,7-trimethylxanthine, 1,3,7-trimethyl-2,6-dioxopurine, or 3,7-dihydro-1,3,7-trimethyl-l*H*-purine-2,6-dione and has been referred to as a purine alkaloid.

Caffeine is odourless and has a characteristic bitter taste. It is a white powder (density ($d^{18/4}$) 1.23) moderately soluble in organic solvents and water. However, its solubility in water is considerably increased at higher temperatures (1% (w/v) at 15 °C and 10% at 60 °C). Its melting point is 234–239 °C and the temperature of sublimation at atmospheric pressure is 178 °C. Caffeine is a very weak base, reacting with acids to yield readily hydrolyzed salts, and relatively stable in dilute acids and alkali. Caffeine forms unstable salts with acids and is decomposed by strong solutions of caustic alkali.

In aqueous solution, caffeine is nonionized at physiological pH. Dimers as well as polymers have been described. The solubility of caffeine in water is increased by the formation of benzoate, cinnamate, citrate, and salicylate complexes. In plants, chlorogenic acid, coumarin, isoeugenol, indolacetic acid, and anthocyanidin have been shown to complex with caffeine.

Caffeine exhibits an ultraviolet absorption spectrum with a maximum at 274 nm and an absorption coefficient of 9700 in aqueous solution. Upon crystallization from water, silky needles are obtained containing 6.9% water (a 4/5 hydrate).

Determination

Caffeine has traditionally been identified in foods by ultraviolet spectrophotometry of an organic solvent extract after suitable cleanup by column chromatography. Such methods tend to be laborious and may be subject to interference from other ultraviolet-absorbing compounds. Recently, high-performance liquid chromatography has been more extensively used. This technique, often in conjunction with solid phase extraction, can provide accurate data for the determination of caffeine in foods and physiological samples.

Absorption, Distribution, and Elimination

Following oral ingestion, caffeine is rapidly and virtually completely absorbed from the gastrointestinal tract into the bloodstream. Mean plasma concentrations of 8–10 mg l^{-1} are observed

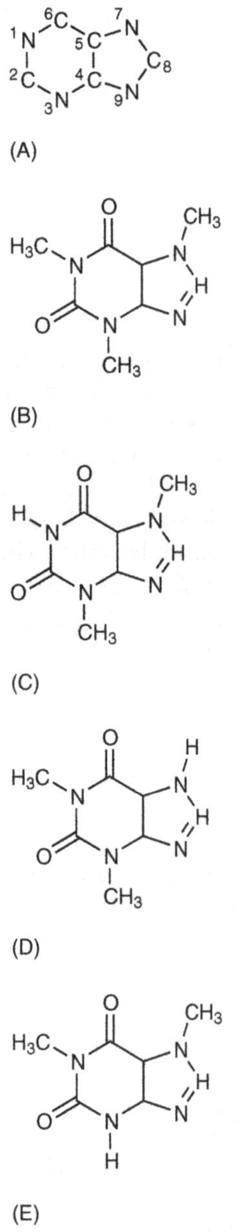

Figure 1 Chemical structures of caffeine and the dimethylxanthines. (A) Purine ring nomenclature according to E. Fischer; (B) caffeine; (C) theobromine; (D) theophylline; (E) paraxanthine. From Dews (1984).

following oral or intravenous doses of 5–8 mg kg^{-1}. The plasma kinetics of caffeine can be influenced by a number of factors, including the total dose of caffeine, the presence of food in the stomach, and low pH values of drinks, which can modify gastric emptying. Caffeine enters the intracellular tissue water and is found in all body fluids: cerebrospinal fluid, saliva, bile, semen, breast milk, and umbilical cord blood. A higher fraction of the ingested dose of caffeine is recovered in sweat compared to urine. The fraction of caffeine bound to plasma protein varies from 10 to 30%.

There is no blood–brain barrier and no placental barrier limiting the passage of caffeine through tissues. Therefore, from mother to fetus and to the embryo, an equilibrium can be continuously maintained.

The elimination of caffeine is impaired in neonates because of their immature metabolizing hepatic enzyme systems. For example, plasma half-lives of 65–103 h in neonates have been reported compared to 3–6 h in adults and the elderly.

Gender, exercise, and thermal stress have no effect on caffeine pharmacokinetics in men and women. Cigarette smoking increases the elimination of caffeine, whereas decreases have been observed during late pregnancy or with the use of oral contraceptives and in patients with liver diseases. Drug interactions leading to impaired caffeine elimination are frequently reported.

There is no accumulation of caffeine or its metabolites in the body and less than 2% of caffeine is excreted unchanged in the urine. Some rate-limiting steps in caffeine metabolism, particularly demethylation into paraxanthine that is selectively catalyzed by *CYP1A2*, determine the rate of caffeine clearance and the dose-dependent pharmacokinetics in humans.

Important kinetic differences and variations in the quantitative as well as qualitative metabolic profiles have been shown between species, thus making extrapolation from one species to another very difficult. All of the metabolic transformations include multiple and separate pathways with demethylation to dimethyl- and monomethylxanthines, formation of dimethyl- and monomethylurates, and ring opening yielding substituted diaminouracils (**Figure 2**). The reverse biotransformation of theophylline to caffeine is demonstrated not only in infants but also in adults.

From metabolic studies, an isotopic caffeine breath test has been developed that detects impaired liver function using the quantitative formation of labeled carbon dioxide as an index. From the urinary excretion of an acetylated uracil metabolite, human acetylator phenotype can be easily identified and the analysis of the ratio of the urinary concentrations of other metabolites represents a sensitive test to determine the hepatic enzymatic activities of xanthine oxidase and microsomal 3-methyl demethylation, 7-methyl demethylation, and 8-hydroxylation. Quantitative analyses of paraxanthine urinary metabolites may be used as a biomarker of caffeine intake. Fecal excretion is a minor elimination route, with recovery of only 2–5% of the ingested dose.

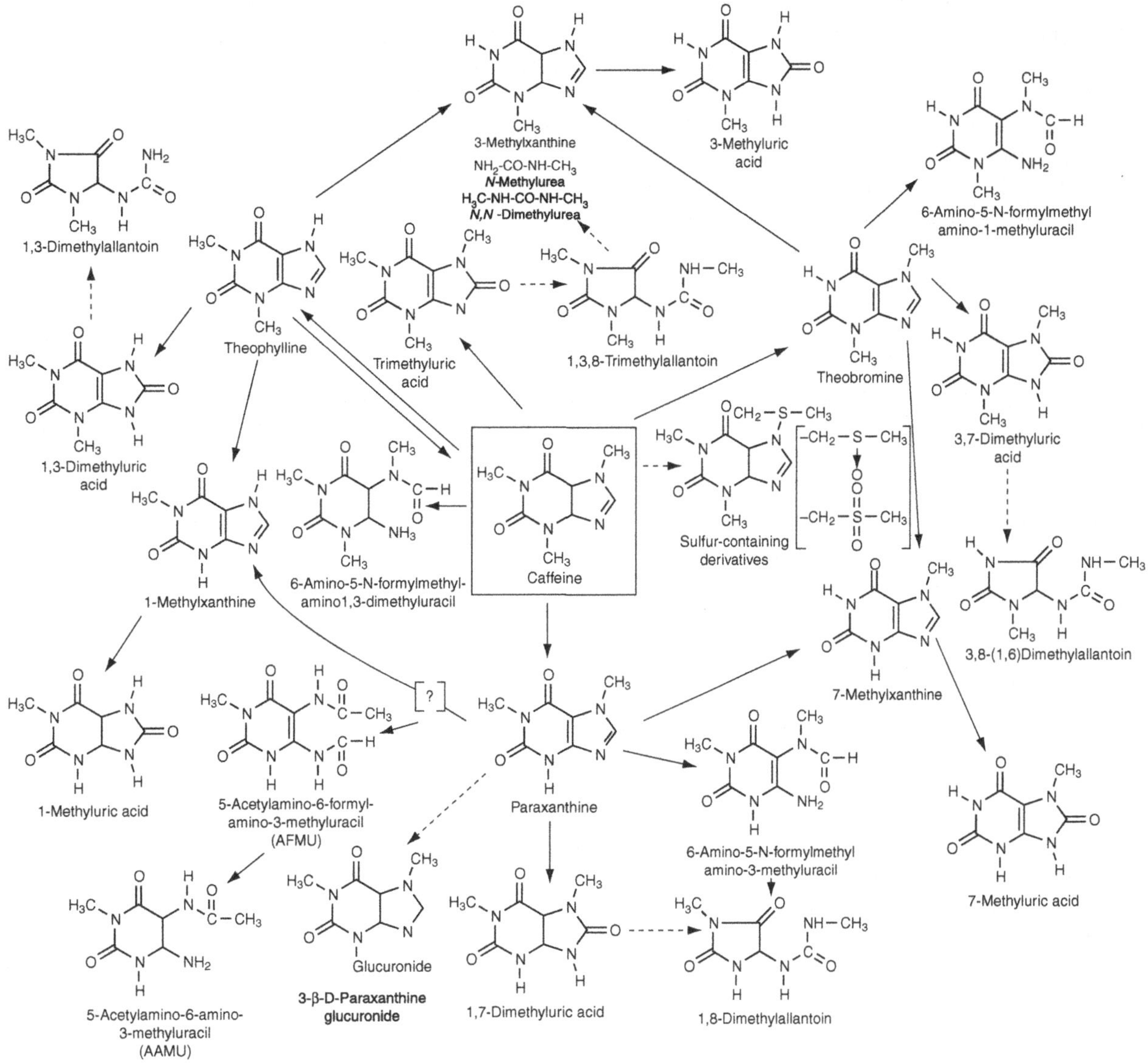

Figure 2 Metabolic pathways of caffeine in the human (⟶), the rat (---➤) and the mouse (---➤). From Garattini (1993).

Physiological and Pharmacological Properties

Because the physiological and pharmacological properties of caffeine represent the cumulative effects of not only the parent compound but also its metabolites, it is quite possible that effects attributed to caffeine *per se* are in fact mediated by one or more of its metabolites. It must also be noted that most of the knowledge about caffeine's effects has been derived from acute administration to fasted subjects submitted to a period of caffeine abstinence in order to ensure low plasma caffeine concentrations. It is thus difficult to extrapolate the results to the usual pattern of caffeine consumption in which most people consume it at different intervals throughout the day and over periods of years.

Effects on the Central Nervous System

Animal experiments have shown caffeine-mediated effects at the neuroendocrine level, such as increased serum corticosterone and β-endorphin and decreased serum growth hormone and thyrotropin, but it is expected that habitual human consumption has only marginal or inconsistent neuroendocrine effects. Caffeine is described as a central nervous system (CNS) stimulant, and the increased formation and release of neurotransmitters such as catecholamines, serotonin, γ-aminobutyric acid, norepinephrine, and acetyl-choline have been reported.

Behavioral effects can be observed in humans after acute and moderate doses of 1–5 mg kg^{-1} of caffeine. In these studies, the subjects felt more alert and active with improved cognitive function, including vigilance, learning, memory, and mood state. It was claimed that they would be better able to cope with their jobs when bored or fatigued and after night work and sleep deprivation. Population-based studies of the effect of caffeine intake on cognition showed a positive trend, especially among elderly women. Comparative studies on regular and deprived caffeine consumers suggest that reversal of caffeine withdrawal is a major component of the effects of caffeine on mood and performance.

A dose-dependent delay in sleep onset is found as well as a decrease in total sleep time and an impairment of sleep quality characterized by an increased number of spontaneous awakenings and body movements. In premature infants, sleep organization appears to be unaffected by treatment with 5 mg/kg/day caffeine to prevent apnoea.

The observation that sensitive subjects are more likely to have trembling hands is considered to be a CNS effect and not a direct effect on muscle. Caffeine doses higher than 15 mg kg^{-1} induce headaches, jitteriness, nervousness, restlessness, irritability, tinnitus, muscle twitchings, and palpitations. These symptoms of chronic excessive caffeine intake are part of the criteria used to make the diagnosis of caffeinism. The same symptoms have been reported in adults on abrupt cessation of caffeine use.

With 100–200 mg kg^{-1} doses, mild delirium appears, followed by seizures and death. Although tolerance with low doses led to a pleasant stimulation, alertness, and performance benefits, on withdrawal, headache, drowsiness, fatigue, and anxiety were reported.

Epidemiology and laboratory studies suggest beneficial effects of caffeine consumption in the development of Parkinson's disease and the mechanisms involved may be mediated through adenosine A$_{2A}$ receptors. The role of these receptors in neuronal injury and degeneration, as well as in other diseases such as Alzheimer's disease, has important therapeutic potential but needs further investigation.

Effects on the Cardiovascular System

Caffeine produces a direct stimulation of myocardial tissue leading to an increase in the rate and force of contraction. This direct cardiac effect can be inhibited by a depressant effect on the heart via medullary vagal stimulation. These opposing effects may explain why bradycardia, tachycardia, or no change can be observed in individuals receiving similar doses of caffeine. The traditional clinical view that caffeine induces arrhythmias in humans has not been confirmed by controlled experimental studies.

Caffeine decreases peripheral resistance by direct vasodilatation and increases blood flow to a small extent. This effect results from the relaxation of smooth muscle of blood vessels. For coronary arteries, vasodilatation is also observed *in vitro*, but the effects of caffeine in human coronary arteries *in vivo* are unknown. Different effects of caffeine on circulation can be observed in different vascular beds and, for example, the treatment of migraine headaches by caffeine is mediated through the vasoconstriction of cerebral arteries. It has also been shown that caffeine is capable of attenuating postprandial hypotension in patients with autonomic failure.

The observed cardiovascular effects consist of a 5–10% increase in both mean systolic and diastolic blood pressure for 1–3 h. A significant association was found between caffeine-related increase in systolic blood pressure and caffeine-related increase in pain tolerance. However, in contrast to the acute pressor effect reported, several epidemiological studies showed that habitual caffeine intake lowers blood pressure. Heart rate is decreased by 5–10% during the first hour, followed by an increase above baseline during the next 2 h. These effects are not detectable in regular coffee drinkers, suggesting that a complete tolerance can be developed. The tolerance to chronic caffeine intake can explain contradictory results reported in the literature. A few studies suggest that caffeine is partly responsible for the homocysteine-raising effect of coffee. This effect is associated with increased risk of cardiovascular disease, but it is uncertain whether this relation is causal.

Epidemiological studies designed to establish a relationship between caffeine intake and the incidences of myocardial infarction, mortality from ischaemic heart disease, or cerebrovascular accidents have provided conflicting results and have failed to establish a significant correlation.

Effects on Renal Functions

In humans, the administration of a single dose of 4 mg kg^{-1} caffeine increases the urinary excretion of sodium, calcium, magnesium, potassium, chloride, and urine volume. The mechanism of this mild diuresis has been attributed to an increase in renal blood flow, an increased glomerular filtration, and a decrease in tubular reabsorption of sodium ions and other ions. Although these effects appeared more pronounced for a higher acute dose of $10 \, mg \, kg^{-1}$, a review concluded that caffeine consumption stimulates a mild diuresis similar to water. There was no evidence of a fluid–electrolyte imbalance as well as disturbed thermoregulation, and caffeine was not detrimental to exercise performance or health.

Tolerance to the diuretic action of caffeine was demonstrated more than 50 years ago and was shown to develop on chronic caffeine intake so that the clinical significance of hypokalemia and calciuria is difficult to evaluate. Although controversial, some epidemiological studies have implicated caffeine in the increased risk for poor calcium retention. For calcium intakes lower than 750 mg per day, increased rate of bone loss and lower bone density were reported. However, it has been suggested that the effect on bone of high caffeine intake requires a genetic predisposition toward osteoporosis. In individuals who ingest calcium recommended daily allowances, there is no evidence of any effect of caffeine on bone status and calcium economy.

Effects on the Respiratory System

In caffeine-naive subjects, a dose of $4 \, mg \, kg^{-1}$ increases the mean respiratory rate. This effect is not found in chronic caffeine ingestion. Several mechanisms have been suggested, such as an increase in pulmonary blood flow, an increased supply of air to the lungs due to the relaxation of bronchiolar and alveolar smooth muscle, an increase in sensitivity of the medullary respiratory center to carbon dioxide, stimulation of the central respiratory drive, an improved skeletal muscle contraction, and an increase in cardiac output.

At higher doses ($7 \, mg \, kg^{-1}$), caffeine ingested by trained volunteers alters ventilatory and gas exchange kinetics during exercise, leading to a transient reduction in body carbon dioxide stores.

Effects on Muscles

Caffeine has been shown to have a bronchial and smooth muscle relaxant effect and to improve skeletal muscle contractility. Significant increases in hand tremor and forearm extensor electromyogram were observed in human subjects after the ingestion of $6 \, mg \, kg^{-1}$ of caffeine. This effect is more likely due to a CNS stimulatory effect than to direct action on the muscle fibers. Skeletal muscle fatigue can be reversed by high concentrations of caffeine obtained only *in vitro* but not *in vivo*.

Effects on the Gastrointestinal System

Caffeine relaxes smooth muscle of the biliary and gastrointestinal tracts and has a weak effect on peristalsis. However, high doses can produce biphasic responses, with an initial contraction followed by relaxation. Caffeine seems to have no effect on the lower oesophageal sphincter. The increase in both gastric and pepsin secretions is linearly related to the plasma levels obtained after the administration of a dose of $4–8 \, mg \, kg^{-1}$. In the small intestine, caffeine modifies the fluid exchange from a net absorption to a net excretion of water and sodium.

The role of caffeine in the pathogenesis of peptic ulcer and gastrointestinal complaints remains unclear, and no association has been found in clinical and epidemiological studies.

Effects on Energy Metabolism

Acute administration of caffeine produces a 5–25% increase in the basal metabolic rate. Inactive subjects exhibit a greater increase in resting metabolic rate than do exercise-trained subjects. It is concluded that endurance training seems to result in a reduced thermogenic response to a caffeine challenge.

These modifications of energy metabolism were associated with significant increases in serum free fatty acids, glycerol, and lactate concentrations, whereas inconsistent findings were reported for blood glucose levels. Acute administration of caffeine was shown to decrease insulin sensitivity and to impair glucose tolerance, possibly as a result of elevated plasma epinephrine. However, it is not understood why a large and long-term epidemiological study associated significant lower risks for type 2 diabetes in both men and women with total caffeine intake. The lipolytic effect is generally explained by the inhibition of phosphodiesterase, the release of catecholamine, or adenosine receptor antagonism. The increased availability of free fatty acids and their oxidation may have a glycogen-sparing effect. However, increasingly more results do not support the hypothesis that caffeine improves endurance performance by stimulating lipolysis, and some of the ergogenic effects in endurance exercise performance may occur directly at the skeletal muscle and CNS levels. In addition, this effect may be suppressed by the simultaneous ingestion of a high-carbohydrate meal, which is a common practice prior to competition.

Despite the controversy among scientists concerning the ergogenic potential of caffeine on sport performance, it is accepted that caffeine will not improve performance during short-term, high-intensity work, whereas an increase in both work output and endurance in long-term exercise is expected. Most studies also show that the duration and the magnitude of the ergogenic effect of caffeine are greater in nonusers than in users.

Based on the assumption that caffeine may enhance athletic performance, the International Olympic Committee defined an upper concentration limit of $12\,\mu g/ml$ in urine samples, above which an athlete was disqualified. However, in the World Anti-Doping Agency Executive Committee Meeting (September 2003), it was observed that the stimulant effect of caffeine is obtained at levels lower than 12. As a consequence, caffeine was removed from the 2004 list of prohibited substances because athletes must be allowed to behave like other people in society and may thus be allowed to drink coffee.

Safety and Toxicology

The acute oral LD_{50} (dose sufficient to kill one-half of the population of tested subjects) of caffeine is more than $200\,mg\,kg^{-1}$ in rats, $230\,mg\,kg^{-1}$ in hamsters and guinea pigs, $246\,mg\,kg^{-1}$ in rabbits, and $127\,mg\,kg^{-1}$ in mice. The sensitivity of rats to the lethal effects of caffeine increases with age, and higher toxicity is observed in male than in female rats.

Vomiting, abdominal pain, photophobia, palpitations, muscle twitching, convulsions, miosis, and unconsciousness were described in several reports of nonfatal caffeine poisonings in children who ingested $80\,mg\,kg^{-1}$ caffeine. In several fatal accidental caffeine poisonings, cold chills, stomach cramps, tetanic spasms, and cyanosis were reported. The likely lethal dose in adult humans has been estimated to be approximately $10\,g$, which corresponds roughly to $150–200\,mg\,kg^{-1}$. With daily doses of $110\,mg\,kg^{-1}$ given via intragastric cannula to female rats over 100 days, hypertrophy of organs such as the salivary gland, liver, heart, and kidneys was reported. Caffeine also induced thymic and testicular atrophy. Developmental and reproductive toxicity was associated with high, single daily doses of caffeine. The no-effect level for teratogenicity is $40\,mg\,kg^{-1}$ caffeine per day in the rat, although delayed sternebral ossification can be observed at lower doses. This effect has been shown to be reversed in the postnatal period. Available epidemiological evidence suggests that maternal caffeine consumption does not cause morphological malformation in the fetus. Caffeine intake has been linked with reduced fetal size in some studies, particularly when intake was more than $600\,mg$ per day, whereas others have not shown an impact on growth. High daily levels given as divided doses in rats were less toxic than when given as a single dose, in which case reduced fetal body weight was the only effect observed.

Caffeine at high concentration levels has mutagenic effects in bacteria and fungi and causes chromosomal damage in vitro. However, there is consensus that caffeine is not mutagenic in higher animals.

An epidemiological study showed no chromosomal aberrations in lymphocytes of normal, caffeine-exposed people, and other studies reported an increased frequency of micronucleated blood cells and the absence of mutagenic compounds in urine. In long-term studies, caffeine was shown to have no carcinogenic potential in rodents. Caffeine has not been classified as carcinogenic in animals or humans by the International Agency for Research on Cancer.

Therapeutic Uses

The most extensively investigated and most firmly established clinical application of caffeine is the control of neonatal apnoea in premature infants. The respirogenic properties of theophylline were first reported, and caffeine is increasingly being used as a substitute for theophylline because of its wider therapeutic index. For infants with a body weight of $2.5\,kg$, the therapeutic loading doses varied from 5 to $30\,mg\,kg^{-1}$, followed by a maintenance dose of $3\,mg\,kg^{-1}$ per day. Plasma caffeine levels must be controlled carefully to reach $10–20\,mg\,l^{-1}$.

Because of the bronchial muscle relaxant effect, caffeine is used in chronic obstructive pulmonary disease and for the treatment of asthma. The use of caffeine in the treatment of children with minimal brain dysfunction, to increase the duration of electroconvulsive therapy-induced seizure, for allergic rhinitis, as well as for atopic dermatitis has also been described. Recently, caffeine has been used as a diagnostic test for malignant hyperthermia and in the diagnosis of neuroleptic malignant syndrome, a complication of neuroleptic therapy.

Caffeine is found in many drug preparations, both prescription and over-the-counter. Caffeine is present in drugs used as stimulants, pain relievers, diuretics, and cold remedies. When used as an analgesic adjuvant, the potency of the analgesic drug is significantly enhanced by the addition of caffeine.

Although caffeine has been shown to promote thermogenesis in humans, it is no longer allowed as an ingredient in weight-control products in the US market because long-term clinical studies demonstrate that it does not help those wishing to lose weight.

Biochemical Mechanisms of Action

The physiological and pharmacological properties of caffeine cannot be explained by a single biochemical mechanism. Three principal hypotheses have been investigated to explain the diverse actions of caffeine.

The first biochemical effect described was the inhibition of phosphodiesterase, the enzyme that catalyzes the breakdown of cyclic adenosine $3',5'$-phosphate (cAMP). Caffeine was shown to increase cAMP concentrations in various tissues. This inhibition occurs at large concentrations (millimolar range) and is of limited importance with regard to the physiological effects of caffeine at levels at which it is normally consumed.

Calcium translocation is the second mechanism frequently suggested from experiments using skeletal muscles. However, high concentrations of caffeine are also necessary to modify intracellular calcium ion storage.

In the plasma, increased levels of β-endorphin, epinephrine, norepinephrine, corticosterone, ACTH, renin, and angiotensin I and decreased levels of growth hormone, thyroxine, triiodothyronine, and thyrotropin were reported with high caffeine doses. The mechanisms responsible for these various effects are largely unknown, and the mediation of adenosine receptors is suggested. The antagonism of benzodiazepine at the receptor level is observed at lower caffeine concentrations ($0.5–0.7$ mM) than those required for phosphodiesterase inhibition.

The third mechanism, antagonism of the endogenous adenosine, is the most plausible mode of action because caffeine exerts its antagonism at micromolar levels. Its main metabolite, paraxanthine, is as potent as caffeine in blocking adenosine receptors. Caffeine is more potent at A_{2A} receptors and less potent at A_3 receptors compared to A_1 and A_{2B} receptors. An upregulation of adenosine receptor is the postulated biochemical mechanism of caffeine tolerance.

Adenosine receptor antagonism appears to be the mechanism that explains most of the effects of caffeine on CNS activity, intestinal peristalsis, respiration, blood pressure, lipolysis, catecholamine release, and renin release. However, some effects, such as opiate antagonism or effects that are similar to those of adenosine, must be mediated by other mechanisms, such as the potentiation by caffeine of inhibitors of prostaglandin synthesis.

See also: **Sports Nutrition**.

Further Reading

Armstrong LE (2002) Caffeine, body fluid–electrolyte balance and exercise performance. *International Journal of Sport Nutrition and Exercise Metabolism* 12: 205–222.

Arnaud MJ (1987) The pharmacology of caffeine. *Progress in Drug Research* 31: 273–313.

Clarke RJ and Macrae R (eds.) (1988) Physiology. In *Coffee*, vol. 3. London: Elsevier.

Clarke RJ and Vitzhum OG (eds.) (2001) *Coffee. Recent Developments*. London: Blackwell Science.

Debry G (1994) *Coffee and Health*. Paris: John Libbey Eurotext.

Dews PB (ed.) (1984) *Caffeine*. Berlin: Springer-Verlag.

Dews PB, O'Brien CP, and Bergman J (2002) Caffeine: Behavioural effects of withdrawal and related issues. *Food and Chemical Toxicology* 40: 1257–1261.

Garattini S (ed.) (1993) *Caffeine, Coffee and Health*. New York: Raven Press.

Graham TE (2001) Caffeine and exercise, metabolism, endurance and performance. *Sports Medicine* 31: 785–807.

James JE (1991) *Caffeine and Health*. London: Academic Press.

Lorist MM and Tops M (2003) Caffeine, fatigue, and cognition. *Brain and Cognition* 53: 82–94.

Nawrot P, Jordan S, Eastwood J *et al.* (2003) Effects of caffeine on human health. *Food Additives and Contaminants* 20: 1–30.

Schmitt JAJ (2001) *Serotonin, Caffeine and Cognition. Psychopharmacological Studies in Human Cognitive Functioning*. Maastricht, The Netherlands: Neuropsych.

Snel J and Lorist MM (eds.) (1998) *Nicotine, Caffeine and Social Drink, Behaviour and Brain Function*. Amsterdam: Harwood Academic.

World Health Organization–International Agency for Research on Cancer (1991) *IARC Monographs on the Evaluation of Carcinogenic Risks to Humans: Coffee, Tea, Mate, Methylxanthines and Methylglyoxal*, vol. 51. Lyon, France: WHO–IARC.

CALCIUM

L H Allen, University of California at Davis, Davis, CA, USA

J E Kerstetter, University of Connecticut, Storrs, CT, USA

Calcium is an essential nutrient. Although most of the calcium in the body is found in bones and teeth, the other 1% has critical, life-sustaining functions. Most people in the world, including those in industrialized countries, fail to consume the recommended amounts of calcium, which will ultimately result in poor bone health and increase the risk of osteoporosis. Adequate calcium intake is critical to the achievement of peak bone mass in the first several decades of life, the retention of bone during middle adulthood, and the minimization of bone loss during the last several decades. Without adequate intake, the intestine, bone, and renal systems have intricate ways of retaining more calcium and normalizing serum calcium levels. These three primary tissues of calcium homeostasis (intestine, bone, and kidneys) are dynamic in their handling of calcium, reacting to dietary intake, physiological need, or disease processes. This article discusses calcium absorption, regulation, function, metabolism, and excretion as well as the changes in calcium physiology during the lifespan.

Absorption and Transport

Intake and Distribution

The dietary intake of calcium in the United States is approximately 20 mmol (600–1200 mg) per day unless supplements are consumed. Approximately 73% of dietary calcium is supplied from milk products, 9% from fruits and vegetables, 5% from grains, and the remaining 12% from all other sources. Approximately 25% of women take a nutritional supplement that contains calcium, but supplement use by men and children is much lower.

Approximately 25–50% of dietary calcium is absorbed and delivered to the exchangeable calcium pool. Of the 25–30 mol (1000–1200 g) of calcium in the body, 99% is found in the skeleton and teeth. The remaining 1% is in the blood, extracellular fluid, muscle, and other tissues. The extracellular pool of calcium turns over 20–30 times per day in adults, whereas bone calcium turns over every 5 or 6 years. A remarkably large amount is filtered through the kidneys, approximately 250 mmol (10 000 mg) per day, of which approximately 98% is reabsorbed, so that urinary excretion of the mineral is only 2.5–5 mmol (100–200 mg) per day (**Figure 1**).

Intestinal Calcium Absorption

The efficiency of dietary calcium absorption depends on two major factors: its interaction with other dietary constituents and physiological/pathological factors. Dietary factors that reduce the total amount of calcium absorbed by the intestine include phosphate, oxalate, phytate, fiber, and very low calcium intakes, whereas those that increase absorption include protein (or specific amino acids, lysine and arginine) and lactose in infants. The physiological/pathological factors that decrease intestinal calcium absorption include low serum $1,25(OH)_2$ vitamin D (the form of the vitamin that effects calcium absorption), chronic renal insufficiency, hypoparathyroidism, aging, and vitamin D deficiency, whereas increased absorption is observed during growth, pregnancy, primary hyperparathyroidism, sarcoidosis, and estrogen and growth hormone administration. The interindividual variability in intestinal calcium absorption is very high for reasons that are not entirely clear. On tightly controlled diets, a homogenous group of subjects can have intestinal calcium absorptions ranging from 10 to 50%.

Dietary calcium is complexed to food constituents such as proteins, phosphate, and oxalate, from which it needs to be released prior to absorption. The role of gastric acid (or the lack thereof induced by commonly used proton pump inhibiting drugs) in intestinal calcium absorption is not well established, although achlorhydria can impair absorption in the fasted state.

Calcium crosses the intestinal mucosa by both active and passive transport. The active process is saturable, transcellular, and occurs throughout the

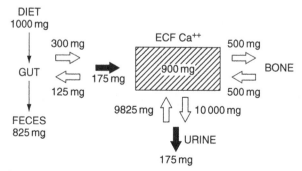

Figure 1 Daily calcium turnover.

small intestine. The transcellular pathway is a multistep process, starting with the entry of luminal calcium into the enterocyte (possibly via a calcium channel) and translocation of calcium from the microvillus border of the apical plasma membrane to the basolateral membrane followed by extrusion out of the enterocyte. Calbindin, a calcium binding protein that is regulated by the hormonal form of vitamin D, $1,25(OH)_2D_3$, affects every step in the movement of calcium through the enterocyte, including entry into the cell, movement in the cell interior, and transfer into the lamina propria. Although details of the movement of calcium through intestinal cells are still under investigation, it appears that the vitamin D-dependent calcium binding protein calbindin-D_{9k} and the plasma membrane calcium-pumping ATPase 1b (PMCA1b) are critical transport molecules in the cytoplasm and basolateral membrane, respectively. The active transport pathway is predominant at lower levels of calcium intake, and it becomes more efficient in calcium deficiency or when intakes are low and also when calcium requirements are high during infancy, adolescence, and pregnancy. It becomes less efficient in vitamin D-deficient individuals and in elderly women after menopause.

The passive transport pathway is nonsaturable and paracellular. It occurs throughout the small intestine and is unaffected by calcium status or parathyroid hormone (PTH). It is relatively independent of $1,25(OH)_2D_3$, although this metabolite has been found by some investigators to increase the permeability of the paracellular pathway. A substantial amount of calcium is absorbed by passive transport in the ileum due to the relatively slow passage of food through this section of the intestine. The amount of calcium absorbed by passive transport will be proportional to the intake and bioavailability of calcium consumed.

Fractional calcium absorption increases in response to low intake but varies throughout life. It is highest during infancy (60%) and puberty (25–35%), stable at approximately 25% in adults, and then declines with age (by approximately 2% per decade after menopause). There is little difference in calcium absorption efficiency between Caucasians and African Americans. The lower urinary calcium and better calcium conservation in African Americans probably contributes to their higher bone mineral density.

Storage

The skeleton acts as the storage site for calcium. Bone calcium exists primarily in the form of hydroxyapatite ($Ca_{10}(PO_4)_6(OH)_2$), and this mineral comprises 40% of bone weight. In the short term, the release of calcium from bone serves to maintain serum calcium concentrations. In the longer term, however, persistent use of skeletal calcium for this purpose without adequate replenishment will result in loss of bone density. The storage of very small amounts of calcium in intracellular organelles and its subsequent release into cytosol acts as an intracellular signal for a variety of functions.

Between 60 and 80% of the variance in peak bone mass is explained by genetics, including polymorphisms in the vitamin D–receptor gene and in genes responsible for insulin-like growth factor-1 (IGF-1) and collagen production.

Metabolism and Excretion

Regulation by Hormones

The concentration of ionized calcium in serum is closely regulated because it has profound effects on the function of nerves and muscles, blood clotting, and hormone secretion. The principal regulators of calcium homeostasis in humans and most terrestrial vertebrates are PTH and the active form of vitamin D, $1,25(OH)_2$ vitamin D_3 (**Figure 2**).

PTH is a single-chain polypeptide that is released from the parathyroid when there is a decrease in the calcium concentration in extracellular fluid. The calcium-sensing receptor (acting as the thermostat for calcium) is found on the parathyroid gland, where it detects small perturbations in serum ionized calcium. The decline in serum calcium induces an increase in PTH secretion. PTH has the effect of restoring extracellular calcium concentrations by stimulating the resorption of bone to release

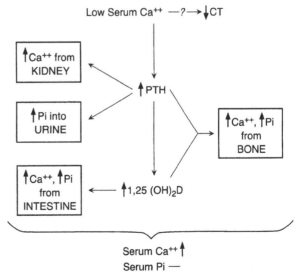

Figure 2 Hormonal regulation of calcium metabolism.

calcium, by increasing the renal reabsorption of calcium, and by enhancing the renal conversion of $25(OH)D_3$ to the active, hormonal form of the vitamin, $1,25(OH)_2$ vitamin D_3. The active form of vitamin D then increases the synthesis of intestinal calcium binding protein (CaBP), leading to more efficient intestinal calcium absorption. PTH release is inhibited when serum calcium and $1,25(OH)_2$ vitamin D_3 increase or when serum phosphate is decreased. The highly regulated interactions among PTH, calcium, $1,25(OH)_2$ vitamin D_3, and phosphate maintain blood calcium levels remarkably constant despite significant changes in calcium intake or absorption, bone metabolism, or renal functions. The extracellular calcium concentration is the most important regulator of PTH secretion and occurs on a minute-by-minute basis. Acute PTH administration leads to release of the rapidly turning over pool of calcium near the bone surface. Chronic administration of PTH increases osteoclast cell number and activity. Interestingly and paradoxically, intermittent PTH administration is anabolic, increasing formation of trabecular bone. In the kidney, PTH has three major functions: It increases calcium reabsorption, inhibits phosphate reabsorption, and enhances the synthesis of the active form of vitamin D. All of these actions are designed to defend against hypocalcemia.

There are two sources of vitamin D: the diet (where it is found as the fortificant vitamin D_2 or natural D_3) or synthesis in skin during exposure to ultraviolet radiation (sunlight). The vitamin enters the circulation and is transported on a vitamin D binding protein to the liver, where it is hydroxylated to 25(OH) cholecalciferol, which leaves the liver, is bound again to the binding protein in the circulation, and enters the kidney where it is hydroxylated again to $1,25(OH)_2D_3$, the most active metabolite of the vitamin. The primary biological effect of $1,25(OH)_2D_3$ is to defend against hypocalcemia by increasing the efficiency of intestinal calcium absorption and by stimulating bone resorption. $1,25(OH)_2D_3$ interacts with the vitamin D receptor on the osteoblasts, and via RANKL/RANK it stimulates the maturation of osteoclasts that function to dissolve bone, releasing calcium into the extracellular space. The recently discovered RANK ligand, a member of the tumor necrosis factor superfamily, and its two receptors (RANK and osteoprotegerin) are pivotal regulators of osteoclastic bone resorption, both *in vivo* and *in vitro*. More of the active metabolite is produced during calcium deficiency or after a low calcium intake in order to restore serum calcium by increasing intestinal calcium absorption, renal calcium reabsorption, and bone turnover.

Serum vitamin D concentrations decline in winter and are generally related to vitamin D intake and sunlight exposure. When serum $25(OH)D_3$ concentrations decline below 110 nmol/l, PTH levels increase, contributing to the bone loss that occurs in vitamin D deficiency and that is evident in northern Europe, the United States, Japan, and Canada during winter months. Rickets is becoming a more recognized health problem, particularly in infants of African American mothers who are not taking vitamin D supplements or consuming adequate amounts of vitamin D-fortified milk and who are exclusively breast-feeding their infants. In the US national nutrition survey conducted in the 1990s, 42% of African American women had low 25(OH) vitamin D concentrations in plasma. Thus, vitamin D deficiency is more prevalent than once believed, and it is particularly a risk for the elderly due to their reduced capacity for synthesizing vitamin D precursors in their skin, in those who are infirm and/or in nursing homes or living at more northern or southern latitudes, or in other situations in which the skin is not exposed to sunlight. The result of vitamin D deficiency is normal serum calcium and elevated PTH and alkaline phosphatase. The secondary hyperparathyroidism causes increased osteoclastic activity, calcium loss from bone, and ultimately bone loss.

Several other hormones also affect calcium metabolism. Notably, estrogens are necessary for the maintenance of balance between bone resorption and accretion. The decrease in serum estrogen concentrations at approximately the time of menopause is the primary factor contributing to the elevated rate of bone resorption that occurs at this stage of life and that is the primary contributory factor to osteoporosis. Estrogen treatment will reduce bone resorption within a few weeks and subsequently lead to higher serum concentrations of PTH and $1,25(OH)_2D_3$ and improved intestinal absorption and renal reabsorption of calcium. Testosterone also inhibits bone resorption, and lack of this hormone can cause osteoporosis in men. Glucocorticoids, sometimes used to treat conditions such as osteoid arthritis, inflammatory bowel disease, and asthma, inhibit both osteoclastic and osteoblastic activity, impair collagen and cartilage synthesis, and reduce calcium absorption. Consequently, excessive bone loss often results from glucocorticoid treatment or occurs when excessive amounts of the hormone are secreted, such as in Cushing's disease. Oral calcium supplements should be considered for patients receiving exogenous glucocorticoids. Thyroid hormones stimulate bone resorption so that bone abnormalities occur in both hyper- and hypothyroidism. Growth hormone stimulates cartilage formation, the formation of $1,25(OH)_2D$, and intestinal calcium absorption. Insulin stimulates collagen production by osteoblasts and impairs the renal reabsorption of calcium.

Excretion

Ionized calcium in the plasma is freely filtered by the kidney so that very large amounts enter the kidney each day, but 99.8% of this calcium is reabsorbed throughout the nephron. Regulated active transport occurs in the distal convoluted tubule and involves vitamin D, CaBP, and PTH. Typically, approximately 2.5–6 mmol (100–240 mg) of calcium is excreted in urine daily.

Dietary calcium has a relatively small impact on urinary calcium (e.g., only 6–8% of an increase in dietary calcium intake will appear in the urine). The major food components that affect urinary calcium are protein, phosphorus, caffeine, and sodium. For each 50-g increment in dietary protein, approximately 1.5 mmol (60 mg) of additional calcium is lost in urine. The higher amounts of phosphorus consumed concurrently with a high-protein diet can blunt, but not eliminate, this phenomenon. Dietary phosphorus (as well as intravenously administered phosphorus) increases PTH synthesis and subsequently stimulates renal calcium reabsorption and reduces the urinary excretion of calcium. Caffeine causes a reduction in renal reabsorption of calcium and a subsequently increased loss of urinary calcium soon after it is consumed. It has been shown repeatedly in animals and humans that dietary sodium, in the form of salt (NaCl), increases urinary calcium excretion. On average, for every 100 mmol (2300 mg) of sodium excreted in urine, there is an approximately 0.6–1 mmol (24–40 mg) loss of calcium in free-living healthy populations of various ages. Because most of the urinary calcium is of bone origin, it is commonly hypothesized that those nutrients or food components that are hypercalciuretic are also detrimental to the skeleton. On the other hand, thiazide medications are hypocalciuric and, as such, may have modest positive effects on bone.

Metabolic Functions

The most obvious role of calcium is to provide structural integrity and strength in bones and teeth. Approximately 99% of the total body calcium content is used for this purpose. Bone also serves as a reservoir of calcium that can be drawn upon when serum calcium concentrations decline. The remaining 1% of the body's calcium is contained in blood, extracellular space, muscle, and other tissues, in which calcium concentrations are kept relatively constant. The maintenance of constant serum calcium concentrations at approximately 2.5 mmol/l is critical for a number of cellular functions.

The extracellular concentration of calcium is in the 10^{-3} M range, whereas in the cytosol it is approximately 10^{-6} M. Almost all of the intracellular calcium is bound within organelles such as the nucleus, endoplasmic reticulum, and vesicles. Cytosolic calcium concentrations are very low and influenced greatly by release of some calcium from cellular organelles. Therefore, a small change in the release of calcium from intracellular sites or transport across the cell membrane results in a relatively large change in cytosolic calcium concentration. Binding of a hormone or a growth factor to a plasma membrane receptor increases inositol triphosphate release, which in turn increases the free intracellular calcium concentration. The ionized calcium then binds to calmodulin, followed by a conformation change in the protein to trigger cellular events such as muscle contraction, nerve conduction, cell movement and differentiation, cell division, cell-to-cell communication, and secretion of hormones such as insulin. In these roles, calcium acts as an intracellular messenger.

Calcium may play a role in energy regulation and risk of obesity. Dietary calcium regulation of circulating $1,25(OH)_2D_3$ in turn regulates the concentration of calcium in adipocytes. When adipocyte intracellular calcium concentration increases, this promotes the expression of lipogenic genes, and fat breakdown is reduced leading to accumulation of lipid in adipocytes. Through this pathway, low-calcium diets appear to promote fat deposition, whereas high-calcium intakes afford some protection from obesity.

Changes in Calcium Metabolism during the Life Span

The total body calcium content of the newborn infant is approximately 0.75 mol (30 g), which increases during growth to approximately 1000 g in adult women and 1200 g in adult men. This represents an average daily accumulation of approximately 2.5–3.7 mmol (100–150 mg) from infancy to adulthood.

The efficiency of calcium absorption is highest during infancy (approximately 60%), and the amount absorbed from breast milk does not appear to be affected by calcium consumed in solid foods. During the growth spurt of adolescence, calcium retention and accretion increase to peak at approximately 200–300 mg per day in girls and boys, respectively. It involves the action of growth hormone, IGF-1, and sex steroids. The onset of menstruation in girls is associated with a rapid decline in bone formation and resorption. Intestinal calcium absorption is predictably more efficient during the growth spurt and also decreases subsequently. Importantly, it is thought that calcium intakes during the period of growth can affect the peak bone mass achieved and therefore influence the amount of bone mineral remaining when osteoporosis begins in later life. Bone mass may continue to accumulate up to approximately age 30 years, although the amount gained is relatively small after age 18 years.

During pregnancy, a relatively small amount of calcium, approximately 625–750 mmol, is transported to the fetus. Most of this calcium is thought to be obtained through greater efficiency of maternal intestinal calcium absorption, possibly induced by increases in $1,25(OH)_2D_3$ production. For this reason, a higher calcium intake during pregnancy is probably not required.

Most studies have reported that there is no increase in intestinal calcium absorption during lactation even when dietary intake of the mineral is relatively low. Changes in biochemical markers and kinetic studies using isotopes indicate that the source of much of the calcium secreted in breast milk is the maternal skeleton, as well as more efficient renal reabsorption and subsequently lower urinary excretion of the mineral. Bone calcium is restored at the end of lactation as the infant is weaned, when ovarian function returns and menstruation resumes. At this time, intestinal calcium absorption increases, urinary calcium remains low, and bone turnover rates decline to normal levels. There is no strong evidence that lactation per se or maternal calcium intake during lactation affect later risk of osteoporosis in women. Thus, there is no strong rationale for increasing maternal calcium intake during lactation. Breast milk calcium concentration is relatively unaffected by maternal intake, and it remains stable throughout lactation.

Menopause begins a period of bone loss that extends until the end of life. It is the major contributor to higher rates of osteoporotic fractures in older women. The decrease in serum estrogen concentrations at menopause is associated with accelerated bone loss, especially from the spine, for the next 5 years, during which approximately 15% of skeletal calcium is lost. The calcium loss by women in early menopause cannot be prevented unless estrogen therapy is provided. Calcium supplements alone are not very helpful in preventing postmenopausal bone loss. Upon estrogen treatment, bone resorption is reduced and the intestinal calcium

absorption and renal reabsorption of calcium are both increased. Similarly, amenorrheic women have reduced intestinal calcium absorption, high urinary calcium excretion, and lower rates of bone formation (compared to eumenorrheic women). In both men and women, there is a substantial decline in intestinal absorption of calcium in later life.

Calcium Deficiency

When calcium absorption is chronically low, because of low intakes, poor bioavailability, or conditions that impair intestinal absorption, there is a decrease in the serum ionized calcium concentration. This in turn stimulates the release of PTH, which returns serum calcium to normal by increasing renal calcium reabsorption, stimulating the renal production of $1,25(OH)_2D_3$, and inducing bone reabsorption. The result of long-term calcium deficiency is accelerated bone loss in older individuals or the inability to fully achieve peak bone mass in younger individuals.

Dietary Sources

Food Sources

The majority of dietary calcium in industrialized countries comes from milk products; one serving (i.e., 250 ml milk or yogurt or 40 g cheese) contains approximately 7.5 mmol (300 mg). Nondairy sources (fruits, vegetables, and grain products) supply approximately 25% of total calcium. When substantial amounts of grains are consumed, for example, in breads or as maize products, these can be important sources, although the calcium in cereals tends to be less bioavailable than that in dairy products. Other foods high in calcium include tofu set with a calcium salt, kale, broccoli, and, increasingly, calcium-fortified juices and cereals. No matter what the source, a high percentage of people in both industrialized and less wealthy countries fail to meet recommended guidelines for optimal calcium intake.

Bioavailability

Several dietary constituents decrease the bioavailability of calcium in food. Increasing fiber intake by, for example, replacing white flour by whole wheat flour in a typical Western diet has long been associated with negative calcium balance even when calcium intakes meet recommended levels. Likewise, the fiber in fruits and vegetables can cause negative calcium balance. In cereals, phytic acid is the main constituent of fiber that binds calcium, making it unavailable for absorption. The fermentation of bread during leavening reduces phytate content substantially, making calcium more bioavailable. In fruits and vegetables, the uronic acids in hemicellulose are strong calcium binders, as is the oxalic acid present in high concentrations in foods such as spinach. Calcium bioavailability from beans is approximately half and that from spinach approximately one-tenth of the bioavailability from milk. In contrast, calcium absorption from low-oxalate vegetables, such as kale, broccoli, and collard greens, is as good as that from milk. The difference in calcium absorption between the various forms of supplements is not large.

Dietary fat does not affect calcium absorption except in individuals with diseases that impair fat malabsorption (e.g., short bowel syndrome, celiac disease, and pancreatitis). In these conditions, the calcium forms an insoluble and unabsorbable 'soap' with the unabsorbed fat in the alkaline lumen of the small intestine, potentially resulting in impaired bone mineralization. In addition, the luminal calcium is not available to precipitate the oxalates, meaning that the free oxalates will be hyperabsorbed leading to increased risk for renal oxalate stones. Neither dietary phosphorus nor a wide range of phosphorus-to-calcium ratios affect intestinal calcium absorption in very low-birth-weight infants and adults.

Lactose improves calcium absorption in young infants, in whom absorption of calcium is predominantly by passive transport. In adults, the presence of lactose in the diet has little effect on the efficiency of calcium absorption.

Effects of High Calcium Intakes

Calcium can inhibit the absorption of both heme iron (found in meat, fish, and poultry) and non-heme iron. The mechanism by which this occurs remains controversial, but the inhibition probably occurs within the mucosal cells rather than in the intestinal lumen. This interaction is of concern because calcium supplements are taken by many women who may have difficulty maintaining adequate iron stores. Approximately 300–600 mg of calcium, as a supplement or in foods, reduces the absorption of both heme and non-heme iron by approximately 30–50% when consumed in the same meal. The inhibitory effect on iron absorption is inversely related to iron status so that it is relatively unimportant above a serum ferritin concentration of approximately 50–60 μg/l. Thus, consideration should be given to monitoring the iron status of menstruating women with low iron stores who take calcium supplements. There is no inhibitory effect when calcium and iron supplements

are consumed together in the absence of food, and inhibition may be less with calcium citrate.

In the past, it was common to restrict dietary calcium in patients with a history of calcium oxalate stones. However, recent data suggest that a severe calcium restriction in patients with oxalate stones is not only ineffective but also can lead to bone demineralization. For the prevention of recurrent stone formation, a diet restricted in oxalate, sodium, and animal protein is probably most effective. Only if absorptive hypercalciuria is present should a moderate calcium restriction be imposed.

Long-term consumption of approximately 1500–2000 mg calcium per day is safe for most individuals, although there will be some reduction in the efficiency of iron absorption. However, higher intakes from supplements (62.5 mmol or 2.5 g per day) can result in milk–alkali syndrome (MAS), with symptoms of hypercalcemia, renal insufficiency, metabolic alkalosis, and severe alterations in metabolism. Based on risk of developing MAS, the upper limit for calcium intake is 2500 mg per day for adults and children.

See also: **Vitamin D**: Physiology, Dietary Sources and Requirements; Rickets and Osteomalacia.

Further Reading

Bronner F (1992) Symposium: Current concepts of calcium absorption. *Journal of Nutrition* 122: 641–686.

Heaney RP (2003) How does bone support calcium homeostasis? *Bone* 33: 264–268.

Institute of Medicine (1997) *Dietary Reference Intakes for Calcium, Phosphorus, Magnesium, Vitamin D and Fluoride.* Washington, DC: National Academy Press.

Prentice A (2000) Calcium in pregnancy and lactation. *Annual Reviews in Nutrition* 20: 249–272.

Prentice A (2004) Diet, nutrition and the prevention of osteoporosis. *Public Health Nutrition* 7: 227–243.

Specker BL (2004) Nutrition influences bone development from infancy through toddler years. *Journal of Nutrition* 134: 691S–695S.

Wasserman RH and Fullmer CS (1995) Vitamin D and intestinal calcium transport: Facts, speculations and hypotheses. *Journal of Nutrition* 125: 1971S–1979S.

Weaver CM and Heaney RP (1999) Calcium. In: Shils ME, Olson JA, Shike M *et al.* (eds.) *Modern Nutrition in Health and Disease.* Philadelphia: Lea & Febiger.

Zemel MB and Miller SL (2003) Dietary calcium and dairy modulation of adiposity and obesity risk. In *Primer on the Metabolic Bone Diseases and Disorders of Mineral Metabolism,* 5th edn. Washington, DC: American Society for Bone and Mineral Research.

CARBOHYDRATES

Contents

Requirements and Dietary Importance

C L Stylianopoulos, Johns Hopkins University, Baltimore, MD, USA

Introduction

Carbohydrates are an important energy source in the human diet. They generally supply about 45% of the energy requirement in developed countries and up to 85% in developing countries. Carbohydrates have been considered a fundamental source of nourishment and inexpensive and versatile staple of the diet.

The type and composition of dietary carbohydrates varies greatly among different food products. Dietary carbohydrates can be predominantly found in the form of sugar (monosaccharides and disaccharides) and starch or nonstarch polysaccharides. Furthermore, in the food industry they can be used in the form of hydrolyzed cornstarch, high-fructose corn syrups, modified starches, gums, mucilages, and sugar alcohols.

The current global emphasis for healthy eating focuses on increasing carbohydrate consumption, particularly in the form of whole grains, fruit, and vegetables. Epidemiological and clinical studies have shown a positive association between carbohydrate consumption and reduced risk of chronic disease and certain types of cancer.

Dietary Sources and Intakes

The major sources of carbohydrates are cereals, accounting for over 50% of carbohydrate consumed in both developed and developing countries, followed by sweeteners, root crops, pulses, vegetables, fruit, and milk products. Carbohydrate and nutrient intake in general can be estimated using data from food production and balance sheets, household surveys, and individual assessments (**Table 1**). **Figure 1** shows the trends in carbohydrate consumption by food group as a percentage of total carbohydrate in developed and developing countries, obtained from food balance data in 1994.

Sugars

The term 'sugar' includes monosaccharides and disaccharides. The most common monosaccharides are glucose (or dextrose), fructose, and galactose. Glucose is found in fruit, honey, maple syrup, and vegetables. Glucose is also formed from sucrose hydrolysis in honey, maple syrup and invert sugar, and from starch hydrolysis in corn syrups. The properties of glucose are important for improving food texture, flavor, and palatability. Glucose is the major cell fuel and the principal energy source for the brain. Fructose is found in honey, maple sugar, fruit, and vegetables. Fructose is also formed from sucrose hydrolysis in honey, maple syrup, and invert sugar. It is commonly used as a sweetener in soft drinks, bakery products, and candy in the form of high-fructose corn syrups. Galactose is found primarily in milk and dairy products.

Table 1 Approaches for determination of trends in nutrient consumption worldwide

Approach	Advantages	Disadvantages
Food production	Figures available for every crop	Affected by agricultural practices, weather conditions, external forces
Food balance sheets	Figures available for every food item	Inadequate to determine food waste and spoilage
Household surveys	Figures close to actual food consumption	Inadequate to determine food consumption outside the home, food waste, and spoilage
Individual assessments	Figures close to actual food consumption	Data not available for all countries Diverse methods of assessment

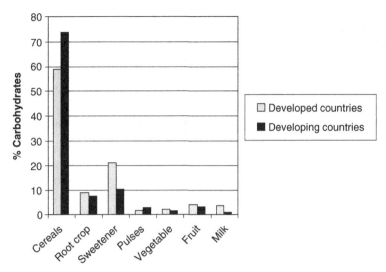

Figure 1 Trends in energy consumption by carbohydrate food group as a percentage of total carbohydrate in developed and developing countries, obtained from food balance data in 1994. Data obtained from FAO/WHO (1998). Carbohydrates in human nutrition. Report of a joint FAO/WHO expert consultation. *FAO Food and Nutrition Papers* 19 **66**: 1–140.

The most common disaccharides are sucrose, lactose, and maltose. Sucrose is mostly found in sugar cane and beet, and in lesser amounts in honey, maple sugar, fruit, and vegetables. The properties of sucrose are important in improving viscosity, sweetness, and flavor of baked foods, ice cream, and desserts. Maltose is formed from starch digestion. It is also produced from the germination of grain for malt liquors. Lactose is found in milk and dairy products, and is not as sweet as glucose or sucrose.

In the second part of the twentieth century, sugar intake increased markedly in the US, because of increased consumption of added sugars in beverages and foods. According to the US Food Supply Data, consumption of added sugars has increased from 27 teaspoons/person/day in 1970 to 32 teaspoons/person/day in 1996, which represents a 23% increase. Soft drinks are the most frequently used form of added sugars, and account for one-third of total sugar intake. In Europe the trend of sugar consumption has been a steady one.

Polysaccharides

Starch Starch is the most important and abundant food polysaccharide. Starch is predominantly derived from plant seed, such as wheat, maize, rice, oats, and rye, and from plant roots, such as potatoes. Legumes and vegetables also contribute to the starch content of the diet. Bread and pasta are popular forms of starch, while tropical starchy foods, such as plantains, cassava, sweet potatoes, and yams are increasingly contributing to carbohydrate intake. Starch accounts for 20–50% of total

energy intake, depending on the total carbohydrate consumption.

Nonstarch Nonstarch polysaccharides (NSP), formerly referred to as 'dietary fiber,' can either be soluble or insoluble and are mainly derived from cereals, especially wholegrain. Wheat, rice, and maize contain predominantly insoluble NSP, while oats, rye, and barley contain predominantly soluble NSP. Vegetables are also a source of NSP and contain equal amounts of insoluble and soluble NSP. Intakes of NSP range from about $19\,\mathrm{g\,day^{-1}}$ in Europe and North American countries to $30\,\mathrm{g\,day^{-1}}$ in rural Africa.

Health Effects of Carbohydrates

Carbohydrates are stored in the human body as glycogen mainly in the liver and muscle. The human body has a limited storage capacity for carbohydrates compared to fat. The total amount of carbohydrates stored in tissues and circulating in the blood as glucose is approximately $7.56\,\mathrm{MJ}$ (1800 kcal). Diets high in carbohydrate ensure adequate glycogen storage available for immediate energy utilization. Carbohydrates are the preferred energy source for the human brain and have an important role in reducing protein breakdown when energy intake is inadequate.

Dietary carbohydrates are absorbed in their hexose form (glucose, fructose, galactose) and provide $15.6\,\mathrm{kJ\,g^{-1}}$ ($3.75\,\mathrm{kcal\,g^{-1}}$) of energy. Although sugars and polysaccharides provide similar amounts of energy, they differ in their physiological and metabolic properties. The effects of carbohydrate-containing foods on blood glucose levels during digestion and absorption are variable, depending on the type of dietary carbohydrate. Postprandial glucose response is reduced when glucose absorption is slow. Glycemic index (GI) is used for the quantification of blood glucose response after carbohydrate consumption. GI is the area under the curve of the blood glucose increase 2 h after carbohydrate ingestion of a set amount of a particular food (e.g., 50 g) compared to the blood glucose increase 2 h after ingestion of the same amount of a reference food (white bread or glucose). GI is influenced significantly by the carbohydrate types and physical determinants of digestion rate (intact versus ground grains, cooked versus uncooked food, and soluble fiber content). Carbohydrate ingestion in the presence of fat and protein reduces the GI of a meal. The GI of carbohydrate-containing meals has been linked to several health outcomes. The role of carbohydrates in health is a growing area of research and has received a great amount of interest in the past decade.

Carbohydrates and Nutrient Density

Increased sugar consumption has generated concern in recent years because of the potential to displace the micronutrient content of the diet by increasing 'empty calories' and energy intake. There is some evidence that essential nutrient intake decreases with increasing total sugar intake. However, sugar intake has not been shown to accurately predict micronutrient ingestion. Moderate intakes of sugar coincide with sufficient nutrient intake. The risk of low micronutrient status is increased for individuals with a diet high in sugars and low in total energy intake, as in the case of children or people on restrictive diets. Data analysis on food intake of preschool children suggests that the intake of some micronutrients (calcium, zinc, thiamin, riboflavin, and niacin) is inversely related to sugar intake. However, the dilutional effects of sugars may be somewhat distorted by the fact that some rich sources of added sugars are also fortified with micronutrients, as in the case of breakfast cereals. The Dietary Reference Intake (DRI) Panel on Macronutrients, using national food intake data, reported that a clear dilutional effect on micronutrient intake starts when sugar intake approaches 25% of total calories. The American Heart Association dietary guidelines stress the consumption of fruit, vegetables, grains, and complex carbohydrates so that micronutrient requirements are met by whole rather than supplemented foods.

Several human studies have demonstrated that diets rich in NSP may reduce the bioavailability of minerals, such as iron, calcium, and zinc. Nevertheless, this effect is more likely due to the presence of phytate, which inhibits the absorption of those minerals, than the NSP content of the diet.

Carbohydrates and Obesity

Several studies have been conducted to establish an association between sugar ingestion and total energy intake. There have been consistent reports of a negative association between sugar intake and body mass index in adults and children. However, this observation could be confounded by the correlation of dietary fat and obesity, since high-fat diets are usually low in carbohydrates. Some ad libitum dietary studies have shown that diets low in sugar are associated with weight loss, maybe as a result of reduced calorie intake. Nevertheless, in human metabolic studies, no effect on weight or energy expenditure was observed when carbohydrate was replaced by fat or protein in isocaloric diets.

Foods high in sugars or GI are highly palatable and it has been suggested that they create a potential risk for energy overconsumption and weight gain. However, there is no evidence to support this claim or confirm the role of GI in body weight regulation. Foods high in sugar have high energy density and thus decreasing their consumption can assist in weight reduction. On the contrary, foods rich in NSP are bulky and have less energy density and as a result induce greater satiety when ingested. It follows that diets rich in NSP may be useful for obesity prevention, since they prevent energy overconsumption. However, there is no evidence to indicate that increasing the carbohydrate content of a low-energy diet facilitates weight loss.

The consumption of sugar-sweetened soft drinks may contribute to weight gain because of the low satiety of liquid foods. Short-term human studies have shown that sugar-sweetened soft drink consumption does not result in a decrease of total energy intake. Thus, sugar-sweetened soft drinks can significantly increase the total caloric intake and result in weight gain. Consumption of these drinks has been associated with childhood obesity.

Carbohydrate and Cardiovascular Disease

Dietary factors influence the risk factors, such as obesity, diabetes, and hyperlipidemia, that lead to the development of cardiovascular disease (CVD). A diet rich in carbohydrates in the form of whole grain cereals, fruit, and vegetables may assist in the reduction of saturated fat and may increase the antioxidant content of the diet, thus reducing the risk of heart disease. On the contrary, a high intake of carbohydrates (>65% of total calories), especially in the form of refined sugars and starch, may increase serum triacylglycerol levels and adversely affect plasma lipoprotein profile. Short-term studies show a consistent relationship between sugar consumption and elevation of triacylglycerol levels as well as a decrease in plasma high-density lipoprotein (HDL) levels, which could result in increased atherosclerosis and heart disease risk. However, longitudinal cohort studies have failed to show a consistent association of sugar consumption with CVD, mainly because of the confounding factors associated with increased heart disease risk.

Certain NSP (for example β glycans) have been shown to reduce low-density lipoprotein (LDL) and total cholesterol levels on a short-term basis. Therefore, a protective effect for CVD has been shown with consumption of foods high in NSP. This protective effect has not been duplicated with NSP supplements. Furthermore, no long-term effect has been established.

High-GI diets have been shown to slightly increase hemoglobin A1c, total serum cholesterol and triacylglycerols, and decrease HDL cholesterol and urinary C-peptide in diabetic and hyperlipidemic individuals. In addition, low-GI diets have been shown to decrease cholesterol and triacylglycerol levels in dyslipidemic individuals. There are insufficient studies performed on healthy individuals and further research on the role of GI in lipid profile and CVD risk factors is warranted.

Carbohydrates and Type 2 Diabetes

There is little evidence from prospective studies to support a positive association between total dietary carbohydrate consumption and risk of type 2 diabetes. Some recent evidence suggests that rapidly digested refined sugars, which have a high GI, may increase the risk of type 2 diabetes. Short-term studies have shown that decreasing the GI of a meal can improve glucose tolerance and insulin sensitivity in healthy people. Furthermore, the substitution of high-GI with low-GI carbohydrates can decrease postprandial glucose and insulin levels. Some epidemiological studies have demonstrated a protective effect of NSP consumption against type 2 diabetes.

Carbohydrates and Dental Caries

The quantity and frequency of sugars in the diet play a significant role in the development of dental caries. Their digestion by salivary amylase provides an acid environment for the growth of bacteria in the mouth, thus increasing the rate of plaque formation. Sucrose is the most cariogenic of the sugars, followed by glucose, fructose, and maltose. The milk sugars (lactose and galactose) are considerably less cariogenic. There is no epidemiological evidence to support a cariogenic role of polysaccharide foods with no added sugars.

Dental caries is a multifaceted disease, affected not only by the frequency and type of sugar consumed, but also by oral hygiene and fluoride supplementation and use. Despite the increase in sugar consumption, the incidence of dental caries has decreased worldwide because of the increased use of fluoride and improvement in oral hygiene.

Carbohydrate and Cancer

Case-control studies have shown that colorectal cancer risk increases with high intakes of sugar-rich foods, while other studies have failed to prove such a relationship. Thus, there is insufficient evidence to support the role of sugar in the risk for colorectal cancer. On the contrary, carbohydrate consumption in the form of fruit, vegetables, and cereals has been shown to be protective against colorectal cancer.

Carbohydrate foods are a good source of phytoestrogens, which may protect against breast cancer. However, studies related to carbohydrate intake and breast cancer have been inconsistent and are insufficient to establish an association between carbohydrates and breast cancer risk.

The Health Professionals Follow-up Study showed a negative association of prostate cancer risk with high fructose intake. Additional data on the role of sugar consumption on prostate cancer risk is lacking. Some evidence suggests that increased fiber intakes are related to decreased prostate cancer risk.

Carbohydrates and Gastrointestinal Health

High intakes of NSP, in the range of 4–32 g day^{-1}, have been shown to contribute to the prevention and treatment of constipation. Population studies have linked the prevalence of hemorrhoids, diverticular disease, and appendicitis to NSP intakes, although there are several dietary and lifestyle confounding factors that could directly affect these relationships. High-carbohydrate diets may be related to bacterial growth in the gut and subsequent reduction of acute infective gastrointestinal disease risk.

Low-Carbohydrate Diets

The recent trend of weight loss diets promotes some level of carbohydrate restriction and increased protein consumption. Some examples are Dr Atkins

New Diet Revolution, The South Beach Diet, and The Carbohydrate Addict's Diet. This dietary advice is contrary to that proposed by governmental agencies (US Department of Agriculture/Department of Health Services, National Institutes of Health) and nongovernmental organizations (American Dietetic Association, American Heart Association, American Diabetes Association, and American Cancer Society).

There is consistent evidence that weight loss in low-carbohydrate diets is triggered by negative energy balance resulting from low caloric intake, and that it is not a function of macronutrient composition. There is no scientific evidence to suggest that low-carbohydrate diets are more metabolically efficient than restricted calorie conventional diets. Several studies have shown that low-carbohydrate diets result in weight loss because of reduced caloric intake.

Low-carbohydrate diets promote the lipolysis of stored triacylglycerols known as ketosis, reduce glucose and insulin levels, and suppress appetite. As a result, there is an increase in blood uric acid concentration. Some studies have shown that the consumption of high amounts of nondairy protein results in a decline in kidney functions in individuals with mildly compromised kidney function. However, no such effect has been shown in individuals with normal kidney functions. Furthermore, low-carbohydrate diets can have side effects such as bad taste, constipation, diarrhea, dizziness, headache, nausea, thirst, and fatigue.

Low-carbohydrate diets lack essential vitamins and minerals because of inadequate consumption of fruit, vegetables, and grains, and require supplementation to achieve nutritional adequacy. Controlled trials of low-carbohydrate diets are necessary to establish long-term effectiveness and adverse health effects or benefits.

Requirements and Recommendations

According to the new definition of the expert panel appointed by the Institute of Medicine of the National Academies of Science (IOM), dietary reference intakes (DRIs) are defined as a set of reference values for nutrient intake, and include the estimated average requirement (EAR), recommended dietary allowance (RDA), adequate intake (AI), and tolerable upper intake level (UL). EAR refers to the average daily intake value of a nutrient that is estimated to fulfill the needs of healthy people in a particular lifestage or group. RDA refers to the minimum daily intake that fulfills the need of almost all healthy people in a particular lifestage or group. AI refers to the observed intake of a particular group of healthy people, and is used when there is lack of scientific experimentation for the determination of the EAR or the RDA. UL refers to the maximum daily intake level of a nutrient that is not likely to pose an adverse health effect for almost all people.

The DRIs for carbohydrate consumption of individual groups and lifestages are outlined in **Table 2**. These values are based on the average minimum amount of glucose needed for brain function. A UL for carbohydrates was not set because no studies have shown that excessive consumption of carbohydrates has a detrimental effect on health. Based on the dilutional effect of added sugars on micronutrients, the expert panel suggests a maximal intake of less than 25% of energy from added sugars. Total sugar intake can be decreased by limiting foods high in added sugars and consuming naturally occurring sugar products, like milk, dairy products, and fruit.

The IOM does not specify dietary requirements or recommendations for NSP consumption, but has provided recommended intakes for fiber, which includes NSP. The DRIs for total fiber consumption of individual groups and lifestages are outlined in

Table 2 Carbohydrate requirements and recommendations (DRIs)

Age group/Life stage	EAR (g day^{-1})		RDA (g day^{-1})		AI (g day^{-1})
	Males	Females	Males	Females	
Infants (0–6 months)					60
Infants (6–12 months)					95
Children (1–18 years)	100	100	130	130	
Adults (>18 years)	100	100	130	130	
Pregnancy		135		175	
Lactation		160		210	

DRIs, dietary reference intakes; EAR, estimated average requirement; RDA, recommended dietary allowance; AI, adequate intake.-
Data from Institute of Medicine of the National Academies (2002) *Dietary Reference Intakes for Energy, Carbohydrate, Fiber, Fat, Fatty Acids, Cholesterol, Protein, Amino Acids.* Washington, DC: The National Academies Press.

Table 3 Total fiber recommendations (DRIs)

Age group/Lifestage	AI (g day^{-1})	
	Males	Females
Children (1–3 years)	19	19
Children (4–8 years)	25	25
Children (9–13 years)	31	26
Children (14–18 years)	38	26
Adults (19–50 years)	38	25
Adults (>51 years)	30	21
Pregnancy		28
Lactation		29

DRIs, dietary reference intakes; AI, adequate intake.Data from Institute of Medicine of the National Academies (2001) *Dietary Reference Intakes for Energy, Carbohydrate, Fiber, Fat, Fatty Acids, Cholesterol, Protein, Amino Acids*. Washington, DC: The National Academies Press.

Table 3. It has not been shown that a high fiber intake has a harmful effect in healthy individuals. Therefore, a UL for fiber has not been set.

There is insufficient evidence to support a recommendation by the IOM for the consumption of low-GI foods or the replacement of high-GI foods, like bread and potatoes. Although several studies propose adverse effects of high-GI carbohydrates and beneficial effects of low-GI foods, a recommendation on consumption of low-GI foods is a major dietary change that requires substantial scientific evidence. Therefore, a UL based on GI is not set.

The 1998 report of the Food and Agriculture Organization (FAO) and the World Health Organization (WHO) regarding the role of carbohydrates in human nutrition recommends the consumption of at least 55% of total energy in the form of carbohydrates from a variety of sources. The committee proposes that the majority of carbohydrates consumed should originate from NSP, principally from cereals, vegetables, legumes, and fruit. Furthermore, it suggests that free sugars should be restricted to less than 10% of total energy. This report recognizes that there is no direct causal link between sugar consumption and chronic disease. However, sugars significantly increase the energy density of the human diet and high-sugar drinks have been associated with childhood obesity.

A 2002 report of the American Heart Association suggests the restriction of sugar consumption. This report recognizes that there are no beneficial effects of increased sugar consumption. On the contrary, some studies suggest that it may have adverse health effects. In order to enhance the nutrient density and reduce the energy density of the diet, increased consumption of high-sugar foods should be avoided.

See also: **Carbohydrates**: Resistant Starch and Oligosaccharides. **Dietary Fiber**: Role in Nutritional Management of Disease.

Further Reading

Anderson GH and Woodend D (2003) Consumption of sugars and the regulation of short-term satiety and food intake. *American Journal of Clinical Nutrition* 78(supplement): 843S–849S.

Brody T (1999) *Nutritional Biochemistry*, 2nd edn, pp. 57–192 and 457–475. San Diego: Academic Press.

Eastwood M (2003) *Principles of Human Nutrition*, 2nd edn pp. 195–212, 418–426 and 456–509. Oxford: Blackwell.

FAO/WHO (1998) Carbohydrates in human nutrition. Report of a joint FAO/WHO expert consultation. *FAO Food and Nutrition Papers 19* **66**: 1–140.

Groff JL and Gropper SS (2000) *Advanced Nutrition and Human Metabolism*, 3rd edn, pp. 70–115. ch. 4. Belmont: Wadsworth.

Howard BV and Wylie-Rosett J (2002) Sugar and cardiovascular disease. A statement for healthcare professionals from the Committee on Nutrition of the Council on Nutrition, Physical Activity, and Metabolism of the American Heath Association. *Circulation* **106**: 523–527.

Institute of Medicine of the National Academies (2002) *Dietary Reference Intakes for Energy, Carbohydrate, Fiber, Fat, Fatty Acids, Cholesterol, Protein, Amino Acids*. Washington, DC: The National Academies Press.

James WPT (2001) European diet and public health: the continuing challenge. *Public Health and Nutrition* **4**: 275–292.

Johnson RK and Frary C (2001) Choose beverages and foods to moderate your intake of sugars: the 200 dietary guidelines for Americans – what's all the fuss about? *Journal of Nutrition* **131**: 2766S–2771S.

Levin RJ (1999) Carbohydrates. In: Shils ME, Olson JA, Shike M, and Ross AC (eds.) *Modern Nutrition in Health and Disease*, 9th edn, pp. 49–65 ch. 3. Media: Lippincott Williams & Wilkins.

Ruxton CHS, Garceau FJS, and Cottrell RC (1999) Guidelines for sugar consumption in Europe: is a quantitative approach justified? *European Journal of Clinical Nutrition* **53**: 503–513.

Saris WHM (2003) Sugars, energy metabolism, and body weight control. *American Journal of Clinical Nutrition* 78(supplement): 850S–857S.

Schlenker ED (2003) Carbohydrates. In: Williams SR and Schlenker ED (eds.) *Essentials of Nutrition and Diet Therapy*, 8th edn, pp. 47–65. St. Louis: Mosby.

Schlenker ED (2003) Digestion, Absorption, and Metabolism. In: Williams SR and Schlenker ED (eds.) *Essentials of Nutrition and Diet Therapy*, 8th edn, pp. 23–45. St. Louis: Mosby.

Touger-Decker R and van Loveren C (2003) Sugars and dental caries. *American Journal of Clinical Nutrition* 78(supplement): 881S–92S.

Relevant Websites

http://www.usda.gov – US Department of Agriculture and US Department of Health and Human Services (2000) Nutrition and your health: dietary guidelines for Americans, 5th edn.

Resistant Starch and Oligosaccharides

A Laurentin, Universidad Central de Venezuela, Caracas, Venezuela
C A Edwards, University of Glasgow, Glasgow, UK

Introduction

In recent years, there has been increasing interest in those carbohydrates that escape absorption in the small intestine and enter the colon, where they may have specific health benefits due to their fermentation by the colonic microflora and their effect on gut physiology. This entry considers the definition, classification, dietary sources, methods of analysis, colonic fermentation, and health benefits of both resistant starch and oligosaccharides, and compares them with those of dietary fiber.

Resistant Starch

Definition

In 1992, a concerted action of European researchers defined resistant starch as "the sum of starch and the products of starch degradation not absorbed in the small intestine of healthy individuals." This concept completely changed our understanding of the action of carbohydrates in the diet because up until the early 1980s, it was thought that starches were completely digested and absorbed in the human small intestine. Three important considerations are attached to this physiological definition. First, resistant starch is made up not only of high-molecular weight polymers but also can include dextrins, small oligosaccharides, and even glucose, all derived from digested starch that escapes absorption. Second, resistant starches reach the human large intestine where they are metabolized by the complex colonic microflora. Finally, the actual amount of resistant starch in a food (i.e., the amount reaching the colon) depends on the physiology of the individual and it may be affected by age.

Classification and Dietary Sources

Food starches can be classified according to the way they are metabolized by the human small intestine into those that are rapidly digested, those that are slowly digested, and those that are resistant to digestion. Similarly, resistant starch has been classified into three types: physically inaccessible starch, resistant starch granules, and retrograded starch (**Table 1**).

Table 1 Classification of resistant starch

Food source	Type[a]	Content in food (g per 100 g)	Contribution to total RS intake
Cereal products containing whole grains or grain fragments	RS$_1$	1–9	Minor
Brown breads			
Legumes			
Pastas			
Unripe bananas	RS$_2$	17–75	Very little
Uncooked potatoes			
High amylose starches			
Bread	RS$_3$	1–10	Major
Cornflakes			
Cooked cooled potatoes			
Legumes			
Amylose–lipid complex	Others	Not known	Unknown
Modified starches			

[a]RS$_1$, physically inaccessible starch; RS$_2$, resistant granules; RS$_3$, retrograded starch.

Physically inaccessible starch (RS$_1$) Type I resistant starch is physically inaccessible and is protected from the action of α-amylase, the enzyme that hydrolyzes the breakdown of starch in the human small intestine. This inaccessibility is due to the presence of plant cell walls that entrap the starch, for example, in legume seeds and partially milled and whole grains. RS$_1$ can also be found in highly compact processed food like pasta. The RS$_1$ content is affected by disruption of the food structure during processing (e.g., milling) and, to some extent, by chewing.

Resistant granules (RS$_2$) Starch granules are plant organelles where starch is produced and stored. Each plant has characteristic starch granules that differ in size, shape, amylose to amylopectin ratio, crystalline to amorphous material ratio, starch supramolecular architecture, and amylose–lipid complexes, amongst other features. It is believed that combinations of these factors make some granules more resistant to the attack of digestive enzymes than other granules. Type II resistant starch is found in unripe bananas, uncooked potatoes, and high amylose starches. RS$_2$ disappears during cooking, especially in water, because a combination of water and heat make the starch gelatinize, giving more access to amylases.

Table 2 Classification of modified starches

Starch	Modifying agent	Physicochemical characteristic	Use in food
Pregelatinized	Extrusion Drum drying	Soluble in cold water	Cake and instant products
Derivatized	Acetyl Hydroxypropyl Phosphate	Stable at freeze-thawing cycles	Canned and frozen food
Cross-linked	Epiclorhydrine Trimetaphosphate	Stable at higher temperatures, extreme pH, and higher shear forces	Meat sauce thickeners Instant soup Weaning infant food Dressings
Dextrinized	Acid hydrolysis Oxidizing agents Irradiation Heat (pyrodextrins) Amylolytic enzymes	Soluble in cold water Lower or nil viscosity	Chewing gums Jelly Syrups

Retrograded starch (RS$_3$) Type III resistant starch is the most abundant of the resistant starches present in food. It is formed during usual food processing by cooking and then cooling. When starch is cooked in an excess of water, it gelatinizes, i.e., the granular structure is disrupted, the granule swells, and amylose leaks out of the amylopectin matrix. Then, when the food is cooled down, amylose (and more slowly amylopectin) recrystallizes to a new ordered and more compact structure (process known as retrogradation), which decreases access for digestive enzymes. RS$_3$ production can be affected by the amylose to amylopectin ratio, amount of water, and temperature during cooking, and the number of repeated cooking and cooling cycles. Retrograded starch can be found in bread, some brands of corn flakes, cooked-cooled potatoes, and legumes.

Others sources of resistant starch In recent years, amylose–lipid complex and modified starches have also been recognized as other sources of resistant starches (Table 1). Amylose–lipid complexes occur when fatty acids (12–18 carbons) are held within the helical structure of amylose. They are formed naturally during starch biosynthesis, but may also be produced during cooking. Lipids may interfere with amylose retrogradation, impairing the production of retrograded starch during processing. However, these complexes themselves have lower digestibility than cooked starch.

As well as naturally resistant starch complexes, there are different types of modified starches that are manufactured by the food industry for a variety of reasons. They can be defined as native starches that have been submitted to one or more physical, chemical, or enzymatic treatments promoting granular disorganization, polymer degradation, molecular rearrangements, oxidation, or chemical group

addition. Modified starches can be classified into four main categories accordingly to their main physicochemical characteristic: pregelatinized, derivatized, cross-linked, and dextrinized starches (Table 2). However, they usually are known as physically, chemically, or enzymatically modified starch because of the way they are produced (Table 3). The digestibility of these modified starches is variable and depends on the type and extent of the treatment. Some authors have proposed a new category, type IV resistant starch, to include chemically modified starches. Indeed, it has

Table 3 Methods of modified starch production

Treatment	Modification	Description
Physically modified	Pregelatinization	Starch paste is precooked and dried by extrusion or drum drying
	Dextrinization	Starch polymers are hydrolyzed to smaller molecules by irradiation
Chemically modified	Derivatization[a]	Lateral groups are added to starch lateral chains
	Cross-linking[a]	Multifunctional groups are used to link two different starch molecules together
	Dextrinization	Starch polymers are hydrolyzed by oxidizing agents, acid hydrolysis, pyrodextrinization
Enzymatically modified	Dextrinization	Starch polymers are hydrolyzed to smaller molecules by incubation with amylases

[a]Double-derived starches are produced by combination of these two processes.

been shown that cross-linked starches have a 15–19% decrease in *in vitro* digestibility when compared with their native starches, and hydroxypropylated starch is only 50% digestible. However, pregelatinized starches produced by drum drying and extrusion have a 3–6% and 5–11% decrease in digestibility, respectively. Part but not all of this reduction in digestibility is due to the formation of retrograded starch; therefore, physically modified starches should also be considered as a category of resistant starch.

In addition to the starch properties already described, several starchy foods (for instance, cereals and legumes) have antinutritional factors, such as lectins, tannins, phytates, and enzyme inhibitors (both protease and amylase inhibitors). Amylase inhibitors present in raw pulses may reduce the activity of amylase in the human small intestine. However, most of these factors, especially enzyme inhibitors, are inactivated during food processing and cooking.

Analysis

The definition of resistant starch is based on its physiological behavior in the human small intestine, i.e., resistant starch is a heterogeneous group of molecules from small monosaccharides to large polymers with different molecular weight, degree of polymerization, and supramolecular architecture. This complexity makes it difficult to quantify accurately. All *in vitro* methods therefore need to be corroborated against *in vivo* models; however, *in vivo* models are also very difficult to validate.

In general, *in vitro* methods try to imitate human small intestine digestion using different sample preparation (i.e., milling, chewing, etc.), sample pretreatment (i.e., simulation of oral or stomach digestion), sample treatment (i.e., different enzymes mixtures), sample post-treatment (i.e., different resistant starch solubilizing agents and enzyme mixtures), and incubation conditions (i.e., shaking/stirring, pH, temperature, time) (**Table 4**). The choice of each of these multiple factors represents a huge analytical problem because not only a compromise between physiological conditions and analytical handling has to be achieved, but also because the resistant starch content values must be in agreement with *in vivo* data.

On the other hand, in human *in vivo* methods, samples of digested food that reach the end of the small intestine are taken for analysis, either from ileostomy patients (i.e., where the large intestine has been removed) or from healthy volunteers using special cannulas in the ileum. Animals can also be employed for *in vivo* experiments, such as gnotobiotic (i.e., germ-free) and pseudognotobiotic (i.e., antibiotic treated) rats. In these cases, colonic bacterial

fermentation is absent or suppressed by antibiotics and it is assumed that what reaches the end of the small intestine appears in feces. The main difficulty with these methods is that *in vivo* starch digestion may occur during the whole transit through the small intestine, which varies between individuals and the type of meal consumed. Moreover, these studies are difficult to perform in healthy volunteers and the physiological significance of using ileostomy patients is debatable, for example, it may not relate to infants and children who have decreased digestive capacity.

The initial *in vitro* assays were adapted from the enzymatic-gravimetric method used for dietary fiber assessment, but could only measure RS_3. Soon new approaches to assess other types of resistant starch were developed. The Berry method, for instance, measures both RS_3 and RS_2 using an exhaustive incubation (16 h) of milled sample with α-amylase and pullulanase, following by centrifugation to separate the insoluble residue, which contains the resistant starch. This residue is treated with KOH to disperse retrograded and native starches, which are then hydrolyzed to glucose with amyloglucosidase. Finally, released glucose is quantified by a colorimetric assay. The Berry method has been subsequently modified by Faisant *et al.* and Goñi *et al.*: the pullulanase was eliminated from the enzyme mixture and a pretreatment with pepsin added to decrease starch-protein interactions (**Table 4**).

Other methods have been developed to assess all types of resistant starch. Indeed, the Englyst method was developed to assess all nutritionally important starch fractions, such as rapidly digestible and slowly digestible starches, along with the three types of resistant starches described above. In this method, resistant starch fractions are estimated altogether by difference between total and digestible starches. Sample preparation is kept to a minimum in an attempt to mimic the way food is consumed. After pretreatment with pepsin, the sample is incubated with a mixture of amyloglucosidase, invertase, and pancreatic enzymes for 2 h. Glucose released is then used to estimate the digestible starch. Next, total starch is measured as glucose released after solubilization of the nondigestible fractions with KOH, followed by amyloglucosidase hydrolysis. The Englyst method also allows evaluation of RS_1, RS_2, and RS_3. The main problem with this method is its low reproducibility, especially between laboratories, because of the technical difficulties involved. Two other methods include chewing by volunteer subjects as sample preparation. In the Muir method, for instance, the chewed sample is sequentially treated with pepsin and an amyloglucosidase–pancreatic amylase mixture to obtain the nondigestible fraction, which is then boiled with Termamyl (a thermostable

Table 4 Comparison between different methods to measure resistant starch *in vitro*

Method	Sample		Pretreatment	Treatment	Post-treatment	Treatment incubation	Types of RS measured[a]
	Preparation						
Berry (1986)	Milling		None	Pancreatic α-amylase and pullulanase	KOH[b] Amyloglucosidase	Shaking for 16 h at 37°C, pH 5.2	Sum of RS$_2$ and RS$_3$
Faisant *et al.* (1995)	Same as above		Same as above	Same as above, but without pullulanase	Same as above	Same as above, but pH 6.9	Same as above
Goñi *et al.* (1996)	Same as above		Pepsin	Same as above	Same as above	Same as above	Same as above
Englyst *et al.* (1992)	Minced or as eaten		Pepsin	Pancreatic α-amylase, amyloglucosidase, and invertase	Same as above	Shaking for 2 h at 37°C, pH 5.2	RS$_1$, RS$_2$, RS$_3$, and total RS
Muir & O'Dea (1992)	Chewing		Salivary α-amylase then pepsin	Pancreatic α-amylase and amyloglucosidase	Thermostable α-amylase Dimethyl sulfoxide[b] Amyloglucosidase and pancreatic α-amylase	Stirring for 15 h at 37°C, pH 5.0	Total RS
Akerberg *et al.* (1998)	Same as above		Same as above	Same as above	KOH[b] Thermostable α-amylase Amyloglucosidase	Stirring for 16 h at 40°C, pH 5.0	Same as above
McCleary & Monaghan (2002)	Milling		None	Same as above	KOH[b] Amyloglucosidase	Shaking for 16 h at 37°C, pH 6.0	Sum of RS$_2$ and RS$_3$

[a]RS, resistant starch; RS$_1$, physically inaccessible starch; RS$_2$, resistant granules; RS$_3$, retrograded starch.
[b]KOH and dimethyl sulfoxide are used as resistant starch solubilizing agents.

α-amylase) and solubilized with dimethyl sulfoxide followed by another amyloglucosidase–pancreatic amylase mixture step to yield finally glucose. The Akerberg method is similar to the Muir method, but it includes other steps that permit the estimation of available starch and dietary fiber along with resistant starch (**Table 4**).

Recently, the most commonly used *in vitro* methods were extensively evaluated and a simplified version was proposed (McCleary method). Here, samples are treated with an amyloglucosidase–pancreatic amylase mixture only and the insoluble residue, after washing with ethanol, is dispersed with KOH, followed by the amyloglucosidase step to yield glucose. This protocol has been accepted by AOAC International (AOAC method 2002.02) and the American Association of Cereal Chemists (AACC method 32-40) (**Table 4**).

Regarding the quantification of the resistant fractions in modified starches, care must be taken because some nondigestible fractions are soluble in water and they can be lost during washing steps. This is particularly important with pregelatinized starches and pyrodextrins. One suitable way to look at the impact of the modification on the starch availability is measure total starch before and after the modification.

Dietary Intake

It is very difficult to assess resistant starch intake at present, because there are not enough data on the resistant starch content of foods. In addition, as the resistance of the starch to digestion depends on the method of cooking and the temperature of the food as eaten, the values gained from looking at old dietary intake data may be misleading. Despite this, an average value for resistant starch intake across Europe has been estimated as $4.1\,g\,day^{-1}$. Figures comparable with this estimation have been made in other countries, for instance, Venezuela ($4.3\,g\,day^{-1}$). It is very difficult to separate the benefits of slowly, but completely, digestible starches from those that are resistant. In some groups like small children, whose small intestinal digestive capacity is reduced, the very same food may provide more starch that is resistant to digestion than it would in normal adults.

Quantification of modified starch intake is even more difficult. First, food labels do not usually provide information about the nature of the modification used. Second, the commonly used method to estimate resistant starch can underestimate any nondigestible fractions that became soluble in water because of the modification. At present, there is no data available on how much modified starch is eaten.

Fermentation in the Colon

The main nutritional properties of resistant starch arise from its potential fermentation in the colon. The diverse and numerous colonic microflora ferments unabsorbed carbohydrates to short-chain fatty acids (SCFA), mainly acetate, propionate and butyrate, and gases (H_2, CO_2, and CH_4). Acetate is the main SCFA produced (50–70%) and is the only one to reach peripheral circulation in significant amounts, providing energy for muscle and other tissues. Propionate is the second most abundant SCFA and is mainly metabolized by the liver, where its carbons are used to produce glucose (via gluconeogenesis). Propionate has also been associated with reduced cholesterol and lipid synthesis. Finally, butyrate is mainly used as fuel by the colonic enterocytes, but has been shown *in vitro* to have many potential anticancer actions, such as stimulating apoptosis (i.e., programed cell death) and cancer cell differentiation (i.e., increasing expression of normal cell function), and inhibiting histone deacetylation (this protects the DNA). Resistant starch fermentation has been shown to increase the molar proportion of butyrate in the colon.

The main physiological effects of digestion and fermentation of resistant starch are summarized in **Table 5**. However, most of these effects have been observed with a resistant starch intake of around $20-30\,g\,day^{-1}$, which represents from 5 to 7 times the estimated intake for the European population.

Oligosaccharides

Definition and Classification

Oligosaccharides are carbohydrate chains containing 3–10 sugar units. However, some authors also include carbohydrates with up to 20 residues or even disaccharides. Oligosaccharides can be made of any sugar monomers, but most research has been carried out on fructooligosaccharides (e.g., oligofructose) and galactooligosaccharides (e.g., raffinose, human milk oligosaccharides). Few oligosaccharides are hydrolyzed and absorbed in the small intestine (e.g., maltotriose), but nearly all enter the colon intact (nondigestible oligosaccharides). **Table 6** shows several examples of oligosaccharides (and disaccharides, for comparison purposes), their chemical structure, and source.

Table 5 Physiological effects of resistant starch intake

Energy	$8-13\,kJ\,g^{-1}$; cf. $17\,kJ\,g^{-1}$ for digestible starches
Glycemic and insulinemic response	Depends on food, e.g., legumes (high in RS_1) and amylose-rich starchy foods (which tend to produce RS_3 on cooking) increase glucose tolerance, but cornflakes and cooked potatoes, both with high and similar glycemic indexes, have different resistant starch content
Lipid metabolism	Decreases plasma cholesterol and triacylglyceride levels in rat, but not in humans
Fermentability	Complete, although some RS_3 are more resistant
SCFA production	Increased production, especially butyrate
CO_2 and H_2 production	Occurs
Colonic pH	Decreased, especially by lactate production
Bile salts	Deoxycholate, a secondary bile salt with cytotoxic activity, precipitated due to the low pH
Colon cell proliferation	Stimulated in proximal colon, but repressed in distal colon; may be mediated by butyrate
Fecal excretion	At high dose, fecal bulk increases due to an increase in bacteria mass and water retention
Transit time	Increased intestinal transit at high dose
Nitrogen metabolism	Increased bacterial nitrogen and biomass
Minerals	May increase calcium and magnesium absorption in large intestine
Disease prevention	Epidemiological studies suggest prevention against colorectal cancer and constipation

Dietary Sources and Intake

The first source of oligosaccharides in the human diet is mother's milk, which contains approximately $12\,g\,l^{-1}$. In human breast milk, there are over 100 different oligosaccharides with both simple and complex structures. They are composed of galactose, fucose, sialic acid, glucose, and N-acetylglucosamine. Most are of low molecular weight, but a small proportion are of high molecular weight. Ninety per cent of breast milk oligosaccharides are neutral; the remainder are acidic. Interestingly, the nature of these oligosaccharide structures is determined by the mother's blood group. These oligosaccharides may have important function in the small intestine, where they can bind to the mucosa or to bacteria, interfering with pathogenic bacterial attachment and thus acting as anti-infective agents. As they are nondigestible, they enter the colon and may act as

a major energy for the colonic microflora and promote the growth of typical lactic acid bacteria that are characteristic of the normal breast-fed infant. More recently, oligosaccharides have been added to some infant formulas to mimic the actions of those in human milk. Recently, several studies have shown that these promote the growth of bifidobacteria in feces and make the stools more like those of breast-fed infants in terms of consistency, frequency, and pH.

In adults, the main dietary sources of oligosaccharides are chicory, artichokes, onions, garlic, leeks, bananas, and wheat. However, much research has been carried out on purified or synthetic oligosaccharide mixtures, mostly fructooligosaccharides derived from inulin. The normal dietary intake of oligosaccharides is difficult to estimate, as they are not a major dietary component. Around $3\,g\,day^{-1}$ has been suggested in the European diet. However, with the increasing information on the health benefits of isolated oligosaccharide sources (see below) they are being incorporated into functional foods.

Analysis

In general, oligosaccharides are a less heterogeneous group of compounds than resistant starches. Almost all nondigestible oligosaccharides (some fructooligosaccharides are an exception) are soluble in 80% (v/v) ethanol solution, which makes them relatively easy to isolate from insoluble components. Liquid chromatography, more specifically high-performance anion exchange chromatography (HPAEC), has been extensively employed not only to separate mixtures of different oligosaccharides, but also to separate, identify, and quantify individual carbohydrate moieties after appropriate hydrolysis of the oligosaccharide to its individual monomers. A more comprehensive study of the oligosaccharide structure can be achieved using more sophisticated techniques, like nuclear magnetic resonance and mass spectrometry. However, from a nutritional viewpoint, where simpler methods are needed for quality control and labeling purposes, HPAEC is usually applied to quantify the monomers (and dimers) present before and after hydrolysis of the studied oligosaccharide with appropriate enzymes and then the oligosaccharide level is worked out by difference.

Fermentation in the Colon and Health Benefits

Most oligosaccharides escape digestion in the small intestine and are fermented by the colonic bacteria. They are rapidly fermented resulting in a low pH and have been shown to increase the

Table 6 Chemical structure and source of sugars and oligosaccharides

Common name	Simplified structure[a]	Source	NDO[b]
Sugars (disaccharides)			
Lactose	Galβ1 → 4Glc	Milk, milk products	No
Maltose	Glcα1 → 4Glc	Glucose syrups, hydrolysis of starch	No
Sucrose	Fruβ2 → 1Glc	Table sugar	No
Cellobiose	Glcβ1 → 4Glc	Hydrolysis of cellulose	Yes
Trehalose	Glcα1 → 1Glc	Mushrooms, yeast	No
Melibiose	Galα1 → 6Glc	Hydrolysis of raffinose	Yes
Gentiobiose	Glcβ1 → 6Glcβ	Plant pigments, like saffron	Yes
Trisaccharides			
Maltotriose	Glcα1 → 4Glcα1 → 4Glc	Glucose syrups, hydrolysis of starch	No
Umbelliferose	Galα1 → 2Glcα1 → 2Fruβ	Plant tissues	Yes
Raffinose	Galα1 → 6Glcα1 → 2Fruβ	Legume seeds	Yes
Planteose	Galα1 → 6Fruβ2 → 1Glc	Plant tissues	Yes
Sialylα(2–3)lactose	NeuAcα2 → 3Galβ1 → 4Glc	Human milk	Yes
Tetrasaccharides			
Stachyose	Galα1 → 6Galα1 → 6Glcα1 → 2Fruβ	Legume seeds	Yes
Lychnose	Galα1 → 6Glcα1 → 2Fruβ1 → 1Gal	Plant tissues	Yes
Isolychnose	Galα1 → 6Glcα1 → 2Fruβ3 → 1Gal	Plant tissues	Yes
Sesamose	Galα1 → 6Galα1 → 6Fruβ2 → 1Glc	Plant tissues	Yes
Pentasaccharides			
Verbacose	Galα1 → 6Galα1 → 6Galα1 → 6Glcα1 → 2Fruβ	Plant tissues	Yes
Lacto-*N*-fucopentaose I	Fucα1 → 2Galβ1 → 3GlcNAcβ1 → 3Galβ1 → 4Glc	Human milk	Yes
Lacto-*N*-fucopentaose II	Galβ1 → 3[Fucα1 → 4]GlcNAcβ1 → 3Galβ1 → 4Glc	Human milk	Yes
Fructans			
Oligofructose	[Fruβ2 → 1]Fruβ2 → 1Glc with 1–9 [Fruβ2 → 1] residues	Hydrolysis of inulin or synthesis from sucrose	Yes
Inulin (polysaccharide)	[Fruβ2 → 1]Fruβ2 → 1Glc with 10–64 [Fruβ2 → 1] residues	Artichokes	Yes

[a]Fru, D-fructose; Fuc, L-fucose; Gal, D-galactose; Glc, D-glucose; GlcNAc, *N*-acetylglucosamine; NeuAc, *N*-acetylneuraminic acid (or sialic acid).
[b]NDO, nondigestible oligosaccharides.

survival of so-called probiotic organisms, i.e., lactobacilli and bifidobacteria. Probiotic bacteria have been show to have strain-specific effects, including reduction in duration of rotavirus and other infective diarrhea and reduction in symptoms of atopic eczema. They may also have some anticarcinogenic effects, but these have not been demonstrated in human *in vivo* studies. This action of oligosaccharides to promote the growth of bifidobacteria and lactobacilli defines them as prebiotics. Some studies are now investigating the synergistic effects of probiotics mixed with prebiotics. These mixtures are termed synbiotics. In addition to these actions, some oligosaccharides have similar health benefits to fermentable dietary fiber and resistant starch by increasing colonic fermentation, production of SCFA (especially butyrate), and reduction in colonic pH.

Resistant Starch, Oligosaccharides, or Just Dietary Fiber?

There has been much debate of the definition of dietary fiber and in particular whether it should include carbohydrates other than nonstarch polysaccharides. Recently, the American Association of Cereal Chemists (AACC) proposed a new definition of dietary fiber, which would include both oligosaccharides and resistant starch as well as associated plant substances. This new definition would also require complete or partial fermentation and demonstration of physiological effects such as laxation, and reduction in blood glucose or blood cholesterol. A similar approach to include beneficial physiological effects is also proposed by the Food and Nutrition Board of the US Institute of Medicine.

Table 7 The physiological effects of resistant starch, oligosaccharides, and dietary fiber

Physiological effect	Resistant starch	Oligosaccharides	Dietary fiber
Energy supply	$8–13\,kJ\,g^{-1}$	$8–13\,kJ\,g^{-1}$	$8–13\,kJ\,g^{-1}$
Increased glucose tolerance	Some foods	No	Some NSP[a]
Decreased plasma cholesterol and triacylglyceride levels	No	Not known	Some NSP
Fermentability	Complete	Complete	Variable
Production of SCFA	Yes	Yes	Yes
Increased butyrate production	High	High	Variable
CO_2 and H_2 production	Yes	Yes	Variable
Decreased fecal pH	Yes	Yes	Some NSP
Decreased production of deoxycholate	Yes	Yes	Some NSP
Increased colonocyte proliferation	Yes	Yes	Yes
Increased fecal bulk	At high dose	No	Variable
Faster whole gut transit time	At high dose	No	Yes
Increased bacterial nitrogen and biomass	Yes	Yes	Yes
Reduced mineral absorption in small intestine	No	No	Some NSP
Increased mineral absorption in large intestine	Yes	Yes	Some NSP
Possible prevention of colorectal cancer	Yes	Not known	Yes

[a]NSP, nonstarch polysaccharide.

Thus, it is being increasingly recognized that oligosaccharides, resistant starch, and nonstarch polysaccharides are very similar especially in their effects on gut physiology and colonic fermentation. A comparison of their actions is summarized in **Table 7**. This inclusion of resistant starch and oligosaccharides in the definition of dietary fiber could have major implications for food labeling.

See also: **Dietary Fiber**: Physiological Effects and Effects on Absorption; Potential Role in Etiology of Disease; Role in Nutritional Management of Disease. **Microbiota of the Intestine**: Prebiotics.

Further Reading

Blaut M (2002) Relationship of prebiotics and food to intestinal microflora. *European Journal of Nutrition* 41(supplement 1): i11–i16.

Bornet FRJ, Brouns F, Tashiro Y, and Duvillier V (2002) Nutritional aspects of short-chain fructooligosaccharides: natural occurrence, chemistry, physiology and health implications. *Digestive and Liver Disease* 34(supplement 2): S111–S120.

Champ M, Langkilde A-M, Brouns F, Kettlitz B, and Collet YL (2003) Advances in dietary fibre characterisation. 1. Defini-

tion of dietary fibre, physiological relevance, health benefits and analytical aspects. *Nutrition Research Reviews* 16: 71–82.

Delzenne NM (2003) Oligosaccharides: state of the art. *Proceedings of the Nutrition Society* 62: 177–182.

DeVries JW (2003) On defining dietary fibre. *Proceedings of the Nutrition Society* 62: 37–43.

Ghisolfi J (2003) Dietary fibre and prebiotics in infant formula. *Proceedings of the Nutrition Society* 62: 183–185.

Greger JL (1999) Non-digestible carbohydrates and mineral bioavailability. *Journal of Nutrition* 129(supplement S): 1434S–1435S.

Kunz C, Rudloff S, Baier W, Klein N, and Strobel S (2000) Oligosaccharides in human milk: Structural, functional, and metabolic aspects. *Annual Review of Nutrition* 20: 699–722.

McCleary BV (2003) Dietary fibre analysis. *Proceedings of the Nutrition Society* 62: 3–9.

Roberfroid M (2002) Functional food concept and its application to prebiotics. *Digestive and Liver Disease* 34(supplement 2): S105–S110.

Roberfroid MB (2003) Inulin and oligofructose are dietary fibres and functional food ingredients. In: Kritchevsky D, Bonfield CT, and Edwards CA (eds.) *Dietary Fiber in Health and Disease: 6th Vahouny Symposium*, pp. 161–163. Delray Beach, FL: Vahouny Symposium.

Topping DL, Fukushima M, and Bird AR (2003) Resistant starch as a prebiotic and synbiotic: state of the art. *Proceedings of the Nutrition Society* 62: 171–176.

CAROTENOIDS

Contents
Chemistry, Sources and Physiology
Epidemiology of Health Effects

Chemistry, Sources and Physiology

B K Ishida and G E Bartley, Agricultural Research
Service, Albany, CA, USA

Published by Elsevier Ltd.

Chemistry

Structure

Most carotenoids are 40-carbon isoprenoid compounds called tetraterpenes. Isoprenoids are formed from the basic five-carbon building block, isoprene (**Figure 1**). In nature, carotenoids are synthesized through the stepwise addition of isopentenyl diphosphate (IPP) units to dimethylallyl diphosphate (DMAPP) to form the 20-carbon precursor geranylgeranyl diphosphate (GGPP). Two molecules of GGPP are combined to form the first carotenoid in the biosynthetic pathway, phytoene, which is then desaturated, producing 11 conjugated double bonds to form lycopene, the red pigment in ripe tomato fruit (**Figure 1**). Nearly all other carotenoids can be derived from lycopene. Lycopene can be cyclized on either or both ends to form α- or β-carotene, and these in turn can be oxygenated to form xanthophylls such as β-cryptoxanthin, zeaxanthin, or lutein (**Figure 1** and **Figure 2**). Carotenoids having fewer than 40 carbons can result from loss of carbons within the chain (nor-carotenoids) or loss of carbons from the end of the molecule (apocarotenoids). Longer carotenoids, homocarotenoids (C45–C50), are found in some bacterial species. The alternating double bonds along the backbone of carotenoid molecules form a polyene chain, which imparts unique qualities to this group of compounds. This alternation of single and double bonds also allows a number of geometrical isomers to exist for each carotenoid (**Figure 1**). For lycopene, the theoretical number of steric forms is 1056; however, when steric hindrance is considered, that number is reduced to 72. In nature most carotenoids are found in the all-*trans* form although mutants are known in plants, e.g., *Lycopersicon esculentum* (Mill.) var. Tangerine tomato, and eukaryotic algae that produce

poly-*cis* forms of carotenoids. The mutant plant is missing an enzyme, carotenoid isomerase (CRTISO), which catalyzes the isomerization of the *cis* isomers of lycopene and its precursors to the all-*trans* form during biosynthesis. Light can also cause *cis* to *trans* isomerization of these carotenoids depending upon the surrounding environment. The isomeric form determines the shape of the molecule and can thus change the properties of the carotenoid affecting solubility and absorbability. *Trans* forms of carotenoids are more rigid and have a greater tendency to crystallize or aggregate than the *cis* forms. Therefore, *Cis* forms may be more easily absorbed and transported. End groups such as the β or ε rings of α-carotene and β-carotene and the amount of oxygenation will also affect carotenoid properties.

Chemical Properties

In general, carotenoids are hydrophobic molecules and thus are soluble only in organic solvents, having only limited solubility in water. Addition of hydroxyl groups to the end groups causes the carotenoid to become more polar, affecting its solubility in various organic solvents. Alternatively, carotenoids can solubilize in aqueous environments by prior integration into liposomes or into cyclic oligosaccharides such as cyclodextrins.

In general, carotenoid molecules are very sensitive to elevated temperatures and the presence of acid, oxygen, and light when in solution, and are subject to oxidative degradation.

Electronic Properties

What sets carotenoids apart from other molecules and gives them their electrochemical properties is the conjugated double bond system. In this alternating double and single bond system, the π-electrons are delocalized over the length of the polyene chain. This polyene chain or chromophore imparts the characteristic electronic spectra and photophysical and photochemical properties to this group of molecules. The highly delocalized π-electrons require little energy to reach an excited state so that light energy can cause a transition.

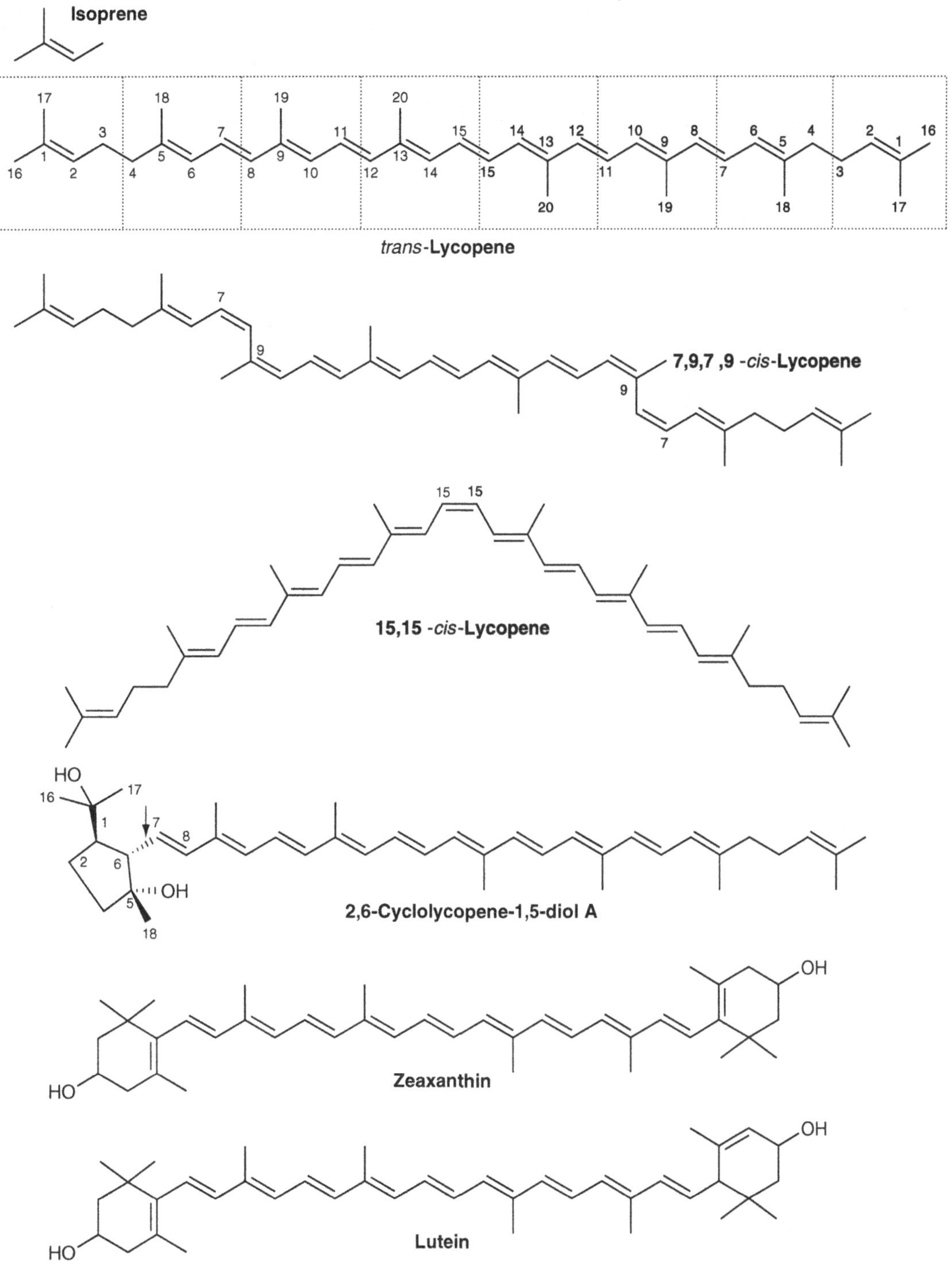

Figure 1 Carotenoid structures. Lycopene is shown with numbered carbons. The down arrow on 2,6-cyclolycopene-1,5-diol A indicates the only difference from the B isomer.

The length of the conjugated polyene or chromophore affects the amount of energy needed to excite the π-electrons. The longer the conjugated system, the easier it is to excite, so longer wavelengths of light can be absorbed. The result is that phytoene, having three conjugated double bonds is colorless, and phytofluene, having five, is colorless, but fluoresces green under UV light. Zetacarotene has seven, absorbs light at ∼400 nm and appears yellow, while neurosporene has nine, absorbs light at ∼451, and appears orange, and lycopene has eleven conjugated double bonds,

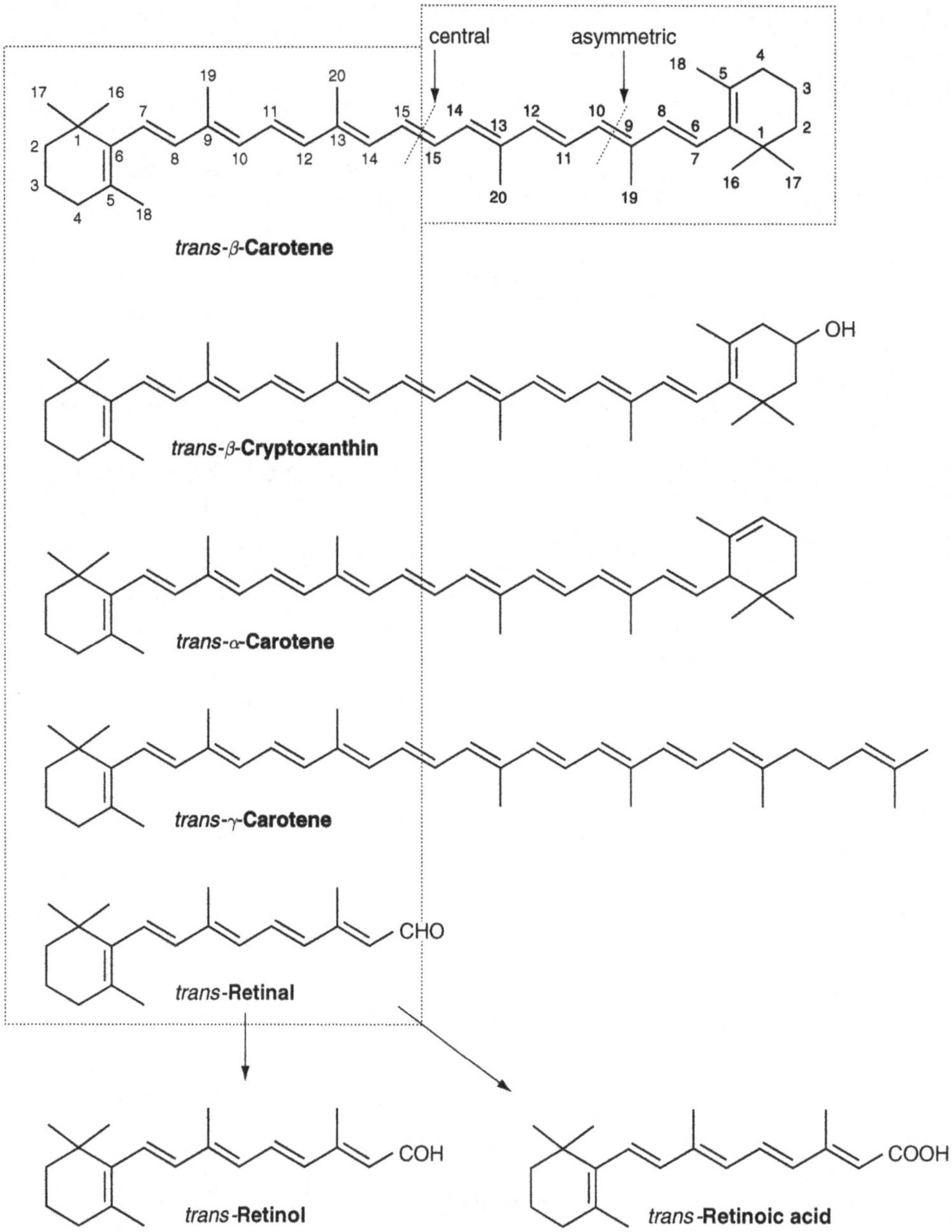

Figure 2   Provitamin A carotenoids. Dotted lines indicate the provitamin A moiety.

absorbs at ~472, and appears red. The polyene chain also allows transfer of singlet or triplet energy.

Reactions

Light and Chemical Energy

The basic energy-transfer reactions are assumed to be similar in plants and animals, even though environments differ. Excess light can cause excitation of porphyrin molecules (porphyrin triplets). These triplet-state porphyrin molecules can transfer their energy to oxygen-forming singlet oxygen, $^1O_2$. Singlet oxygen can damage DNA and cause lipid peroxidation, thereby killing the cell. Carotenoids, having nine or more conjugated double bonds, can prevent damage by singlet oxygen through: (1) transfer of triplet energy from the excited porphyrin to the carotenoid, forming a carotenoid triplet, which would be too low in energy for further transfer and would simply dissipate as heat; or (2) singlet oxygen energy could transfer to the carotenoid, also forming a triplet carotenoid, dissipating heat, and returning to the ground state. This ability to quench sensitized triplets has been useful in treating protoporphyria (PP) and congenital erythropoietic porphyria (CEP) in humans. Porphyrias are disorders resulting from a defect in heme biosynthesis. Precursor porphyrins accumulate and can be sensitized to the singlet state and drop to the lower triplet state. The triplet state is longer-lived and thus more likely to react with other molecules such as oxygen to form singlet oxygen, which can cause cellular damage. Because β-carotene can transfer and dissipate either sensitized triplet or singlet oxygen energy it has been used to treat these disorders.

Light absorption and possibly scavenging of destructive oxygen species by the xanthophylls lutein and zeaxanthin are also important in the macula of the primate eye. Lutein and two isomers of zeaxanthin are selectively accumulated in the macula, creating a yellow area of the retina responsible for high visual acuity (smaller amounts are also found in the lens). Both carotenoids absorb light of about 450 nm 'blue light,' thus filtering light to the light receptors behind the carotenoid layer in the macula. Filtering blue light can reduce oxidative stress to retinal light receptors and chromatic aberration resulting from the refraction of blue light. A similar filter effect may occur in the lens, but the concentration of the xanthophylls is much lower, and further protection occurs with age when the lens yellows. Whether scavenging of destructive oxygen species by these carotenoids is useful here is unproven, but the retina is an area of higher blood flow and light exposure than other tissues.

Cleavage to Vitamin A

Provitamin A carotenoids are sources of vitamin A. Of the 50–60 carotenoids having provitamin A activity, β-carotene, β-cryptoxanthin, and α-carotene are the major sources of vitamin A nutrition in humans, β-carotene being the most important (**Figure 2**). Vitamin A (retinol) and its derivatives retinal and retinoic acid perform vital functions in the vertebrate body. Retinal (11-*cis* retinal) combined with opsin functions in the visual system in signal transduction of light reception. Retinol and retinoic acid function in reproduction (spermatogenesis), growth regulation (general development and limb morphogenesis), and cell differentiation. Provitamin A activity requires at least one unsubstituted β-ionone ring, the correct number and orientation of methyl groups along the polyene backbone, and the correct number of conjugated double bonds, preferably in the *trans*-isomer orientation. Two pathways for the formation of retinal from β-carotene have been proposed. First, central cleavage by which β-carotene 15,15′-mono- or dioxygenase catalyzes β-carotene cleavage to form two

molecules of retinal, which can then be converted to retinol or retinoic acid (**Figure 2**). Some debate on the mechanism of the β-carotene central cleavage enzyme still exists, but evidence leans towards activity as a monooxygenase, not a dioxygenase. Alternatively, in the eccentric cleavage pathway β-carotene can be cleaved at any of the double bonds along the polyene backbone (other than the 15-15′double bond). Products of these reactions (apocarotenals) are then further metabolized to retinoic acid and retinol. An asymmetric cleavage enzyme has recently been cloned that cleaves β-carotene at the 9′-10′-double bond to form β-ionone and β-apo-10′-carotenal. The discovery of this enzyme indicates at least some eccentric cleavage occurs in vertebrates. This eccentric cleavage process has been proposed to occur during more oxidative conditions, while central cleavage would predominate under normal physiological conditions. Central cleavage is considered to be the major pathway because of the scarcity of eccentric cleavage products detected *in vivo*.

Radical Reactions

Excess amounts of radicals, molecules having unpaired electrons, e.g., peroxyls (ROO$^\bullet$), can be created in tissues exogenously, e.g., by light exposure, or endogenously, e.g., by overexercising. Radicals react with lipids, proteins, and DNA causing damage, which possibly contributes to disease symptoms and aging. The special properties of the polyene chain make carotenoids susceptible to electrophilic attack, resulting in formation of resonance-stabilized radicals that are less reactive.

Three possible reactions can occur with carotenoids.

1. Adduct formation (CAR + R$^\bullet$ → R-CAR$^\bullet$); these products should be stable because of resonance in the polyene structure. If the radical were a lipid peroxyl, this reaction (CAR + ROO$^\bullet$ → ROO-CAR$^\bullet$) would prevent further propagation (chain-breaking).
2. Hydrogen atom abstraction (CAR + R$^\bullet$ → CAR$^\bullet$ + RH), where a hydrogen atom is taken from the carotenoid allylic to the polyene chain, leaving a resonance-stabilized carotenoid radical.
3. Electron transfer (CAR + R$^\bullet$ → CAR$^{\bullet +}$ + R$^-$), which has been reported in plant and cyanobacterial photosystems using laser flash photolysis of Photosystem II.

In many cases, the products formed are colorless, thus revealing the bleaching effect of many oxidants on carotenoids. Further oxidation of the carotenoid or carotenoid radical can occur as in studies of soybean (*Glycine max*) and recombinant pea (*Pisum sativum*) lipoxygenase-mediated cooxidation of carotenoids and polyunsaturated fatty acids. Approximately 50 breakdown products of β-carotene were detected. This large number of products seems to indicate a random attack along the polyene chain of β-carotene by a linoleoylperoxyl radical. Studies using potassium permanganate, a metalloporphyrin (a P450 enzyme center mimic), and autooxidation have been performed with lycopene, resulting in formation of a number of apo-lycopenals and apo-lycopenones. However, only two metabolites of lycopene have been identified in human plasma, 2,6-cyclolycopene-1,5 diols A and B (**Figure 1**). Additionally, seven metabolites of the carotenoids lutein and zeaxanthin have been detected in human tissues.

Prooxidant Behavior

The ability to quench singlet oxygen, porphyrin triplet energies, and free radical reactions are examples of the antioxidant nature of carotenoids. An *in vitro* study showed that, at low partial pressures of oxygen (pO_2), β-carotene consumed peroxy radicals efficiently as in: $CAR + ROO^{\bullet} \rightarrow CAR^{\bullet+} + ROO^{-}$. At higher pO_2, however, β-carotene became a prooxidant through autooxidation. Recently, experiments in intact murine normal and tumor thymocytes showed that β-carotene lost its antioxidant potency at higher pO_2, and the effect was more pronounced in tumor cells. It is still unclear, however, whether some effects of carotenoid behavior at higher pO_2 are due to prooxidant activity or simply lack of antioxidant ability. Prooxidant effects of β-carotene have also been used to explain results from intervention trials of β-carotene supplementation in diets of smokers or individuals suffering from asbestosis where the incidence of carcinogenesis was higher in those individuals taking the β-carotene supplement. Generation of deleterious oxidation products from β-carotene reaction with reactive oxygen species in tobacco smoke or as a result of asbestosis has been proposed. Interference with retinoid signaling was also considered. However, whether those effects were due to prooxidant behavior or lack of antioxidant ability is still unclear.

Dietary Sources

Carotenoids cannot be synthesized by humans; therefore they must be obtained from dietary sources. These are primarily highly pigmented red, orange, and yellow fruits and vegetables. The carotenoid lycopene is red; however, not all red fruits and vegetables contain lycopene. For example, the red in strawberries, apples, and cherries is a result of their anthocyanin content; whereas, tomatoes, watermelon, and pink grapefruit derive their red color from lycopene. The carotenoids

β-carotene, β-cryptoxanthin, lutein, zeaxanthin, and violaxanthin are yellow to orange, and phytoene and phytofluene are colorless. Green, leafy vegetables also contain carotenoids, whose colors are masked by the green color of chlorophyll. **Table 1** lists carotenoids

Table 1 Carotenoid content (μg per g fresh weight) of fresh fruit and vegetables

Carotenoid	Concentration (μg per g fresh weight)	Source
Lycopene	380–3054	Gac (*Momordica cochinchinensis*, Spreng) aril
	179–483	Autumn olive (*Elaeagnus umbellate*)
	27–200	Tomato
	23–72	Watermelon
	53	Guava
	19–40	Papaya
	8–33	Grapefruit, pink
β-Carotene	101–770	Gac aril
	49–257	Carrot, orange
	16–216	Cantaloupe
	15–92	Kale
	0.5–92	Sweet potato
	47–89	Spinach
	46	Turnip greens
	26–64	Apricot
	22–58	Gac mesocarp
	3–70	Tomato
	42	Squash, butternut
	40	Swiss chard
	14–34	Mango
	33	Collards
	4–10	Grapefruit, pink
	0.51–1.2*	Orange (*blood)
Lutein	64–150	Kale
	6–129	Mango
	108	Parsley
	39–95	Spinach
	33–51	Collards
	15–28	Broccoli
	27	Chinese cabbage
	26	Watercress
	25	Pepper, orange
	24	Squash, butternut
	1–7	Tomato
Zeaxanthin	16–85	Pepper, orange
	43	Gou Qi Zi (*Lycium barabarum*)
	9	Gac aril
	22	Pepper, red
	7	Watercress
	1–5	Spinach
	5	Parsley
	5	Japanese persimmon
	1–3	Kale
	3	Squash, butternut
	0.4	Broccoli
	0.03–0.5	Tomato

Continued

Table 1 Continued

Carotenoid	Concentration (µg per g fresh weight)	Source
Lutein + zeaxanthin	71–3956	Kale
	119	Spinach
	84	Turnip greens
	26	Lettuce
	24	Broccoli
	21	Squash, zucchini
	16	Brussel sprouts
	8	Japanese persimmon
	7	Watercress
	6	Beans, green snap
	5	Tangerine
β-Cryptoxanthin	22	Pepper, sweet red
	14	Japanese persimmon
	11	Starfruit
	0.7–9	Pepper, chili
	2–8	Pepper, orange
	0.5–5	Tangerine
	4	Cilantro
	1.4	Papaya
	1	Watermelon
α-Carotene	20–206	Carrot
	8	Squash, butternut
	2	Collards
	1	Tomato
	0.7–0.9	Beans, green snap
	0.5	Swiss chard

found in fruits and vegetables. Smaller amounts are also available from animal sources such as ocean fish and dairy products. The pink color of salmon, for example, is derived from the xanthophylls, astaxanthin and canthaxanthin, which they obtain from eating small crustaceans and krill. Lutein imparts its yellow-orange color to eggs, and milk, butter, and cheese contain retinols and β-carotene. Carotenoids, such as lutein from marigolds and bixin (red color) from annatto, are also used widely as colorants in processed foods to make them more attractive.

Concentrations of carotenoids in fruit and vegetable sources vary, resulting from differences in conditions under which they are grown (temperature, amount of sunlight, degrees of stress from extremes in climate such as drought, heat, and cold), genotype, and maturity or ripeness. The carotenoid content in animal sources depends upon amounts contained in animal feeds and seasons of the year, which affect the availability of carotenoid-containing plants eaten by grazing animals.

Human diets and tissues contain six carotenoids in significant amounts (listed in **Table 1**). Lycopene is typically the carotenoid consumed in greatest amounts in Western diets. Per capita intakes in Europe and North America average from 1.6 to more than 18 mg lycopene per day. More than 85% of the lycopene in North American diets comes from tomato products, which also contain significant amounts of other carotenoids (α- and β-carotene and lutein/zeaxanthin), as well as vitamins C, A, and E, and potassium and folic acid. (Flavonoids are also found in tomato skin; thus, cherry tomatoes contain higher concentrations.) In the US, the annual per capita consumption of tomatoes by 1999 averaged about 17.6 pounds of fresh and 72.8 pounds of processed tomatoes.

Effects of Storage and Processing

Carotenoids are susceptible to oxidative degradation and isomerization resulting from storage and processing conditions. These reactions result in both loss of color and biological activity and formation of often unpleasant volatile compounds. Degradation occurs upon exposure to oxygen and is accelerated by the presence of substances such as metals, enzymes, unsaturated lipids, and prooxidants; exposure to light; and conditions that destroy cell wall and ultrastructural integrity. Heating can promote isomerization of the naturally occurring all-*trans* to various *cis* isomers. This process then affects bioavailability of the carotenoid. Processing also affects bioavailability by macerating tissues, destroying or weakening cell ultrastructure, denaturing or weakening complexes with proteins, and cleaving ester linkages, thereby releasing carotenoids from the food matrix.

Processed foods are frequently fortified with carotenoids to increase nutritive value and/or enhance attractiveness. For example, annatto, an extract from the seeds of the *Bixa orella* tree, containing the carotenoids bixin and norbixin, is added to butter, margarine, and processed cheese to give a yellow-orange color to these products. Tomato oleoresin is added to processed tomato products, increasing lycopene content while enhancing their attractive red color.

Physiology

Digestion

Numerous factors affect the intestinal absorption of carotenoids. Digestion of food in the stomach increases accessibility of carotenoids for absorption by maceration in HCl and digestive enzymes. The acidic environment of the stomach helps to disrupt cell walls and other cellular ultrastructure of raw fruits and vegetables and causes further breakdown of cooked foods to release carotenoids from food matrices in which they are contained or bound.

Carotenoids in green leafy vegetables are found in chloroplasts; those in fruit are located in chromoplasts. Absorption studies comparing plasma levels of β-carotene and retinol after consuming fruit vs. green leafy vegetables showed that β-carotene is more efficiently absorbed from fruit, indicating that chloroplasts (or the bonds linking chloroplast proteins and carotenoids) are more resistant to disruption in the digestive tract than chromoplasts. Thus, the location of a carotenoid in the cell affects its accessibility.

Carotenoid isomerization can occur in the acidic gastric milieu. Lycopene present in fruits and vegetables occurs almost exclusively as the all-*trans* isomer, but is converted to *cis* isomers, which seem to be more bioavailable. Plasma and tissue profiles show that *cis* isomers make up more than 50% of the total lycopene present. On the other hand, studies show that no *trans/cis* isomerization of β-carotene occurs in the stomach. In fact, evidence has been found for transfer of a significant portion of both β- and α-carotene to the fat phase of the meal in the stomach, which would increase bioavailability of these carotenoids for absorption. No studies are available relating isomerization to bioavailability of other carotenoids.

Absorption and Transport

Because carotenoids are hydrophobic molecules, they are associated with lipophilic sites in cells, such as bilayer membranes. Polar substituents such as hydroxyl groups decrease their hydrophobicity and their orientation with respect to membranes.

Lycopene and β-carotene are aligned parallel to membrane surfaces to maintain a hydrophobic environment, whereas the more polar xanthophylls lutein and zeaxanthin become oriented perpendicular to membrane surfaces to keep their hydroxyl groups in a more hydrophilic environment. These differences can affect the physical nature of a membrane as well as its function. Carotenoids can form complexes with proteins, which would aid them in moving through an aqueous environment. They can also interact with hydrophobic regions of lipoproteins. Carotenoproteins have been found mainly in plants and invertebrates, but intracellular β-carotene-binding proteins have been found in bovine liver and intestine and in livers of the rat and ferret. In addition, a xanthophyll-binding protein has been found in human retina and macula. Carotenoids are also present in nature as crystalline aggregates (lycopene in chromoplasts) or as fine dispersions in aqueous media (β-carotene in oranges).

In the intestinal lumen (**Figure 3**) where carotenoids are released from the food matrix, cleavage of carotenoproteins and fatty acid esters by carboxylic ester hydrolase, which is secreted by the pancreas, can occur. Carotenoids are then solubilized into lipid micelles. These hydrophobic compounds are thus more efficiently absorbed when accompanied by at least a small amount of fat. The amount of fat for optimal carotenoid absorption seems to differ among carotenoids. For example, lutein esters require more fat for optimal absorption than β-carotene. These differences have not been quantified for each carotenoid. In addition, the presence of a nonabsorbable, fat-soluble component was shown to

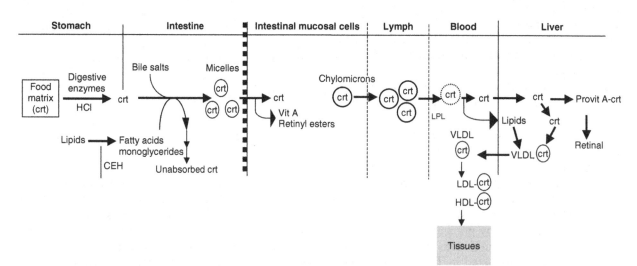

Figure 3 Factors affecting digestion, absorption, metabolism, and transport of carotenoids. crt, carotenoids; CEH, carboxylic ester hydrolase, secreted by the pancreas; LPL, lipoprotein lipase; VLDL, very low-density lipoprotein; LDL, low-density lipoprotein; HDL, high-density lipoprotein.

decrease carotenoid absorption. Sucrose polyester, a nonabsorbable fat replacer decreased carotenoid levels in plasma after ingestion by 20–120%. The extent of this inhibition depends upon the amount of nonabsorbable compound ingested, as well as the particular carotenoid under consideration. The mechanism for this inhibition is apparently similar to the action of fiber, i.e., sequestration. The type of fat that is ingested along with carotenoids will also affect carotenoid absorption. As macerated food passes into the intestinal lumen, carotenoids freed from the food matrix then become incorporated into micelles, consisting of free fatty acids, monoglycerides, phospholipids, and bile acids. Many other factors can affect intestinal absorption such as micelle size, phospholipid composition, solubilization of carotenoids into mixed micelles, and concentration of available bile salts, among others.

The presence of other carotenoids can affect the absorption of carotenoids into intestinal mucosal cells, since carotenoids can compete for absorption or facilitate the absorption of another. Data on carotenoid interactions are not clear. Human studies show that β-carotene decreases lutein absorption, while lutein has either no effect or a lowering effect on β-carotene absorption. Although not confirmed in humans, the inhibitory effect of lutein on β-carotene absorption might be partly attributed to the inhibition of the β-carotene cleavage enzyme by lutein shown in rats. Beta-carotene also seemed to lower absorption of canthaxanthin, whereas canthaxanthin did not inhibit β-carotene absorption. Studies showed that β-carotene increased lycopene absorption, although lycopene had no effect on β-carotene. Alpha-carotene and cryptoxanthin show high serum responses to dietary intake compared to lutein. In addition, *cis* isomers of lycopene seem to be more bioavailable than the all-*trans*, and selective intestinal absorption of all-*trans* β-carotene occurs, as well as conversion of the 9-*cis* isomer to all-*trans* β-carotene. It is clear, then, that selective absorption of carotenoids takes place into the intestinal mucosal cell.

Another complicating factor in the intestinal mucosal cell is the partial conversion of provitamin A carotenoids (β- and α-carotenes and cryptoxanthin) to vitamin A (primarily to retinyl esters). Therefore, in absorption studies these metabolic reactions must be accounted for in measuring intestinal transport. Nonprovitamin A carotenoids such as lycopene, lutein, and zeaxanthin are incorporated intact, although some cleavage can occur. Earlier studies on rats indicated that lycopene and β-carotene are absorbed by passive diffusion. However, recent evidence from the kinetics of β-carotene transport through Caco-2 cell monolayers indicates the involvement of a specific epithelial transporter that facilitates absorption.

In the intestinal mucosa, both carotenoids and retinyl esters are incorporated into chylomicrons and secreted into the lymph for transport to blood. In blood, lipoprotein lipase rapidly degrades the chylomicrons, and the liver sequesters the resulting carotenoid-containing fragments. The liver then secretes carotenoids back into the bloodstream in association with hepatic very low-density lipoproteins (VLDL). Most carotenoids in fasting plasma are carried by low-density lipoproteins (LDL) and high-density lipoproteins (HDL). Seventy-five per cent of the hydrocarbon carotenoids, e.g., lycopene and β-carotene, are associated with LDL, the rest is associated with HDL and, in smaller amounts, with VLDL. More polar carotenoids such as lutein and zeaxanthin are found equally distributed between HDL and LDL. After ingestion, carotenoids first appear in the bloodstream in chylomicrons, resulting from excretion from intestinal mucosal cells (4–8 h). HDL carotenoid levels peak in the circulation between 16 and 28 h; LDL carotenoid levels peak between 24 and 48 h. The bloodstream then transports carotenoids to different tissues (e.g., liver, prostate gland, fat, ocular macula) where they are sequestered by various mechanisms.

Distribution and Impact on Health

In general, carotenoid concentrations in serum reflect concentrations contained in the food that is ingested. Carotenoids have been found in various human organs and tissues. These include human liver, lung, breast, cervix, skin, and adipose and ocular tissues. The major storage organs are adipose tissue (probably because of its volume) and the liver. Tissues containing large amounts of LDL receptors seem to accumulate high levels of carotenoids, probably as a result of nonspecific uptake by lipoprotein carriers. Preferential uptake, however, is indicated in some cases. For example, unusually high concentrations of phytoene in the lung, ζ-carotene and phytofluene in breast tissue, lycopene in the prostate and colon, lycopene, β-carotene, and phytofluene in cervical tissue, and lutein and zeaxanthin in ocular tissues have been found.

The epidemiological findings that the ingestion of tomato and tomato products is strongly correlated with a reduced risk of several types of cancer, particularly prostate cancer, has stimulated a great deal of research on the protective effects of lycopene. Lycopene is the most efficient biological antioxidant. Hence, it has been assumed that it is this antioxidant activity that is responsible for the protection against prostate cancer. However, a recent study in which carcinogenesis was induced in rats using N-methyl-N-nitrosourea showed that a diet containing whole tomato powder inhibited development of prostate cancer, but the same diet to which pure synthetic lycopene was added instead did not. These results indicate that lycopene alone was ineffective in reducing the incidence of prostate cancer. Therefore, either some other element in the tomato powder was the effective agent or the effect was obtained by lycopene working in concert with other tomato constituents. Obviously, more studies are required to determine which elements contained in tomato are responsible for the protective effect.

The finding that lutein and zeaxanthin are accumulated in the macula lutea of the eye has led to the hope that dietary supplementation might reduce the risk of age-related macular degeneration (AMD), which affects the central portion of the retina and is the most common cause of irreversible blindness in the Western world. Some studies have indicated benefits of diets supplemented with lutein and zeaxanthin from spinach in preventing AMD; others found no significant correlation between plasma levels of these carotenoids and reduced risk of AMD. Lutein, zeaxanthin, and a zeaxanthin stereoisomer 3R, 3'S(=meso)-zeaxanthin form the yellow pigment of the macula lutea. 3R, 3'S(=meso)-zeaxanthin is not found in either food or plasma in significant amounts. Also notable is that, in most food consumed in large quantities, the concentration of lutein is much greater than that of zeaxanthin (e.g., see **Table 1**, spinach, kale, broccoli, tomato). The yellow pigment of the macula is located in the center of the macula, covering the central fovea and overlapping the avascular zone. This location would allow the pigment to shield the photoreceptors from blue light. An environmental factor that seems to play a role in the development of age-related macular degeneration is ocular exposure to sunlight, in particular a history of exposure to blue light in the preceding 20 years. Light has been shown to induce oxidative damage in the presence of photosensitizers. Macular carotenoids are distributed in a pattern that is particularly advantageous. The two stereoisomers of zeaxanthin are concentrated in the central area and lutein in higher concentrations in the more peripheral regions. The lutein:zeaxanthin ratio in the center of the macula is about 0.8, in the peripheral regions about 2.4, but in plasma between 4 and 7. Therefore, the macula is able to concentrate lutein and zeaxanthin, change concentration ratios that are normally found in plasma, and invert the ratio to achieve higher zeaxanthin concentrations in the center of the macula

lutea. The exact mechanism for this accumulation is not known; however, a specific membrane-associated, xanthophyll-binding protein was recently isolated from the human retina.

Carotenoids are believed to play a significant role in protecting skin from oxidative damage. *In vivo* measurements in humans of lycopene, β-, ζ-, γ-, and α-carotenes, lutein and zeaxanthin, phytoene, and phytofluene have shown that carotenoid concentrations are correlated with the presence or absence of skin cancer and precancerous lesions. Carotenoids are also believed to protect against several other types of cancer, cardiovascular diseases, and cataract formation and aid in immune function and gap-junction communication between cells, which is believed to be a protective mechanism related to their cancer-preventative activities.

Conclusions

Numerous studies indicate that carotenoids and their metabolites play a role in combating degradative reactions that are harmful to human health. Most of these functions seem to be related to their antioxidant nature and ability to dissipate energy from light and free radical-generating reactions. Obviously much research is still required to shed light onto mechanisms involved in these protective functions. Other fascinating roles in nature are also being discovered, for example, the signaling of apparent good health and consequently good potential parenting in birds by the red coloration of beaks, which seems to serve as an attractant to prospective mates.

See also: **Carotenoids**: Epidemiology of Health Effects. **Vitamin A**: Biochemistry and Physiological Role.

Further Reading

Borel P (2003) Factors affecting intestinal absorption of highly lipophilic food microconstituents (fat-soluble vitamins, carotenoids and phytosterols). *Clinical Chemistry and Laboratory Medicine* 41: 979–994.

Britton G (1995) Structure and properties of carotenoids in relation to function. *FASEB Journal* 9: 1551–1558.

Britton G, Liaaen-Jensen S, and Pfander H (eds.) (1995) *Carotenoids: Isolation and Analysis* vol. 1A and *Spectroscopy*, vol. 1B Basel, Boston, Berlin: Birkhäuser Verlag.

During A and Harrison EH (2004) Intestinal absorption and metabolism of carotenoids: insights from cell culture. *Archives of Biochemistry and Biophysics* 430: 77–78.

Frank HA, Young AJ, Britton G, and Cogdell RJ (1999) *The Photochemistry of Carotenoids*, (*Advances in Photosynthesis*, vol. 8). Dordrecht: Kluwer Academic Publishers.

Holden JM, Eldridge AL, Beecher GR, Buzzard IM, Bhagwat S, Davis CS, Douglass LW, Gebhardt S, Haytowitz D, and Schakel S (1999) Carotenoid content of U.S. foods: An update of the database. *Journal of Food Composition and Analysis* 12: 169–196.

Isler O (1971) *Carotenoids*. Basel: Birkhäuser-Verlag.

Khachik F, Carvalho L, Bernstein PS, Muir GJ, Zhao D-Y, and Katz NB (2002) Chemistry, distribution, and metabolism of tomato carotenoids and their impact on human health. *Experimental Biology and Medicine* 227: 845–851.

Krinsky NI, Mayne ST, and Sies H (eds.) (2004) *Carotenoids in Health and Disease* (Oxidative Stress and Disease Series vol. 15). New York: Marcel Dekker.

Rodriguez-Amaya B (1999) In *A Guide to Carotenoid Analysis in Foods*. Washington, DC: ILSI Press.

Schalch W (2001) Possible contribution of lutein and zeaxanthin, carotenoids of the macula lutea, to reducing the risk for age-related macular degeneration: a review. *HKJ Ophthalmology* 4: 31–42.

Yeum K-J and Russell RM (2002) Carotenoid bioavailability and bioconversion. *Annual Review of Nutrition* 22: 483–504.

Epidemiology of Health Effects

S A Tanumihardjo and Z Yang, University of Wisconsin-Madison, Madison, WI, USA

Introduction

The colors of many fruits and vegetables are due to a class of compounds known as carotenoids. Over 600 carotenoids have been identified in nature. Humans are unique in that they can assimilate carotenoids from the foods that they eat whereas many other animals do not. Thus, carotenoids are an important class of phytochemicals. Phytochemicals are compounds derived from plants that may or may not have nutritional value. While many carotenoids circulate in humans, the most commonly studied ones are β-carotene, α-carotene, β-cryptoxanthin, lycopene, lutein, and zeaxanthin (**Figure 1**). The nutritional significance of carotenoids is that some are used by the body to make vitamin A. Indeed, approximately 50 carotenoids can be converted by the body into vitamin A and are known as provitamin A carotenoids. The three most abundant provitamin A carotenoids in foods are β-carotene, α-carotene, and β-cryptoxanthin. Provitamin A carotenoids, especially β-carotene, provide less than one-half of the vitamin A supply in North America but provide more than one-half in Africa and Asia.

Dietary recommendations for the intake of specific carotenoids have not been established due to lack of an adequate evidence base. To date, carotenoids are not considered essential nutrients. Dietary recommendations for vitamin A exist: 900 retinol activity equivalents (RAE) for men and 700 RAE for women. An RAE is equivalent to 1 μg of retinol. The recommendations for infants and children are less and range from 300 to 600 RAE depending on age. Consumers need to eat sufficient amounts of carotenoid-rich fruits and vegetables to meet their daily vitamin A requirement, and to achieve optimal dietary carotenoid intake to lower the risk of certain chronic diseases. In 2001, the Institute of Medicine revised the amount of carotenoids needed to provide vitamin A from foods as being approximately 12 μg of β-carotene or 24 μg of other provitamin A carotenoids to yield 1 RAE. Currently, high-dose pharmacological supplementation with carotenoids is not advised. Despite this, a tolerable upper intake level, the maximum daily amount of a nutrient that appears to be safe, has not been established for any individual carotenoid; however, supplemental β-carotene at 20 mg day^{-1} or more is contraindicated for use in current heavy smokers by the European Commission.

Because many factors affect the assimilation of carotenoids from foods (**Figure 2**), conversion factors need to be considered. This is especially important when most sources of vitamin A are from provitamin A carotenoids in the population. Bioavailability of preformed vitamin A, i.e., retinol and retinyl esters, is not a major concern because 80–95% of them are absorbed. However, foods that are high in preformed retinol (liver, eggs, and fortified milk) are not necessarily consumed by everybody. When discussing carotenoids from food, four terms need to be defined (see **Table 1**):

- bioaccessibility refers to how much carotenoid can be extracted from the food and is available for absorption;
- bioavailability is how much carotenoid is absorbed from the food and is available for physiological function;
- bioconversion relates to the provitamin A carotenoids and is defined as the amount of retinol that is formed from absorbed provitamin A carotenoids; and
- bioefficacy encompasses all of the biological processing of provitamin A carotenoids and is the amount of retinol formed from the amount of carotenoid contained in the food.

The study of carotenoid bioefficacy from foods is important in international health as the most frequently consumed sources of vitamin A are fruit and vegetables. A 100% bioefficacy means that 1 μmol of dietary β-carotene provides 2 μmol of retinol in the body; however, 100% bioefficacy does

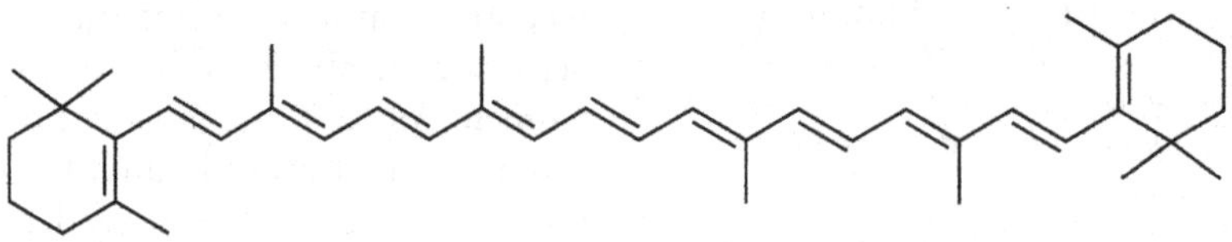

β-Carotene

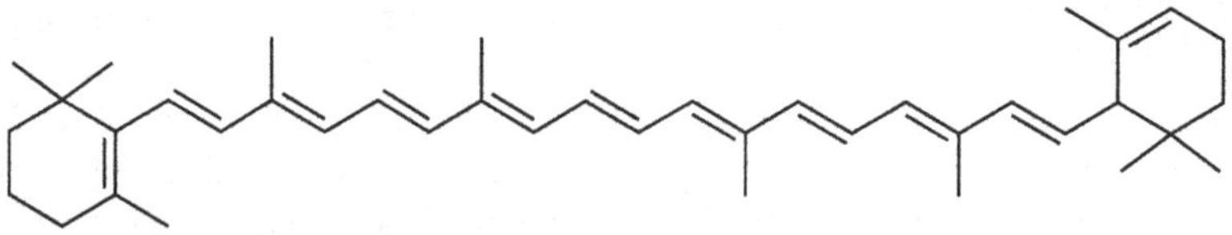

α-Carotene

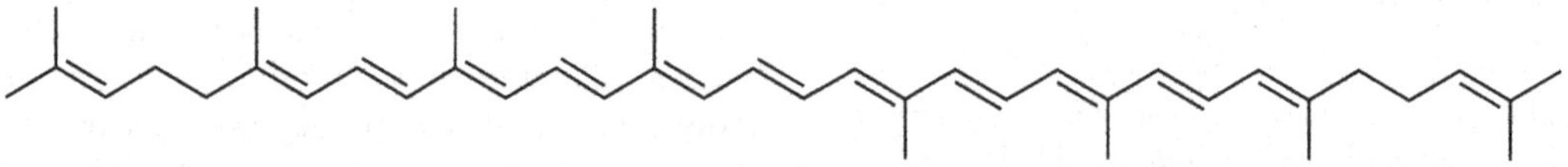

Lycopene

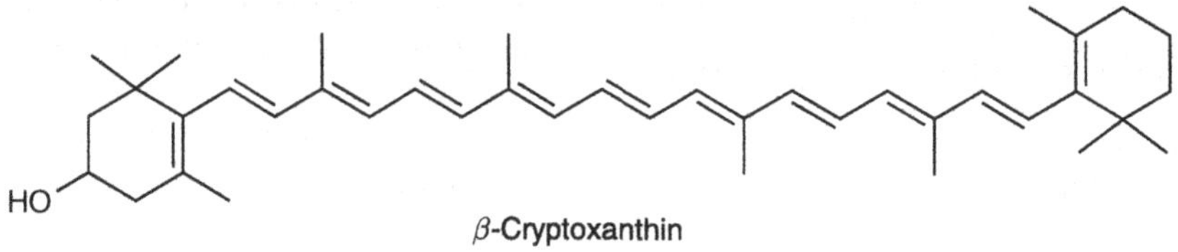

β-Cryptoxanthin

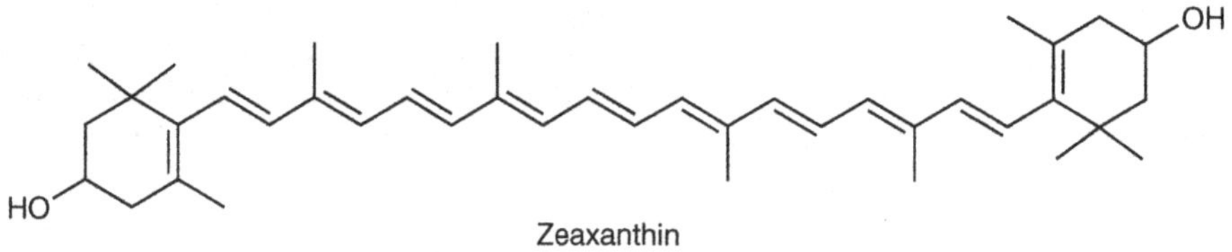

Zeaxanthin

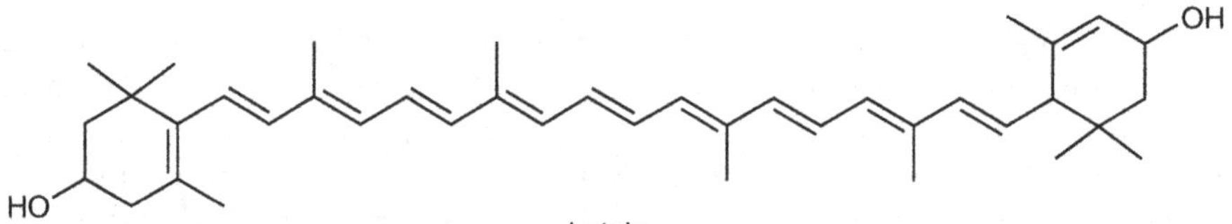

Lutein

Figure 1 The structures of the most common carotenoids found in the human body. Three of them, β-carotene, α-carotene and β-cryptoxanthin, can be used by the body to make vitamin A. All carotenoids are antioxidants found in fruits and vegetables.

not actually occur in the process of digestion and carotenoid uptake by the body.

Once in the body, carotenoids can act as potent antioxidants, which are substances that neutralize free radicals formed from the natural metabolic processes of cells. Free radicals damage tissues and cells through oxidative processes. While free radical formation is a natural process in the body, environmental factors such as smoking and pollution can increase free radical load and thus disease risk. Carotenoids may counter these influences by functioning as an antioxidant and quenching oxygen-containing free radicals. In high- and low-density lipoproteins and cell membranes, carotenoids may also regenerate the antioxidant form of vitamin E as well as protect vitamin E from oxidation.

At the whole-body level, some population studies have indicated that certain carotenoids from either dietary intake or blood concentration data are associated with better immune response, lower rates of age-related macular degeneration (AMD) and cataract, as well as lower risk for certain cancers and cardiovascular disease. β-Carotene may increase immunological functions by enhancing lymphocyte

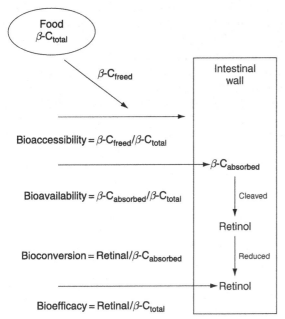

Figure 2 A schematic outlining the path of β-carotene (β-C) as it moves out from the food into the intestinal wall. The definition of terms associated with understanding β-carotene release, absorption, and conversion to retinol are illustrated: bioaccessibility, bioavailability, bionconversion, and bioefficacy. (Reproduced with permission from Tanumihardjo SA (2002) Factors influencing the conversion of carotenoids to retinol: Bioavailability to bioconversion to bioefficacy. *International Journal of Vitamin and Nutrition Research* **72**: 40–45.)

Table 1 Terms that are associated with the β-carotene vitamin A value of foods and subsequent utilization as retinol

Term	Definition	100%
Bioaccessibility	$\dfrac{\beta\text{-Carotene freed}}{\beta\text{-Carotene in food}}$	$\dfrac{1\,\mu\text{mol freed}}{1\,\mu\text{mol in food}}$
Bioavailability	$\dfrac{\beta\text{-Carotene absorbed}}{\beta\text{-Carotene in food}}$	$\dfrac{1\,\mu\text{mol absorbed}}{1\,\mu\text{mol in food}}$
Bioconversion	$\dfrac{\text{Retinol formed}}{\beta\text{-Carotene absorbed}}$	$\dfrac{2\,\mu\text{mol formed}}{1\,\mu\text{mol absorbed}}$
Bioefficacy	$\dfrac{\text{Retinol formed}}{\beta\text{-Carotene in food}}$	$\dfrac{2\,\mu\text{mol formed}}{1\,\mu\text{mol in food}}$

proliferation independent of its provitamin A functions. The associations between specific carotenoids and decreased risk of various diseases are summarized in **Table 2**.

Blood levels of specific carotenoids are often used as biomarkers of fruit and vegetable intake to strengthen or replace dietary intake data. A wide variation in analytical methods exists and standardization between laboratories does not routinely occur. Nonetheless, higher blood concentrations have been favorably correlated with certain disease states. For example, vitamin A and carotenoid concentrations in serum were measured in middle-aged women who later developed breast cancer. Median concentrations of β-carotene, lycopene, lutein, and total carotenoids were significantly lower in women with breast cancer compared with case-control women who had not developed breast cancer. In contrast, vitamin A concentrations were either not different or showed a mixed response between cohorts, suggesting that carotenoids may be protective against breast cancer. Furthermore, the Nurses' Health Study, which included a cohort of over 83 000 women, also showed a significant inverse association between dietary β-carotene intake and breast cancer risk. This was especially strong for premenopausal women with a family history of breast cancer or high alcohol consumption. However, other prospective studies have had mixed results.

Hydrocarbon Carotenoid: β-Carotene

β-Carotene is one of the most widely studied carotenoids – for both its vitamin A activity and its abundance in fruits and vegetables. Epidemiological studies have often pointed to an abundance of carotenoids in the diet being protective against many diseases. Diets rich in fruits and vegetables are recommended to reduce the risk of cardiovascular disease and some forms of cancer. However, when β-carotene is removed from the plant matrix and administered as a supplement, these benefits

Table 2 A summary of epidemiologic and/or clinical studies where carotenoids and a significant association to a specific disease risk has been shown in at least one study[a]

Carotenoid	Cardiovascular disease	Cataract	Macular degeneration	Lung cancer	Prostate cancer
β-Carotene	Yes	–	–	Yes[b]	–
α-Carotene	Yes	–	–	Yes	–
β-Cryptoxanthin	–	–	–	Yes	–
Lycopene	Yes	–	–	Yes	Yes
Lutein/zeaxanthin	Yes	Yes	Yes	Yes	–

[a]For a more complete discussion of the association of specific carotenoids to disease please refer to: Krinsky NI, Mayne SI, and Sies H, (eds.) (2004) *Carotenoids in Health and Disease*. New York: Marcel Dekker.
[b]The opposite finding has been observed in clinical trials.

sometimes disappear. For example, because lung cancer is the leading cause of cancer death in many developed countries, the β-Carotene and Retinol Efficacy Trial (CARET) in the 1990s set out to test whether β-carotene conferred protection against cancer. CARET was based on a number of observational studies that showed high levels of β-carotene from food sources were protective against lung cancer. However, the CARET trial was halted for showing an increased risk for lung cancer in the treatment group over the control. Subsequent studies in ferrets showed that the amounts of β-carotene commonly consumed from fruit and vegetables were protective against lung damage but higher amounts, equivalent to those in CARET, increased the formation of abnormal tissue in the lung.

A similar outcome was observed among smokers in the α-Tocopherol β-Carotene (ATBC) Study Group. Although evidence clearly exists showing an association between β-carotene and enhanced lung function, as in the CARET study, the ATBC trial also found an increase in lung cancer rates among smokers. It is plausible that the lung cancer had already been initiated in the smokers and supplementation with β-carotene could not prevent the development of cancer. The ATBC study also showed an increased incidence of angina pectoris, a mild warning sign of heart disease characterized by chest pain, among heavy smokers. This may have been due to low blood levels of vitamin C in the study group leading to the inability of the individuals to quench β-carotene radicals, but this relationship requires more research.

In both the CARET and ATBC intervention trials, much higher doses of β-carotene were used than could be obtained from the diet, and the blood levels attained were two to six times higher than the 95th percentile level of β-carotene in a survey of a representative sample of the US population. Thus, it remains unclear whether β-carotene is a procarcinogen or an anticarcinogen. The associations for lower disease risk observed in epidemiologic studies may reflect other protective dietary agents or an interaction between dietary components. Furthermore, people with higher intake of fruits and vegetables may have healthier lifestyles that contribute to their lower risk of chronic diseases. The higher disease risk observed in the clinical trials may be correlated with the use of high doses of β-carotene where the mechanisms have not yet been identified, the limited duration of treatment, and/or the timing of the interventions was too late for cancers that were already present due to a history of heavy smoking. More research on β-carotene's biological actions is needed to explore the mechanisms involved. Current

consensus is that the beneficial effects of β-carotene are associated with dietary consumption, whereas the harmful effects in some subpopulations are with pharmacological supplements.

Another explanation for a lack of a beneficial outcome with β-carotene supplementation may be that not all people respond to the same degree to β-carotene treatment, some being low- or non-responders. Some researchers believe that individuals who do not respond to β-carotene supplementation may be better at converting it to vitamin A. Blood response to β-carotene supplementation is also inversely related to body mass index (BMI), which may be due to increased sequestration of lipophilic β-carotene by the larger amount of fat stores present in people with larger BMI. This theory may not hold true as individuals with larger BMIs do not necessarily have a high body fat percentage, but rather increased lean muscle mass.

Excellent food sources of β-carotene include carrots, winter squash, red-orange sweet potato, and various types of dark green leafy vegetables. No deficiency or toxicity has been observed from dietary β-carotene intake, although very rarely high intakes can be associated with yellow pigmentation of the skin as carotenoids are stored in adipose tissue. Supplements containing β-carotene are common. In the Women's Health Initiative, the largest observational/intervention study in postmenopausal women to date, approximately 50% reported using a supplement containing β-carotene. This trial included both a clinical trial and observational study involving more than 160 000 women. The Physicians' Health Study II also included β-carotene as one of its interventions to determine the balance of risks and benefits of this carotenoid with cancer, cardiovascular disease, and eye disease.

Hydrocarbon Carotenoid: α-Carotene

α-Carotene, another carotenoid frequently present in food, also has provitamin A activity. Based on its structure, it is only converted to one molecule of biologically active retinol after central cleavage. Like other carotenoids, it has antioxidant and possibly anticarcinogenic properties, and may enhance immune function as well. Some, but not all, epidemiological studies observed that higher α-carotene intake was associated with lower risk of cardiovascular disease and cancer, whereas others did not. Clinical trials to test α-carotene influences in humans have not been conducted to date. This is probably because α-carotene is usually associated with ample amounts of β-carotene when found in fruits and vegetables and singling out α-carotene is difficult.

α-Carotene's concentration is especially high in orange carrots. Low or high dietary intake of α-carotene alone has not been associated with any specific disease outcome or health condition.

Xanthophyll: β-Cryptoxanthin

β-Cryptoxanthin is one of the lesser known carotenoids that also has provitamin A activity and appears to have a protective health role. Several epidemiological studies suggest that dietary β-cryptoxanthin is associated with lower rates of lung cancer and improved lung function in humans. A large prospective study on dietary intake and cancer, which included an interview on dietary habits and life style, identified β-cryptoxanthin as protective against lung cancer after correcting for smoking. However, the beneficial effects for β-cryptoxanthin suggested by these results could be merely an indicator for other antioxidants and/or a measure of a healthy life style that are more common in people with high dietary intakes of β-cryptoxanthin. In tissue culture, β-cryptoxanthin has a direct stimulatory effect on bone formation and an inhibitory effect on bone resorption. Studies of these beneficial effects in humans have not been conducted.

No deficiency or toxicity has been observed from dietary β-cryptoxanthin intake. The best food sources for β-cryptoxanthin are oranges, papaya, peaches, and tangerines. Tropical fruit intake is directly proportional to β-cryptoxanthin blood concentrations.

Hydrocarbon Carotenoid: Lycopene

Lycopene, while having no provitamin A activity, is a potent antioxidant with twice the activity of β-carotene for quenching singlet oxygen and 10 times the antioxidant activity of α-tocopherol in some model systems. The antioxidant potential of food chemicals varies widely according to location in the body and the presence of other body chemicals. The primary sources of dietary lycopene are tomatoes and tomato products. Epidemiological evidence shows an inverse association between lycopene consumption and the incidence and development of certain cancers. This association is especially strong for prostate cancer, which is the most common cancer among men in Western countries and the second leading cause of cancer death in American men. Prostate cancer rates in Asian countries are much lower, but appear to be increasing rapidly. Lycopene is localized in prostate tissue. The current consensus is that a high consumption of tomatoes or high circulating concentrations of lycopene are associated with a 30–40% risk reduction for prostate cancer, especially the most aggressive forms. Recent studies in rats show that tomato products are more protective against prostate cancer than isolated lycopene.

Epidemiologic studies have also observed lower rates of bladder, cervical, and breast cancers as well as cancers of the gastrointestinal tract among people with high intake of lycopene. The discovery of significant concentrations of lycopene in specific tissues in the body, i.e., plasma, testes, adrenal glands, liver and kidney, suggests that lycopene may play a role in these tissues.

While the body of evidence seems strong, several studies have found either no or weak associations between lycopene consumption and disease. Some of this may be explained by the fact that blood lycopene concentrations were much lower in these studies than in those that showed a beneficial effect. Thus, future dietary based studies need to include blood sampling to further define the range of blood concentrations of lycopene in the population, ideally with method standardization so that studies can be directly compared. The prostate cancer association is usually stronger for cooked tomato products rather than raw tomatoes or total lycopene intake. This too supports the idea that it is the whole food, with a broad array of nutrients and nonnutritive bioactive components, that is important for overall health rather than isolated compounds. It is possible that the beneficial effects of tomatoes are increased by preparing a concentrated product that enhances the nutrient bioavailability, as processed and cooked tomatoes are more closely associated to decreased risk of disease than either raw tomatoes or tomato juice.

Because lycopene is a potent antioxidant, it may be protective against heart disease by slowing down the oxidation of polyunsaturated fats in the low-density lipoprotein particles in the blood. Epidemiological and clinical studies show that higher blood lycopene concentrations are associated with lower risk and incidence of cardiovascular disease. Higher fat stores of lycopene have also been associated with lower risk of myocardial infarction. The most profound protective effect is in nonsmokers. The evidence for protective cardiovascular effects is compelling, as studies have shown a 20–60% improvement in cardiovascular parameters with higher blood concentrations of lycopene. Furthermore, higher intake of fruits and vegetables is associated with better lung function. In particular, high tomato intake is associated with higher timed expiratory volume.

The major food source of lycopene globally is tomatoes and tomato products. In the US, more than 80% of dietary lycopene comes from tomatoes. Other sources include watermelon, pink grapefruit, and red carrots.

Xanthophylls: Lutein and Zeaxanthin

The structural isomers lutein and zeaxanthin are non-provitamin A carotenoids that are also measurable in human blood and tissues. Lutein and zeaxanthin have been identified as the xanthophylls that constitute the macular pigment of the human retina. The relative concentration of lutein to zeaxanthin in the macula is distinctive. Zeaxanthin is more centralized and lutein predominates towards the outer area of the macula. A putative xanthophyll-binding protein has also been described, which may explain the high variability among people to accumulate these carotenoids into eye tissues. Increased lutein intake from both food sources and supplements is positively correlated with increased macular pigment density, which is theorized to lower risk for macular degeneration. AMD is the leading cause of irreversible blindness in the elderly in developed countries. AMD adversely affects the central field of vision and the ability to see fine detail. Some, but not all, population studies suggest lower rates of AMD among people with higher levels of lutein and zeaxanthin in the diet or blood. Possible mechanisms of action for these carotenoids include antioxidant protection of the retinal tissue and the macular pigment filtering of damaging blue light.

Free radical damage is also linked to the development of cataracts. Cataracts remain the leading cause of visual disability in the US and about one-half of the 30–50 million cases of blindness throughout the world. Although cataracts are treatable, blindness occurs because individuals have either chosen not to correct the disease or do not have access to the appropriate medical treatment. Several epidemiological studies have shown inverse associations between the risk of cataracts and carotenoid intake. However, these studies also present inconsistencies with regard to the different carotenoids and their association with cataract risk. Lutein and zeaxanthin are found in the lens and are thought to protect cells in the eye against oxidative damage, and consequently prevent formation of cataracts. However, to date, there is no evidence that any carotenoid supplement can protect against cataract development. Eating plenty of fruits and vegetables, good sources of many antioxidants including carotenoids, is a preventative measure for many diseases.

Because lutein and zeaxanthin may be involved in disease prevention, much needs to be learned regarding human consumption of these carotenoids. One complicating factor that requires better understanding is the bioavailability of lutein from food sources and supplements. The food matrix is an important factor influencing lutein bioavailability and the amount and type of food processing generally influences the bioavailability of all carotenoids. For example, the processing of spinach does not affect bioavailability of lutein, but it does enhance that of β-carotene. Such studies have been conducted with lutein supplements and/or foods containing lutein fed to human subjects. In humans, lutein from vegetables seems to be more bioavailable than β-carotene; however, this may be partially explained by bioconversion of β-carotene to vitamin A. Competition between carotenoids, such as lutein and β-carotene, for incorporation into chylomicra has been noted in humans consuming vegetables and supplements. The amount of fat consumed with the lutein source also affects bioavailability, as higher fat increases the bioavailability of lipid-soluble carotenoids. Decreased plasma lutein concentrations are noted when alcohol is consumed, but the mechanism is poorly defined.

Lutein may also protect against some forms of cancer and enhance immune function. Lutein may work in concert with other carotenoids such as β-carotene to lower cancer risk due to their antimutagenic and antitumor properties. Because of these potential health benefits, lutein supplements are sold commercially and incorporated into some multivitamins. However, the amount provided in multivitamins (about 10–20% of the level in an average diet) is likely to be too low for a biological influence. Levels of lutein available as a single supplement vary widely and neither benefit nor safety of lutein supplements has been adequately studied. Major dietary sources of both lutein and zeaxanthin in the diet include corn, green leafy vegetables, and eggs. Lutein tends to be the predominant isomer in foods. Lutein supplements are often derived from marigold flowers.

Summary

Most of the epidemiological evidence points to carotenoids being a very important class of phytochemicals. While some of the effects may be attributable to a diet high in fruits and vegetables, and an overall healthy lifestyle, the presence of specific carotenoids localized in different areas of the human body lend evidence to their overall importance in the human diet. As methods are developed to assess carotenoid levels noninvasively in humans, large-scale studies that determine carotenoid levels in blood, skin, and the eye may lead to a better understanding of their importance in human health and disease prevention. Additional epidemiologic studies to further strengthen the associations that have been observed in populations are needed.

It must be kept in mind that study design and statistical analyses vary across published work and no one study can give conclusive evidence. An integrated multidisciplinary approach to study the functions and actions of carotenoids in the body is necessary to understand fully the role of carotenoids in health and disease prevention. This includes comparisons of carotenoids in whole fruits and vegetables and their effect on human health and well being. High fruit and vegetable intake is associated with a decreased risk of cancer, cardiovascular disease, diabetes, AMD, and osteoporosis. Removing any one class of phytochemicals from the intricate matrix of the whole plant may not give the same beneficial outcome in terms of human health. Considering that the average intake of fruits and vegetables is still less than that recommended by health professionals, programs that promote the consumption of more fruit and vegetables may be more effective at preventing disease in the long-term than using individual pharmacological carotenoid supplements.

A question that remains is whether or not carotenoids can be considered nutrients. A variety of phytochemicals contained in fruits and vegetables including carotenoids are assumed to be needed for optimal health and reduction of chronic disease risk, but have not been classified as nutrients. Indeed, in 2000, the Institute of Medicine was unable to recommend a daily reference intake for any carotenoid. Several factors have been defined that categorize substances as nutrients: substances that must be obtained from the diet because the body cannot synthesize the active form, and are used in the body for growth, maintenance, and tissue repair. In addition, to being classified as a nutrient, further studies must be done to determine the essentiality of the substance and its specific function in the body. Other criteria for defining a nutrient include concentration in specific tissues, consumption, and/or supplementation resulting in tissue concentration increases and improved tissue function. Lastly, a daily established dosage needs to be defined and a biomarker identified to assess status.

A large body of observational studies suggests that high blood concentrations of carotenoids obtained from food are associated with chronic disease risk reduction. However, there is little other evidence of their specific role in the body. Lutein and zeaxanthin are the only carotenoids found in a specific tissue (the macular region of the retina) that seem to have a specific function. Providing lutein in the diet increases macular pigment in humans. Animal studies show that a diet low in lutein can deplete macular pigment, but the influence on the health of the eye is not yet well understood. To further our understanding, large randomized prospective intervention trials need to be conducted to explore the essentiality of lutein supplementation for reducing ocular disease risk in humans. Thus, to date, no one specific carotenoid has been classified as an essential nutrient.

See also: **Antioxidants**: Diet and Antioxidant Defense; Observational Studies; Intervention Studies. **Carotenoids**: Chemistry, Sources and Physiology. **Coronary Heart Disease**: Prevention. **Lycopenes and Related Compounds. Phytochemicals**: Epidemiological Factors. **Supplementation**: Dietary Supplements.

Further Reading

Alves-Rodrigues A and Shao A (2004) The science behind lutein. *Toxicology Letters* 150: 57–83.

Christen WG, Gaziano JM, and Hennekens CH (2000) Design of Physicians' Health Study II – a randomized trial of beta-carotene, vitamins E and C, and multivitamins, in prevention of cancer, cardiovascular disease, and eye disease, and review of results of completed trials. *Annals of Epidemiology* 10: 125–134.

Giovannucci E (2002) A review of epidemiologic studies of tomatoes, lycopene, and prostate cancer. *Experimental Biology of Medicine* 227: 852–859.

Hwang ES and Bowen PE (2002) Can the consumption of tomatoes or lycopene reduce cancer risk? *Integrative Cancer Therapies* 1: 121–132.

Institute of Medicine, Food and Nutrition Board (2000) *Dietary Reference Intakes for Vitamin C, Vitamin E, Selenium, and Carotenoids*. Washington, DC: National Academy Press.

Johnson EJ (2002) The role of carotenoids in human health. *Nutrition in Clinical Care* 5: 56–65.

Krinsky NI, Landrum JT, and Bone RA (2003) Biologic mechanisms of the protective role of lutein and zeaxanthin in the eye. *Annual Review of Nutrition* 23: 171–201.

Krinsky NI, Mayne SI, and Sies H (eds.) (2004) *Carotenoids in Health and Disease*. New York: Marcel Dekker.

Mares-Perlman JA, Millen AE, Ficek TL, and Hankinson SE (2002) The body of evidence to support a protective role for lutein and zeaxanthin in delaying chronic disease. *Journal of Nutrition* 132: 518S–524S.

Rapola JM, Virtamo J, Haukka JK *et al.* (1996) Effect of vitamin E and beta-carotene on the incidence of angina pectoris. A randomized, double-blind, controlled trial. *Journal of the American Medical Association* 275: 693–698.

Tanumihardjo SA (2002) Factors influencing the conversion of carotenoids to retinol: Bioavailability to bioconversion to bioefficacy. *International Journal of Vitamin and Nutrition Research* 72: 40–45.

The Alpha-Tocopherol Beta Carotene Cancer Prevention Study Group (1994) The effect of vitamin E and beta carotene on the incidence of lung cancer and other cancers in male smokers. *New England Journal of Medicine* 330: 1029–1035.

CHOLINE AND PHOSPHATIDYLCHOLINE

X Zhu and S H Zeisel, University of North Carolina at Chapel Hill, Chapel Hill, NC, USA

Introduction

Choline, an essential nutrient for humans, is consumed in many foods. It is part of several major phospholipids (including phosphatidylcholine – also called lecithin) that are critical for normal membrane structure and function. Also, as the major precursor of betaine it is used by the kidney to maintain water balance and by the liver as a source of methyl groups for the removal of homocysteine in methionine formation. Finally, choline is used to produce the important neurotransmitter acetylcholine (catalyzed by choline acetyltransferase in cholinergic neurons and in such non-nervous tissues as the placenta). Each of these functions for choline is absolutely vital for the maintenance of normal function.

Although there is significant capacity for biosynthesis of the choline moiety in the liver, choline deficiency can occur in humans. Male adults deprived of dietary choline become depleted of choline in their tissues and develop liver and muscle damage. Premenopausal women may not be sensitive to dietary choline deficiency (unpublished data). No experiments have been conducted to determine if this occurs in similarly deprived pregnant women, infants, and children.

Endogenous Formation of Choline Moiety as Phosphatidylcholine

Unless eaten in the diet, choline can only be formed during phosphatidylcholine biosynthesis through the methylation of phosphatidylethanolamine by phosphatidylethanolamine N-methyltransferase (PEMT) using S-adenosylmethionine as the methyl donor. This enzyme is most active in the liver but has been identified in many other tissues including brain and mammary gland. At least two isoforms of PEMT exist: PEMT1, localized to the endoplasmic reticulum and generating the majority of PEMT activity, and PEMT2, which resides on mitochondria-associated membranes. Both enzymes are encoded by the same gene but differ either because of post-translational modification or alternative splicing. This gene is very polymorphic and functional

SNPs (single nucleotide polymorphisms) in humans may exist and, if so, would influence dietary requirements for choline. In mice in which this gene is knocked out, the dietary requirement for choline is increased and they get fatty liver when eating a normal choline diet. Estrogen induces greater activity of PEMT perhaps explaining why premenopausal women require less choline in their diets. In addition to formation of choline, this enzyme has an essential role in lipoprotein secretion from the liver.

Choline, Homocysteine, and Folate are Interrelated Nutrients

Choline, methionine, methyltetrahydrofolate (methyl-THF), and vitamins B_6 and B_{12} are closely interconnected at the transmethylation metabolic pathways that form methionine from homocysteine. Perturbing the metabolism of one of these pathways results in compensatory changes in the others. For example, as noted above, choline can be synthesized *de novo* using methyl groups derived from methionine (via S-adenosylmethionine). Methionine can be formed from homocysteine using methyl groups from methyl-THF, or using methyl groups from betaine that are derived from choline. Similarly, methyl-THF can be formed from one-carbon units derived from serine or from the methyl groups of choline via dimethylglycine. When animals and humans are deprived of choline, they use more methyl-THF to remethylate homocysteine in the liver and increase dietary folate requirements. Conversely, when they are deprived of folate, they use more methyl groups from choline, increasing the dietary requirement for choline. There is a common polymorphism in the gene for methyltetrahydrofolate reductase that increases dietary requirement for folic acid; 15–30% of humans have this mutation. In mice in which this gene is knocked out, the dietary requirement for choline is increased and they get fatty liver when eating a normal choline diet.

Choline in Foods

Choline, choline esters, and betaine can be found in significant amounts in many foods consumed by humans (see **Figure 1** and **Figure 2**); some of the choline and betaine is added during processing (especially in the preparation of infant formula).

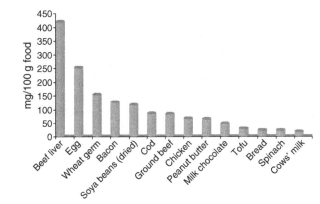

Figure 1 Total choline content of some common foods. Foods, which had been prepared as normally eaten, were analyzed for choline, phosphocholine, glycerophosphocholine, phosphatidylcholine, and sphingomyelin content using an HPLC mass spectrometric method. (Modified from Zeisel SH, Mar M-H, Howe JC, and Holden JM (2003) Concentrations of choline-containing compounds and betaine in common foods. *Journal of Nutrition* 133: 1302–1307.)

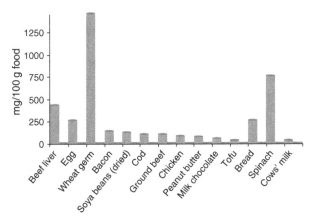

Figure 2 Total choline plus betaine content of some common foods. For methyl donation choline must be converted to betaine, thus the methyl donor capacity is best expressed as total choline and betaine content, assayed as in **Figure 1**. Several vegetable and grain products contain significant amounts of betaine (Modified from Zeisel SH, Mar M-H, Howe JC, and Holden JM (2003) Concentrations of choline-containing compounds and betaine in common foods. *Journal of Nutrition* 133: 1302–1307.)

Though the different esters of choline have different bioavailability, it is likely that choline in all forms is fungible; therefore, total choline content is probably the best indicator of food choline content. Betaine should also be considered, as it spares the use of choline for methyl donation.

A number of epidemiologic studies have examined the relationship between dietary folic acid and cancer or heart disease. It may be helpful to also consider choline intake as a confounding factor because folate and choline methyl donation can be interchangeable.

Table 1 Recommended adequate intakes (AI) for choline

Population	Age	AI (mg day⁻¹)
Infants	0–6 months	125
	6–12 months	150
Children	1 through 3 years	200
	4 through 8 years	250
	9 through 13 years	375
Males	14 through 18 years	550
	19 years and older	550
Females	14 through 18 years	400
	19 years and older	425
Pregnancy	All ages	450
Lactation	All ages	550

From Institute of Medicine, National Academy of Sciences USA (1998) Dietary reference intakes for folate, thiamin, riboflavin, niacin, vitamin B₁₂, panthothenic acid, biotin, and choline, vol. 1. Washington DC: National Academy Press.

Dietary Recommendations

The Institute of Medicine, USA National Academy of Sciences, recommended an adequate intake (I) of 550 mg/70 kg body weight for choline in the diet. This amount may be influenced by gender, and it may be influenced by pregnancy, lactation, and stage of development (**Table 1**).

Amino acid-glucose solutions used in total parenteral nutrition of humans lack choline. The lipid emulsions that deliver extra calories and essential fatty acids during parenteral nutrition contain choline in the form of lecithin (20% emulsion contains 13.2 mmol l⁻¹). Humans treated with parenteral nutrition require 1–1.7 mmol of choline-containing phospholipid per day during the first week of parenteral nutrition therapy to maintain plasma choline levels.

Human milk, which contains approximately 200 mg l⁻¹ choline and choline esters, is an especially good source of choline. An infant consuming 500 ml breast milk in a day ingests 50 mg choline. Human milk is not a static food; its choline composition changes over time postnatally. The choline composition of infant formulas can differ greatly from that present in human milk. It is essential that variations in the bioavailability and utilization of choline, phosphocholine, glycerophosphocholine, and lecithin in milk be considered when milk substitutes are developed.

Functional Effects of Varying Choline in the Diet

Fatty Liver

The triacylglycerol (TG) produced by the liver is mainly delivered to other tissues as very low-density lipoprotein (VLDL) of which lecithin is a required component. In choline deficiency, the diminished ability of liver cells to synthesize new lecithin molecules results in the intracellular accumulation of TG. Treating malnourished patients with high-calorie total parenteral nutrition (TPN) solutions that contain little or no choline will deplete choline stores and cause fatty liver and hepatic dysfunction that can be reversed by treatment with phosphatidylcholine.

Liver Cell Death

When deprived of dietary choline, healthy male subjects have diminished plasma concentrations of choline and phosphatidylcholine, and they develop liver cell death (elevated plasma alanine aminotransferase). In similarly deprived animal models, the liver cell death is caused by apoptosis, a regulated form of cell suicide. In an ongoing study of choline deficiency in humans, muscle cell death (elevated plasma creatine phosphokinase, MM form) has also been noted.

Liver Cancer

Dietary deficiency of choline in rodents causes development of hepatocarcinomas in the absence of any known carcinogen. Choline is the only single nutrient for which this is true. It is interesting that choline-deficient rats not only have a higher incidence of spontaneous hepatocarcinoma but also are markedly sensitized to the effects of administered carcinogens. Several mechanisms are suggested for the cancer-promoting effect of a choline-devoid diet. A progressive increase in cell proliferation that is related to regeneration after parenchymal cell death occurs in the choline-deficient liver. Cell proliferation and its associated increased rate of DNA synthesis could be the cause of the heightened sensitivity to chemical carcinogens. Methylation of DNA is essential to the regulation of expression of genetic information, and the undermethylation of DNA observed during choline deficiency (despite adequate dietary methionine) may be responsible for carcinogenesis. Choline-deficient rats experience increased lipid peroxidation in the liver. Lipid peroxides in the nucleus are a possible source of free radicals that could modify DNA and cause carcinogenesis. Choline deficiency activates protein kinase C signaling, usually involved in growth factor signaling in hepatocytes. Finally, a defect in cell suicide (apoptosis) mechanisms may contribute to the carcinogenesis of choline deficiency.

Kidney Function

Renal function is compromised by choline deficiency, which leads to abnormal concentrating ability, free-water reabsorption, sodium excretion, glomerular filtration rate, renal plasma flow, and gross renal hemorrhage. The deterioration in renal function may be related to changes in acetylcholine release by nerves that regulate blood flow to the kidney. Additionally, the renal glomerulus uses the choline-metabolite betaine as an osmolyte to assist cells in maintaining their volume in the presence of concentrated salts in urine.

Brain Development

During the fetal and neonatal period, the availability of choline to tissues fluctuates because of the varied dietary intake of choline among neonates and the slower oxidation of choline during the first weeks of life. However, ensured availability of this amine appears to be vital to infants because organ growth, which is extremely rapid in the neonate, requires large amounts of choline for membrane biosynthesis. Choline is also particularly important during the neonatal period because it appears to change brain function. There are two sensitive periods in rat brain development during which treatment with choline produces long-lasting enhancement of spatial memory that is lifelong and has been detected in elderly rats. The first occurs during embryonic days 12–17 and the second, during postnatal days 16–30. Choline supplementation during these critical periods elicits a major improvement in memory performance at all stages of training on a 12-arm radial maze.

The choline-induced spatial memory facilitation correlates with altered distribution and morphology of neurons involved in memory storage within the brain, with biochemical changes in the adult hippocampus and with electrophysiological changes in the adult hippocampus. It also correlates with changes in proliferation, apoptosis, and migration of neuronal precursor cells in the hippocampus during fetal brain development. When pregnant rats were treated with varying levels of dietary choline between day 12 and 18 of gestation, it was found that choline deficiency significantly decreased the rate of mitosis in the neuroepithelium of fetal brain adjacent to the hippocampus. An increased number of apoptotic cells were found in the region of the dentate gyrus of choline-deficient hippocampus compared to controls. Modulation of dietary choline availability changed the distribution and migration of precursor cells produced on embryonic day 16 in the fimbria, primordial dentate gyrus, and Ammon's horn of the fetal hippocampus. Choline deficiency also decreased the migration of newly proliferating cells from the neuroepithelium into the lateral septum, thus indicating that the sensitivity of fetal brain to choline availability is not restricted to the hippocampus. The expression of TOAD-64 protein, an early neuronal differentiation marker, increased in the hippocampus of choline-deficient day E18 fetal brains compared to controls. These findings show that dietary choline availability during pregnancy alters the timing of mitosis, apoptosis, migration, and the early commitment to neuronal differentiation by progenitor cells in fetal brain hippocampus and septum, two regions known to be associated with learning and memory.

A disruption in choline uptake and metabolism during neurulation produces neural tube defects in mouse embryos grown *in vitro*. Exposing early somite staged mouse embryos *in vitro* with an inhibitor of choline uptake and metabolism, 2-dimethylaminoethanol (DMAE) causes craniofacial hypoplasia and open neural tube defects in the forebrain, midbrain, and hindbrain regions. Embryos exposed to an inhibitor of phosphatidylcholine synthesis, 1-O-octadecyl-2-O-methyl-rac-glycero-3-phosphocholine (ET-18-OCH$_3$) exhibit similar defects or expansion of the brain vesicles and a distended neural tube at the posterior neuropore as well as increased areas of cell death. Thus, choline like folic acid is important during neural tube closure.

Are these findings in rats likely to apply to humans? We do not know. Human and rat brains mature at different rates; rat brain is comparatively more mature at birth than is the human brain, but in humans synaptogenesis may continue for months after birth. Are we varying the availability of choline when we substitute infant formulas for human milk? Does choline intake in infancy contribute to variations in memory observed between humans? These are good questions that warrant additional research.

Brain Function in Adults

It is unlikely that choline acetyltransferase in brain is saturated with either of its substrates, so that choline (and possibly acetyl-CoA) availability determines the rate of acetylcholine synthesis. Under conditions of rapid neuronal firing acetylcholine release by brain neurons can be directly altered by dietary intake of choline. Based on this observation, choline has been used as a possible memory-improvement drug. In some patients with Alzheimer's disease, choline or phosphatidylcholine has beneficial effects, but this effect is variable. Both verbal and visual memory may be impaired in other patients who require long-term intravenous feeding and this may be improved with choline supplementation.

Measurement of Choline and Choline Esters

Radioisotopic, high-pressure liquid chromatography, and gas chromatography/isotope dilution mass spectrometry (GC/IDMS) methods are available for measurement of choline. However, these existing methods are cumbersome and time consuming, and none measures all of the compounds of choline derivatives. Recently, a new method has been established for quantifying choline, betaine, acetylcholine, glycerophosphocholine, cytidine diphosphocholine, phosphocholine, phosphatidylcholine, and sphingomyelin in liver, plasma, various foods, and brain using liquid chromatography/electrospray ionization-isotope dilution mass spectrometry (LC/ESI-IDMS).

Acknowledgments

Supported by the National Institutes of Health (DK55865, AG09525, DK56350).

See also: **Folic Acid**. **Vitamin B$_6$**.

Further Reading

Albright CD, Tsai AY, Friedrich CB, Mar MH, and Zeisel SH (1999) Choline availability alters embryonic development of the hippocampus and septum in the rat. *Brain Research. Developmental Brain Research* 113: 13–20.

Buchman AL, Dubin M, Jenden D, Moukarzel A, Roch MH, Rice K, Gornbein J, Ament ME, and Eckhert CD (1992) Lecithin increases plasma free choline and decreases hepatic steatosis in long-term total parenteral nutrition patients. *Gastroenterology* 102: 1363–1370.

da Costa KA, Badea M, Fischer LM, and Zeisel SH (2004) Elevated serum creatine phosphokinase in choline-deficient humans: mechanistic studies in C2C12 mouse myoblasts. *Am J Clin Nutr* 80: 163–70.

Institute of Medicine, National Academy of Sciences USA (1998) *Dietary Reference Intakes for Folate, Thiamin, Riboflavin, Niacin, Vitamin B12, Panthothenic Acid, Biotin, and Choline*, vol. 1. Washington DC: National Academy Press.

Koc H, Mar MH, Ranasinghe A, Swenberg JA, and Zeisel SH (2002) Quantitation of choline and its metabolites in tissues and foods by liquid chromatography/electrospray ionization-isotope dilution mass spectrometry. *Analytical Chemistry* 74: 4734–4740.

Meck WH and Williams CL (1997) Simultaneous temporal processing is sensitive to prenatal choline availability in mature and aged rats. *Neuroreport* 8: 3045–3051.

Montoya DA, White AM, Williams CL, Blusztajn JK, Meck WH, and Swartzwelder HS (2000) Prenatal choline exposure alters hippocampal responsiveness to cholinergic stimulation in adulthood. *Brain Research. Developmental Brain Research* 123: 25–32.

Niculescu MD and Zeisel SH (2002) Diet, methyl donors and DNA methylation: interactions between dietary folate, methionine and choline. *Journal of Nutrition* 132: 2333S–2335S.

Zeisel SH and Blusztajn JK (1994) Choline and human nutrition. *Annual Review of Nutrition* 14: 269–296.

Zeisel SH, daCosta K-A, Franklin PD, Alexander EA, Lamont JT, Sheard NF, and Beiser A (1991) Choline, an essential nutrient for humans. *FASEB Journal* 5: 2093–2098.

Zeisel SH, Mar M-H, Howe JC, and Holden JM (2003) Concentrations of choline-containing compounds and betaine in common foods. *Journal of Nutrition* 133: 1302–1307.

COPPER

X Xu, S Pin, J Shedlock and Z L Harris, Johns Hopkins Hospital and School of Medicine, Baltimore, MD, USA

Introduction

Transition metals occupy a special niche in aerobic physiology: as facile electron donors and acceptors, they are essential participants in oxidation/reduction reactions throughout the cell. These unique properties of transition metals are largely dependent on the electronic configuration of the electrons in the outer shell and in the penultimate outer shell. These metals can exist in different oxidation states, which is critical for their usefulness as catalysts. However, it is during these same committed reactions essential for aerobic metabolism that toxic reactive oxygen species can be generated. As such the transition metals are chaperoned as they traffic through the body and are regulated tightly. Subtle disruptions of metal homeostasis culminate in disease and death. Iron, copper, and zinc are the most abundant and well-studied transition metals. Copper is the oldest metal in use: copper artifacts dating back to 8700BC have been found. The physiology, requirements, and dietary sources of copper are described here with an emphasis on the role of copper in human health and disease.

Copper, as a trace metal, can be found in all living cells in either the oxidized Cu(II) or reduced Cu(I) state. Copper is an essential cofactor for many enzymes critical for cellular oxidation. These include: cytochrome *c*-oxidase, which is essential for mitochondrial respiration as the terminal enzyme in the electron transport chain; superoxide dismutase, a potent antioxidant defense mechanism; tyrosinase, which is critical for melanin production; dopamine B-hydroxylase, a prerequisite for catecholamine production; lysyl oxidase, which is responsible for collagen and elastin cross-linking; ceruloplasmin, a ferroxidase/metallo-oxidase; hephaestin, a ferroxidase/metallo-oxidase; and peptidylglycine α-amidating monooxygenase, a peptide processor (**Table 1**). Mice that lack the copper transport protein Ctr1 are embryonic lethal, which confirms the importance of copper in enzyme function and normal cellular homeostasis.

Copper Homeostasis

Dietary intake of copper is approximately 5 mg day^{-1} with an equivalent amount being excreted by bile in stool. Approximately 2 mg day^{-1} are directly absorbed across the gastrointestinal tract daily and incorporated into blood, serum, liver, brain, muscle, and kidney. An equal amount is excreted and maintains the sensitive copper balance (**Figure 1**). The main sources of copper are seeds, grains, nuts, beans, shellfish, and liver (**Table 2**). Drinking water no longer contributes significantly. When copper pipes were commonly used for

Table 1 Mammalian copper enzymes

Enzyme	Function
Cytochrome *c*-oxidase	Mitochondrial respiration
cu,zn-Superoxide dismutase	Antioxidant defense
Tyrosinase	Melanin production
Dopamine B-hydroxylase	Catecholamine production
Lysyl oxidase	Collagen and elastin cross-linking
Ceruloplasmin	Ferroxidase/metallo-oxidase
Hephaestin	Ferroxidase/metallo-oxidase
PAM	Peptide processing

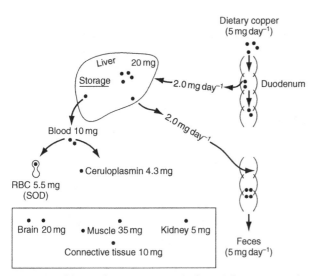

Figure 1 Mammalian copper metabolism: daily copper cycle including oral absorption, tissue distribution, and excretion. Values are for adult men (mg day⁻¹). An equal amount of copper is absorbed and excreted to maintain copper balance.

Table 2 Copper content of various foods

Food	Copper concentration (μg wet wt)	Size of typical serving (g)	Copper/ serving (mg g⁻¹)
Fish	0.61	120	0.070
Turkey	0.71	120	0.090
Chicken	0.34	120	0.040
Hamburger	0.95	120	0.110
Roast beef	0.82	120	0.100
Steak	1.2	120	0.140
Sheep liver	157.05	120	18.850
Pork liver	141.14	120	16.940
Egg	0.8	40	0.030
Single sliced cheese	0.43	120	0.050
Whole wheat	1.07	30	0.030
Scallops	6.08	120	0.030
Clams	7.39	120	0.730
Crab	1.75	120	0.890
Shrimp	1.75	120	0.210
Oysters	2.89	120	0.350
Smoked oysters	15	120	1.800
Mussels	4.75	120	0.570
Lobster	36.6	120	4.390
Candy bar	1.18	15	0.020
Milk	0.33	120	0.040
Peas	2.38	120	0.290
Soy beans	109	120	0.130
Applesauce (can)	0.2	120	0.020
Avocado	1.68	120	0.200
Raisins	1.68	30	0.050
Peanut butter	8.53	30	0.260

plumbing, copper toxicity was a more recognized phenomenon.

It is difficult to define specific dietary copper requirements because of the lack of suitable indices to assess copper status. As such, knowledge of factors affecting the bioavailability of dietary copper is limited. Ceruloplasmin contains 95% of the copper found in serum and is frequently used as a marker of copper status. However, ceruloplasmin levels vary with pregnancy and inflammation and ceruloplasmin mRNA is regulated by estrogen, infection, and hypoxia among other factors. Currently, investigators are searching for genetic biomarkers in intestinal, liver, and lymphocyte cells that respond to copper levels and may serve as better markers of copper status. Whole-body copper metabolism is difficult to study in human subjects. However, isotopic tracers and kinetic modeling have added a dimension to what can be learned in humans by direct measurement. These studies suggest that the efficiency of copper absorption varies greatly, depending on dietary intake. Mechanisms regulating total body copper seem to be strong, given the relatively small and constant body pool, but they are not yet well understood. Changes in efficiency of absorption help to regulate the amount of copper retained by the body. In addition, endogenous excretion of copper into the gastrointestinal tract depends heavily on the amount of copper absorbed. When dietary copper is high and an excess is absorbed, endogenous excretion increases, protecting against toxic accumulation of copper in the body. When intake is low, little endogenous copper is excreted, protecting against copper depletion. Regulation is not sufficient with very low amounts of dietary copper (0.38 mg day⁻¹) and appears to be delayed when copper intake is high.

Recommended Intakes

The Tolerable Upper Intake Limit (UL) for adults is 10 mg daily, based on degree of liver damage associated with intake. UL for children vary with age: 1–3 years/1 mg daily, 4–8 years/3 mg daily, 9–13 years/ 5 mg daily, 14–18 years/8 mg daily (irrespective of pregnancy or lactation status). UL for children under the age of 1 year are not possible to establish. There are no official recommended daily allowances (RDAs) for copper in children. The RDA for adult males and females is a daily intake of 0.9 mg. Measurements of the dietary requirements for copper in adult men have shown the requirement to range from about 1.0 to 1.6 mg daily. A review of nutrient intakes in the US from 1909 to 1994 confirms

Table 3 Recommended dietary allowances for copper (mg day^{-1})

Age	RDA (daily)
Infants	
<6 months	0.2 (30 mcg/kg)
6–12 months	0.2–0.3 (24 mcg/kg)
Children	
1–3 years	0.34
4–8 years	0.44
9–13 years	0.7
14–18 years	0.89
Adult	
19+ years	0.9
Pregnant women	1
Nursing women	1.3

that intake varied between 1.5 mg day^{-1} (1965) to 2.1 mg day^{-1} (1909). These trends reflect a diet higher in copper-rich potatoes and grain predominating in 1909 versus a decline in potato popularity in 1965. Daily intake recommendations for children vary with age (see **Table 3**). Persons who consume diets high in zinc and low in protein are at risk of copper deficiency. High intakes of dietary fiber apparently increase the dietary requirement for copper. Diets in Western countries provide copper below or in the low range of the estimated safe and adequate daily dietary intake. Copper deficiency is usually a consequence of low copper stores at birth, inadequate dietary copper intake, poor absorption, elevated requirements induced by rapid growth, or increased copper losses.

Bioavailability

The issue of bioavailability from food sources and the interactions between food groups and copper availability remains a critical question. Lonnerdal *et al.* demonstrated that heat treatment of cows' milk formula decreases the copper bioavailability. Transitional complexes form in the milk upon heating that have a similar configuration to copper and thereby directly inhibit copper absorption. High doses of zinc also reduce copper bioavailability, as does combined iron and zinc supplementation. The dilemma is how to prepare an infant formula containing adequate copper, iron, and zinc that will meet the RDA for copper. Other nutrients dramatically affect copper absorption from foods. Soy protein-based diets promote less copper retention in tissues than lactalbumin-based diets. However, it is unclear if this effect is solely due to the soy protein composition or to the higher zinc in these soy-based formulas. In animals, phytate causes a drop in serum copper but human stable isotope studies reveal no

effect on copper absorption in adult men. Patients with low copper indices need to be evaluated for the copper content of their diets, other foods ingested at the same time, and other mineral supplements that may be given.

Absorption and Excretion

Dietary copper is absorbed across the small intestine. It diffuses through the mucous layer that covers the wall of the bowel via the divalent metal transporter DMT1. Copper is thus released into the serum and presumably is transported bound to either albumin or histidine to the multiple sites that require copper or to storage tissues. The liver is the primary storage organ for copper followed by muscle and bone. Not all of the copper ingested is absorbed and gastrointestinal cells that hold on to the excess copper are 'sloughed' when the lining of the gut is turned over every 24–48 hs. Copper bound to albumin or histidine enters the hepatocyte via the high-affinity mammalian copper transporter, hCtr1. Initially identified in yeast by functional complementation studies, this protein has subsequently been cloned in mice and humans. Human Ctr1 has a high homology to the yeast proteins Ctr1 and Ctr3 involved in high-affinity copper uptake. The N-terminus of the protein is rich in histidine and methionine residues, which presumably bind the copper and move it into the cell. Characterization of hCtr1 confirms its localization on the plasma membrane consistent with its role as a copper transporter. *In vitro* work has also identified a vesicular perinuclear distribution for hCtr1 that is copper concentration dependent. Redistribution of the hCtr1 suggests that under different copper states, copper moves through the membrane transporter and into a vesicular compartment for further 'assignment' within the cell. hCtr2, a low-affinity copper uptake transporter, has also been identified. This low-affinity copper transporter is unable to complement the respiratory defect seen in yeast strains lacking copper transport capabilities. Once inside the cell, copper has one of four fates: (1) bind to and be stored within a glutathione/metallothionein pool; (2) bind to CCS, the copper chaperone for Cu, Zn - SOD; (3) bind to cox 17 for delivery to mitochondrial cytochrome *c*-oxidase; or (4) bind to HAH1 (human Atox1 homolog) for subsequent copper delivery to either the Wilson disease P-type ATPase or the Menkes' P-type ATPase. Copper from HAH1 is incorporated into ceruloplasmin, the most abundant serum cuproprotein, within the trans golgi network (TGN). How the protein unfolds within the TGN to accept copper and how the copper is incorporated into ceruloplasmin is still under study. Ceruloplasmin is then secreted into the serum, and any excess copper not incorporated into ceruloplasmin is recycled in vesicles containing either the Wilson disease P-type ATPase or Menkes' P-type ATPase, and excreted into bile or stored in the liver. Recent characterization of a new protein, Murr1, suggests that this protein regulates copper excretion into bile such that mutations in the Murr1 gene are associated with normal copper uptake but severe defects in exporting copper from hepatocytes.

Approximately 15% of the total copper absorbed is actually transported to tissues while the remaining 85% is excreted. Of that copper pool, 98% is excreted in bile with the remaining 2% eliminated in the urine. The liver is the predominant organ responsible for regulating copper homeostasis at the level of excretion. Whereas copper import is highly conserved between yeast and humans, copper export in vertebrates involves a complex vesicular system that culminates in a lysosomal excretion pathway 'dumping' copper into the bile for elimination. At steady state, the amount of copper excreted into the biliary system is directly proportional to the hepatic copper load. In response to an increasing copper concentration within the hepatocyte, biliary copper excretion increases. There is no enterohepatic recirculation of copper and once the unabsorbable copper complex is in bile it is excreted in stool. Localization studies reveal redistribution of the ATP7b from the TGN to a vesicular compartment that migrates out to the biliary epithelium in response to increasing copper concentrations. Alternatively, under conditions of copper deficiency, the ATP7b remains tightly incorporated with the TGN for maximal copper incorporation into ceruloplasmin.

The highly homologous Wilson disease P-type ATPase (ATP7b) and the Menkes's P-type ATPase (ATP7a) differ only in their tissue expression and both function to move copper from one intracellular compartment to another. The ATP7a is predominantly located in the placenta, blood–brain barrier, and gastrointestinal tract and hence any mutation in the Menkes's P-type ATPase results in a copper deficiency in the fetus, brain, and tissues. In contrast, the Wilson's disease P-type ATPase is expressed in the liver and mutations in this culminate in profound copper overload of the liver because of the inability to shuttle copper into the trans golgi network for incorporation into ceruloplasmin. The excess copper is stored in the liver and eventually leaks out in the serum where it is deposited within sensitive tissues: the eye and brain. The psychiatric

illnesses ascribed to Wilson's disease are a result of hepatocyte-derived copper 'leaking' out of the liver and accumulating within the basal ganglia. Similarly, Kayser-Fleischer rings arise from copper deposition in the cornea. The toxic copper in the liver eventually results in cirrhosis and hepatic fibrosis as a result of oxyradical damage. Menkes's syndrome has an incidence of 1:300 000 while Wilson's disease has an incidence of 1:30 000. Expression of these diseases may differ considerably among affected family members.

The recognition of a novel disorder of iron metabolism associated with mutations in the copper-containing protein ceruloplasmin revealed an essential role for ceruloplasmin as a ferroxidase and regulator of iron homeostasis. Patients and mice lacking the serum protein ceruloplasmin have normal copper kinetics: normal absorption, distribution, and copper-dependent activity. These data suggest that although under experimental conditions ceruloplasmin may donate copper, ceruloplasmin is not a copper transport protein. The six atoms of copper are incorporated into three type 1 coppers, one type 2 copper, and a type 3 copper. The type 1 coppers provide the electron shuttle necessary for the concomitant reduction of oxygen to water that occurs within the trinuclear copper cluster comprised of the type 2 and type 3 copper. This reaction is coupled with the oxidation of a variety of substrates: amines, peroxidases, iron, NO, and possibly copper. The recent observation that Fet3, the yeast ceruloplasmin homolog, also has critical cuprous oxidase activity in addition to ferroxidase activity has prompted renaming some of the multicopper oxidases (ceruloplasmin, Fet3, hephaestin) as 'metallo-oxidases' rather than ferroxidases.

Copper Deficiency

Reports of human copper deficiency are limited and suggest that severe nutrient deficiency coupled with malabsorption is required for this disease state to occur. Infants fed an exclusive cows' milk diet are at risk for copper deficiency. Cows' milk not only has substantially less copper than human milk but the bioavailability is also reduced. High oral intake of iron or zinc decrease copper absorption and may predispose an individual to copper deficiency. Other infants at risk include those with: (1) prematurity secondary to a lack of hepatic copper stores; (2) prolonged diarrhea; and (3) intestinal malabsorption syndromes. Even the premature liver is capable of impressive copper storage. By 26 weeks' gestational age the liver already has 3 mg of copper stored. By 40 weeks' gestational age, the hepatic liver has 10–12 mg copper stored with the majority being deposited in the third trimester. Iron and zinc have been shown to interfere with copper absorption and further complicate the picture of copper deficiency. The most frequent clinical manifestations of copper deficiency are anemia refractory to iron treatment, neutropenia, and bone demineralization presenting as fractures.

The anemia is characterized as hypochromic and normocytic with a reduced reticulocyte count, hypoferremia, and thrombocytopenia. Bone marrow aspirate reveals megaloblastic changes and vacuolization of both erythroid and myeloid progenitor lineages. It is believed that a profound copper deficiency results in a multicopper oxidase deficient state and as such bone marrow demands are unmet by the lack of ferroxidase activity. Bone abnormalities are common and manifest as osteoporosis, fractures, and epiphyseal separation. Other manifestations of copper deficiency include hypopigmentation, hypotonia, growth arrest, abnormal cholesterol and glucose metabolism, and increased rate of infections.

Multiple factors associated with copper deficiency are responsible for the increased rate of infection seen. Most copper-deficient patients are malnourished and suffer from impaired weight gain. The immune system requires copper to perform several functions. Recent research showed that interleukin 2 is reduced in copper deficiency and is probably the mechanism by which T-cell proliferation is reduced. These results were extended to show that even in marginal deficiency, when common indexes of copper are not affected by the diet, the proliferative response and interleukin concentrations are reduced. The number of neutrophils in human peripheral blood is reduced in cases of severe copper deficiency. Not only are they reduced in number, but their ability to generate superoxide anion and kill ingested microorganisms is also reduced in both overt and marginal copper deficiency. This mechanism is not yet understood.

Copper Excess

Excess copper is the result of either excessive copper absorption or ineffective copper excretion. The most common diseases associated with copper excess are: (1) Wilson's disease, a genetic disease resulting in mutations in the Wilson's disease P-type ATPase and excessive hepatocyte copper accumulation; (2) renal disease, in patients on hemodialysis due to kidney failure when dialysate solutions become contaminated with excess copper; and (3) biliary obstruction. Excessive use of copper supplements may also contribute to copper toxicity and is clinically manifested by severe anemia, nausea and vomiting, abdominal pain, and diarrhea.

Copper toxicosis can rapidly progress to coma and death if not recognized. Current management of most diseases associated with copper toxicity includes a low-copper diet, a high-zinc diet (competitively interferes with copper absorption), and use of copper chelators such as penicillamine and trientine. Affected individuals should have their tap water analyzed for copper content and drink demineralized water if their water contains more than 100 μg/liter. Given that the liver is the most significant copper storage organ, any activity that can affect hepatic cellular metabolism needs to be monitored. Hence, alcohol consumption is strongly discouraged.

There are reports of chronic copper exposure resulting in toxic accumulation. Fortunately, these events appear to be geographically restricted. Indian childhood cirrhosis (ICC), also known as Indian infantile cirrhosis or idiopathic copper toxicosis, has been associated with increased copper intake from contaminated pots used to heat up infant milk. The milk is stored and warmed in brass (a copper alloy) or copper containers. It is interesting to note that the increased copper absorption alone is not critical for disease formation but rather this occurs in infants that already have prenatal liver copper stores in excess of adult values. How the neonatal liver is able to compartmentalize this toxic metal so effectively is unknown. Perhaps in ICC, this delicate balance is disrupted. Tyrolean liver disease, occurring in the Austrian Tyrol, despite having a Mendelian pattern of inheritance suggestive of an autosomal recessive trait, appears related to use of copper cooking utensils. However, recent reports describe how a persistent percentage of the German population remains susceptible to copper toxicosis despite adjustments in cooking utensils. Perhaps a genetic susceptibility exists in this population that has yet to be determined.

Conclusion

Adult copper homeostasis rests on the foundation of an adequate copper balance in early life. Copper deficiency, either due to inadequate intake or abnormal absorption, may result. While the clinical stigmata of severe copper deficiency are easy to identify, the subtle changes in neurobehavioral development associated with mild copper deficiency are unknown. Given the high copper concentration in the brain, one could postulate that critical copper deficiency during development could lead to significant central nervous system deficits. Recent evidence suggesting that copper metabolism may be involved as an epigenetic factor in the development of Alzheimer's disease (AD) highlights the importance of balance. In this scenario, elevated central nervous system copper, as seen in AD, may initiate increased oxyradical formation and hasten damage. In fact, some are advocating that serum copper might be a good biomarker for AD. Copper is an essential trace metal critical for normal development. The goal of future studies will be to develop sensitive biomarkers for copper status. Only with these tools can we adequately assess copper status and treat copper-deficient and copper excess states appropriately.

See also: **Zinc**: Physiology.

Further Reading

Araya M, Koletzko B, and Uauy R (2003) Copper deficiency and excess in infancy: developing a research agenda. *Journal of Pediatric Gastroenterology and Nutrition* 37: 422–429.

Bush Al and Strozyk D (2004) Serum copper: A biomarker for Alzheimer disease. *Archives of Neurology* 61: 631–632.

Gitlin JD (2003) Wilson disease. *Gastroenterology* 125: 1868–1877.

Klein CJ (2002) Nutrient requirements for preterm infant formulas. *Journal of Nutrition* 132: 1395S–1577S.

Lutter CK and Dewey KG (2003) Proposed nutrient composition for fortified complimentary foods. *Journal of Nutrition* 133: 3011S–3020S.

Prohaska JR and Gybina AA (2004) Intracellular copper transport in mammals. *Journal of Nutrition* 134: 1003–1006.

Rees EM and Thiele DJ (2004) From aging to virulence: forging connections through the study of copper homeostasis in eukaryotic microorganisms. *Current Opinion in Microbiology* 7: 175–184.

Schulpis KH, Karakonstantakis T, Gavrili S *et al.* (2004) Maternal-neonatal serum selenium and copper levels in Greeks and Albanians. *European Journal of Clinical Nutrition* 1: 1–5.

Shim H and Harris ZL (2003) Genetic defects in copper metabolism. *Journal of Nutrition* 133: 1527S–1531S.

Tapiero H, Townsend DM, and Tew KD (2003) Trace elements in human physiology. Copper. *Biomedicine & Pharmacotherapy* 57: 386–398.

Uauy R, Olivares M, and Gonzalez M (1998) Essentiality of copper in humans. *American Journal of Clinical Nutrition* 67(S): 952S–959S.

Wijmenga C and Klomp LWJ (2004) Molecular regulation of copper excretion in the liver. *Proceedings of the Nutrition Society* 63: 31–39.

CORONARY HEART DISEASE

Contents
Lipid Theory
Prevention

Lipid Theory

D Kritchevsky, Wistar Institute, Philadelphia, PA, USA

Introduction

Arteriosclerosis is a group of conditions characterized by thickening and stiffening of the arterial wall. Atherosclerosis is characterized by the formation of atheromas (lipid-laden plaques) in medium to large arteries. These are associated with calcifications of the arterial wall along with other changes. Eventually, the arterial lumen is reduced and the restricted blood flow due to these changes leads to clinical symptoms. Over the years there have been varying theories about the development of arterial lesions and these theories become more complex as our biochemical and molecular biological skills and knowledge increase.

Arterial fatty streaks are ubiquitous in humans and appear early in life. The fatty streak is comprised of lipid-rich macrophages and smooth muscle cells. Macrophages that accumulate lipid and are transformed into foam cells may be involved in the transformation of the fatty streak to an atherosclerotic lesion. In susceptible persons the fatty streaks may progress to fibrous plaques. Fibrous plaques, at their core, consist of a mixture of cholesterol-rich smooth muscle and foam cells. This core may contain cellular debris, cholesteryl esters, cholesterol crystals, and calcium. The fibrous cap consists of smooth muscle and foam cells, collagen, and lipid. The final stage in this process is the complicated plaque, which can obstruct the arterial lumen. Rupture of the cap may lead to clot formation and occlusion of the artery.

There are several theories of atherogenesis and these may eventually be shown to be interactive. The lipid hypothesis suggests that persistent hyperlipidemia leads to cholesterol accumulation in the arterial endothelium. Hypercholesterolemia may activate protein growth factors, which stimulate smooth muscle cell proliferation.

The lipid infiltration hypothesis proposes that elevated LDL levels increase LDL infiltration which, in turn, increases uptake of epithelial cells, smooth muscle cells, and macrophages. This cascade leads to cholesterol accumulation and, eventually, atheroma formation. The endothelial injury may arise from the action of oxidized lipid.

The endothelial injury hypothesis may help to explain the focal distribution of atheromas, which is not adequately accounted for by the lipid hypothesis. The endothelial injury hypothesis asserts that plaque formation begins when the endothelial cells that cover fatty streaks separate thus exposing the underlying lesion to the circulation. This may lead to smooth muscle proliferation, stimulated by circulating mitogens, or may cause platelet aggregation leading to mural thrombosis.

Another hypothesis relating to atherogenesis is the response-to-injury hypothesis. In this hypothesis the injury may be due to mechanical factors, chronic hypercholesterolemia, toxins, viruses, or immune reactions: these increase endothelial permeability, and lead to monocyte adherence to the epithelium or infiltration and platelet aggregation or adherence at the site of the injury. Injury releases growth factors that stimulate proliferation of fibrous elements in the intima. These growth factors may arise from the endothelial cell, monocyte, macrophages, platelet, smooth muscle cell, and T cell. They include epidermal growth factor, insulin-like growth factors, interleukins 1 and 2, platelet-derived growth factors, transforming growth factors α and β, and tumor necrosis factors α and β, among others. Monocytes and smooth muscle cells carry the 'scavenger' receptor, which binds oxidized but not native low-density lipoprotein (LDL) in a nonsaturable fashion. Uptake of oxidized LDL converts macrophages and smooth muscle cells into foam cells. Another theory of atherogenesis suggests that it begins as an immunological disease, which starts by an autoimmune reaction against the heat stress protein, hsp60. There have been suggestions that oxidized LDL may be an underlying cause of arterial injury.

The term 'atherosclerosis' is derived from the Greek words *athere*, meaning gruel, and *skleros*, meaning hardening. The term was coined by Marchand in 1904 to describe the ongoing process beginning with the early lipid deposits in the arteries to the eventual hardening. The World Health Organization (WHO) definition describes atherosclerosis as a 'variable combination of changes in the intima of the arteries involving focal accumulation of lipids and complex carbohydrates with blood and its constituents accompanied by fibrous tissue formation, calcification, and associated changes in the media' – a decidedly more complex concept than attributing it all to the dietary cholesterol.

Discussions of the etiology of heart disease always describe it as a life-style disease and list a number of risk factors, which include family history, hypercholesterolemia, hypertension, obesity, and cigarette smoking. Having listed these factors, discussion generally reverts to blood cholesterol and its control.

The fasting blood plasma of a healthy individual is a clear, straw-colored liquid, which may contain 400–800 mg of lipids per 100 ml. This clear solution, which is high in lipids, is made possible by the water-soluble complex of lipids with protein, the lipoproteins. A generalized view of lipoprotein metabolism is provided in **Figure 1**. The existence of soluble lipid–protein

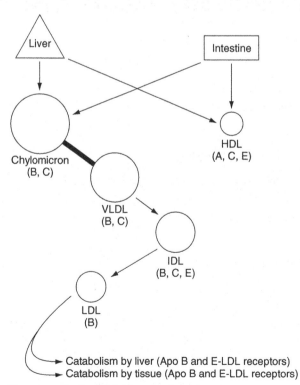

Figure 1 Outline of lipid metabolism. Letters in parentheses refer to apolipoproteins (apo). HDL, high-density lipoprotein; VLDL, very-low-density lipoprotein; IDL, intermediate-density lipoprotein; LDL, low-density lipoprotein.

complexes in serum was suggested about a century ago. Precipitation of a lipoprotein from horse serum was achieved in 1929 and classes of lipoproteins were adduced from studies using moving boundary electrophoresis. The critical experiments were carried out by Gofman and his group in the 1950s. They demonstrated that classes of lipoprotein complexes could be identified by their flotation characteristics in the analytical ultracentrifuge. These complexes were separable because they possessed different hydrated densities and they were defined initially by Svedberg units of flotation (S_f). The lipoproteins vary in chemical composition and although it is common to provide tables describing lipoprotein composition, the values are generally average values. This is so since the lipoproteins exist in a dynamic state exchanging their lipid components with those of tissues or other lipoproteins. Since identification is made according to a physical property, i.e., hydrated density, it is evident that different agglomerates of lipid and protein may have similar hydrated densities. In general, the lipoproteins are a series of macromolecules that, as they progress from low to high density, display decreasing triacylglycerol content and increasing cholesteryl ester, phospholipid, and protein.

Table 1 describes the major lipoproteins. Their chemical composition is described in **Table 2**.

As research continues and as analytical methodology becomes more precise we find a higher resolution of some lipoprotein classes and better definition of their roles. One example is lipoprotein (a) (lp(a)), first described in 1963. Lipoprotein (a) is an LDL whose normal apoprotein (apo B) is linked to an additional protein, apoprotein a, via a disulfide bridge. Lipoprotein (a) interferes with normal fibrinolysis leading to an increased prevalence of blood clots, and is thought to present an especially high risk for myocardial infarction. Characteristics and functions of lipoproteins are described in **Table 3**.

Table 2 Plasma lipoprotein composition

Lipoprotein	Composition (wt%)				
	FC	CE	TAG	PL	PROT
Chylomicron	1	3	90	4	2
VLDL	7	14	55	16	8
IDL	6	22	30	24	18
LDL	7	48	5	20	20
HDL	4	15	4	27	50

FC, free cholesterol; CE, cholesteryl ester; TAG, triacylglycerol; PL, phospholipid; PROT, protein; VLDL, very-low-density lipoprotein; IDL, intermediate-density lipoprotein; LDL, low-density lipoprotein; HDL, high-density lipoprotein.

Molecular size influences the ease with which LDL particles can enter the arterial wall. Diabetic rabbits have greatly elevated plasma lipid levels but display surprisingly little atherosclerosis. The reason for this apparent discrepancy is that the lipoproteins of diabetic rabbits are rather large in size and do not penetrate the artery. Since 1982 we have known of an array of LDL particles ranging from small and dense to large and comparatively light. An LDL pattern characterized by an excess of small, dense particles is associated with a threefold increased risk of myocardial infarction, independent of age, sex, or body weight. Commonly, LDL is known as the 'bad' cholesterol and high-density lipoprotein (HDL) as the 'good' cholesterol. These recent findings indicate the presence of 'good, bad' cholesterol and 'bad, good' cholesterol.

Among the apolipoproteins, polymorphism of apoprotein E apparently dictates a subject's chances for successful treatment of lipidemia. The apoE alleles are designated as E2, E3, and E4. The most common pattern (55%) is homozygosity for E3, which gives rise to the E3/E3 phenotype. The next most common phenotype is E3/E4 (26%). The least frequently observed phenotype is E2/E (1%), which is often associated with type III hyperlipoproteinemia. There is some evidence suggesting that subjects bearing the E4 allele have higher levels of LDL than those with the E3/E3 pattern; they may also be more

Table 1 Major plasma lipoproteins

Lipoprotein class	Size (nm)	Mol. wt	Density (g ml^{-1})	Electrophoretic mobility	Origin	Major apoproteins
Chylomicron	100–400	10^6–10^7	<0.95	Origin	Intestine	A-I, B-48, C-II, C-III, E
VLDL	40–70	5×10^3	0.95–1.006	Prebeta	Liver	B-100, C-II, C-III, E
IDL	30–40	4.5×10^3	1.006–1.019	Between prebeta and beta	Catabolism of VLDL	B-100, C-II, C-III, E
LDL	22.5–27.5	2×10^3	1.019–1.063	Beta	Catabolism of VLDL and IDL	B-100
HDL	7.5–10	0.4×10^3	1.063–1.210	Alpha	Liver, intestine	A-I, A-II, C-II, C-III, E

VLDL, very-low-density lipoprotein; IDL, intermediate-density lipoprotein; LDL, low-density lipoprotein; HDL, high-density lipoprotein.

Table 3 Characteristics and functions of major apolipoproteins

Apolipoprotein	Lipoprotein	(Approximate molecular weight (kD))	Source	(Average plasma) concentration (mg dL^{-1})	(Physiologic) function
A-1	HDL, chylomicrons	28	Liver, intestine	100–120	Structural apoprotein of HDL, cofactor for LCAT
A-II	HDL, chylomicrons	17	Intestine, liver	35–45	Structural apoprotein of HDL, cofactor for hepatic lipase
A-IV	HDL, chylomicrons	46	Liver, intestine	10–20	Unknown
Apo (a)	Lp(a)	600	Liver	1–10	Unknown
B-48	Chylomicrons	264	Intestine	Trace	Major structural apoprotein, secretion and clearance of chlylomicrons
B-100	VLDL, LDL	550	Liver	100–125	Ligand for LDL receptor, structural apoprotein of VLDL and LDL
C-I	Chylomicrons, VLDL, HDL	5.80	Liver	6–8	Cofactor for LCAT
C-II	Chylomicrons, VLDL, HDL	9.10	Liver	3–5	Cofactor for LCAT
C-III	Chylomicrons, VLDL, HDL	8.75	Liver	12–15	Inhibitor of LPL, involved in lipoprotein remnant uptake
E-2	Chylomicrons, VLDL, HDL	35	Liver, peripheral tissues	4–5	Ligand for cell receptor
E-3	Chylomicrons, VLDL, HDL	35	Liver, peripheral tissues	4–5	Ligand for cell receptor
E-4	Chylomicrons, VLDL, HDL	35	Liver, peripheral tissues	4–5	Ligand for cell receptor

HDL, LDL, VLDL, high-, low-, and very-low-density lipoprotein; LCAT, lecithin-cholesterol acyltransferase; LPL, lipoprotein lipase.

prone to Alzheimer's disease. **Tables 4** and **5** list primary and secondary dyslipoproteinemias.

Cholesterol and Cholesterolemia

In 1913 Anitschkow showed that it was possible to establish atherosclerosis in rabbits by feeding cholesterol. Since then virtually all research on atherosclerosis has centered on cholesterol – circulating cholesterol and dietary cholesterol. The epidemiological data suggest a role for dietary fat, and hypercholesterolemia has been established as a principal risk factor for atherosclerosis. The lipid hypothesis was developed from the data obtained in the Framingham study, which suggested a curvilinear relationship between risk of atherosclerosis and plasma or serum cholesterol levels. However, studies of actual cholesterol intake as it affects cholesterol levels have yielded equivocal results.

Several studies have shown that the addition of one or two eggs to their daily diet did not influence serum cholesterol levels of free-living subjects. Data from the Framingham study show no correlation between cholesterol intake and cholesterol level. So we are left with the anomalous situation that blood cholesterol is an indicator of susceptibility to coronary disease but it is relatively unaffected by dietary

cholesterol. It is of interest to point out that we are also seeing a correlation between low plasma or serum cholesterol levels and noncoronary death.

The type of fat in the diet has a strong influence on serum or plasma cholesterol levels. Rabbits fed saturated fat develop more severe atherosclerosis than do rabbits fed unsaturated fat. In 1965 the groups of Keys and Hegsted independently developed formulae for predicting changes in cholesterol levels based on changes in the diet. Their formulae were based upon changes in quantity of saturated and unsaturated fat and in dietary cholesterol, but the last value makes a very small contribution to the overall number. The Keys formula is:

$$\Delta C = 1.35(2\Delta S - \Delta P) + 1.5\Delta Z$$

where ΔC represents the change in cholesterol level, ΔS and ΔP represent changes in levels of saturated and unsaturated fat, and Z is the square root of dietary cholesterol in mg per 1000 kcal of diet. The Hegsted formula is:

$$\Delta C_P = 2.16\Delta S - 1.65\Delta P + 0.168\Delta C_D + 85$$

where ΔC_P is change in plasma cholesterol and ΔC_D is change in dietary cholesterol in mg per 1000 kcal.

Table 4 The primary dyslipoproteinemias

Type	Changes in plasma		Apparent genetic disorder	Biochemical defect
	Lipids	Lipoproteins		
I	TAG ↑	CM ↑	Familial LPL deficiency	Loss of LPL activity
II-a	C ↑	LDL ↑	Familial hypercholesterolemia	Deficiency of LDL receptor and activity
II-b	C ↑, TAG ↑	LDL, VLDL ↑	Familial combined hyperlipidemia	Unknown
III	C ↑, TAG ↑	β-VLDL ↑	Familial type III hyperlipidemia	Defect in TAG-rich remnant clearance
IV	TAG ↑	VLDL ↑	Familial hypertriacylglycerolemia	VLDL synthesis ↑, catabolism ↓
V	TAG ↑, C ↑	VLDL ↑, CM ↑	Familial type V hyperlipoproteinemia	Lipolysis of TGA-rich LP ↓, Production of VLDL TAG ↑
Hyper Lp(a)	C ↑	Lp(a) ↑	Familial hyper apo(a) lipoproteinemia	Inhibits fibrinolysis
Hyperapobeta-lipoproteinemia	TAG ↑	VLDL, LDL ↑	Familial type V hyperlipoproteinemia	CETP deficiency
Familial hypobeta-lipoproteinemia	C ↓, TAG ↓	CM ↓, VLDL ↑, LDL ↓	?	Inability to synthesize apo B-48 and apo B-100
A-beta-lipoproteinemia	C ↓, TAG ↓	CM ↓, VLDL ↓, LDL ↓	?	Apo B-48 and apo B-100 not secreted into plasma
Hypo-alphalipoproteinemia	C ↓, TAG ↓	HDL ↓	?	LCAT deficiency
Tangier disease				Apo A-I ↓, apo C-III ↓
Fish eye disease				Abnormal apo A-I, and apo A-II metabolism

C, cholesterol; CM, chylomicrons; CETP, cholesteryl ester transfer protein; HDL, LDL, VLDL, high-, low-, and very-low-density lipoprotein; LCAT, lecithin-cholesterol acyltransferase; LPL, lipoprotein lipase; TAG, triacylglycerol.

Table 5 Secondary dyslipoproteinemias

Type	Associated disease	Lipoproteins elevated	Apparent underlying defect
I	Lupus erythematosis	Chylomicrons	Circulating LPL inhibitor
II	Nephrotic syndrome, Cushing's syndrome	VLDL and LDL	Overproduction of VLDL particles, defective lipolysis of VLDL triglycerides
III	Hypothyroidism, dysglobulinemia	VLDL and LDL	Suppression of LDL receptor activity, overproduction of VLDL triglycerides
IV	Renal failure, diabetes mellitus, acute hepatitis	VLDL	Defective lipolysis of triglyceride-rich VLDL due to inhibition of LPL and HL
V	Noninsulin dependent diabetes	VLDL	Overproduction and defective lipolysis of VLDL triglycerides

HDL, LDL, VLDL, high-, low, and very-low-density lipoprotein; HL, hepatic lipase; LPL, lipoprotein lipase.

Both studies found that changes in dietary stearic acid did not fit the formula. Since those formulae were introduced a number of newer formulae have appeared, which provide a coefficient for every individual fatty acid, but the original formulae are still used most frequently. Under metabolic ward conditions it has been shown that lauric ($C_{12:0}$), myristic ($C_{14:0}$), and palmitic ($C_{16:0}$) acids raise both LDL and HDL cholesterol levels, and that oleic ($C_{18:1}$) and linoleic ($C_{18:2}$) acids raise HDL and lower LDL levels slightly. Thus, the type of fat is the determining factor in considering dietary fat effects on serum cholesterol. Experiments in which subjects were fed low or high levels of cholesterol in diets containing high or low ratios of saturated to polyunsaturated fat have been reported. When the fat was homologous, changing from low to high dietary cholesterol raised serum cholesterol concentration by 2%. However, even under conditions in which low levels of cholesterol were fed, changing from saturated to unsaturated fat raised serum cholesterol levels by 10% or more.

In nature most, but not all, unsaturated fatty acids are in the *cis* configuration. The major source of fats containing *trans* unsaturated fatty acids (*trans* fats) in the diet of developed nations is hydrogenated fat, such as is present in commercial margarines and cooking fats. Interest in *trans* fat effects on atherosclerosis and cholesterolemia was first evinced in the 1960s. In general, *trans* fats behave like saturated fats and raise serum cholesterol levels, but have not been found to be more atherogenic than saturated fats in studies carried out in rabbits, monkeys, and swine. Studies have also shown that *trans* fat effects may be relatively small if the diet contains sufficient quantities of essential fatty acids.

Studies, clinical and epidemiological, on the influence of *trans* unsaturated fats on the risk of coronary heart disease have continued. The evidence is that *trans* fats may influence the chemical indicators of heart disease risk but final proof must rest on verification by clinical trial. The concerns relative to *trans* fat effects have led to recommendations that the levels of *trans* fats present in the diet be reduced as much as possible. The availability of *trans*-free margarines and other fats may render the entire argument obsolete.

Protein

The type of protein in the diet also influences cholesterolemia and atherosclerosis. In animal studies in which the sole source of protein is of animal or plant origin, the former is more cholesterolemic than atherogenic. However, a 1:1 mix of animal and plant protein provides the higher-grade protein of animal protein and the normocholesterolemic effects of plant protein. The results underline the need for a balanced diet.

Fiber

Dietary fiber may influence lipidemia and atherosclerosis. Substances designated as insoluble fibers (wheat bran, for instance) possess laxative properties but have little effect on serum lipid levels. Soluble fibers (gel-forming fibers such as pectin or guar gum) influence lipidemia and glycemia. Oat bran, which contains β-glucans, which are soluble fibers, will lower cholesterol levels despite its designation.

Variations in Cholesterol Levels

Ignoring the differences of technique involved in cholesterol measurement in the laboratory – variations that are amenable to resolution – there are physiological considerations that should be recognized. Age, gender, genetics, adiposity, and personality traits can affect cholesterol levels, as can

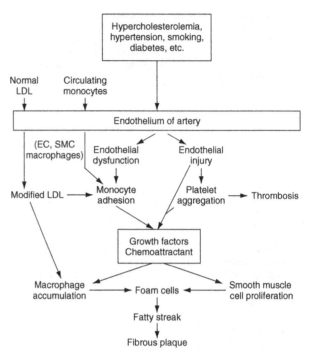

Figure 2 Factors involved in formation of the atherosclerotic plaque.

diseases unrelated to coronary disease. Stress (job stress, deadlines, examinations) can lead to increased cholesterol levels.

A definite seasonal variation in cholesterol levels (usually higher in winter months) has been seen in a number of studies. Scientists from the National Institutes of Health in the US carried out one of the finest studies in this area. They examined carefully the data from the 10 American Lipid Research Clinics. They observed that the etiology of their findings was unknown but they found the total and LDL cholesterol levels varied inversely with length of day. The level of HDL cholesterol varied much less, but its variation was correlated directly with ambient temperature. The foregoing does not reduce the importance of measuring cholesterol levels but makes it important to take into consideration the subjects' physical and mental state as well as time of year.

Figure 2 attempts to summarize the many factors now considered to play a role in the formation of the atherosclerotic plaque.

See also: **Coronary Heart Disease**: Prevention. **Fatty Acids**: *Trans* Fatty Acids.

Further Reading

Ginsburg HN (1998) Lipoprotein physiology. *Endocrinology Metabolism Clinics of North America* 27: 503–519.

Gold P, Grover S, and Roncari DAK (eds.) (1992) *Cholesterol and Coronary Heart Disease – The Great Debate.* Park Ridge, NJ: CRC Press.

Libby P (2002) Inflammation in atherosclerosis. *Nature* **420**: 868–874.

Lusis AJ (2000) Atherosclerosis. *Nature* **407**: 233–241.

McNamara (2000) Dietary cholesterol and atherosclerosis. *Biochimica Biophysica Acta* **1529**: 310–320.

Nicolosi RJ, Kritchevsky D, and Wilson TA (1999) Pathobiology of hypercholesterolemia and atherosclerosis. In: Rippe JM (ed.) *Lifestyle Management and Prevention of Cardiovascular Disease*, pp. 25–39. London: Blackwell Science Press.

Ross R (1999) Atherosclerosis – an inflammatory disease. *New England Journal of Medicine* **340**: 115–126.

Tabas T (2002) Cholesterol in health and disease. *Journal of Clinical Investigation* **110**: 583–589.

Velican C and Velican D (1989) *Natural History of Coronary Atherosclerosis*. Boca Raton, FL: CRC Press.

White RA (1989) *Atherosclerosis and Arteriosclerosis.* Boca Raton, FL: CRC Press.

Prevention

K Srinath Reddy, All India Institute of Medical Sciences, New Delhi, India

Introduction

Coronary heart disease (CHD) is the leading cause of death in the world. While it is well established as the foremost contributor to mortality in most developed countries, it is also a major and rapidly rising cause of death in many developing countries. Global health transitions, which have seen substantial changes in age-specific coronary mortality rates across the world, in the past half a century, have also been associated with changes in nutrition, which explain a large part of the rise or fall of CHD-related death rates.

Diet and nutrition have been extensively investigated as risk factors for CHD. Many dietary factors have been linked directly to an increased or decreased risk of CHD or to major established risk factors of CHD like high blood pressure, disordered blood fats (dyslipidemia), diabetes and metabolic syndrome, overweight and obesity, and also to emerging risk factors like inflammatory markers and homocysteine. Nutrition influences atherogenesis, thrombosis, and inflammation – all of which are interconnected pathways that lead to CHD.

Observational epidemiological studies and clinical trials have contributed to a wide body of knowledge of the role that some nutrients (like saturated and *trans* fats, salt, and refined carbohydrates) play in increasing the risk of CHD and of the protective effect of other nutrients (such as fruit and vegetables, polyunsaturated fats, nuts, and fish) against CHD. This knowledge has been successfully applied both in public health and in clinical practice to reduce the risk of CHD in populations as well as in individuals. The present state of that knowledge, as relevant to prevention of CHD, is summarized below.

Global Trends in CHD as a Reflection of Nutrition Transition

Coronary heart disease accounted for 7.2 million deaths in 2002, which forms a large fraction of not only the total number of deaths worldwide due to cardiovascular diseases (16.6 million) but also of the global total number of deaths from any cause (57 million). While age-specific coronary mortality rates have declined in the industrial countries over the past three decades, the absolute burdens of CHD continue to be high. CHD death rates are rising in the developing countries, where about half of these deaths occur below the age of 70 years. In Eastern and Central Europe CHD mortality rates rose sharply in the 1980s and 1990s and have only recently shown signs of stabilization, albeit at high levels.

These changes in CHD mortality rates have accompanied well-documented or clearly discernible shifts in the nutritional state of the populations. The decline of CHD mortality in Western and Northern Europe was linked to a reduction in the consumption of unhealthy fats (saturated fats and *trans* fats) and salt as well as an increased consumption of fruits and vegetables. This is best documented in The Netherlands and Finland. Similarly, the recent decline of CHD mortality in Poland was explained by the increase in fruit and vegetable consumption and growing substitution of vegetable fats for animal fats. Similar evidence of a favorable nutrition transition preceding the decline in CHD mortality rates is available from other developed countries like the US, Canada, Australia, and New Zealand.

The developing countries have, however, witnessed a recent transition in the opposite direction. China, for example, has experienced a large increase in fat consumption over the past two decades, accompanied by a progressive rise in the mean plasma cholesterol levels of the population as well as in the CHD mortality rates. Other developing countries are also increasingly adopting unhealthy dietary patterns that augment the risk of CHD.

Understanding the Links between Nutrition and CHD

The pathogenesis of CHD is mediated through the interconnected pathways of atherogenesis (fat deposition in the walls of the coronary arteries to form plaques), thrombosis (blood clotting over disrupted plaques) and inflammation (which initially damages the blood vessel walls and continues to destabilize the plaques). Nutrition has a major role in influencing each of these pathways and often provides the connecting link between them.

Major coronary risk factors include an abnormal blood lipid profile (especially plasma cholesterol and its subfractions), high blood pressure, and diabetes. Overweight and obesity (both the general and central patterns) are also associated with an increased risk of CHD. Nutrition has a powerful influence on all of these risk factors, with an unhealthy diet pattern tending to elevate them and a healthy diet pattern reducing the levels of risk. Diet becomes especially important in the context of the metabolic syndrome (a complex of central obesity, high blood pressure, dyslipidemia, and glucose intolerance), an entity which is being increasingly identified as a major risk factor for CHD. Nutrition is also linked to the propensity to develop cardiac arrhythmias, in the setting of CHD, and is an important predictor of sudden cardiac death. These links between dietary patterns and several specific nutrients not only manifest as fat deposition in the arteries, plaque growth, plaque instability, and thrombosis but are evident much earlier in the natural history of CHD, as endothelial dysfunction (inability of the arteries to dilate normally), elevated levels of inflammatory markers (such as C reactive protein), and increased intimal medial thickness of arterial walls. These precede and predict the clinical manifestation of CHD.

Nutrients and CHD

Dietary Fats: Cholesterol

The relationship between dietary fats and cardiovascular disease (CVD), especially CHD, has been extensively investigated, with strong and consistent associations emerging from a wide body of evidence accrued from animal experiments, as well as observational studies, clinical trials, and metabolic studies conducted in diverse human populations. This relationship was initially considered to be mediated mainly through the atherogenic effects of plasma lipids (total cholesterol, lipoprotein fractions, and triglycerides). The effects of dietary fats on

thrombosis and endothelial function as well as the relationship of plasma and tissue lipids to the pathways of inflammation have been more recently understood. Similarly, the effects of dietary fats on blood pressure have also become more evident through observational and experimental research.

Cholesterol in the blood and tissues is derived from two sources: diet and endogenous synthesis. Dairy fat and meat are major dietary sources. Dietary cholesterol raises plasma cholesterol levels. Although both high-density lipoprotein (HDL) and low-density lipoprotein (LDL) fractions increase, the effect on the total/HDL ratio is still unfavorable, but small. The upper limit for dietary cholesterol intake has been prescribed, in most guidelines, to be $300\,\mathrm{mg\,day^{-1}}$. However, as endogenous synthesis is sufficient to meet the physiological needs, there is no requirement for dietary cholesterol and it is advisable to keep the intake as low as possible. If intake of dairy fat and meat are controlled, then there is no need for severe restriction of egg yolk intake, although some limitation remains prudent.

Saturated Fatty Acids (SFAs)

The relationship of dietary saturated fat to plasma cholesterol levels and to CHD was graphically demonstrated by the Seven Countries Study involving 16 cohorts, in which saturated fat intake explained up to 73% of the total variance in CHD across these cohorts. In the Nurses' Health Study, the effect of saturated fatty acids was much more modest, especially if saturates were replaced by carbohydrates. The most effective replacement for saturated fatty acids in terms of CHD prevention is by polyunsaturated fatty acids (PUFAs). This agrees with the outcome of large randomized clinical trials, in which replacement of saturated and *trans* fats by polyunsaturated vegetable oils effectively lowered CHD risk.

Trans-Fatty Acids (*t*-FAs)

t-FAs (*Trans*-Fatty Acids) are geometrical isomers of unsaturated fatty acids that assume a saturated fatty acid-like configuration. Partial hydrogenation, the process used to create *t*-FAs, also removes essential fatty acids such as LA (Linoleic Acid) and ALNA (Alpha Linolenic Acid). Metabolic studies have demonstrated that *t*-FAs render the plasma lipid profile even more atherogenic than SFAs, by not only elevating LDL cholesterol to similar levels but also decreasing HDL cholesterol. As a result, the ratio of LDL cholesterol to HDL cholesterol is significantly higher with a *t*-FA diet (2.58) than with a SFA diet (2.34) or an oleic acid diet (2.02). This greatly enhances the risk of CHD. Evidence that intake of *t*-FAs increases the risk of CHD initially became available from large population-based cohort studies in the US and in an elderly Dutch population. Eliminating *t*-FAs from the diet would be an important public health strategy to prevent CHD. Since these are commercially introduced agents into the diet, policy measures related to the food industry practices would be required along with public education. *t*-FAs have been eliminated from retail fats and spreads in many parts of the world, but deep-fat fried fast foods and baked goods are a major and increasing source.

Monounsaturated Fatty Acids (MUFAs)

The only nutritionally important MUFA is oleic acid, which is abundant in olive and canola oils and also in nuts. The epidemiological evidence related to MUFAs and CHD is derived from studies on the Mediterranean diet (see below), as well as from the Nurses' Health Study and other similar studies in the US.

Polyunsaturated Fatty Acids (PUFAs)

PUFAs are categorized as *n*-6 PUFAs (mainly derived from linoleic acid) and *n*-3 PUFAs (mainly present in fatty fish and also derived from alpha-linoleic acid). Clinical trials, in which *n*-6 PUFAs (containing linoleic acid) were substituted for SFAs showed a greater impact on reduction of both plasma cholesterol and CHD risk, in contrast to trials where low-fat diets were employed.

Much of the epidemiological evidence related to *n*-3 PUFAs is derived from the study of fish consumption in populations or interventions involving fish diets in clinical trials. Fish oils were, however, used in a large clinical trial of 11 300 survivors of myocardial infarction. After 3.5 years of follow-up, the fish oil group (1 g day^{-1}) had a statistically significant 20% reduction in total mortality, 30% reduction in cardiovascular death, and 45% decrease in sudden death.

The Lyon Heart Study in France incorporated an *n*-3 fatty acid (alpha-linolenic acid) into a diet that was altered to develop a 'Mediterranean diet' intervention. In the experimental group, plasma ALNA and EPA (Eicosapentenoic Acid) increased significantly and the trial reported a 70% reduction in cardiovascular mortality at 5 years. Total and LDL cholesterol were identical in the experimental and control groups, suggesting that thrombotic and perhaps arrhythmic events may have been favorably influenced by *n*-3 PUFAs. Since the diet altered many other variables, such as fiber and antioxidants

(by increasing fruit and vegetable consumption), direct attribution of benefits to *n*-3 PUFAs becomes difficult to establish.

The proportions of SFAs, MUFAs, and PUFAs as constituents of total fat intake and total energy consumption have engaged active attention, in view of the strong relationship of these fatty acids to the risk of CHD. The reduction of SFAs in the diet has been widely recommended, but its replacement has been an area of debate, as to whether the place of reduced SFAs should be taken by MUFAs, PUFAs, or carbohydrate. Both MUFAs and PUFAs improve the lipoprotein profile, although PUFAs are somewhat more effective. In view of this, several recent dietary recommendations suggested that SFAs should be kept below 10% of daily energy intake (preferably reduced to 7–8%), MUFAs should be increased to 13–15%, and PUFAs raised to 7–10% of daily energy, with the total fat contributing to less than 30% of all calories consumed. These may need to be adjusted for populations who consume less quantities of total fat, so as to ensure an adequate intake of MUFAs and PUFAs even under those circumstances. The emphasis is now shifting from the quantity of fat to the quality of fat, with growing evidence that even diets with 30–35% fat intake may be protective if the type of fats consumed are mostly from the MUFA and PUFA categories. Enhancing the nutritional quality of dietary fat consumption, to provide greater cardiovascular protection, may be attempted by decreasing the sources of saturated fats and eliminating *t*-FAs in the diet, increasing the consumption of foods containing unsaturated fatty acids (both MUFAs and PUFAs), and decreasing dietary cholesterol consumption.

Carbohydrates

Diets which are high in refined carbohydrates appear to reduce HDL cholesterol levels and increase the fraction of small dense LDL, both of which may impact adversely on vascular disease. This dyslipidemic pattern is consistent with the elevation of plasma triglycerides and is typical of the 'metabolic syndrome.' Carbohydrate diets with high glycemic index might adversely impact on glucose control, with associated changes in plasma lipids, and have been linked to an increased risk of CHD.

Fiber

Most soluble fibers reduce plasma total and LDL cholesterol concentrations, as reported by several trials. Fiber consumption strongly predicts insulin levels, weight gain, and cardiovascular risk factors like blood pressure, plasma triglycerides, LDL and

HDL cholesterol, and fibrinogen. Several large cohort studies in the US, Finland, and Norway have reported that subjects consuming relatively large amounts of whole-grain cereals have significantly lower rates of CHD.

Antioxidants

Though several cohort studies showed significant reductions in the incidence of cardiac events in men and women taking high-dose vitamin E supplements, large clinical trials failed to demonstrate a cardioprotective effect of vitamin E supplements. Beta-carotene supplements also did not provide protection against CHD and, in some trials, appeared to increase the risk.

Folate

The relationship of folate to CVD has been mostly explored through its effect on homocysteine, which has been put forward as an independent risk factor for CHD. Reduced plasma folate has been strongly associated with elevated plasma homocysteine levels and folate supplementation has been demonstrated to decrease those levels. Data from the Nurses' Health Study in the US showed that folate and vitamin B_6, from diet and supplements, conferred protection against CHD (fatal and nonfatal events combined) and suggested a role for their increased intake as an intervention for primary prevention of CHD. Recommendations related to folate supplementation must, however, await the results of ongoing clinical trials. Dietary intake of folate through natural food sources may be encouraged in the meanwhile, especially in individuals at a high risk of arterial or venous thrombosis and elevated plasma homocysteine levels.

Flavonoids and Other Phytochemicals

Flavonoids are polyphenolic antioxidants, which occur in a variety of foods of vegetable origin, such as tea, onions, and apples. Data from several prospective studies indicate an inverse association of dietary flavonoids with CHD. The role of these and other phytochemicals (such as plant stanols and sterols) in relation to CHD needs to be elucidated further.

Sodium and Potassium

High blood pressure (HBP) is a major risk factor for CHD. The relative risk of CHD, for both systolic and diastolic blood pressures, operates in a continuum of increasing risk for rising pressure but the absolute risk of CHD is considerably modified by coexisting risk factors (such as blood lipids and diabetes), many of which are also influenced by diet. A cohort study in Finland observed a 51% greater risk of CHD mortality with a 100 mmol increase in 24-h urinary sodium excretion. Several clinical trials have convincingly demonstrated the ability of reduced sodium diets to lower blood pressure. A meta-analysis of long-term trials suggests that reducing daily salt intake from $12\,\mathrm{g\,day^{-1}}$ to $3\,\mathrm{g\,day^{-1}}$ is likely to reduce CHD by 25% (and strokes by 33%). Even more modest reductions would have substantial benefits (10% lower CHD for a 3-g salt reduction). The benefits of dietary potassium in lowering blood pressure have been well demonstrated but specific effects on CHD risk have not been well studied. Keeping the dietary sodium:potassium ratio at a low level is essential to avoid hypertension.

Food Items

Fruits and Vegetables

A systematic review reported that nine of ten ecological studies, two of three case–control studies, and six of sixteen cohort studies found a significant protective association for CHD with consumption of fruits and vegetables or surrogate nutrients. In a 12-year follow-up of 15 220 male physicians in the US, men who consumed at least 2.5 servings of vegetables per day were observed to have a 33% lower risk for CHD, compared with men in the lowest category (<1 serving per day). A follow-up study of NHANES (National Health and Nutrition Examination Survey), a large national survey in the US, also reported a coronary protective effect of regular fruit and vegetable intake. Persons who consumed fruits and vegetables 3 or more times a day were at 24% lower risk than those who consumed less than one portion a day. A global study of risk factors of CHD in 52 countries (INTERHEART) also reported low consumption of fruit and vegetables to be a major risk factor, across all regions.

Fish

In the UK diet and reinfarction trial, 2-year mortality was reduced by 29% in survivors of a first myocardial infarction in those receiving advice to consume fatty fish at least twice a week. A meta-analysis of 13 large cohort studies suggests a protective effect of fish intake against CHD. Compared with those who never consumed fish or did so less than once a month, persons who ate fish had a lower risk of CHD (38% lower for 5 or more times a week, 23% lower for 2–4 times a week, 15% lower for once a week, and 11% lower for 1–3 times a month). Each $20\,\mathrm{g\,day^{-1}}$ increase in fish consumption was related to a 7% lower risk of CHD.

Nuts

Several large epidemiological studies, the best known among them being the Adventist Health Study, demonstrated that frequent consumption of nuts was associated with decreased risk of CHD. The extent of risk reduction ranged from 18% to 57% for subjects who consumed nuts more than 5 times a week compared to those who never consumed nuts. An inverse dose–response relationship was demonstrated between the frequency of nut consumption and the risk of CHD, in men as well as in women. Most of these studies considered nuts as a group, combining many types of nuts (walnuts, almonds, pistachio, pecans, macadamia nuts, and legume peanuts).

Soy

Soy is rich in isoflavones, compounds that are structurally and functionally similar to estrogen. Several animal experiments suggest that intake of these isoflavones may provide protection against CHD, but human data on efficacy and safety are still awaited. Naturally occurring isoflavones, isolated with soy protein, reduced the plasma concentrations of total and LDL cholesterol without affecting the concentrations of triglycerides or HDL cholesterol in hypercholesterolemic individuals.

Dairy Products

Dairy consumption has been correlated positively, in ecological studies, with blood cholesterol as well as coronary mortality. Milk consumption correlated positively with coronary mortality rates in 43 countries and with myocardial infarction in 19 regions of Europe.

Alcohol

The relationship of alcohol to overall mortality and cardiovascular mortality has generally been J-shaped, when studied in Western populations in whom the rates of atherothrombotic vascular disorders are high. The protective effect of moderate ethanol consumption is primarily mediated through its effect on the risk of CHD, as supported by more than 60 prospective studies. A consistent coronary protective effect has been observed for consumption of 1–2 drinks per day of an alcohol-containing beverage but heavy drinkers have higher total mortality than moderate drinkers or abstainers, as do binge drinkers.

Composite Diets and CHD

The Mediterranean diet

The traditional Mediterranean diet has been described to have eight components:

1. high monounsaturated-to-saturated fat ratio;
2. moderate ethanol consumption;
3. high consumption of legumes;
4. high consumption of cereals (including bread);
5. high consumption of fruits;
6. high consumption of vegetables;
7. low consumption of meat and meat products; and
8. moderate consumption of milk and dairy products.

Most of these features are found in many diets in that region. The characteristic component is olive oil, and many equate a Mediterranean diet with consumption of olive oil.

A secondary prevention trial of dietary intervention in survivors of a first recent myocardial infarction (the Lyon Heart study), which aimed to study the cardioprotective effects of a 'Mediterranean type' of diet, actually left out its most characteristic component, olive oil. The main fat source was rapeseed oil. Vegetables and fruits were also increased in the diet. On a 4-year follow-up, the study reported a 72% reduction in cardiac death and nonfatal myocardial infarction. The risk of overall mortality was lowered by 56%. Large cohort studies in Greece and in several elderly European population groups have also recently reported a protective effect against CHD and better over all survival in persons consuming a Mediterranean type of diet. The protection was afforded by the composite diet rather than by any single component. Improvement in metabolic syndrome and reduction of inflammatory markers has also been observed with this diet, which may explain part of the protection against CHD.

DASH Diets

A composite diet, employed in the Dietary Approaches to Stop Hypertension (DASH) trials, has been found to be very effective in reducing blood pressure in persons with clinical hypertension as well as in people with blood pressure levels below that threshold. This diet combines fruits and vegetables with food products that are low in saturated fats. The blood pressure lowering effect is even greater when the DASH diet is modified to reduce the sodium content. Though the effects on CHD prevention have not been directly studied, the blood pressure and lipid-lowering effects of the low salt-DASH diet are likely to have a substantial impact on CHD risk.

Vegetarian Diets

A reduced risk of CVD has been reported in populations of vegetarians living in affluent countries and in case–control comparisons in developing countries. Reduced consumption of animal fat and increased consumption of fruit, vegetables, nuts, and cereals may underlie such a protective effect. However, 'vegetarian diets' *per se* need not be healthful. If not well planned, they can contain a large amount of refined carbohydrates and t-FAs, while being deficient in the levels of vegetable and fruit consumption. The composition of the vegetarian diet should, therefore, be defined in terms of its cardioprotective constituents.

Prudent versus Western Patterns

In the Health professionals follow-up study in the US, a prudent diet pattern was characterized by higher intake of vegetables, fruits, legumes, whole grains, fish, and poultry, whereas the Western pattern was defined by higher intake of red meat, processed meat, refined grains, sweets and dessert, French fries, and high-fat dairy products. After adjustment for age and other coronary risk factors, relative risks, from the lowest to the highest quintiles of the prudent pattern score, were 1.0, 0.87, 0.79, 0.75, and 0.70, indicating a high level of protection. In contrast, the relative risks, across increasing quintiles of the western pattern, were 1.0, 1.21, 1.36, 1.40, and 1.64, indicating a mounting level of excess risk. These associations persisted in subgroup analyses according to cigarette smoking, body mass index, and parental history of myocardial infarction.

Japanese Diet

The traditional Japanese diet has attracted much attention because of the high life expectancy and low CHD mortality rates among the Japanese. This diet is low in fat and sugar and includes soy, seaweeds, raw fish, and a predominant use of rice. It has been high in salt, but salt consumption has recently been declining in response to Japanese Health Ministry guidelines.

Prevention Pathways

The powerful relationship of specific nutrients, food items and dietary patterns to CHD has been persuasively demonstrated by observational epidemiological studies (which indicate the potential for primary prevention in populations) and by clinical trials (which demonstrate the impact on secondary prevention in individuals).

Atherosclerotic vascular diseases (especially CHD) are multifactorial in origin. Each of the risk factors operates in a continuous manner, rather than across an arbitrary threshold. When multiple risk factors coexist, the overall risk becomes multiplicative. As a result of these two phenomena, the majority of CHD events occurring in any population arise from any individuals with modest elevations of multiple risk factors rather than from the few individuals with marked elevation of a single risk factor.

These phenomena have two major implications for CHD prevention. First, it must be recognized that a successful prevention strategy must combine population-wide interventions (through policy measures and public education) with individual risk reduction approaches (usually involving counseling and clinical interventions). Second, diet is a major pathway for CHD prevention, as it influences many of the risk factors for CHD, and can have a widespread impact on populations and substantially reduce the risk in high-risk individuals. Even small changes in blood pressure, blood lipids, body weight, central obesity, blood sugar, inflammatory markers, etc., can significantly alter the CHD rates, if the changes are widespread across the population. Modest population-wide dietary changes can accomplish this, as demonstrated in Finland and Poland. At the same time, diet remains a powerful intervention to substantially reduce the risk of a CHD-related event in individuals who are at high risk due to multiple risk factors, prior vascular disease, or diabetes.

A diet that is protective against CHD should integrate: plenty of fruits and vegetables ($400–600\,g\,day^{-1}$); a moderate amount of fish (2–3 times a week); a small quantity of nuts; adequate amounts of PUFAs and MUFAs (together constituting about 75% of the daily fat intake); low levels of SFAs (less than 25% of the daily fat intake); limited salt intake (preferably less than $5\,day^{-1}$); and restricted use of sugar. Such diets should be culturally appropriate, economically affordable, and based on locally available foods.

National policies and international trade practices must be shaped to facilitate the wide availability and uptake of such diets. Nutrition counseling of individuals at high risk must also adopt these principles while customizing dietary advice to specific needs of the person. CHD is eminently preventable, as evident from research and demonstrated in practice across the world. Appropriate nutrition is a major pathway for CHD prevention and must be used more widely to make CHD prevention even more effective at the global level.

See also: **Antioxidants**: Diet and Antioxidant Defense; Observational Studies; Intervention Studies. **Coronary Heart Disease**: Lipid Theory. **Dietary Fiber**: Role in Nutritional Management of Disease. **Fatty Acids**: Monounsaturated; Omega-3 Polyunsaturated; Omega-6 Polyunsaturated; Saturated. **Fish. Folic Acid. Potassium. Sodium**: Physiology; Salt Intake and Health. **Vegetarian Diets**.

Further Reading

Appel LJ, Moore TJ, Obarzanek E *et al.* (1997) A clinical trial of the effects of dietary patterns on blood pressure. DASH Collaborative Research Group. *New England Journal of Medicine* 336: 1117–1124.

De Lorgeril M, Salen P, Martin JL *et al.* (1999) Mediterranean diet, traditional risk factors, and the rate of cardiovascular complications after myocardial infarction: final report of Lyon Diet Heart Study. *Circulation* 99: 779–785.

He FJ and MacGregor GA (2003) How far should salt intake be reduced? *Hypertension* 42: 1093–1099

He K, Song Y, Daviglus ML *et al.* (2004) Accumulated evidence on fish consumption and coronary heart disease mortality: a meta-analysis of cohort studies. *Circulation* 109: 2705–2711.

INTERSALT Cooperative Research Group (1988) INTERSALT: an international study of electrolyte excretion and blood pressure. Results for 24 hr urinary sodium and potassium excretion. *British Medical Journal* 297: 319–328.

Kris-Etherton P, Daniels SR, Eckel RH *et al.* (2001) Summary of the scientific conference on dietary fatty acids and cardiovascular health: conference summary from the nutrition committee of the American Heart Association. *Circulation* 103: 1034–1039.

Ness AR and Powles JW (1997) Fruit and vegetables, and cardiovascular disease: a review. *International Journal of Epidemiology* 26: 1–13.

Reddy KS and Katan MB (2004) Diet, nutrition and the prevention of hypertension and cardiovascular diseases. *Public Health and Nutrition* 7: 167–186.

Sacks FM, Svetkey LP, Vollmer WM *et al.* (2001) Effects on blood pressure of reduced dietary sodium and the Dietary Approaches to Stop Hypertension (DASH) diet. DASH-Sodium Collaborative Research Group. *New England Journal of Medicine* 344: 3–10.

Seely S (1981) Diet and coronary disease. A survey of mortality rates and food consumption statistics of 24 countries. *Medical Hypotheses* 7: 907–918.

Trichopoulou A, Costacou T, Bamia C, and Trichopoulos D (2003) Adherence to a Mediterranean diet and survival in a Greek population. *New England Journal of Medicine* 348: 2599–2608.

Verschuren WMM, Jacobs DR, Bloemberg BP *et al.* (1995) Serum total cholesterol and long-term coronary heart disease mortality in different cultures. Twenty-five year follow-up of the Seven Countries Study. *JAMA* 274: 131–136.

World Health Organization (2003) Diet, nutrition and the prevention of chronic diseases. *Technical Report Series* 916: 1–149.

World Health Organization (2002) *The World Health Report 2002. Reducing Risks, Promoting Healthy Life*. Geneva: WHO.

Yusuf S, Hawken S, Ounpuu S *et al.* (2004) INTERHEART study Investigators. Effect of potentially modifiable risk factors associated with myocardial infarction in 52 countries (the INTERHEART study): case-control study. *Lancet* 364: 937–952.

DIETARY FIBER

Contents

Physiological Effects and Effects on Absorption

I T Johnson, Institute of Food Research, Norwich, UK

Introduction

It has long been recognized that both animal feedstuffs and human foods contain poorly digestible components, which do not contribute to nutrition in the classical sense of providing essential substances or metabolic energy. With the development of scientific approaches to animal husbandry in the nineteenth century, the term 'crude fiber' was coined to describe the material that remained after rigorous nonenzymic hydrolysis of feeds. During the twentieth century, various strands of thought concerning the virtues of 'whole' foods, derived from plant components that had undergone only minimal processing, began to converge, leading eventually to the dietary fiber hypothesis. Put simply, this states that the nondigestible components of plant cell walls are essential for the maintenance of human health.

In the early 1970s the physician and epidemiologist Hugh Trowell recognized that the crude fiber figures available at the time for foods had little physiological significance and were of no practical value in the context of human diets. He was amongst the first to use the term dietary fiber to describe the 'remnants of plant cell walls resistant to hydrolysis (digestion) by the alimentary enzymes of man.' This definition was later refined and given the more quantitative form: "The sum of lignin and the plant polysaccharides that are not digested by the endogenous secretions of the mammalian digestive tract." This definition paved the way for the development of analytical methods that could be used to define the fiber content of human foods. Broadly, these techniques are based on enzymic removal of the digestible elements in food, followed by either gravimetric analysis of the residue ('Southgate' and Association of Analytical Chemists (AOAC) methods), which results in the retention of some undigested starch, or chemical analysis ('Englyst' method), which enables a more precise separation of starch from the structural polysaccharides of the cell wall. In the latter case, the cell wall components are defined as 'nonstarch polysaccharides' (NSP). Whatever analytical approach is used, both 'dietary fiber' and nonstarch polysaccharides are shorthand terms for large and complex mixtures of polysaccharides. The components of such mixtures vary widely among foods and they often share few properties other than resistance to digestion in the small intestine. A summary of the main types of plant cell polysaccharides contained in the general definition of dietary fiber is given in **Table 1**.

In recent years this problem has been made more complex in some ways because of the explosion of interest in functional foods for gastrointestinal health. These often contain high levels of novel oligo- and polysaccharides, which might perhaps be regarded as analogs of dietary fiber. Fructose oligosaccharides, which are nondigestible but highly fermentable, are now often added to foods as prebiotic substrates for the colonic microflora. Such materials may not fit the original definition of dietary fiber, but it is certainly not helpful to exclude them from the contemporary concept, which needs to expand to accommodate modern developments.

Table 1 Major components of dietary fiber

Food source	Polysaccharides and related substances
Fruits and vegetables	Cellulose, xyloglucans, arabinogalactans, pectic substances, glycoproteins
Cereals	Cellulose, arabinoxylans, glucoarabinoxylans, β-D-glucans, lignin, and phenolic esters
Legume seeds	Cellulose, xyloglucans, galactomannans, pectic substances
Manufactured products	Gums (guar gum, gum arabic), alginates, carrageenan, modified cellulose gums (methyl cellulose, carboxymethyl cellulose)

Table 2 A Comparison of values for nonstarch polysaccharides and dietary fiber

Food source	Nonstarch Polysaccharides (Englyst method)	Total dietary fiber (AOAC method)
White bread	2.1	2.9
Brown bread	3.5	5.0
Wholemeal bread	5.0	7.0
Green vegetables	2.7	3.3
Potatoes	1.9	2.4
Fresh fruit	1.4	1.9
Nuts	6.6	8.8

Data modified from McCance and Widdowson's (2002) *The Composition of Foods*, 6th Edition, Cambridge: Royal Society of Chemistry.

The presence of large undigested cell wall fragments, finely dispersed particulates, or soluble polysaccharides can alter physiological processes throughout the gut. The effects of different fiber components depend upon their varied physical and chemical properties during digestion, and also upon their susceptibility to degradation by bacterial enzymes in the colon. The complex nature of the various substances covered by the general definition of dietary fiber means that a single analytical value for the fiber content of a food is a poor guide to its physiological effects. This article will review the main mechanisms of action of resistant polysaccharides in the alimentary tract and their implications for human health.

Sources and Types of Dietary Fiber

The main sources of dietary fiber in most Western diets are well characterized, and high-quality data are available for both food composition and dietary intakes. This is not always true for diets in developing countries, however, and this problem bedevils attempts to investigate the importance of fiber by making international comparisons of diet and disease. Another problem is that different analytical approaches give slightly different values for the dietary fiber content of foods, and do not reflect the physical and chemical properties of the different polysaccharide components. The use of enzymic hydrolysis to determine the 'unavailable carbohydrate' content of foods was refined by Southgate, and his technique was used for the 4th edition of the UK standard food tables, *The Composition of Foods* published in 1978. The 6th edition, published in 2002, contains values for nonstarch polysaccharides, derived using the Englyst technique, but recommends use of AOAC methods for food labeling purposes. A comparison of values for nonstarch polysaccharides and dietary fiber values obtained by the AOAC method is given in **Table 2**.

In the UK about 47% of dietary fiber is obtained from cereal products, including bread and breakfast cereals. The level of cell wall polysaccharides in a product made from flour depends on the extraction rate, which is the proportion of the original grain present in the flour after milling. Thus a 'white' flour with an extraction rate of 70% usually contains about 3% NSP, whereas a 'wholemeal' flour with an extraction rate of 100% contains about 10% NSP. The terms 'soluble' and 'insoluble' fiber have been coined in order to partially overcome the problem of the lack of correspondence between the total analytical value for fiber and the physical properties of the measured polysaccharides. By adopting the Englyst technique for the separation and chemical analysis of nonstarch polysaccharides it is possible to specify both the soluble and insoluble fiber content of foods. Some representative values for soluble and insoluble fiber in cereal foods are given in **Table 3**, and those for fruits and vegetables, which provide a further 45% of the fiber in UK diets, are given in **Table 4**.

Fiber in the Digestive Tract

The primary function of the alimentary tract is to break down the complex organic macromolecules of which other organisms are composed into smaller molecules, which can then be selectively absorbed into the circulation by specialized mucosal epithelial cells. Food is conveyed progressively through the alimentary tract, stored at intervals, and broken down mechanically as required, by a tightly controlled system of rhythmic muscular contractions. The digestive enzymes are released into the lumen at the appropriate stages to facilitate the decomposition of carbohydrates, proteins, and complex lipids. By definition, the polysaccharides that comprise

Table 3 Soluble and insoluble nonstarch polysaccharides in some cereal products and nuts

Food source	Nonstarch polysaccharides (g per 100 g fresh weight)		
	Total NSP	Soluble NSP	Insoluble NSP
Sliced white bread	1.5	0.9	0.6
Sliced brown bread	3.6	1.1	2.5
Wholemeal bread	4.8	1.6	3.2
Spaghetti	1.2	0.6	0.6
Rye biscuits	11.7	3.9	7.8
Cornflakes	0.9	0.4	0.5
Crunchy oat cereal	6.0	3.3	2.7
Walnuts	3.5	1.5	2.0
Hazelnuts	6.5	2.5	4.0
Peanuts	6.2	1.9	4.3
Brazil nuts	4.3	1.3	3.0

Data modified from Englyst HN, Bingham SA, Runswick SS, Collinson E, and Cummings JH (1989) Dietary fibre (non-starch polysaccharides) in cereal products. *Journal of Human Nutrition and Dietetics* **2**: 253–271 and Englyst HN, Bingham SA, Runswick SS, Collinson E, Cummings JH (1989) Dietary fibre (non-starch polysaccharides) in fruit vegetables and nuts. *Journal of Human Nutrition and Dietetics* **1**: 247–286.

Table 4 Soluble and insoluble nonstarch polysaccharides in some vegetables and fruits

Food source	Nonstarch polysaccharides (g per 100 g fresh weight)		
	Total NSP	Soluble NSP	Insoluble NSP
Apples (Cox)	1.7	0.7	1.0
Oranges	2.1	1.4	0.7
Plums	1.8	1.2	0.6
Bananas	1.1	0.7	0.4
Potatoes	1.1	0.6	0.5
Sprouts	4.8	2.5	2.3
Peas (frozen)	5.2	1.6	3.6
Carrots	2.5	1.4	1.1
Courgettes	1.2	0.6	0.6
Runner beans	2.3	0.9	1.4
Baked beans	3.5	2.1	1.4
Tomato	1.1	0.4	0.7
Lettuce	1.2	0.6	0.6
Onion	1.7	0.9	0.8
Celery	1.3	0.6	0.7

Data modified from Englyst HN, Bingham SA, Runswick SS, Collinson E, and Cummings JH (1989) Dietary fibre (non-starch polysaccharides) in fruit vegetables and nuts. *Journal of Human Nutrition and Dietetics* **1**: 247–286.

dietary fiber are not digested by endogenous enzymes, though they are often fermented to a greater or lesser degree by bacterial enzymes in the large intestine.

The Mouth and Pharynx

The earliest stages of digestion begin in the mouth, where food particles are reduced in size, lubricated with saliva, and prepared for swallowing. The saliva also contains the digestive enzyme salivary amylase, which begins the hydrolysis of starch molecules. Cell wall polysaccharides are an important determinant of food texture, and they exert an indirect effect on the degree of mechanical breakdown of plant foods prior to swallowing. Hard foods tend to be chewed more thoroughly than soft ones, and hence the presence of dietary fiber in unrefined foods may begin to regulate digestion at a very early stage.

The Stomach

The first delay in the transit of food through the digestive tract occurs in the stomach, where large food fragments are further degraded by rigorous muscular activity in the presence of hydrochloric acid and proteolytic enzymes. The need to disrupt and disperse intractable food particles and cell walls appears to delay the digestive process significantly. For example, the absorption of sugar from whole apples is significantly slower than from apple juice. Similarly, the rate at which the starch is digested and absorbed from cubes of cooked potato has been shown to be much slower when they are swallowed whole than when they are chewed normally. Thus, simple mechanical factors can limit the rate at which glucose from carbohydrate foods enters the circulation.

The Small Intestine

The small intestine is the main site of nutrient absorption, and it is in fact the largest of the digestive organs in terms of surface area. The semi-liquid products of gastric digestion are released periodically into the duodenum, and then propelled downstream by peristaltic movements, at about 1 cm per minute. The hydrolysis of proteins, triglycerides, and starch continues within the duodenum and upper jejunum, under the influence of pancreatic enzymes. The final stages of hydrolysis of dietary macromolecules occur under the influence of extracellular enzymes at the mucosal surface. The released products are absorbed into the circulation, along with water and electrolytes, via the specialized epithelial cells of the intestinal villi. Muscular activity in the small intestinal wall, together with rhythmic contractions of the villi, ensures that the partially digested chyme is well stirred. In adults, the first fermentable residues from a meal containing complex carbohydrates enter the colon approximately 4.5 h after ingestion. When a solution containing indigestible sugar is swallowed without food it reaches the colon about 1.5 h earlier than when the same material is added to a solid meal containing dietary fiber. The presence of solid food residues slows transit, probably by delaying gastric emptying and perhaps also by increasing the viscosity of the chyme so that it tends to resist the peristaltic flow. Soluble polysaccharides such as guar gum, pectin, and β-glucan from oats increase mouth to cecum transit time still further.

In creating the dietary fiber hypothesis, Trowell's principal interest was its role in the prevention of metabolic disorders. In particular, he believed that dietary fiber was a major factor in the prevention of diabetes mellitus, which, he argued, was probably unknown in Western Europe prior to the introduction of mechanized flour milling. In earlier times the near-universal consumption of unrefined carbohydrate foods would have ensured that intact indigestible cell wall polysaccharides were present throughout the upper alimentary tract during digestion. This, according to Trowell and others, favored slow absorption of glucose, which in turn placed less strain upon the ability of the pancreas to maintain glucose homeostasis. There is no doubt that type 2 diabetes has become more common in Western countries as prosperity, and an excess of energy consumption over expenditure, has grown. It is not established that rapid absorption of glucose due to consumption of refined starches is a primary cause of diabetes, but the control of glucose assimilation is certainly a key factor in its management. Cell wall polysaccharides influence the digestion and absorption of carbohydrates in a variety of ways, and are a major determinant of the 'glycemic index,' which is essentially a quantitative expression of the quantity of glucose appearing in the bloodstream after ingestion of a carbohydrate-rich food. To calculate the index, fasted subjects are given a test meal of the experimental food containing a standardized quantity of carbohydrate. The change in concentration of glucose in the blood is then measured over a period of time. The ratio of the area under the blood-glucose curve in response to the test meal to that produced by an equal quantity of a standard reference food is then calculated and expressed as a percentage. When glucose is used as the standard, most complex starchy foods have glycemic indices lower than 100%.

The physical resistance of plant cell walls during their passage through the gut varies considerably from one food to another. Cell walls that remain intact in the small intestine will impede the access of pancreatic amylase to starch. This is particularly true of the cells of legume seeds, which have been shown to retain much of their integrity during digestion. Legume-based foods such as lentils and chilli beans have glycemic indices that are amongst the lowest of all complex carbohydrate foods. Even when enzymes and their substrates do come into contact, the presence of cell wall polysaccharides may slow the diffusion of hydrolytic products through the partially digested matrix in the gut lumen. These effects of dietary fiber on carbohydrate metabolism emphasize once more that physiological effects cannot be predicted from simple analytical values for total fiber, because they are consequences of cellular structure, rather than the absolute quantity of cell wall polysaccharides within the food.

Many studies on postprandial glycemia have been conducted using isolated fiber supplements such, as pectin or guar gum added to glucose test-meals or to low-fiber sources of starch. They demonstrate that, contrary to Trowell's original hypothesis, wheat bran and other insoluble cell wall materials have little effect on glucose metabolism. However, certain soluble polysaccharides, such as guar gum, pectin, and oat β-glucan, which form viscous solutions in the stomach and small intestine, do slow the absorption of glucose. Highly viscous food components may delay gastric emptying and inhibit the dispersion of the digesta along the small intestine, but the primary mechanism of action appears to be suppression of convective stirring in the fluid layer adjacent to the mucosal surface. The rapid uptake of monosaccharides by the epithelial cells tends to reduce the concentration of glucose in this boundary layer, so that absorption from the gut lumen becomes rate-limited by the relatively slow process of diffusion. The overall effect is to delay the assimilation of glucose and hence suppress the glycemic response to glucose or starchy foods in both healthy volunteers and in people with diabetes. A similar mechanism probably inhibits the reabsorption of cholesterol and bile salts in the distal ileum and this may account for the ability of some viscous types of soluble dietary fiber such as guar gum and β-glucan to reduce plasma cholesterol levels in humans.

One of the main reasons for developing analytical methods to distinguish between soluble and insoluble components of dietary fiber was to provide a means of assessing the capacity of fiber-rich foods to influence carbohydrate and lipid metabolism. There is evidence that diets that provide 30–50% of their fiber in the form of soluble polysaccharides are associated with lower cholesterol levels and better glycemic control than diets that contain mostly insoluble fiber. Several officially recognized sets of guidelines for patients with impaired glucose metabolism and its complications (syndrome X) now specifically recommend a high intake of carbohydrate foods that are rich in soluble fiber.

Some of the interactions between cell wall polysaccharides and other food components in the small intestine are much more specific. There has been considerable interest over a number of years in the possibility that the polysaccharides and complex phenolic components of cell walls contain polar groups that could interact with and bind ionized species in the gastrointestinal contents, thereby reducing their availability for absorption. Intraluminal binding of heavy metals, toxins, and carcinogens might be a valuable protective mechanism, but binding of micronutrients could seriously compromise nutritional status.

Interactions of this type can be shown to occur *in vitro*, and studies with animals and human ileostomists suggest that charged polysaccharides such as pectin can displace cations into the colon under experimental conditions. However, there is little objective evidence that dietary fiber *per se* has much of an adverse effect on mineral metabolism in humans. Indeed, highly fermentable polysaccharides and fructose oligosaccharides have recently been shown to promote the absorption of calcium and magnesium in both animal and human studies. The mechanism for the effect is not entirely clear, but it is probably a consequence of fermentation acidifying the luminal contents of the colon and enhancing carrier-mediated transport of minerals across the colonic mucosa.

In unprocessed legume seeds, oats, and other cereals phytate (myo-inositol hexaphosphate) is often present in close association with cell wall polysaccharides. Unlike the polysaccharides themselves, phytate does exert a potent binding effect on minerals, and has been shown to significantly reduce the availability of magnesium, zinc, and calcium for absorption in humans. Phytate levels in foods can be reduced by the activity of endogenous phytase, by hydrolysis with exogenous enzymes, or by fermentation. Dephytinized products may therefore be of benefit to individuals at risk of suboptimal mineral status. However, there are indications from animal and *in vitro* studies that phytate is an anticarcinogen that may contribute to the protective effects of complex fiber-rich foods. The overall significance of phytate in the diet therefore requires further assessment in human trials.

The Large Intestine

Microorganisms occur throughout the alimentary tract but in healthy individuals their numbers and diversity are maintained within strict limits by the combined effects of intraluminal conditions, rapid transit, and host immunity. The colon and rectum, however, are adapted to facilitate bacterial colonization, and the typical adult human colonic microflora has been estimated to contain about 400 different bacterial species. The largest single groups present are Gram-negative anaerobes of the genus *Bacteroides*, and Gram-positive organisms including bifidobacteria, eubacteria, lactobacilli, and clostridia. However, a large proportion of the species present cannot be cultured *in vitro* and are very poorly characterized.

The proximal colon, which receives undigested food residues, intestinal secretions, and the remnants of exfoliated enterocytes from the distal ileum, contains around 200 g of bacteria and substrates in a semiliquid state. These conditions are ideal for bacterial fermentation. Most of the bacteria of the human colon utilize carbohydrate as a source of energy, although not all can degrade polysaccharides directly. Many that are ultimately dependent upon dietary carbohydrate residues for energy are adapted to utilize the initial degradation products of the polysaccharide utilizers, rather than the polymers themselves. It has been estimated that somewhere between 20 and 80 g of carbohydrate enter the human colon every day, about half of which is undigested starch. Around 30 g of bacteria are produced for every 100 g of carbohydrate fermented.

Apart from dietary fiber, there are three major sources of unabsorbed carbohydrate for the colonic microflora. Perhaps the most important is resistant starch, which consists of retrograded starch polymers and starch granules enclosed within intact plant cell walls. Nondigestible sugars, sugar alcohols, and oligosaccharides such as fructooligosaccharides and galactooligosaccharides occur only sparingly in most plant foods, but they are now of great commercial interest because they can be used as prebiotics to selectively manipulate the numbers of bifidobacteria in the human colon. Endogenous substrates including mucus are also important for the colonic microflora. Mucus is an aqueous dispersion of a complex group of glycoproteins containing oligosaccharide side-chains, which are a major source of fermentable substrates. Even when the colon is surgically isolated and has no access to exogenous substrates it still supports a complex microflora.

The beneficial effects of dietary fiber on the alimentary tract were emphasized by another of the founders of the dietary fiber hypothesis, Denis Burkitt, who based his arguments largely on the concept of fecal bulk, developed as a result of field observations in rural Africa, where cancer and other chronic bowel diseases were rare. His hypothesis was that populations consuming the traditional rural diets, rich in vegetables and cereal foods, produced bulkier, more frequent stools than persons eating the refined diets typical of industrialized societies. Chronic constipation was thought to cause straining of abdominal muscles during passage of stool, leading to prolonged high pressures within the colonic lumen and the lower abdomen. This in turn was thought to increase the risk of various diseases of muscular degeneration including varicose veins, hemorrhoids, hiatus hernia, and colonic diverticulas. Colorectal neoplasia was also thought to result from infrequent defecation, because it caused prolonged exposure of the colonic epithelial cells to mutagenic chemicals, which could initiate cancer. Burkitt's overall hypothesis for the beneficial effects of fecal bulk has never really been refuted, and epidemiological evidence continues to support a protective role of fiber against colorectal cancer, particularly within Europe. However, the origins of intestinal neoplasia are now known to be far more complex than Burkitt was able to envisage, and there is little evidence to suggest a direct causal link between chronic constipation and colorectal cancer. Indeed, in one recent prevention trial, the risk of recurrence of colorectal polyps was slightly increased by prolonged supplementation with a bulk laxative based on one specialized source of cell wall polysaccharides.

Whatever the relationship to disease, it is certainly true that the consumption of dietary fiber is one major determinant of both fecal bulk and the frequency of defecation (bowel habit). However, the magnitude of the effect depends upon the type of fiber consumed. Soluble cell wall polysaccharides such as pectin are readily fermented by the microflora, whereas lignified tissues such as wheat bran tend to remain at least partially intact in the feces. Both classes of dietary fiber can contribute to fecal bulk but by different mechanisms. The increment in stool mass caused by wheat bran depends to some extent on particle size, but in healthy Western populations it has been shown that for every 1 g of wheat bran consumed per day, the output of stool is increased by between 3 and 5 g. Other sources of dietary fiber also favor water retention. For example, isphagula, a mucilaginous material derived from *Psyllium*, is used pharmaceutically as a bulk laxative. Soluble polysaccharides such as guar and oat β-glucan are readily fermented by anaerobic bacteria, but solubility is no guarantee of fermentability, as is illustrated by modified cellulose gums such as methylcellulose, which is highly resistant to

degradation in the human gut. Fermentation reduces the mass and water-holding capacity of soluble polysaccharides considerably, but the bacterial cells derived from them do make some contribution to total fecal output. Thus, although all forms of dietary fiber are mild laxatives, the single analytical measurement of total fiber content again provides no simple predictive measure of physiological effect.

Although fermentation of fiber tends to reduce its effectiveness as a source of fecal bulk, it has other very important benefits. The absorption and metabolism of short-chain fatty acids derived from carbohydrate fermentation provides the route for the recovery of energy from undigested polysaccharides. Butyrate functions as the preferred source of energy for the colonic mucosal cells, whilst propionate and acetate are absorbed and metabolized systemically. There continues to be much debate about the importance of butyrate for the colon. *In vitro*, butyrate causes differentiation of tumor cells, suppresses cell division, and induces programed cell death (apoptosis). These effects are thought likely to suppress the development of cancer, but it is not yet entirely clear whether they also occur in the intact intestine. Research continues on the importance of butyrate and other short-chain fatty acids for human health.

The other major breakdown products of carbohydrate fermentation are hydrogen, methane, and carbon dioxide, which together comprise flatus gas. Excess gas production can cause distension and pain in some individuals, especially if they attempt to increase their fiber consumption too abruptly. In most cases, however, extreme flatus is probably caused more by fermentation of oligosaccharides such as stachyose and verbascose, which are found principally in legume seeds, rather than the cell wall polysaccharides themselves.

Conclusion

Several decades of research have confirmed that cell wall polysaccharides modify physiological mechanisms throughout the alimentary tract. Delayed absorption of glucose and lipids in the small intestine makes an important contribution to metabolic control in type 2 diabetes, and certain types of hypercholesterolemia, respectively. Any loss of carbohydrates to the colon will lead to increased fermentative activity, and through this pathway, most of the unabsorbed energy will be recovered as short-chain fatty acids. Unfermented cell wall polysaccharides and increased bacterial mass contribute to fecal bulk. All these established physiological effects, coupled with the possibility of using oligosaccharides as prebiotics to modify the colonic microflora, have greatly stimulated interest in nondigestible carbohydrates amongst food manufacturers and consumers in the past few years. There is little to suggest that conventional sources of fiber compromise micronutrient metabolism in otherwise healthy individuals, but the possibility of this and other adverse effects needs to be considered, as the use of novel polysaccharides as sources or analogs of dietary fiber, both for conventional products and for functional foods, continues to expand.

See also: **Carbohydrates**: Resistant Starch and Oligosaccharides. **Dietary Fiber**: Potential Role in Etiology of Disease; Role in Nutritional Management of Disease. **Functional Foods**: Health Effects and Clinical Applications.

Further Reading

Bell S, Goldman VM, Bistrian BR, Arnold AH, Ostroff G, and Forse RA (1999) Effect of beta-glucan from oats and yeast on serum lipids. *Critical Reviews in Food Science and Nutrition* **39**: 189–202.

Burkitt DP and Trowell HC (eds.) (1975) *Refined Carbohydrate Foods: Some Implications of Dietary Fibre.* London: Academic Press.

Englyst HN, Bingham SA, Runswick SS, Collinson E, and Cummings JH (1989) Dietary fibre (non-starch polysaccharides) in cereal products. *Journal of Human Nutrition and Dietetics* **2**: 253–271.

Englyst HN, Bingham SA, Runswick SS, Collinson E, and Cummings JH (1989) Dietary fibre (non-starch polysaccharides) in fruit vegetables and nuts. *Journal of Human Nutrition and Dietetics* **1**: 247–286.

Englyst HN, Bingham SA, Runswick SS, Collinson E, and Cummings JH (1989) Dietary fibre (non-starch polysaccharides) in fruit vegetables and nuts. *Journal of Human Nutrition and Dietetics* **1**: 247–286.

Food Standards Agency (2002) *McCance and Widdowson's The Composition of Foods,* 6th summary edn Cambridge: The Royal Society of Chemistry.

Johnson IT and Southgate DAT (1994) *Dietary Fibre and Related Substances.* London: Chapman Hall.

Kushi LH, Meyer KA, and Jacobs Jr DR (1999) Cereals legumes and chronic disease risk reduction: Evidence from epidemiologic studies. *American Journal of Clinical Nutrition* **70**: 451S–458S.

McCance and Widdowson's (2002) *The Composition of Foods,* 6th Edition, Cambridge: Royal Society of Chemistry.

Nutrition Society (2003) Symposium on "Dietary Fibre in Health and Disease". *Proceedings of the Nutrition Society* **62**: 1–249.

Scholz-Ahrens KE and Schrezenmeir J (2002) Inulin, oligofructose and mineral metabolism – experimental data and mechanism. *British Journal of Nutrition* **87**(suppl 2): S179–186.

Southgate DAT (1992) *Determination of Food Carbohydrates,* 2nd edn. London: Elsevier Applied Science Publishers.

Potential Role in Etiology of Disease

D L Topping and **L Cobiac**, CSIRO Health Sciences and Nutrition, Adelaide, SA, Australia

Noninfectious diseases cause much morbidity and mortality in developed countries in Europe, the Americas, Asia, and Australasia. They are expected to increase due to an alarming increase in obesity, with its attendant risk of diabetes, coronary heart disease (CHD), and some cancers. Equally important, they are becoming an issue in developing countries through greater affluence. In every case, they have serious negative socioeconomic impacts, and their prevention through appropriate dietary and lifestyle change is the optimal strategy to minimize personal and community costs. This strategy is believed to have contributed substantially to economic growth in countries where it has been applied.

Obesity is a fairly visible problem that tends to overshadow other considerations. Energy intake in excess of expenditure is the root cause of obesity, and dietary carbohydrates are implicated specifically in the development of overweight. Exclusion of carbohydrates is attracting attention as a weight control strategy but this ignores the fact that digestible carbohydrates (including starch) provide the same amount of energy per gram as protein and less than 45% of the energy of fat and 60% of the energy of alcohol. Furthermore, it overlooks the many early comparative population studies that showed that several low-risk groups ate high-starch diets compared to high-risk populations that consumed processed foods high in refined carbohydrates and fat and low in fiber. With time, dietary fiber (rather than the whole diet) received specific attention, and many studies were conducted on the health benefits. This may have contributed to some of the current lack of clarity of the role of fiber and complex carbohydrates in health promotion. It may be compounded by the inadequacy of population data linking fiber (and also starches) to disease processes for important conditions such as colorectal cancer. Only recently have good population data emerged for a protective role for fiber in this condition. This is in marked contrast to the well-established therapeutic and preventive action of fiber in constipation and diverticular disease. Furthermore, it is critical to determine what is meant by the term 'dietary fiber' because other food components may contribute to the major effects ascribed to fiber. This is important when considering the apparent protection conferred by whole grains against disease risk, especially because a health claim is permitted in the United States for their consumption.

Associations between Dietary Fiber and Disease Processes

The early population studies of Walker, Burkitt, and Trowell in Africa in the 1950s showed that serum cholesterol concentrations were low in South African Bantus (at low risk of CHD) who consumed a diet apparently high in fiber and low in fat. Additionally, colon cancer was virtually unknown among the latter, in contrast to white South Africans. Dietary fiber was known to resist digestion by human intestinal enzymes, which helped to explain the greater fecal bulk seen with higher fiber intakes. This was thought to lower colonic exposure to carcinogens through a simple dilution effect with fiber consumption. Subsequently, it was suggested that diabetes may be related to a deficiency of fiber in the diet whereas other epidemiological studies have shown associations between more dietary fiber consumption and lower risk of some of the hormone-dependent cancers (prostate and breast). Many of these observational population studies are limited by their reliance on reported food intakes which may be compromised in turn by food compositional data because the latter can be limited by the analytical methodology used. Multinational comparisons may be affected by the fact that food sources and processing vary between countries. There are other potential confounders. For example, diets high in fiber-rich foods may contain other protective agents (e.g., phyotoestrogens folate and antioxidants) that could be the actual mediators of protection. Finally, some of the experimental studies and human interventions, especially in colorectal cancer, have given ambiguous or negative outcomes due to limitations of study design.

Dietary Fiber, Complex Carbohydrates, and Health Outcomes: A Need for Fiber Equivalents?

Technology has proved to be a significant issue in human fiber research. Early studies were limited by the relatively simple analytical methods then current. These were designed to measure the fiber components of forage consumed by important ruminant farm animals. Forage foods are high in insoluble polysaccharides and contain lignin (which is not a carbohydrate but a complex polyphenolic ether) and look 'fibrous,' so dietary fiber was equated with roughage and was defined as "those structural and exudative components of plants that were resistant to digestion by human gut enzymes." The methods used initially were quite severe and, with increasing sophistication of analytical methodology (notably chromatography), it became apparent that lignin was only a minor component of fiber compared with nonstarch polysaccharides (NSPs). Technological advances have revealed the importance of fractions such as soluble NSPs. As their name suggests, these dissolve in water but not necessarily under gut conditions. Fiber was then redefined as NSPs plus lignin, which has moved the concept of away from the roughage model. Recently, there has been a further substantial revision of the view of what exactly constitutes dietary fiber with the emerging recognition of the contribution of resistant starch (RS) and oligosaccharides (OSs) to 'fiber' action. It was thought that all of dietary starch consumed in cooked foods was digested in the human small intestine. It is becoming clear that this is not so, and that a substantial fraction of ingested starch, RS, escapes from the small intestine and enters the colon of healthy humans. In terms of the dietary polysaccharides entering that viscus, RS may exceed NSPs in quantity and in the range of its actions. Indeed, some populations that were thought to consume high-fiber diets actually eat less than higher risk groups. An example is the native Africans studied by Burkitt and colleagues who eat unrefined diets based on maize but in fact eat less fiber than the high-risk whites.

Unlike NSPs (which are intrinsically resistant to human digestive enzymes), RS is influenced greatly by physiological and physical factors. Thus, raw starches are highly resistant and gelatinized starches (cooked in the presence of water) are much more digestible due to hydration and the loss of granular structure. However, cooling of cooked starchy foods leads to the generation of RS through retrogradation (which is a realignment of the polysaccharide chains). Other factors, including the relative proportions of amylose and amylopectin and the presence of other food components such as NSPs and lipids, influence RS. High-fiber foods tend to be higher in RS, whereas fats can form complexes with starch that resist digestion. Mastication, transit time, and gender can influence the amount of RS, which means that purely chemical determinations probably give an underestimate of the quantity of starch entering the large bowel. Physical breakdown of foods (especially whole grains) may be particularly important because access to upper intestinal digestive enzymes is limited in large particles, especially in the presence of NSPs. RS has been classified into four types based on the main factors that influence its presence, including physical inaccessibility, cooking, and retrogradation (RS types RS_{1-3}). Of particular interest is the emergence of chemically modified starches (RS_4) as RS because these are used widely in food processing.

In the large bowel NSPs and RS are fermented by the microflora, yielding metabolic end products, principally short-chain fatty acids (SCFAs), which may mediate some of the health benefits ascribed to the carbohydrates. Undigested protein (resistant protein) and other nondigested carbohydrates (e.g., OSs) also contribute to large bowel fermentation. These nondigested fractions contribute to dietary fiber via fermentation and could be considered in net dietary fiber intake. This problem could be overcome relatively easily by classifying them (and other non-NSP carbohydrates) as fiber equivalents in which their actions are compared against an agreed standard. This is similar to the situation with other nutrients such as vitamin A, where retinol equivalents include carotenoids, which are retinol precursors. It follows that classifications based on chemical composition alone appear to be quite inadequate if one considers as improved health and diminished disease risk as the most important issues.

Dietary Fiber and the Etiology of Coronary Heart Disease

Population Studies

Consumption of unrefined plant foods has been related to lower risk of CHD for some time, but the hypothesis that dietary fiber (i.e., NSP) intake could protect directly against the disease is relatively recent. The suggestion has been supported by a number of epidemiological studies linking higher intakes with lower risk. Vegetarians who consume more plant foods tend to have lower plasma lipids and blood pressure than age- and gender-matched omnivores. However, the strongest evidence derives not from these studies but from a number of very large cohort studies in several countries showing a consistent protective effect of whole grain consumption and CHD risk. Whole grain cereal consumption has been related to substantially lower risk of CHD in both men and women. The evidence for the latter is considered to be sufficiently strong for the US

Food and Drug Administration to permit a health claim for consumption of whole grain cereal foods and lowering of the risk of CHD. Similar claims are being considered in Europe. However, these relationships are a long way from proving a specific protective effect of dietary fiber. A study of the relationship of long-term intake of dietary fiber by 68 782 women showed a substantial lowering of relative risk of 0.53 for women in the highest quintile of fiber consumption (22.9 g/day) compared with the lowest (11.5 g/day). These intakes are low compared to those recommended by health authorities. Nevertheless, they do support the view that fiber is protective against CHD. Only the effect of cereal fiber was significant; that of fruits and vegetables was not. However, they leave unanswered the question of the relationship of other contributors to the effects of dietary fiber (e.g., RS) and CHD risk.

Potential Mechanisms Indicating a Role in the Etiology of Coronary Heart Disease

The mechanism for risk reduction and the fiber components responsible need resolution. Elevated plasma total and low-density lipoprotein (LDL) cholesterol concentrations are established risk factors for coronary morbidity and mortality. There are abundant human and animal data showing that diets high in soluble fiber lower plasma cholesterol. One population study has shown a significant negative relationship between viscous (soluble) fiber intake and carotid artery atherogensis as measured by intima–media thickness. This association was significant statistically even though average fiber intakes were not particularly high. When dietary fiber intakes have been related to measures of actual disease outcomes, the evidence is less convincing. A protective effect is often observed on univariate analyses, but once confounding variables are added, dietary fiber intake tends not to be a significant independent predictor of risk for developing CHD. However, in one 12-year follow-up study of men and women, a 6-g increase in daily dietary fiber intake was associated with a 25% reduction in the risk of developing CHD. The most likely direct protective role for dietary fiber in CHD etiology is through plasma lipid lowering. The effect appears to be specific for plasma total and LDL cholesterol, and, possibly, triacylglycerols (TAG). Of the main fiber components, soluble NSPs seem to be effective, but insoluble NSPs and RS (and probably OSs) are not. Indeed, it appears that some insoluble NSP preparations, such as wheat bran, may raise plasma cholesterol slightly. There is good evidence from animal and human studies to support a hypocholesterolemic effect of soluble NSPs either in enriched plant fractions (e.g., oat bran) or as natural (e.g., pectins and guar gum) or synthetic isolates (e.g., hydroxypropylmethylcellulose). The magnitude of the effect varies with dose, but reductions of approximately 5–10% at intakes of 6–12 g of NSPs/day appear to be reasonable. This lowering response approaches that seen with certain drugs, such as cholestyramine, used to manage hypercholesterolemia. Some studies have also shown a reduction in TAGs with soluble fibers such as oat bran. However, it is important to recognize that many of the demonstrations of plasma cholesterol lowering by soluble fiber products are against insoluble NSPs such as wheat bran.

There are several hypotheses to explain the NSP action on plasma cholesterol, including enhanced bile acid and neutral sterol excretion, the slowing of fat and cholesterol absorption and direct inhibition of hepatic cholesterol synthesis by propionate formed by large bowel fermentation of NSPs. Whole body cholesterol homoeostasis represents a balance between influx and loss. Cholesterol influx can come from dietary intake and de novo synthesis. Losses occur through the sloughing of epithelial cells and through the fecal excretion of nonabsorbed dietary cholesterol and biliary steroids (bile acids and neutral sterols). Bile acids are generally recovered in the ileum, and those that are not absorbed are excreted in the feces. Any increase in bile acid excretion leads to enhanced hepatic uptake of cholesterol and its conversion to bile acids with a consequent depletion of the plasma cholesterol pool.

It was initially thought that fiber could bind some bile acids selectively, in a similar manner to cholestyramine, an ion exchange resin that binds bile acids. Bile acid binding in vitro by insoluble fiber preparations appears to be an artefact. Cholestyramine is strongly charged, whereas most NSPs with cholesterol-lowering potential are neutral or even acidic (e.g., pectins). Neutrality is not consistent with ionic binding and uronic acid residues would repel bile acids at the pH of the small intestine. The property that appears to mediate the increased steroid excretion is the viscosity in solution. Most (but not necessarily all) NSPs that lower cholesterol form viscous solutions in water. Presumably, bile acids are lost from the ileum through a form of entrapment in a viscous gel. This would also contribute to the loss of cholesterol and the slower digestion of fat seen with ingestion of NSPs. Abundant animal and human data show that feeding soluble NSPs increases fecal steroid excretion. However, the major problem with these relationships is that

although soluble fibers may lower plasma cholesterol, the strongest evidence of a protective effect is for insoluble fibers which do not lower plasma cholesterol. It may be that other components in the grain are actually mediating the effect and fiber is the surrogate marker for their intake.

Dietary Fiber and the Etiology of Cancers—Colon and Rectum

Population Studies

This is one long-standing association that has been surprisingly problematic. Early studies on native Africans who consumed an unrefined diet showed them to have a very low incidence of this cancer. Although subsequent studies have shown a negative association between greater fiber intake and lowered risk, it has proved to be relatively weak. Indeed, in one US study there was no real association between fiber intake and cancer susceptibility. Some of the loss of significance seen in this evaluation may reflect the lack of allowance for confounding variables. For example, in a 6-year follow-up of women, the association between low fiber intake and the incidence of colon cancer disappeared after adjustment was made for meat intake. In another study of men, low fiber intake was an independent risk factor for the incidence of adenomatous polyps during a 2-year follow-up period.

Fruit and vegetable fiber has been consistently associated with a lower risk of colon cancer, but the relationship with cereal fiber is less clear. However, whole grain cereals appear to be protective—a further anomaly in the relationships between plant foods and disease risk. These discrepancies may be in the process of resolution. First, it seems that the early observational data were confounded by the analytical technologies available, and the perception that native populations consuming unrefined diets had high fiber intakes is incorrect. It seems likely that they ate relatively little fiber but had high intakes of RS. Population studies have shown a protective effect of apparent RS intake and colorectal cancer risk. The word 'apparent' is pivotal because there is currently no accepted method for RS determination and thus, there are no reliable data on dietary intakes. There are also issues regarding the intakes of dietary fiber and cancer risk. Part of the problem inherent in the study of colonic cancer is that, in contrast to CHD (in which there are easily measurable risk markers such as plasma cholesterol that can be modified by diet), the only indices for colon cancer are not easily measurable:

the appearance of aberrant crypts, adenomatous polyps, or the disease itself. Hitherto, animal studies have largely been confined to rodents treated with chemical carcinogens (usually dimethylhydrazine), and they suggest that dietary fiber from wheat bran and cellulose may afford greater protection against the development of colon cancer when associated with a low-fat diet compared with soluble NSPs. These data stand in contrast to observational studies but are supported by interventions in humans with familial adenomatous polyposis. These people are at genetically greater risk of colonic cancer and represent one means of assessing risk modification through dietary intervention and monitoring polyp size and frequency through colonoscopy. In the Australian Polyp Prevention Trial, subjects consumed 25 g of wheat bran per day and there was a decrease in dysplasia and total adenoma surface area when the diet was also low in fat. This supports epidemiological studies that show that increased fat and protein intakes increase risk. Other prevention trials have examined the effects of increasing fiber intake on the recurrence of polyps following a polypectomy. In a Canadian study of 201 men and women, a high-fiber, low-fat diet protected against polyp recurrence in women but in men there was actually an increase. A third trial examined the effects of diet on the prevalence of rectal polyps in 64 people with familial polyposis coli who had a total colectomy. Those who received and actually took the high-fiber (22.5 g fiber as a breakfast cereal) showed a reduction in polyps. These data are not conclusive but are reasonably consistent with overall knowledge.

Complex Carbohydrates and Colorectal Cancer

An obvious factor for the inconsistent results of the effect of different intakes of dietary fiber on colorectal cancer is the variation in the analytical methodology used in different studies. There is also increasing evidence that total dietary complex carbohydrates may be as important as fiber. Analysis of stool weight from 20 populations in 12 countries showed that larger stools were correlated with a lower incidence of colon cancer. Intakes of starch and dietary fiber (rather than fiber alone) were the best dietary correlates with stool weight. A subsequent meta-analysis showed that greater consumption of starch (but not of NSPs) was associated with low risk of colorectal cancer in 12 populations. The examination also showed that fat and protein intakes correlated positively with risk. This meta-analysis is probably the first of its kind to

suggest a protective role for starch in large bowel cancer and underscores the need to consider complex carbohydrates as fiber equivalents and not just as NSPs and starch. The need for better information on dietary intake data and risk is underscored by the data from the European Prospective Investigation of Cancer and Nutrition, which showed a substantial reduction in risk with increasing fiber intake. This multinational study is important because it has sufficient power (expressed as a range of fiber intakes and individuals observed) to give confidence in the observations. Follow-up of 1 939 011 person-years throughout 10 countries showed that a doubling of fiber intake from foods could reduce risk by 40%.

Potential Mechanisms Indicating a Role in the Etiology of Colorectal Cancer

Colorectal tumorigenesis is a multistep process. These steps involve a number of genetic alterations that convert a normal epithelium to a hyperproliferative state and then to early adenomas, later adenomas, and, finally, frank carcinoma and metastasis. Fiber may, and probably does, play a role in all of these stages, and several mechanisms have been proposed by which it could play a role in the etiology of the disease (Table 1).

Table 1 Effects of dietary fiber and resistant starch that could impact on the etiology of colorectal cancer

Increased stool bulk (mainly insoluble NSPs)
Decreases transit time, minimizing contact between colonocytes and luminal carcinogens
Reduces exposure through dilution of carcinogens

Binding of bile acids and other potential carcinogens (mainly insoluble NSPs)
Lowers free concentrations of mutagens

Modifying fecal flora and increasing bacterial numbers (soluble and insoluble NSPs and RS)
Decreases secondary bile acids, which are potential carcinogens
Lowers colonic NH_3 (a cytotoxic agent) by fixing nitrogen in the bacterial mass

Lowering fecal pH through SCFA production (NSPs but mainly RS)
Inhibits growth of pH-sensitive, potentially pathogenic species, which may degrade food constituents, and endogenous secretions to potential carcinogens
Lowers absorption of toxic alkaline compounds (e.g., amines)
Lowers solubility of secondary bile acids

Fermentation to SCFAs (NSPs but mainly RS)
Depending on source, raises butyrate which is a preferred substrate for normal colonocytes, and (*in vitro*) promotes a normal cell phenotype, retards the growth of cancer cells, and facilitates DNA repair

NSPs, nonstarch polysaccharides; RS, resistant starch; SCFAs, short-chain Fatty acids.

A number of agents may induce genetic damage in the colonocyte, including mono- and diacylglycerols, nonesterified fatty acids, secondary bile acids, aryl hydrocarbons and other pyrrolytic products of high-temperature cooking, and ammonia and amines and other products of large bowel bacterial protein degradation. One of the simplest protective mechanisms for dietary fiber is purely physical. By increasing fecal bulk, fiber could produce a more rapid transit time as well as act as a diluent and thus reduce exposure to potential mutagenic agents. It is also possible that fiber components could bind mutagens. However, because this appears to be unlikely for bile acids, the same may apply to other carcinogens.

Production of SCFAs by the resident microflora induces a number of general changes in the colonic environment, including a lowering of pH. Case–control studies show that pH is higher in patients with cancer compared to controls but this may reflect altered dietary habits rather than long-term risk. However, at lower pH, basic toxins are ionized while secondary bile acids are less soluble so that the absorption of both would be reduced. The activities of both of the enzymes 7α-dehydroxylase and glucuronidase are decreased at lower pH. These changes would diminish the conversion of primary to secondary bile acids and the hydrolysis of glucuronide conjugates, respectively and thus limit their carcinogenic potential. However, there is consensus that the effects of SCFAs may be rather more specific and mediated through one acid—butyrate. Butyrate is a preferred substrate for normal colonocytes and numerous studies *in vitro* have shown that it has several actions that promote a normal cell phenotype. Cell studies show that butyrate induces hyperacylation of histones, leading to downregulation of gene expression and arrest of proliferation. Other actions include DNA hypermethylation which would have similar effects on tumor cell growth. Butyrate also has favorable effects on apoptosis so that a normal program of cell death is maintained. One marker of a differentiated colonocyte is its ability to produce alkaline phosphatase and butyrate is a powerful promoter of alkaline phosphatase *in vitro*. There is reciprocal downregulation of various oncogenes in colorectal cancer cell lines. These data are very promising for a direct role of butyrate in protecting against colonic cancer but there is an emerging paradox. In the presence of butyrate, there is either increased proliferation or no effect in normal cells but the proliferation of neoplastic cells is reduced. The differentiation of the normal cells is unchanged or suppressed with butyrate but is induced in cancer cells. These differing effects may be explained by neoplastic alterations (perhaps as a result of mutations in oncogenes) in cell signal systems.

It must be emphasized that none of the effects of butyrate *in vitro* have been duplicated *in vivo*, but they are of great promise and supportive evidence continues to accumulate. This is especially true for RS which appears to produce relatively more butyrate than other nondigestible carbohydrates. However, consideration may also need to be given to the existence of interindividual differences in the fermentative capacity of the microflora, the fact that RS from different sources may be fermented to different extents, and the actual colonic site at which fermentation takes place (i.e., whether in the proximal or distal colon).

Inter alia, the data suggest that protection against colorectal cancer is due to several mechanisms and that these can interact. One factor of considerable importance is the issue of overweight which is an independent risk factor for colorectal cancer. Obesity may have to be taken into account much more than has been the case in earlier studies. It appears that some of the effect may be mediated through raised plasma insulin and insulin-like growth factors (which may well be influenced by dietary carbohydrates).

Dietary Fiber and the Etiology of Hormone-Dependent Cancers

Population Studies

Cancers of the breast, endometrium, ovary, and prostate fall into the hormone-dependent classification. An association between hormonal status and cancer risk arose from observations of oestrogen deprivation and breast cancer and testosterone deprivation and prostate cancer. Nutritional influences on breast cancer have been studied extensively and several (but not all) studies show diminished risk with greater intakes of dietary fiber. The situation for other cancers, especially prostate cancer, appears to be rather unclear, but given the commonality of the proposed protective mechanisms, it is reasonable to expect that some linkage may be found. Male vegetarians have been reported to have lower testosterone and oestradiol plasma concentrations compared to omnivores, and inverse correlations of testosterone and oestradiol with fiber intake have been reported.

Potential Mechanisms Indicating a Role in the Etiology of Hormone-Dependent Cancers

There are many published studies that have produced mixed and inconsistent results on the potential mechanisms involved. Dietary fiber could act by reducing circulating concentrations of oestrogen and testosterone. Such an effect would not be unexpected in view of the fact that soluble NSPs can increase bile acid and neutral steroid excretion and fecal steroid outputs are higher in vegetarians than in omnivores. However, one anomaly is the finding that wheat bran (which does not enhance biliary steroid excretion) lowers circulating and urinary oestrogens. It is possible that fiber acts rather differently on hormones than on bile acids and neutral sterols. For example, the colonic flora may be modified so as to increase deconjugation of the sex hormone precursors or their conversion to other metabolites. Direct binding of sex hormones is possible but is subject to the same concerns as were raised for cholesterol reduction. In addition, it is possible that other components in, or associated with, fiber (phytooestrogens or antioxidants) may be responsible for any observed protective effect. Soy phytooestrogens are believed to play a role in lowering the risk of breast cancer in Asian populations. Lycopenes are antioxidant carotenoids from tomatoes, and their intake has been correlated with a lower risk of prostate cancer.

Dietary Fiber, Obesity, and the Etiology of Diabetes

In 1975, Trowell suggested that the etiology of diabetes might be related to a dietary fiber deficiency. This is supported by several key pieces of evidence. Vegetarians who consume a high-fiber lacto-ovo vegetarian diet appear to have a lower risk of mortality from diabetes-related causes compared to nonvegetarians. Consumption of whole grain cereals is associated with a lower risk of diabetes. Importantly, the same dietary pattern appears to lower the risk of obesity, itself an independent risk factor in the etiology of type 2 diabetes. Obesity is emerging as a problem of epidemic proportions in affluent and developing countries. Consumption of whole grain cereal products lowers the risk of diabetes. A report showed that in 91 249 women questioned about dietary habits in 1991, greater cereal fiber intake was significantly related to lowered risk of type 2 diabetes. In this study, glycemic index (but not glycemic load) was also a significant risk factor, and this interacted with a low-fiber diet to increase risk. These results provide epidemiological evidence of a role of fiber in the etiology of diabetes.

Potential Mechanisms Indicating a Role in the Etiology of Diabetes

It can be hypothesized that a reduction in the general and postprandial glycemic and insulinemic response may delay the development of insulin resistance and thus the development of diabetes (NIDDM) although there is very little direct evidence to support this hypothesis. However, diets high in both carbohydrate and dietary fiber have been reported to improve insulin sensitivity. Much of the research in this area has studied the effect of dietary fiber on the management rather than the prevention or etiology of diabetes.

There is good evidence that diminished glucose absorption lowers the insulin response to a meal. The action of fiber in this regard may be through slowing the digestion of starch and other nutrients. It seems that soluble fiber may play a role because large amounts of soluble dietary fiber have been shown to reduce postprandial glucose concentration and insulinemic responses after a single meal in both normal and diabetic subjects. However, the effect appears to be dependent on viscosity rather than on solubility *per se*. The very viscous gum, guar gum, gum tragacanth, and oat gum are all very effective whereas psyllium and some pectins are less viscous and less effective. One suggested mechanism for reducing the glycemic response is an impairment in the convective movement of glucose and water in the intestinal lumen due to the formation of a viscous gel: Glucose is trapped in the gel matrix, such that there is less movement toward the absorptive brush border of the surface of the intestinal wall and the glucose needs to be squeezed out by the intestinal motor activity of the intestine. However, other factors may also be important. There may be some impairment in digestive activity in the lumen, an alteration in hormonal secretion by cells in the gut mucosa, and a reduced gut motility that delays transit time. In the case of whole grains, there is scope for the fiber to interfere with the physical accessibility of starch to small intestinal α-amylase. Clearly, there is also potential for foods of low glycemic index to be high in RS and this does seem to be the case. A specific instance is a novel barley cultivar that exhibits both characteristics. It should be noted that there are reports of a second meal effect (i.e., the dietary fiber ingested at one meal can affect the glucose rise after the subsequent meal). The mechanism for this is unknown.

A Role for Fiber in the Etiology of Other Diseases?

Although much of the earlier observational studies in native African populations were wide ranging, most attention has subsequently focused on CHD and cancer. Probably this is a reflection of the socio-economic importance of these conditions in economically developed societies. However, fiber has a role in the prevention and management of other conditions, but much of the relevant information has come from interventions, not from case–control or cross-sectional studies.

Constipation, diverticular disease, and laxation
Unquestionably, fiber is of direct benefit in relieving the symptoms of constipation and diverticular disease but there is little information about its role in the etiology of these conditions. Numerous interventions have shown that foods high in insoluble NSPs (e.g., certain cereal brans) and some soluble NSP preparations (e.g., psyllium) are very effective at controlling constipation and diverticular disease and enhancing laxation. The actual effect can vary with source. Wheat bran increases undigested residue, and fiber from fruits and vegetables and soluble polysaccharides tend to be fermented extensively and are more likely to increase microbial cell mass. Some NSP (and OS) preparations retain water in the colon. The physical form of the fiber is also important: Coarsely ground wheat bran is a very effective source of fiber to increase fecal bulk, whereas finely ground wheat bran has little or no effect and may even be constipating. RS appears to be a mild laxative and seems to complement the laxative effects of NSPs. The effective dose appears to be approximately 20–30 g of total fiber/day consumed either in food or as a supplement. In addition, animal studies show that NSPs and RS appear to prevent colonic atrophy seen in low-fiber diets. The mechanism of action appears to be greater fecal bulking and fermentation and the generation of SCFAs, which is necessary to prevent atrophy.

Diarrhea   Colonic SCFA absorption stimulates fluid and electrolyte uptake in the colon and thus can assist in reducing diarrhea. Complex carbohydrates may also play a role in modifying the colonic microflora thus reducing the number of pathogens. An etiological role for fiber is unknown, but there is good evidence that RS can act to minimize the fluid losses that occur in serious conditions such as cholera.

Inflammatory bowel diseases (colitis and Crohn's disease)   Clearly, inflammatory conditions have an immune component. In the case of Crohn's disease, there appears to be no established therapeutic or etiological role for fiber. The situation is slightly different for distal ulcerative colitis, in which fiber intake seems unrelated to incidence. However, rectal infusion of SCFAs (especially butyrate) has been reported to lead to remission, so it appears that either the generation of these acids or their delivery to the distal colon may be the issue.

See also: **Coronary Heart Disease**: Prevention. **Dietary Fiber**: Physiological Effects and Effects on Absorption.;

Further Reading

Baghurst PA, Baghurst KI, and Record SJ (1996) Dietary fibre, non-starch polysaccharides and resistant starch—A review. *Food Australia* 48(supplement): S3–S35.

Bingham SA, Day NE, Luben R *et al.* European Prospective Investigation into Cancer and Nutrition (2003) Dietary fibre in food and protection against colorectal cancer in the European Prospective Investigation into Cancer and Nutrition (EPIC): An observational study. *Lancet* 361: 1496–1501.

Ellis PR, Rayment P, and Wang Q (1996) A physico-chemical perspective of plant polysaccharides in relation to glucose absorption, insulin secretion and the entero-insular axis. *Proceedings of the Nutrition Society* 55: 881–898.

Giovannucci E (2001) Insulin, insulin-like growth factors and colon cancer: A review of the evidence. *Journal of Nutrition* 131(supplement 3): 109S–120S.

Olson BH, Anderson SM, Becker MP *et al.* (1997) Psyllium-enriched cereals lower blood total cholesterol and LDL cholesterol, but not HDL cholesterol in hypercholesterolemic adults: Results of a meta-analysis. *Journal of Nutrition* 127: 1973–1980.

Richardson DP (2003) Whole grain health claims in Europe. *Proceedings of the Nutrition Society* 62: 161–169.

Schulze MB, Liu S, Rimm EB *et al.* (2004) Glycemic index, glycemic load, and dietary fiber intake and incidence of type 2 diabetes in younger and middle-aged women. *American Journal of Clinical Nutrition* 80: 243–244.

Slavin JL (2000) Mechanisms for the impact of whole grain foods on cancer risk. *Journal of the American College of Nutrition* 19: 300S–307S.

Stamler J, Caggiula AW, Cutler JA *et al.* (1997) Dietary and nutritional methods and findings: The Multiple Risk Factor Intervention Trial (MRFIT). *American Journal of Clinical Nutrition* 65(1 supplement): 183S–402S.

Topping DL and Clifton PM (2001) Short-chain fatty acids and human colonic function: Roles of resistant starch and nonstarch polysaccharides. *Physiological Reviews* 81: 1031–1064.

Topping DL, Morell MK, King RA *et al.* (2003) Resistant starch and health – *Himalaya* 292, a novel barley cultivar to deliver benefits to consumers. *Starch/stärke* 53: 539–545.

Truswell AS (2002) Cereal grains and coronary heart disease. *European Journal of Clinical Nutrition* 56: 1–14.

Wu H, Dwyer KM, Fan Z *et al.* (2003) Dietary fiber and progression of atherosclerosis: The Los Angeles Atherosclerosis Study. *American Journal of Clinical Nutrition* 78: 1085–1091.

Role in Nutritional Management of Disease

A R Leeds, King's College London, London, UK

Introduction

Dietary Fiber was an unknown phrase to all but a handful of individuals in the early years of the 1970s when a wide range of potential therapeutic applications were suggested by Hugh Trowell, Denis Burkitt, and Alexander Walker. Twenty-five years later there can hardly be an ordinary mortal who has not heard the term, though he may not be able to define it. In some cases the claims remain largely unsubstantiated but in three areas, hyperlipidemia, diabetes, and bowel function, there is sufficient evidence to allow dietary advice to be given.

Hyperlipidemia

Some forms of dietary fiber lower blood lipids, notably total cholesterol and low-density lipoprotein (LDL) cholesterol. The earliest observations on fiber preparations and blood lipids date from the mid 1930s when there was a fairly extensive investigation of the effects of pectin (polygalacturonic acid). The next period of investigation dates from 1974 when extracted and purified dietary fiber preparations such as guar gum – a glucomannan – were tested in normal subjects, diabetics, and hyperlipidemic subjects and were found to lower blood cholesterol when given in sufficient quantities. In very large doses these materials increase fecal excretion of fat and sterol compounds and would be expected to reduce the body bile salt pool. Subsequent work has shown that at lower doses preparations of soluble dietary fiber have a mild cholestyramine-like effect: they bind bile salts rendering them unavailable for reabsorption in the terminal ileum, thus interfering with the normal entero-hepatic cycle of bile salts and depleting the bile salt pool. Total and LDL cholesterol fall as cholesterol is diverted for the resynthesis of lost bile salts. There have been few direct clinical applications of the early experimental work on pectin and guar gum. No pectin compounds have been developed commercially, but there are a few pharmaceutical preparations of guar gum presented primarily as adjuncts to dietary therapy in diabetes rather than for lipid lowering. Dietetic food products containing guar gum have been developed, again for use in controlling diabetes.

Preparations of soluble dietary fiber have been shown to lower blood cholesterol whereas most preparations of predominantly insoluble fiber, such as wheat bran, have little or no effect. The major food sources of soluble fiber are oats, beans, lentils, rye, and barley, and these foods have naturally become the subject of investigations. The addition of oats to the diet in normolipidemic and hyperlipidemic subjects following either their normal diets or where pretreated with low-fat diets has been the subject of extensive research. In sufficient quantity oats, oat products, and oat β-glucan (providing at least 3 g oat β-beta glucan per day) lower blood total cholesterol and LDL cholesterol (usually by 5–10%) while leaving triglycerides and HDL cholesterol largely unchanged. A sufficiently large number of good-quality studies have now been done on oats that the Food and Drug Administration (FDA) has allowed the first ever food-specific health claim: "Soluble fiber from oatmeal, as part of a low saturated fat, low cholesterol diet, may reduce the risk of heart disease." Products that are labeled with this claim must provide at least 0.75 g of soluble fiber (as β-glucan) per serving. When considering the above claim the FDA reviewed 37 studies and found that a sufficient number provided convincing evidence of efficacy. An earlier meta-analysis of some of those trials had shown that the efficacy of oats and oat products was influenced by the initial values of blood cholesterol in the subjects: patients with high starting values (over 6.7 mmol per liter total cholesterol) showed the greatest reductions when treated with oats, while healthy young subjects with low–normal starting values showed little response. There was a dose effect: food products providing more than 3 g soluble fiber per day had a greater blood cholesterol lowering effect than diets that provided less than 3 g per day.

Other soluble fiber-containing products have been shown to lower blood cholesterol. Recent extensive studies on psyllium (*Plantago ovata*) presented both as a pharmaceutical preparation and as a food product (a ready to eat breakfast cereal) have shown blood cholesterol-lowering properties where the dose–effect relationship is such that a useful additional therapeutically meaningful lipid-lowering effect can be achieved by prescribing a daily portion of psyllium-fortified breakfast cereal. Products of this type are now marketed in the US and Australia, and the US FDA has now allowed a food specific health claim for psyllium.

There is also a small literature on the effects of beans on blood lipids and the findings of a blood cholesterol-lowering effect are as expected.

Virtually all of the reports of the effects of soluble fiber products on blood lipids report lowering effects on total cholesterol and LDL cholesterol without any effect on HDL cholesterol or triglycerides – this contrasts with the effects of some drugs that may cause slight rises of triglycerides and falls of HDL cholesterol. The relationship between lowering of blood cholesterol and lowering of risk of heart disease is now generally accepted and a proven lipid-lowering effect is taken to mean a beneficial effect on risk of coronary heart disease. This means that in clinical practice it is perfectly reasonable to include advice on use of foods high in soluble dietary fiber in a lipid-lowering diet, and perfectly proper to emphasize the benefits of oats and oat products. Generally, a high-soluble-fiber diet is more acceptable when the soluble fiber is drawn from smaller quantities of a larger range of foods; thus the diet includes beans, lentils, rye breads, and barley as well as generous use of oats. A range of foods containing mycoprotein and fungal mycelial cell walls (chitin) may also help to lower blood cholesterol.

Diabetes

Diabetes mellitus is characterized by either an absolute or relative lack of insulin, which has short-term and long-term consequences. Diabetic people may develop both microvascular complications (mainly affecting the eyes, kidneys, and nerves) and macrovascular complications (essentially accelerated development of atherosclerosis presenting mainly as heart attack and peripheral vascular disease). Medical management aims to replace the insulin, or modulate its production or efficacy using oral (hypoglycemic) drugs, in a metabolic environment enhanced by good control of diet and body composition. Medical management also aims to achieve early detection of complications and other risk factors for cardiovascular disease by regular testing of blood and urine biochemical variables and blood pressure and by regular physical examination of the eyes, neurological, and cardiovascular systems.

Control of dietary energy intake (in relation to the varying demands for growth, maintenance, physical activity, etc.) remains the key feature of dietary control affecting metabolic fluxes, blood glucose levels, and body weight. Views on the appropriate proportional sources of energy from fat, carbohydrate, and protein have changed enormously over the last century from seriously energy-restricted high-fat diets (with percentage energy from fat as high as 70% raising some doubts about the level of compliance) through to very high-carbohydrate diets (sometimes 60–65% energy from carbohydrate) used in specialist centers in the US. Today, for most diabetic patients in most countries the target is to achieve 50–55% energy from carbohydrate sources. Prior to the 1970s, when the move towards high-carbohydrate diets began, the high fat content of the diet along with less tight blood glucose (and urine glucose) control than is customary today was partly responsible for the high relative mortality from cardiovascular disease seen among diabetic patients. At that time young male diabetics were up to nine times more likely to die from heart attack than matched nondiabetic individuals. Reduction of fat in the diet and achievement of an optimal distribution from saturated, monounsaturated, and polyunsaturated sources (<10%, 10–20%, and no more than 10%, respectively, for patients with diabetes in the UK) remain a major aspect of dietary management of diabetic people in order to reduce the risk of developing coronary heart disease.

Control of blood glucose is critical in order to achieve avoidance of prolonged periods of hyperglycemia, which is associated with glycation of proteins and the risk of development of microvascular complications, and avoidance of hypoglycemia with its attendant risks of coma. In day-to-day practice, the avoidance of hypoglycemia is very important to patients and any new method of achieving normalization of blood glucose profiles is an advance. Dietary fiber offered such an advance from the mid 1970s when some forms (notably isolated polysaccharides such as guar gum, a glucomannan, and pectin, polygalacturonic acid) were shown to reduce the area under the blood glucose and insulin curves after acute test meals. Subsequent long-term (6-week) clinical trials showed that diets high in foods containing soluble dietary fiber, such as beans, oats, and barley, were more effective in reducing the area under the 24-h blood glucose profiles than diets containing more high-fiber foods based on wheat products.

Research in this area led David Jenkins to describe (in 1981) the concept of the 'glycemic index' (GI) which is a numerical expression of the ability of a food to raise blood glucose levels. In practice it is measured by comparing the blood glucose response to a 50-g carbohydrate portion of food with the response to 50 g glucose (in some papers the comparison is with a 50-g carbohydrate portion of bread). The dietary fiber (especially soluble fiber) content of a food slows down the rate of digestion and absorption of starch in foods giving flatter blood glucose responses and a lower GI; however, the structure of the starch (whether amylose or amylopectin) influences its rate of degradation and the extent to which the starch granules are hydrated by processing (including cooking) is also important. The physical structure of the food (particularly the extent to which plant cells are intact), the presence of fat, which may slow gastric emptying, and the presence of some 'antinutrient' substances may all influence the GI. Low-GI diets have been shown in many clinical trials to improve important variables that are secondary indicators of blood glucose control, and to reduce blood lipids. Low-GI diets may be particularly helpful to patients who are frequently troubled by episodes of hypoglycemia though adequate proof of this is still awaited. Low-GI diets are not just relevant to treatment of diabetes but have been shown in two large-scale epidemiological surveys published in 1997 to result in a significant reduction in the risk of development of maturity onset (type 2) diabetes in middle-aged American men and women. Thus, there is good reason to believe that there should be greater emphasis on the GI of diabetic diets and the fiber content, as well as emphasis on GI for those at risk of developing diabetes, especially the older obese person. Expert committees in many developed countries of the world have set target values for dietary fiber intake for diabetic patients (e.., the American Diabetes Association (ADA) recommends 20–35 g day^{-1} total dietary fiber by the AOAC method) and many, especially the Australian Diabetes Association and with the notable exception of the ADA, have recommended an increase in low-GI foods. In 2003 even Diabetes UK (the UK Diabetes Association) noted that there might be merit in taking account of GI in dietary management for those with diabetes. Some physicians believe that the GI of foods is too complex an issue for patients to grasp, but in essence simply requires a partial substitution of bread and potatoes with pasta products, an increased use of high-fiber breakfast cereals including oats, increased use of beans and lentils, and emphasis on the use of temperate fruits (e.g., apples and pears).

Obesity (body mass index (weight in kilograms divided by height in meters squared) in excess of 30 kg m^{-2}) is becoming more prevalent in developing countries and attracts an increased risk of the development of diabetes mellitus; a high proportion of established type 2 diabetics are obese and overweight. In the popular diet book 'The F-Plan Diet,' published in 1982, Audrey Eyton claimed that dietary fiber would help people lose weight by a number of mechanisms including reducing the efficiency of dietary energy absorption and by making people feel full for longer after meals thus having an overall

effect on reducing food intake. At the time of publication these ideas were hypothetical - subsequent investigation has shown that increasing fiber intake two- or threefold by a variety of dietary changes can increase fecal energy losses by 75–100 kcal day^{-1}. Studies on the effects of dietary fiber on postprandial satiety where experimental meals are carefully designed to differ little except for fiber content have given variable results. However, there is a clear effect of fiber on chewing (the number of chews necessary to eat the same energy equivalent of food) where high- and low-fiber types of commonly consumed foods are eaten and this may have an important satiating effect. Clinical trials of high-fiber weight loss regimens have given variable results. Double-blind placebo-controlled trials using pressed barley fiber and pectin tablets compared to a starch control have been undertaken in Scandinavia and have demonstrated statistically significantly greater weight losses in the fiber-treated groups up to 26 weeks of treatment. It seems reasonable to conclude that under some conditions the right kind of high-fiber diet can facilitate weight loss, but may not always do so.

Diabetic people are more likely to have dyslipidemia than nondiabetic people. When control of diabetes is lost, patients may demonstrate gross hypertriglyceridemia due to increased production of very-low-density lipoprotein (VLDL) particles in the liver as a consequence of the increased flux of free fatty acids from the peripheral tissues. At the same time total and LDL cholesterol may be raised. Improvement in diabetic control often achieves normalization of blood lipids, but where hyperlipidemia persists there may be a place for use of dietary fiber, especially soluble fiber, and especially oat β-glucan-containing foods as an adjunct to dietary and pharmacological therapy (see above).

Bowel Disorders

Denis Burkitt first suggested a role for dietary fiber in bowel disorders in 1971. In the intervening period understanding of the normal physiology and pathophysiology of the colon have improved enormously. During the same period methods of analysis have been refined and a distinction is drawn between dietary fiber (as determined by the AOAC gravimetric method) and nonstarch polysaccharide (NSP; determined by GLC analysis of component sugars), and starch not digested in the small gut is now defined as being resistant. Three types of resistant starch have been described. These advances in analysis have helped physiologists appreciate the contributions of various substrates to colonic fermentation and stool bulking.

The intake of dietary fiber (nonstarch polysaccharides) is directly related to the amount of wet stool passed each day in large population groups. An average wet stool weight for the UK is about $105\,g\,day^{-1}$, which corresponds roughly to a nonstarch polysaccharide (Englyst method) intact of $12.5\,g\,day^{-1}$. Nearly half of the members of groups studied in the UK have stool weights of less than $100\,g\,day^{-1}$ below which complaints of constipation are common. Stool weight has been shown to be clearly inversely related to colon cancer incidence in population groups: a mean daily stool weight of $105\,g$ corresponding to a relatively high population colon cancer incidence of about $22\,per\,100\,000$ per annum. An incidence rate of $11\,per\,100\,000$ per annum corresponds to a mean daily stool weight of about $175\,g\,day^{-1}$. This information was used as the numerical basis for calculating the UK's dietary reference value (DRV) for nonstarch polysaccharide (NSP) in the late 1980s. In the UK the population is urged to increase NSP intake by 50% to a population averageof $18\,g\,day^{-1}$ in order to shift the distribution of wet stool weight upwards.

Constipation is generally considered to be infrequent opening of the bowels with straining to pass stools (less than three defecations per week and straining and or the passing of hard stools in more than one in four defecations). Constipation is sometimes caused by other specific disease of either an endocrine nature (e.g., myxoedema – reduced thyroid function) or physical obstructive nature (e.g., colon cancer). Where constipation has developed recently in a previously nonconstipated individual over the age of 40 years colon cancer must be excluded as the cause of the change of bowel habit. In the absence of evidence that the constipation is secondary it is probably due to dietary and life-style factors. The mucosa of the lower colon has a great capacity to desiccate its contents. If the call to stool does not occur or is ignored residual material drys out and individual fecal pellets become smaller. There is experimental evidence to suggest that greater abdominal pressures are needed to expel pellets that are 1 cm in diameter than those that are 2 cm in diameter. Thus, factors that result in the call to stool being ignored, like not allowing sufficient time for defecation after a stimulus such as breakfast or the walk to the station or being unprepared to defecate anywhere except at home (a common characteristic consistent with mammalian behavior), are likely to cause constipation. Simple solutions include going to bed earlier and getting up earlier in the morning, and finding another acceptable location for defecation at the workplace. Increasing fiber in the diet, most easily achieved by making breakfast a high-fiber meal with either high-fiber breakfast cereals or high-fiber breads, will increase stool bulk, shorten transit time (the time for a marker to pass from the mouth and be passed in the stool), and alleviate symptoms in many cases. The importance of exercise in maintaining normal colon function is gradually being recognized – the importance of brisk walking should not be underestimated. However, some specific types of simple constipation have been identified which do not necessarily respond to high-fiber diets. Grossly prolonged transit times reflecting seriously slow colonic motility has been seen particularly in young women and do not respond well to high-fiber diets, and some 'outflow abnormalities,' which sometimes have a basis in abnormal rectal conformation, may also not respond.

Diverticular disease of the colon, characterized by the development of protrusions of mucosa through the bowel wall, is common and usually asymptomatic. It has been shown to be less likely to develop in those following a high-fiber diet, and once acquired can be managed, in many cases, by ensuring an adequate amount of fiber in the diet. Experimentally, various fiber supplements and 'bulking agents' have been shown to reduce the abnormally high peak intracolonic pressures that are characteristic of diverticular disease. Sometimes 10–20 g of coarse wheat bran as a supplement is all that is required, but some patients develop flatulence and distension at least initially. Other fiber supplements such as ispaghula husk (psyllium) may be as effective, without the initial adverse side effects. Sometimes, simple dietary changes to achieve an adequate total daily intake of dietary fiber particularly from wheat-based foods are effective. Diverticulitis (inflammation of the diverticula) is a complication requiring medical management, which will usually include a short period of abstention from food. Many patients remain largely without symptoms once the right 'fiber' regimen has been determined.

The irritable bowel syndrome (IBS) is a 'functional' disorder of the bowel, which is said to affect up to 15% of the population and is characterized by some, but not necessarily all, of a range of symptoms including abdominal pain relieved by constipation, alternating diarrhea and constipation, recurrent abdominal pain, and urgent or frequent defecation. An important part of management is the exclusion of other serious organic disease such as inflammatory bowel diseases. In IBS the gut is abnormally sensitive to distension, and symptoms may be related to or exacerbated by external emotional events. The role of high-fiber diets in IBS has been investigated and not surprisingly is only of benefit in some cases: in those patients in whom the predominant feature is constipation. In some patients high-fiber diets may make their symptoms worse.

In inflammatory bowel disease (IBD) high fiber diets have no special part to play in the management of Crohn's disease where enteral feeding (with formula low-residue, low-fiber preparations) is especially beneficial where there is acute extensive small bowel disease. In ulcerative colitis specific dietary advice is usually unnecessary though fiber supplements may be of benefit in patients whose disease is limited to proctitis (inflammation of the rectum).

The treatment of newly diagnosed colon cancer does not include diet therapy, but treatment of those at increased risk of developing colon cancer by dietary and other means will become increasingly common as more information about the effects of high fiber diets and supplements on colon function becomes available. The critical step in the adenoma-carcinoma sequence in the human large bowel is the enlargement of the small adenoma (which has a low risk of malignant transformation) to a large adenoma (which has a high risk of malignant transformation); dietary factors, including low amounts of fiber in the diet, enhance adenoma growth. Bile acids are strongly linked to adenoma growth and bile acid concentrations in the colon are influenced by dietary fat and dietary fiber. Other effects of fiber may also be protective: bulking the stool and accelerating material through the colon, and provision of substrate for fermentation particularly with production of butyrate, which may have antineoplastic properties. However, despite a great deal of epidemiological and experimental work the potential role of dietary fiber in modulating the risk of colon cancer remains controversial.

See also: **Dietary Fiber**: Physiological Effects and Effects on Absorption; Potential Role in Etiology of Disease.

Further Reading

Committee on Medical Aspects of Food Policy (1991) *Dietary Reference Values for Food Energy and Nutrients for the United Kingdom: Non Starch Polysaccharides*, pp. 61–71. London: HMSO.

Cummings JH (1997) *The Large Intestine in Nutrition and Disease. Danone Chair Monograph.* Brussels: Institute Danone.

Diabetes UK Dietary Guidelines (2003) The implementation of nutritional advice for people with diabetes. *Diabetic Medicine* 20: 786–807.

Food and Agriculture Organization (1998) *Carbohydrates in Human Nutrition.* FAO Food and Nutrition Paper 66. Rome: FAO.

Jenkins DJA *et al.* (2003) The garden of Eden – plant based diets, the genetic drive to conserve cholesterol and its implications for heart disease in the 21st century. *Comparative Biochemistry and Physiology Part A* **136**: 141–151.

Relevant Websites

http://www.fda.gov – FDA health claim for psyllium on reducing risk of heart disease.

http://www.cfsan.fda.gov – FDA health claim for soluble fiber from whole oats and risk of coronary heart disease.

http://www.jhci.org.uk – JHCI final health claim for whole-grain foods and heart health.

http://www.jhci.org.uk – JHCI generic health claim for whole oats and reduction of blood cholesterol.

FATTY ACIDS

Contents

Metabolism

P A Watkins, Kennedy Krieger Institute and Johns Hopkins University School of Medicine, Baltimore, MD, USA

Introduction

Fatty acids and glucose are the primary metabolic fuels used by higher organisms, including man. As such, fatty acids occupy a central position in human nutrition. Fat, carbohydrate, and protein comprise the macronutrients. When nutritionists speak of fat, they are referring mainly to triacylglycerol (triglyceride), which consists of three fatty-acid molecules covalently linked to a backbone of glycerol. Several properties of fatty acids and triacylglycerol make them highly suited to the storage and provision of energy. When a gram of fatty acid is burned as fuel, about 9 kcal of energy is recovered – more than twice that yielded when a gram of carbohydrate or protein is utilized. Unlike carbohydrates, fat can be stored in an anhydrous compact state, allowing the organism to amass large quantities of fuel reserves in times of plenty. This property can have unfortunate consequences in prosperous societies, as evidenced by the increasing incidence of obesity. Fatty acids are also fundamental building blocks for the synthesis of most biologically important lipids, including phospholipids, sphingolipids, and cholesterol esters. They are the precursors of bioactive molecules such as prostaglandins and other eicosanoids. In addition, fatty acids and their coenzyme A derivatives have many metabolic regulatory roles.

Fatty-Acid Nomenclature Conventions

In this article, fatty acids will be identified by their chain length, the number of double bonds present, and the position of the first double bond from the methyl end of the molecule. Thus 14:0 denotes a saturated fatty acid with 14 carbon atoms, 16:1n-9 denotes a monounsaturated fatty acid with 16 carbon atoms in which one double bond occurs nine carbon atoms from the methyl end, and 20:4n-6 denotes a polyunsaturated fatty acid with 20 carbon atoms in which the first of four double bonds is found six carbon atoms from the methyl end. Unless otherwise noted, all double bonds are in the *cis* configuration and double bonds in polyunsaturated fatty acids are separated by a single methylene (–CH_2–) group. The carboxyl carbon atom of any fatty acid is carbon-1. The adjacent carbon atom is referred to as either carbon-2 or the α-carbon; the next is carbon-3 or the β-carbon, and so on. Some examples are shown in **Figure 1**.

Physical Properties of Fatty Acids

Fatty acids are aliphatic organic acids with the fundamental structure $CH_3(CH_2)_nCOOH$, where n can range from zero to more than 26. Thus, fatty acids range from the shortest, acetic acid (2:0), to the very long-chain fatty acids

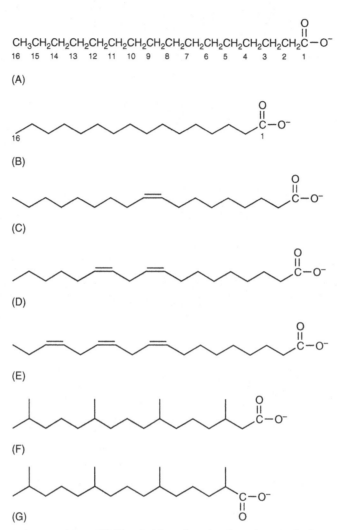

CH₃CH₂CH₂CH₂CH₂CH₂CH₂CH₂CH₂CH₂CH₂CH₂CH₂CH₂CH₂C—O⁻
16 15 14 13 12 11 10 9 8 7 6 5 4 3 2 1

(A)

(B)

(C)

(D)

(E)

(F)

(G)

Figure 1 Fatty-acid structure and nomenclature. (A) Chemical formula and carbon atom numbering system for a 16-carbon saturated fatty acid (16:0). (B) Schematic representation of 16:0. (C) A monounsaturated fatty acid, 18:1*n*-9, showing the double bond nine carbon atoms from the methyl end (carbon 18). (D) The essential *n*-6 fatty acid 18:2*n*-6, where the first double bond is found six carbon atoms from the methyl end. The two double bonds are separated by a methylene (–CH₂–) group. (E) The essential *n*-3 fatty acid 18:3*n*-3, where the first double bond is found three carbon atoms from the methyl end. (F) Phytanic acid, a dietary *β*-methyl-branched-chain fatty acid (3,7,11,15-tetramethyl 16:0). The methyl group on carbon 3 prevents this fatty acid from degradation by *β*-oxidation. (G) Pristanic acid (2,6,10,14-tetramethyl 15:0) is the product of phytanic acid *α*-oxidation, in which a single carbon (carbon 1) is lost. The methyl group on carbon 2 does not preclude subsequent degradation by *β*-oxidation.

containing 26 or more carbon atoms (e.g., 26:0). Although fatty acids with an odd number of carbon atoms exist in nature, most common fatty acids have an even number. The most abundant fatty acids in human lipids and in dietary lipids are the long-chain fatty acids 16:0 (palmitic acid) and 18:1*n*-9 (oleic acid) (**Figure 1**). The hydrophobic nature of the hydrocarbon chain of fatty acids containing more than eight carbon atoms renders them quite insoluble in aqueous media. It has been estimated that for every two additional carbon atoms in the fatty-acid chain its solubility decreases 10-fold.

Owing to the poor solubility of the most abundant fatty acids, free (non-esterified) fatty acids are often found associated with binding and/or transport proteins. Serum albumin has at least six binding sites for fatty acids and is the primary transporter of these molecules through the bloodstream. Several low-molecular-weight fatty-acid binding proteins have been identified and implicated in the intracellular transport of free fatty acids. While free fatty acids can associate with lipophilic cellular and organellar membranes, concentrations of these non-esterified compounds in membranes are typically very low.

Fatty-Acid Activation

Biochemically, fatty acids are rather nonreactive molecules unless they are first activated by thioesterification to coenzyme A (CoA). This reaction is catalyzed by acyl-CoA synthetases (also known as acid : CoA ligases, E.C. 6.2.1.x). The overall acyl-CoA synthetase reaction is

$$RCOOH + ATP + CoA\text{-}SH$$
$$\rightarrow RCO\text{-}S\text{-}CoA + AMP + PPi$$

where PPi is inorganic pyrophosphate, ATP is adenosine triphosphate, and AMP is adenosine monophosphate. Owing to the wide diversity of fatty-acid chain lengths, many enzymes with varied substrate specificities have been identified.

It is estimated that humans have more than 25 enzymes capable of activating fatty acids and/or fatty-acid-like compounds. Acyl-CoA synthetases that activate fatty acids of similar chain lengths often have different tissue-expression patterns and/or different subcellular locations. Thus, each enzyme may direct its fatty-acid substrates into a particular metabolic pathway.

Mitochondrial Fatty-Acid β-Oxidation

To recover their stored energy, fatty acids must be oxidized. Quantitatively, the most important energy-yielding degradation pathway is mitochondrial β-oxidation (**Figure 2**). Fatty acids must first enter cells or tissues. Serum triacylglycerol, usually associated with lipoproteins, is hydrolyzed by lipoprotein lipase located on the capillary endothelium, releasing fatty acids for cellular uptake. In addition, albumin-bound circulating free fatty acids (e.g., produced by the mobilization of adipocyte fat stores) reach the cell surface. Although hydrophobic fatty acids can traverse the plasma membrane by simple diffusion, a role for membrane transport proteins in this process remains controversial. Once inside the cell, fatty acids are thought to be moved to the mitochondria (or other intracellular sites) by intracellular fatty-acid binding proteins.

Acyl-CoA synthetase activity towards long-chain fatty-acid substrates is present in the outer mitochondrial membrane. However, fatty acyl-CoAs do not readily traverse biological membranes such as the inner mitochondrial membrane. A highly sophisticated transport system has evolved to allow tight regulation of fatty-acid entry into the mitochondrion (**Figure 2**). Carnitine palmitoyl transferase 1 (CPT1), located on the inner aspect of the outer mitochondrial membrane, catalyzes a transesterification reaction:

$$\text{fatty acyl-CoA} + \text{carnitine}$$
$$\rightarrow \text{fatty acyl-carnitine} + \text{CoA-SH}$$

Carnitine–acylcarnitine translocase (CACT), located in the inner mitochondrial membrane, carries the fatty acyl-carnitine inside the mitochondrion in exchange for a free carnitine molecule. CPT2, located inside the mitochondrion, then catalyzes the reversal of the CPT1 reaction. Thus, the concerted actions of CPT1, CACT, and CPT2 effectively translocate fatty acyl-CoA across the inner mitochondrial membrane.

Entry of fatty acids into the mitochondrion is regulated by several mechanisms. Although long-chain fatty acids can readily diffuse across the lipophilic inner mitochondrial membrane, the mitochondrial matrix lacks long-chain acyl-CoA synthetase activity. Thus, long-chain fatty acids cannot be activated intramitochondrially to enter the β-oxidation pathway. Control is also exerted extramitochondrially via malonyl-CoA, a cytoplasmic intermediate in fatty-acid biosynthesis and an indicator of high cellular energy status. Malonyl-CoA is a potent inhibitor of CPT1, prohibiting fatty acids from entering the mitochondria to be degraded.

As depicted in **Figure 2**, the four primary enzymes of mitochondrial β-oxidation act on intra-mitochondrial fatty acyl-CoA by sequential dehydrogenation, hydration, dehydrogenation, and thiolytic cleavage reactions. The products are (1) fatty acyl-CoA that has been shortened by two carbon atoms, (2) acetyl-CoA, (3) reduced flavin adenine dinucleotide (FADH$_2$), and (4) reduced nicotinamide adenine dinucleotide (NADH). FADH$_2$ and NADH can directly enter the electron transport chain at complex 2 and complex 1, respectively, yielding about five ATP molecules. Acetyl-CoA can be further degraded to carbon dioxide and water by the tricarboxylic acid cycle, yielding additional reducing equivalents that can enter the electron transport chain and produce ATP. Importantly, the entire β-oxidation process can be repeated using the shortened fatty acyl-CoA as a substrate. This process can be repeated until the entire carbon skeleton of the fatty acid has been degraded to two-carbon acetyl-CoA units. Theoretically, complete oxidation of one molecule of 16:0 (β-oxidation and tricarboxylic acid cycle) will yield more than 160 ATP molecules.

Essentially all cells and tissues can use carbohydrate (glucose) for fuel, and a few (e.g., nerves and erythrocytes) are dependent on this fuel source. An

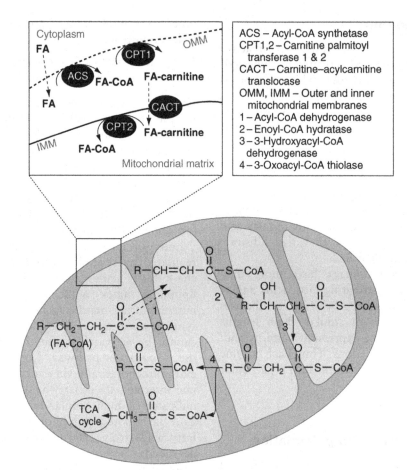

Figure 2 Mitochondrial fatty-acid (FA) β-oxidation pathway. Long-chain fatty acids are activated, converted to carnitine esters, transported across the inner mitochondrial membrane, and re-converted to their CoA thioester once in the mitochondrial matrix. Four sequential mitochondrial enzyme reactions shorten the fatty acyl-CoA (FA-CoA) by two carbon atoms, which are released as acetyl-CoA. The shortened fatty acyl-CoA can undergo additional cycles of degradation until the entire carbon chain has been converted to acetyl-CoA units. $FADH_2$ and NADH, produced in reactions 1 and 3, respectively, can enter the electron transport chain for ATP production. Acetyl-CoA enters the tricarboxylic acid (TCA) cycle, yielding additional NADH and $FADH_2$ for ATP production. Mitochondrial β-oxidation is the primary pathway for recovering the energy stored as triacylglycerol or 'fat'.

important nutritional consideration is that carbon derived from fatty acids via β-oxidation cannot be converted to glucose in net quantities. In the postprandial state, however, most cell types other than nerves and erythrocytes derive the majority of their energy from fatty-acid oxidation under normal physiologic conditions. Some tissues, e.g., skeletal muscle, completely oxidize fatty acids to carbon dioxide and water. Others, e.g., liver, only partially oxidize fatty acids, using the acetyl-CoA product for biosynthethic needs. In particular, liver uses intramitochondrial acetyl-CoA for the synthesis of ketone bodies, acetoacetate and β-hydroxybutyrate (**Figure 3**). Ketone bodies can be oxidized by all tissues except the liver and provide an alternative fuel source during starvation. In particular, nervous tissue can oxidize ketone bodies. During prolonged starvation, increased ketone-body use spares the brain's requirement for glucose.

Peroxisomal Fatty-Acid β-Oxidation

Like mitochondria, peroxisomes contain pathways for the β-oxidation of fatty acids. The mechanism by which fatty acids enter peroxisomes is unclear but does not appear to involve the CPT1–CACT–CPT2 pathway. Long-chain and very-long-chain acyl-CoA synthetase activities are associated with peroxisomes, but it has not been established whether fatty acids or fatty acyl-CoAs traverse the peroxisomal membrane. The basic reactions of peroxisomal β-oxidation resemble those found in mitochondria, but the peroxisomal and mitochondrial enzymes are distinct proteins (**Figure 4**). In fact, peroxisomes contain two sets of β-oxidation enzymes, which appear to function with distinct substrates.

Unlike mitochondria, peroxisomes do not contain an electron transport chain or tricarboxylic acid

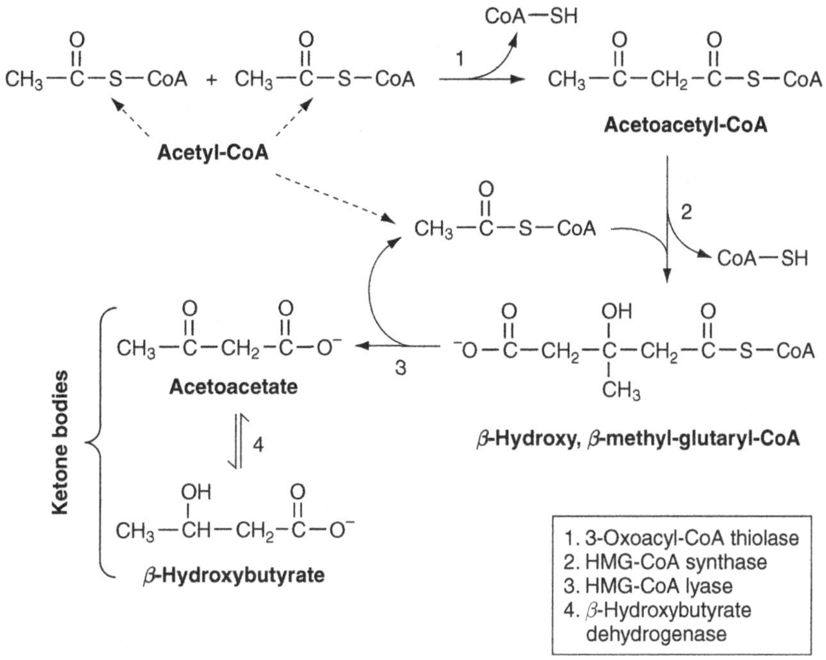

Figure 3 Synthesis of ketone bodies. In the mitochondria of hepatocytes, acetyl-CoA derived from β-oxidation is converted to ketone bodies, primarily acetoacetate and β-hydroxybutyrate, rather than entering the tricarboxylic acid cycle. Two molecules of acetyl-CoA condense in a reversal of the last β-oxidation reaction (3-oxoacyl-CoA thiolase). The product, acetoacetyl-CoA, condenses with another molecule of acetyl-CoA, yielding β-hydroxy, β-methyl-glutaryl-CoA (HMG-CoA), a reaction catalysed by HMG-CoA synthase. Cleavage of HMG-CoA by HMG-CoA lyase yields acetoacetate, regenerating one molecule of acetyl-CoA. Acetoacetate is reversibly reduced to β-hydroxybutyrate via the NAD-dependent enzyme β-hydroxybutyrate dehydrogenase. These ketone bodies can traverse the inner mitochondrial membrane, eventually reaching the bloodstream for ultimate use by the brain and other tissues.

cycle, and, thus, peroxisomal fatty-acid degradation is not directly coupled to energy production. Rather, peroxisomes have a more specialized fatty-acid oxidation role, degrading fatty-acid substrates that cannot be catabolized in mitochondria. Peroxisomes are indispensable for the degradation of very-long-chain fatty acids (containing more than 22 carbon atoms), which are neurotoxic if allowed to accumulate. These fatty acids undergo several cycles of peroxisomal β-oxidation until they are between eight and 10 carbon atoms long, after which they go to the mitochondria for further catabolism. Degradation of xenobiotic fatty acyl-like compounds (e.g., sulphur-substituted fatty acids and many nonsteroidal anti-inflammatory drugs) takes place in peroxisomes. Oxidation of dicarboxylic acids (from the diet or from ω-oxidation) and 2-methyl-branched-chain fatty acids (from the diet or from α-oxidation) also occurs in peroxisomes.

The peroxisomal β-oxidation pathway also fulfils an important biosynthetic role. In the hepatic synthesis of bile acids from cholesterol, the aliphatic side chain, which resembles an α-methyl-branched-chain fatty acid, must be shortened. A single cycle of peroxisomal β-oxidation will remove a three-carbon portion of the side chain, converting the 27-carbon bile acid precursors dihydroxycholestanoic and tri-hydroxycholestanoic acids into the 24-carbon primary bile acids chenodeoxycholate and cholate, respectively.

Fatty-Acid α-Oxidation and ω-Oxidation

Other important fatty-acid catabolic pathways include α-oxidation and ω-oxidation. α-Oxidation is required for degradation of the dietary fatty acid phytanic acid (3,7,11,15-tetramethyl-16:0). This fatty acid cannot be degraded by β-oxidation owing to the methyl group on carbon-3. In the human diet, phytanic acid is obtained from the consumption of ruminant meats, fats, and dairy products. Rumen bacteria hydrolyze chlorophyll, releasing the phytol side chain; phytol is oxidized to phytanic acid and incorporated into triacylglycerol and phospholipids by the animal. Humans typically ingest 50–100 mg of phytanic acid per day. The current view of the α-oxidation pathway, which is found in peroxisomes, is shown in **Figure 5**. After activation to its CoA derivative, phytanoyl-CoA is hydroxylated on the 2-carbon. The next reaction catalyzes the removal of

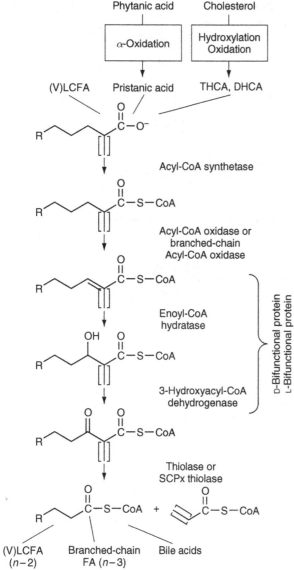

Figure 4 Peroxisomal fatty-acid (FA) β-oxidation pathways. While saturated long-chain fatty acids (LCFA) are preferentially degrade in mitochondria, saturated very-long-chain fatty acids (VLCFA) and some LCFA are shortened by peroxisomal β-oxidation. Degradation of pristanic acid, the product of phytanic acid α-oxidation, and the conversion of the cholesterol-derived 27-carbon bile-acid precursors dihydroxycholestanoic acid (DHCA) and trihydroxycholestanoic acid (THCA) to 24-carbon bile acids also require this pathway. The mechanism by which these substrates enter peroxisomes is unknown. Four enzymatic reactions serve to shorten the substrates by either two (LCFA, VLCFA) or three (pristanic acid, DHCA, THCA) carbon atoms. The 2-methyl group of the latter substrates is shown in brackets. SCPx thiolase refers to the thiolase activity of sterol carrier protein x.

a one-carbon CoA derivative as formyl-CoA. The other product of this reaction is an aldehyde, pristanal, that can be oxidized to form pristanic acid (2,6,10,14-tetramethyl-15:0). This chain-shortening reaction effectively shifts the position of the first

methyl group from carbon-3 (in phytanic acid) to carbon-2 (in pristanic acid). The 2-methyl-branched chain fatty acids can then be degraded further via peroxisomal β-oxidation.

Another mechanism for degradation of fatty acids that cannot undergo β-oxidation is known as ω-oxidation. In this process, the terminal methyl group (referred to as the ω-end) of a fatty-acid chain is oxidized to a carboxylic acid via cytochrome P450 isozymes, particularly the CYP52A family, in the endoplasmic reticulum. The resulting dicarboxylic acids can then be at least partially degraded by β-oxidation from the ω-end, primarily in peroxisomes.

Fatty-Acid *de novo* Synthesis

Much of our need for fatty acids as constituents of phospholipids and other complex lipids is met by the diet. In addition, certain lipogenic tissues are capable of the *de novo* synthesis of fatty acids (**Figure 6**). These tissues include liver (hepatocytes), adipose tissue, and lactating mammary gland. Much of the fatty acids synthesized by all three tissues is incorporated into triacylglycerol. Hepatic synthesis is primarily for export to other tissues (in very low-density lipoproteins), while synthesis in adipocytes and mammary gland is for local storage.

The carbon used for fatty-acid synthesis typically derives from the products of glycolysis. The end product of glycolysis, pyruvate, enters the mitochondria and becomes the substrate for two separate reactions. In one, pyruvate is decarboxylated via the pyruvate dehydrogenase complex, yielding acetyl-CoA. Lipogenic tissues also contain another mitochondrial enzyme, pyruvate carboxylase, which converts pyruvate to the four-carbon acid oxaloacetate (OAA). Acetyl-CoA and oxaloacetate condense to form the six-carbon acid citrate. As citrate accumulates within the mitochondrion, it is exported to the cytoplasm, where it is converted back to oxaloacetate and acetyl-CoA. Cytoplasmic acetyl-CoA is the fundamental building block for *de novo* synthesis of fatty acids.

The first enzyme unique to fatty-acid synthesis is acetyl-CoA carboxylase, which converts the two-carbon substrate acetyl-CoA into the three-carbon product malonyl-CoA. Citrate, in addition to being the precursor of cytoplasmic acetyl-CoA, has a regulatory role. Citrate is an allosteric activator of acetyl-CoA carboxylase and serves as a signal that there is an ample carbon supply for fatty-acid synthesis. As noted above, malonyl-CoA is a potent inhibitor of CPT1. Cytoplasmic

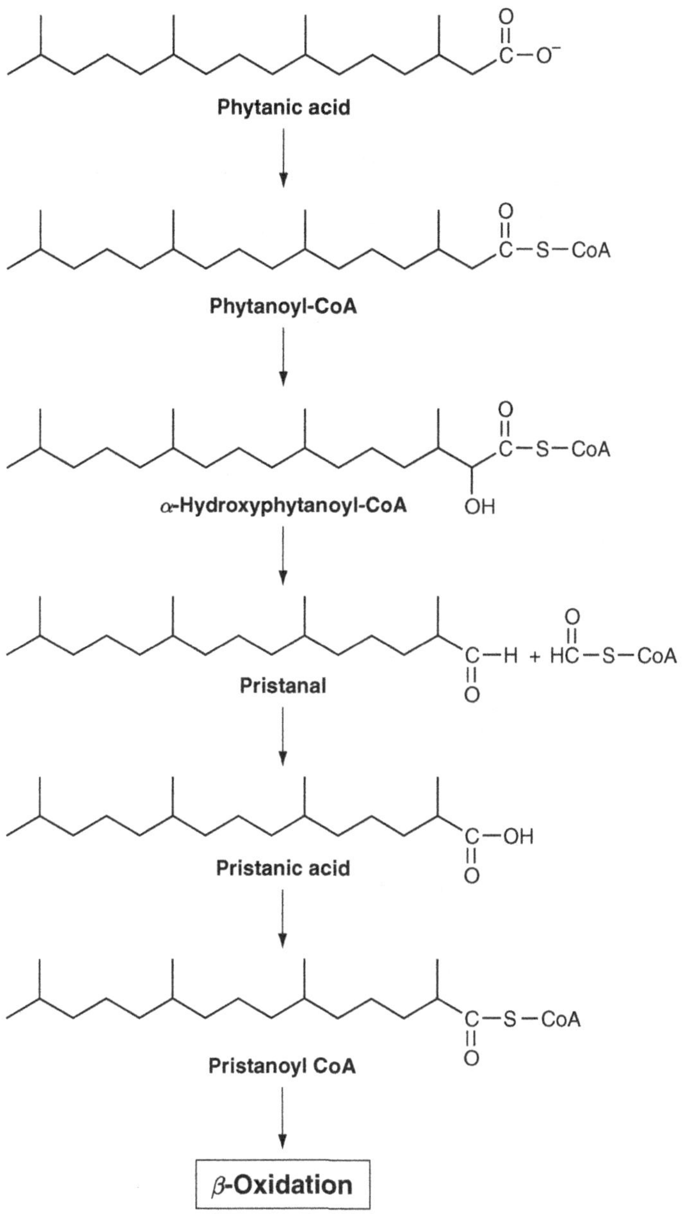

Figure 5 Peroxisomal phytanic acid α-oxidation pathway. The dietary 3-methyl-branched fatty acid phytanic acid is toxic if allowed to accumulate in the tissues. Its 3-methyl group prevents degradation by β-oxidation; therefore, this fatty acid is first shortened by one carbon atom. Like the substrates for peroxisomal β-oxidation, phytanic acid enters peroxisomes by an unknown mechanism. Activated phytanic acid is hydroxylated on carbon 2. Cleavage between carbons 1 and 2 yields a one-carbon CoA compound, formyl-CoA, and an aldehyde, pristanal. After oxidation and reactivation to the CoA derivative, pristanoyl-CoA can be degraded by β-oxidation.

malonyl-CoA levels will be high only when there is significant flux through glycolysis, indicative of a high cellular energy state. Under these conditions, entry of fatty acids into the mitochondria (and subsequent β-oxidation) is prevented. Interestingly, there are two isoforms of acetyl-CoA carboxylase. One is found in the above-named lipogenic tissues. The other is found in many tissues that are not capable of synthesizing fatty acids, e.g., the heart. It is thought that the primary role of the second

isozyme is to regulate mitochondrial fatty-acid β-oxidation by synthesizing malonyl-CoA when cellular energy needs are being met by carbohydrate metabolism.

The subsequent reactions of fatty-acid synthesis in humans are catalyzed by a multienzyme complex, fatty-acid synthase. After binding of one molecule each of acetyl-CoA and malonyl-CoA to unique binding sites within the complex, a condensation reaction occurs in which carbon dioxide is

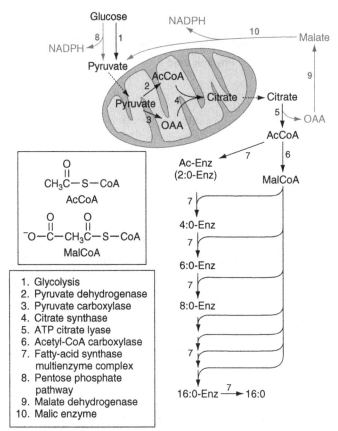

Figure 6 Fatty-acid biosynthesis. Cytoplasmic acetyl-CoA (AcCoA) is the primary substrate for *de novo* fatty-acid synthesis. This two-carbon compound most commonly derives from the glycolytic degradation of glucose, and its formation is dependent upon several reactions in the mitochondria. The mitochondrial enzyme pyruvate carboxylase is found primarily in tissues that can synthesize fatty acids. AcCoA is converted to malonyl-CoA (MalCoA) by acetyl-CoA carboxylase. Using AcCoA as a primer, the fatty-acid synthase multienzyme complex carries out a series of reactions that elongate the growing fatty acid by two carbon atoms. In this process MalCoA condenses with AcCoA, yielding an enzyme-bound four-carbon β-ketoacid that is reduced, dehydrated, and reduced again. The product is enzyme-bound 4:0. This process is repeated six more times, after which 16:0 is released from the complex. The reductive steps require NADPH, which is derived from enzyme reactions and pathways shown in grey. Enz refers to the fatty acid synthase multienzyme complex.

released and an enzyme-bound 4-carbon 3-ketoacid is formed. Subsequent reactions include a reduction step, a dehydration step, and a second reduction step. The intermediates produced in these reactions are similar to those seen in β-oxidation (**Figure 2**), in reverse order. The product (enzyme bound) is the saturated fatty acid 4:0, which can then condense with another molecule of malonyl-CoA to start the process anew. After seven such cycles, the ultimate product is 16:0, which is released from the complex.

The reductive steps in fatty-acid synthesis require reduced nicotinamide adenine dinucleotide phosphate (NADPH). Some NADPH is produced during recycling of the oxaloacetate formed during the cytoplasmic hydrolysis of citrate, described above. Oxaloacetate is first converted to malate (via cytoplasmic malate dehydrogenase). Malate is then decarboxylated to pyruvate in an $NADP^+$-dependent reaction catalyzed by malic enzyme; NADPH is produced in this reaction. NADPH for fatty-acid biosynthesis also comes from reactions in the pentose phosphate pathway (hexose monophosphate shunt).

In several respects, the enzymatic reactions of fatty-acid synthesis are the converse of those in fatty-acid oxidation. However, there are key differences, which are summarized in **Table 1**.

Fatty-Acid Elongation

The primary product synthesized by the *de novo* pathway is 16:0. While 16:0 is an important fatty acid, there is a need to synthesize longer-chain acids. Enzymes for elongation of fatty-acids have been found in membranes of the endoplasmic reticulum

Table 1 Distinctions between fatty-acid β-oxidation and fatty-acid synthesis

	Fatty-acid β-oxidation	Fatty-acid synthesis
Tissues with active pathway	Nearly all tissues except brain, nerve, and erythrocytes	Liver, adipose, and lactating mammary gland
Subcellular location	Mitochondria	Cytoplasm
Redox cofactors	NAD, FAD	NADPH
Acyl-group carrier	CoA	Enzyme-bound acyl carrier protein
Stereochemistry of 3-hydroxy intermediate	L-	D-

and mitochondria. However, these pathways are less well-characterized than that of fatty-acid synthesis. In the endoplasmic reticulum, the reactions involved in fatty-acid elongation are very similar to those of cytoplasmic fatty-acid synthesis. The donor of the added carbon atoms is also malonyl-CoA, indicating that an active acetyl-CoA carboxylase is required for elongation. Whereas the primary reactions of fatty-acid synthesis are found within the fatty-acid synthase multienzyme complex, individual proteins catalyze the four elongation reactions (condensation, reduction, dehydration, and reduction). Like synthesis, elongation in the endoplasmic reticulum requires reducing equivalents in the form of NADPH.

Fatty-acid elongation in mitochondrial membranes is thought to be slightly different from the process in the endoplasmic reticulum. The primary difference is that the donor of elongation units is thought to be acetyl-CoA, not malonyl-CoA. The four elongation reactions are similar, but may require NADH rather than NADPH as source of reducing equivalents. Little is known about how fatty-acid elongation in either the mitochondria or the endoplasmic reticulum is regulated.

Fatty-Acid Unsaturation and the Essential Fatty Acids

Monounsaturated and polyunsaturated fatty acids are extraordinarily important in human health and nutrition. Thus, the insertion of double bonds into the carbon skeleton of a fatty acid is a vital metabolic function. However, humans are in general not capable of inserting double bonds closer than nine carbon atoms from the methyl end of a fatty acid. Thus, we are incapable of the *de novo* synthesis of

two important classes of fatty acids, the *n*-3 fatty acids such as docosahexaenoic acid (22:6*n*-3) and the *n*-6 fatty acids such as arachidonic acid (20:4*n*-6). The *n*-3 fatty acids have proven to be beneficial in the prevention of coronary artery disease. The fatty acid 22:6*n*-3 has been shown to be important for the normal development of the brain and retina, leading some manufacturers to include this fatty acid in their infant formula preparations. The *n*-6 fatty acids are important constituents of membrane lipids. The fatty acid 20:4 is also the well-known precursor of prostaglandins and other bioactive eicosanoids. Since we cannot synthesize these fatty acids *de novo*, we are dependent on the presence of at least some *n*-3 and some *n*-6 fatty acids in the diet. Linoleic acid (18:2*n*-6) and α-linolenic acid (18:3*n*-3) are the precursors of most biologically important *n*-3 and *n*-6 fatty acids; thus, they are referred to as essential fatty acids.

As noted earlier, the most abundant fatty acids in humans include a saturated fatty acid (16:0) and a monounsaturated fatty acid (18:1*n*-9). Humans can readily insert a *cis*-double bond nine carbons from the carboxyl carbon atom of a fatty acid (Δ9) in a reaction catalyzed by stearoyl-CoA desaturase (SCD1; so-named because the preferred substrate is the CoA derivative of 18:0, stearic acid). Because SCD1 is involved in the synthesis of such an abundant fatty acid, 18:1, the importance of this enzyme in metabolism was initially overlooked. However, 18:1 produced by SCD1 appears to be directed specifically towards triacylglycerol synthesis. Mice in which the SCD1 gene is disrupted have decreased adiposity. Furthermore, genetically obese leptin-deficient (ob–/ob–) mice in which the SCD1 gene is also disrupted have significantly reduced body weight compared with ob–/ob– mice, leading to the hypothesis that leptin regulates the synthesis of SCD1. Interestingly, dietary 18:1 seems to be more readily incorporated into lipids other than triacylglycerols, implying that the dietary and the SCD1-produced pools of this fatty acid are metabolically distinct. As with the *n*-3 fatty acids, dietary ingestion of monounsaturated fatty acids such as 18:1 has been associated with benefits to cardiovascular health.

Humans are also capable of inserting *cis*-double bonds either five or six carbon atoms from the carboxyl carbon atom of a fatty acid (Δ5 desaturase and Δ6 desaturase activity, respectively). These activities, when combined with the elongation pathways described above, form a powerful mechanism for synthesis of highly polyunsaturated fatty acids such as 20:4*n*-6 and 22:6*n*-3 from the dietary essential fatty acids. Previously, it was thought that humans also had the ability to insert a double bond four carbon atoms from the carboxyl carbon (Δ4 desaturase activity), as this activity was thought to be necessary for the conversion of 18:3n-3 to 22:6n-3. However, attempts to measure Δ4 desaturase activity experimentally were not successful. It is now thought that, through a series of elongation and desaturation reactions, 18:3n-3 is converted to the penultimate intermediate, 22:5n-3. Rather than using a Δ4 desaturase to complete the synthesis, 22:5n-3 is elongated to 24:5n-3, converted to 24:6n-3 by Δ6 desaturase, and finally chain-shortened to 22:6n-3 by one cycle of peroxisomal β-oxidation.

Fatty Acids as Components of Complex Lipids

Fatty acids are important building blocks for various cellular complex lipids (**Figure 7**). For simplicity, the pathways for incorporation of fatty acids into these lipids are outlined only briefly. More details can be found in any good biochemistry text. In most cases, fatty acyl-CoA and not free

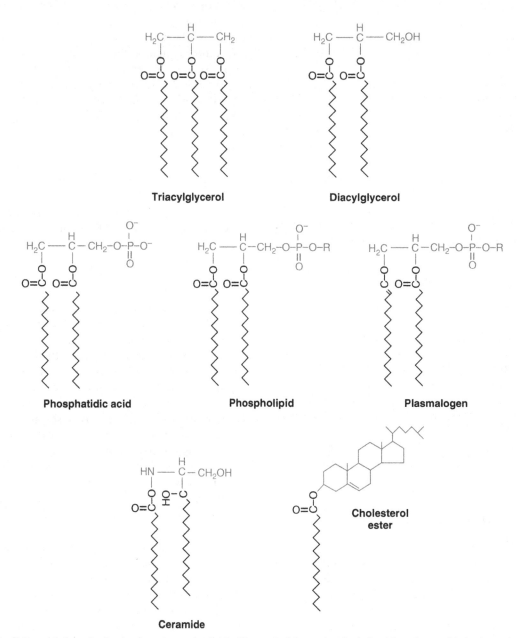

Figure 7 Fatty acids form the basis of most complex lipids. The part of the molecule derived from fatty acids is shown in black, and the part derived from other sources is shown in grey. For phospholipids and plasmalogens, R = choline, ethanolamine, inositol, serine, or a similar head group.

fatty acid participates in these biosynthetic reactions. Nearly all cells synthesize phospholipids, which are essential membrane constituents. Phospholipid synthesis takes place in the endoplasmic reticulum. It begins by fatty acylating the two free hydroxyl groups in α-glycerophosphate, a triose derived from glycolytic intermediates, yielding phosphatidic acid. Various head groups (e.g., choline, ethanolamine, inositol, or serine) can then be linked to the phosphate group. For synthesis of triacylglycerol, this phosphate moiety is removed, yielding diacylglycerol, and a third fatty acyl group is esterified to the free hydroxyl group.

Another type of lipid, the ether-linked phospholipids (e.g., plasmalogens), comprises about 20% of membrane phospholipids (**Figure 7**). Plasmalogen synthesis requires enzymes present in both peroxisomes and the endoplasmic reticulum. These lipids are thought to be part of the cellular defense mechanism against oxidative injury.

Fatty acids are also found esterified to the 3-hydroxyl group of cholesterol (cholesterol esters; ChE). ChE, which are more hydrophobic than free cholesterol, are a transport and storage form of cholesterol. ChE are found in high concentrations in low-density lipoproteins. Intracellular lipid droplets containing ChE are found in steroidogenic tissues and are thought to be a reservoir of cholesterol for steroid-hormone synthesis. The fatty acid most commonly found in ChE is 18:1. It must be activated to its CoA derivative before transfer to cholesterol in a reaction catalyzed by acyl-CoA cholesterol acyltransferase. ChE are also formed within lipoproteins by the transfer of one fatty acyl chain from phosphatidyl choline to cholesterol, a reaction catalyzed by circulating lecithin: cholesterol acyltransferase.

Synthesis of sphingolipids, which include sphingomyelin, ceramides, cerebrosides, and gangliosides, begins by the condensation of palmitoyl-CoA (16:0-CoA) with serine. The amino group of serine is then acylated by a second fatty acyl-CoA to form ceramide; the chain length of the second fatty acid can be variable. Transfer of phosphorylcholine (from the phospholipid phosphatidyl choline) to the hydroxyl group of ceramide yields sphingomyelin. Alternatively, sugars (from sugar nucleotide donors) are added to produce the cerebrosides, gangliosides, and related lipids.

Eicosanoid Synthesis

The fatty acid 20:4n-6 (arachidonic acid) is the precursor of most eicosanoids, which include the prostaglandins, leukotrienes, and thromboxanes.

Because it is an n-6 fatty acid, 20:4 must be derived from dietary lipids or synthesized by elongation and unsaturation of the essential fatty acid 18:2n-6. As with other fatty acids, cellular concentrations of unesterified 20:4 are low. Conversion of 20:4 to eicosanoids begins with an agonist-induced release of the fatty acid from the sn-2 position of membrane phospholipids via the action of phospholipase A2. Unlike most reactions of fatty acids, eicosanoid synthesis appears to use free 20:4 rather than its CoA derivative as the substrate. Cyclooxygenases (COX1 and COX2) catalyze a complex molecular oxygen-requiring reaction that converts 20:4 to prostaglandin G2. This reaction involves carbon atoms in the middle of the acyl chain, rather than the methyl carbon (such as occurs in ω-oxidation) or the carboxyl carbon (such as occurs in nearly all other reactions of fatty acids). Prostaglandin G2 can subsequently be converted to other prostaglandins or to thromboxanes. As these compounds have potent biological effects, including mediation of inflammation, COX inhibitors are an important class of anti-inflammatory drugs. Free 20:4 is also the primary substrate for the enzyme 5-lipoxygenase, which is the first step in the synthesis of leukotrienes.

Fatty Acylation of Proteins

Covalent modification of proteins is a more recently discovered role of fatty acids. Fatty acylation of proteins frequently serves as a means of targeting or anchoring a protein to a membrane. Myristoylation, the addition of 14:0 to a protein, occurs at N-terminal glycine residues after removal of the initiator methionine. This process is generally co-translational and irreversible. N-myristoyl proteins include many signal-transduction-associated proteins, e.g., *src* and ADP-ribosylation factors. The enzyme N-myristoyltransferase catalyzes the reaction and uses 14:0-CoA as substrate.

Palmitoylation, the addition of 16:0 to a protein, is also commonly observed. This modification to the sulfydryl side chain of cysteine residues occurs post-translationally and is reversible. Both membrane-associated proteins and integral membrane proteins can be palmitoylated; examples are ion channels, neurotransmitter receptors, and sonic hedgehog. Protein palmitoyl transferases also use the CoA derivative of the fatty acid as a substrate. Several proteins are modified with both an N-terminal 14:0 and an S-linked 16:0 elsewhere in the protein chain. α-subunits of heterotrimeric G-proteins and endothelial nitric oxide synthase are examples of dually acylated proteins.

Table 2 Vitamins associated with fatty-acid metabolism

Vitamin	Active form	Enzymes	Pathways
Pantothenic acid	CoA	Many enzymes	Most reactions involving fatty acids
Niacin	NAD, NADH, NADP, NADPH	Dehydrogenases; reductases	Many pathways, particularly β-oxidation and fatty-acid synthesis and elongation
Riboflavin	FAD, FADH$_2$	Oxidases	β-Oxidation
Thiamine	Thiamine pyrophosphate	Pyruvate dehydrogenase complex; β-hydroxyphytanoyl-CoA lyase	Fatty-acid synthesis from glucose; phytanic acid β-oxidation
Biotin	Biocytin	Acetyl-CoA carboxylase; pyruvate carboxylase	Fatty-acid synthesis from glucose

There are instances of acylation by fatty acids with chain lengths other than 14 or 16 carbon atoms. One nutritionally important example is the recently identified orexigenic peptide ghrelin. The active form of this 28-amino-acid peptide hormone has the medium-chain fatty acid 8:0 covalently esterified to the hydroxyl group of serine-3. Octanoylated ghrelin is believed to act at the level of the hypothalamus to stimulate appetite, perhaps via neuropeptide Y.

Vitamins and Fatty-Acid Metabolism

Several of the B vitamins are essential for normal fatty-acid metabolism (**Table 2**). Pantothenic acid is a constituent of CoA and is thus required for numerous reactions of fatty acids. Niacin and riboflavin are necessary for the synthesis of oxidized and reduced NAD(P) and FAD, respectively. These compounds play essential roles in fatty-acid oxidation, synthesis, and elongation. Biotin is a constituent of acetyl-CoA carboxylase and pyruvate carboxylase, both of which are involved in the synthesis of fatty acids from glucose. Thiamine is required for activity of the pyruvate dehydrogenase complex, which also participates in fatty-acid synthesis from glucose.

Regulation of Fatty-Acid Metabolism

A few specific aspects of the regulation of fatty-acid metabolism have been described above. More global regulatory mechanisms that deserve mention include those mediated by insulin and glucagon, sterol regulatory element-binding protein (SREBP) 1c, and peroxisome proliferator-activated receptor (PPAR) α. In the fed and fasted states, control of fuel metabolism is mediated to a large extent by insulin and glucagon, respectively. Effects of glucagon are mediated via cyclic adenosine monophosphate (cAMP)-dependent kinases

and serve to decrease flux through glycolysis, thus decreasing the rate of *de novo* fatty-acid biosynthesis and increasing rates of mitochondrial β-oxidation and ketogenesis. Insulin effects are mediated through activation of its receptor tyrosine kinase and are in general opposite to those of glucagon, stimulating glycolysis and fatty-acid synthesis while inhibiting fatty-acid degradation. Insulin and glucagon have both acute and long-term effects on fatty-acid metabolism. The transcription factor SREBP1c is thought to mediate the action of insulin in upregulating genes involved in fatty-acid synthesis. Activation of PPARα on the other hand increases rates of fatty-acid oxidation and ketogenesis. Endogenous ligands for this nuclear receptor are thought to include polyunsaturated fatty acids and branched-chain fatty acids. The PPARs heterodimerize with the retinoid X receptor, and both receptors must be ligand-bound for transcriptional activation. Several mitochondrial, microsomal, and peroxisomal genes associated with fatty-acid catabolism are upregulated via PPARα stimulation.

See also: **Fatty Acids**: Monounsaturated; Omega-3 Polyunsaturated; Omega-6 Polyunsaturated; Saturated; *Trans* Fatty Acids.

Further Reading

Frohnert BI and Bernlohr DA (2000) Regulation of fatty acid transporters in mammalian cells. *Progress in Lipid Research* **39**: 83–107.

Gibbons GF (2003) Regulation of fatty acid and cholesterol synthesis: co-operation or competition? *Progress in Lipid Research* **42**: 479–497.

Gunstone FD, Harwood JL, and Padley FB (eds.) (1994) *The Lipid Handbook*, 2nd edn. London: Chapman & Hall.

Kunau WH, Dommes V, and Schulz H (1995) Beta-oxidation of fatty acids in mitochondria, peroxisomes, and bacteria: a century of continued progress. *Progress in Lipid Research* **34**: 267–342.

McGarry JD and Foster DW (1980) Regulation of hepatic fatty acid oxidation and ketone body production. *Annual Review of Biochemistry* **49**: 395–420.

Numa S (ed.) (1984) *Fatty Acid Metabolism and its Regulation.* New York: Elsevier.

Vance DE and Vance JE (eds.) (2002) *Biochemistry of Lipids, Lipoproteins and Membranes*, 4th edn. New Comprehensive Biochemistry 36. New York: Elsevier.

Wanders RJ, Vreken P, Ferdinandusse S *et al.* (2001) Peroxisomal fatty acid alpha- and beta-oxidation in humans: enzymology, peroxisomal metabolite transporters and peroxisomal diseases. *Biochemical Society Transactions* **29**: 250–267.

Watkins PA (1997) Fatty acid activation. *Progress in Lipid Research* **36**: 55–83.

Monounsaturated

P Kirk, University of Ulster, Coleraine, UK

This article is reproduced from the previous edition, pp. 744–751, © 1998, Elsevier Ltd.

Introduction

Fatty acids are described according to two characteristics: chain length and degree of saturation with hydrogen. Monounsaturated fatty acids (MUFA) have, as the name suggests, only one unsaturated bond attached to the carbon chain. This double bond is fixed in nature and is positioned on the ninth carbon atom counting from the methyl (omega) end of the fatty-acid chain. Four of these MUFA are found in significant quantities in food, the most common being oleic acid ($C_{18:1}$) (Figure 1). This n-9 fatty acid is capable of being synthesized by animals, including humans, but is predominantly incorporated via the diet. While butter and animal fats contain only small amounts of oleic acid, olive oil is a rich source. Olive oil, which comprises up to 70% of the fat intake in Mediterranean diets, is postulated to be effective in decreasing the risk of certain chronic diseases. These include such diseases as coronary heart disease, cancers, and inflammatory disorders, particularly rheumatoid arthritis.

Cholesterol Metabolism

Cholesterol metabolism is of fundamental biological importance. All vertebrates require cholesterol as a precursor for bile acids and hormones, including corticosteroids, sex steroids, and vitamin D. The amount of cholesterol found in tissues greatly exceeds the requirement for production of these hormones and bile acids, and the bulk of this excess is associated with the cell-membrane structure, where it is believed to modulate the physical state of phospholipid bilayers.

Cholesterol circulates in plasma as a component of lipoproteins. There are several distinct classes of plasma lipoprotein, which differ in several respects, including type of apolipoprotein and relative content of triacylglycerol and cholesterol.

Cholesterol transport

Chylomicron remnants deliver dietary cholesterol to the liver. It is then incorporated into very low-density lipoproteins (VLDL), which are secreted in plasma. The VLDL acquire cholesteryl esters and apolipoprotein E (apo E) from high-density lipoproteins (HDL) to produce intermediate-density lipoproteins (IDL), which are rapidly taken up by the liver or are further catabolized into low-density lipoproteins (LDL). These cholesterol-rich LDL particles are catabolized only slowly in human plasma and are therefore present at relatively high concentrations. Elimination of cholesterol from these extrahepatic cells is achieved by the delivery of cholesterol from cell membranes to plasma HDL in the first step of a pathway known as reverse cholesterol transport. This process allows for esterification of cholesterol and its delivery back to the liver.

LDL, HDL, and atherosclerosis

Membrane function is compromised if it contains either too much or too little cholesterol. Epidemiological studies have classified raised plasma cholesterol levels as a risk factor for atherosclerosis, and it is one of the more important predictors of coronary heart disease (CHD). Elevated plasma cholesterol concentration (hypercholesterolemia) is associated with an increased concentration of LDL, owing to either an increased rate of LDL formation or a decrease in the rate at which they are cleared from plasma, and usually a decreased concentration of HDL. Numerous dietary-intervention studies have aimed both to prevent CHD and to reduce total mortality, but almost all have been ineffective.

MUFA and CHD

Many of the trials conducted concentrated on the substitution of polyunsaturated vegetable oils for saturated fat from animal sources and on decreasing the amount of dietary cholesterol. These studies followed the reasoning that fats rich in saturated fatty acids (SFA) raised plasma cholesterol mainly by

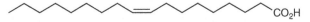

Figure 1 Structure of oleic acid, $C_{18:1}$.

increasing plasma LDL cholesterol levels, and oils rich in polyunsaturated fatty acids (PUFA) lowered plasma cholesterol mainly by decreasing LDL cholesterol. The MUFA were first considered neutral in regard to their influence on plasma cholesterol, but more recent findings suggest a decrease in total LDL cholesterol concentration following substitution of SFA by MUFA. Moreover, clinical trials have also shown that a MUFA-rich diet does not decrease concentrations & HDL, the lipoprotein inversely correlated with CHD.

Although important links exist between cholesterol metabolism and aspects of cell function, other complicating factors must be considered. Cholesterol metabolism is sensitive to the inflammatory response that accompanies most pathological events. Tumor necrosis factor (TNF) reduces LDL and HDL cholesterol levels and inhibits lipoprotein lipase, resulting in a fall in cholesterol and an increase in triacylglycerol levels. These changes may be perpetuated beyond the acute phase if an inflammatory process is present. Cholesterol metabolism is also sensitive to genetic and environmental factors, which may have independent effects on noncardiovascular disease. As a consequence, the relationship between cholesterol levels and the presence or absence of a disease state must be interpreted with caution.

Atherogenesis and Endothelial Dysfunction

Atherosclerosis can be considered as a chronic inflammatory disease, which slowly progresses over a period of decades before clinical symptoms become manifest. The atherogenic process comprises interactions between multiple cell types, which initiate a cascade of events involving alterations in vascular production of autocoids, cytokines, and growth factors. The endothelium, because of its location between blood and the vascular wall, has been implicated in the atherogenic process from the initial stages.

Function of endothelial cells

Owing to the strategic location of the endothelium, it is able to perform many different functions. In addition to acting as a protective barrier, endothelial cells have been shown to play important roles in control of homeostasis, capillary transport, and, more importantly, regulation of the tone of underlying vascular smooth muscle. The endothelium evokes relaxation of these muscle cells, allowing vasodilation via the chemical factor endothelium-derived relaxing factor (EDRF), which has been identified as nitric oxide (NO). The EDRF or NO is vital for maintaining the vasodilatory capacity of vascular muscle and also controls levels of platelet function and monocyte adhesion. Any endothelial injury or dysfunction could therefore be an important factor in atherosclerosis.

Endothelial dysfunction

Decrease in the production, release, or action of NO may lead to enhanced expression of adhesion molecules and chemotactic factors at the endothelial surface. The exact nature of endothelial dysfunction is unknown, although possibilities include a decreased expression of NO synthase, imbalance between the production of endothelium-derived constricting and relaxing factors, production of an endogenous NO synthase inhibitor, and overproduction of oxygen-derived free radicals including O_2^-. The release of the free radical O_2^- from smooth muscle cells is believed to be responsible for the oxidation of LDL cholesterol. Raised cholesterol levels and – more importantly – increased levels of oxidatively modified LDL cholesterol (OxLDL) are considered to be among the most powerful inhibitors of normal endothelial function and hence contribute to the process of atherogenesis.

Lipid peroxidation and atherosclerosis

Lipid peroxidation apparently plays a major role in the pathology of atherosclerosis. Atherosclerosis, which is usually a precondition for CHD, is a degenerative process leading to the accumulation of a variable mixture of substances including lipid in the endothelium of the arteries. This disease is characterized by the formation of a fatty streak and the accumulation of cells loaded with lipid: the foam cells. These cells are believed to arise from white blood cell-derived macrophages or arterial smooth muscle cells. Most of the lipid in the foam cells is in the form of LDL particles. Although research has determined that LDL receptors are responsible for the uptake of LDL by cells, the arterial uptake of LDL, which leads to development of foam cells, occurs by a different pathway. It is only when the LDL particles have undergone oxidative modification that they are available for uptake by macrophages via the scavenger receptor. During the course of oxidative modification, LDL cholesterol acquires various biological properties not present in native LDL that make it a potentially important mediator, promoting atherogenesis. The LDL, once oxidized, becomes cytotoxic and causes local cellular damage to the endothelium. This process, which enhances

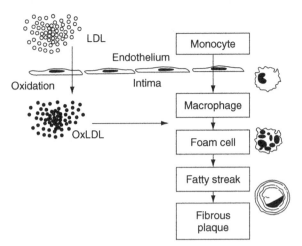

Figure 2 The role of oxidized LDL (OxLDL) in formation of foam cells. Reproduced with permission from Ashwell M (1993) *Diet and Heart Disease – A Round Table of Factors*. London: British Nutrition Foundation.

LDL uptake to generate foam cells, is considered one of the earliest events in atherogenesis (**Figure 2**).

MUFA and atherogenesis

Studies have looked at the oxidizability *in vitro* of LDL using nonphysiological oxidizing conditions to evaluate the susceptibility of LDL to oxidation and hence its atherogenic potential. It is well known that modification of LDL is inhibited by various antioxidants commonly present within plasma LDL particles. More recent studies, however, indicate that raising the ratio of $C_{18:1}$ to $C_{18:2}$ (linoleic acid) may also reduce the susceptibility of LDL to oxidation. The LDL is particularly vulnerable to peroxidation once PUFA form part of the lipoprotein fraction of cell membranes, as these fatty acids have reactive double bonds in their structures. The MUFA are much less easily oxidized as they have only one double bond. This property may confer a protective effect against CHD by generating LDL particles more resistant to oxidation. Further protection may be afforded from MUFA as they do not lower HDL. It is postulated that oxidized HDL, in contrast to oxidized LDL, is not avidly taken up by macrophages but instead inhibits the modification of LDL, thereby substantially decreasing oxidized LDL cellular uptake.

Oxidation of LDL cholesterol is, therefore, clearly linked to damage to the endothelium and hence to the process of atherogenesis. It has, however, more far-reaching effects, as it has also been linked to activation and aggregation of platelets. This process is involved in the production of occlusive thrombosis, which contributes significantly to the fibrous atherosclerotic plaque.

Thrombosis and Fibrinolysis

The importance of thrombosis in causing heart disease is receiving increasing attention. Thrombosis, in contrast to atherosclerosis, is an acute event resulting in the formation of a thrombus or blood clot, which is an aggregate of fibrin, platelets, and red cells. Blood clotting or coagulation is an important process as it is responsible for repairing tissues after injury. Under normal physiological conditions, a blood clot forms at the site of injury. Platelets are attracted to the damaged tissue and adhere to the surface. They are then activated to release substances that attract more platelets, allowing platelet aggregation and triggering coagulation mechanisms.

The coagulation cascade

The process of blood coagulation involves two pathways: the extrinsic and intrinsic pathways (**Figure 3**). The cascade is dependent on a series of separate clotting factors, each of which acts as a catalyst for the next step in the system. The process results in the formation of insoluble fibrin from the soluble protein fibrinogen. This then interacts with a number of blood components, including red blood cells, to form the thrombus. Any damage to the endothelium, therefore, causes platelet aggregation and adherence to the lining of the blood-vessel walls, thereby triggering the coagulation cascade. An imbalance of this process, by increasing the rate of thrombus formation, could increase the risk of CHD, and data have shown that levels of factor VII and fibrinogen are particularly important in balancing the coagulation cascade.

Factor VII and fibrinogen

There is accumulating evidence the factor VII is involved in arterial thrombosis and atherogenesis. The physiology of the factor VII system is intricate, not least since it can potentially exist in several forms. Activation of factor VIIc is generally achieved by tissue factor and initiates blood coagulation by subsequent activation of factors IX and X. It has been further suggested that tissue factor associated with the lipoproteins LDL and VLDL, but not HDL, may possibly generate factor VIIc activity, and a direct relationship is believed to exist between the level of factor VII complex in plasma and the dietary influence on plasma triacylglycerol concentration.

Several mechanisms have been suggested whereby an increase in plasma fibrinogen concentration may be linked to CHD. These include the involvement of fibrinogen and fibrin in the evolution of the atheromatous plaque through fibrin deposition and in

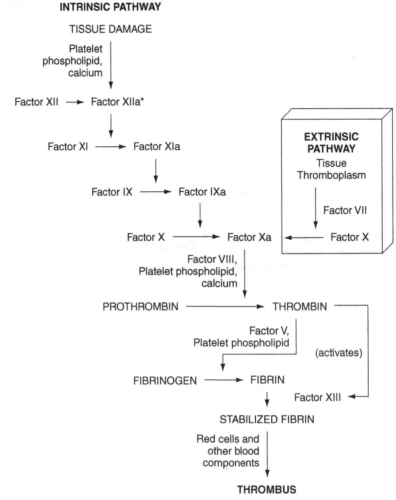

Figure 3 The coagulation cascade; a, active. Reproduced with permission from Buttriss JL and Gray J (1992) *Coronary Heart Disease II, Fact File 8*. London: National Dairy Council. Copyright National Dairy Council.

platelet aggregation through its impact on blood viscosity, which in turn is related to the risk of thrombosis. A mechanism exists to dissolve the thrombus by the breakdown or lysis of the fibrin meshwork (fibrinolysis). Plasminogen, which is generated by plasmin, is the zymosan that ultimately effects fibrinolysis. Failure of the mechanism to activate will cause obstruction of blood vessels and prevent normal blood supply.

Fibrinolysis

Investigators have shown that a decrease in the release of tissue plasminogen activator (tPA) and an elevation of plasminogen activator inhibitor 1 (PAI-1) will reduce fibrinolytic function. It has emerged that triacylglycerol-rich lipoproteins stimulate PAI-1 secretion from endothelial cells, and furthermore it has been shown that OxLDL induces secretion, whereas native LDL has no detectable

effect. Lipoprotein (a) (Lp(a)) has also been linked with a decrease in fibrinolysis. Lp(a) is an LDL-like particle consisting of the protein apo(a). It is believed that apo(a) competes with plasminogen and plasmin for binding to fibrin, thus interfering with fibrinolysis; LDL and Lp(a) may represent, therefore, an important link between thrombotic and lipid mechanisms in atherogenesis.

MUFA and thrombosis

Results from animal studies have shown an elevation in platelet activation and hence greater risk of thrombosis as a result of feeding saturated fat. Platelet aggregation thresholds, however, decrease when total fat intake is decreased or when dairy and animal fats are partially replaced with vegetable oils rich in PUFA. These studies failed, however, to keep the intakes of SFA and total fat constant. More recent work has shown that, in fact, diets high in

PUFA significantly increase platelet aggregation in animals, compared with MUFA-rich diets. The changes in fatty-acid composition may affect blood clotting because the increase in PUFA allows for oxidation of LDL. As previously mentioned, OxLDL is cyto-toxic, and this can cause endothelial damage leading to the activation of platelets, generation of factor VII, and hence thrombus formation. Increased dietary intakes of MUFA may also increase the rate of fibrinolysis by lowering levels of LDL cholesterol and reducing the susceptibility of LDL to oxidation, thereby affecting both PAI-1 secretion and apo(a) activity.

It must be noted that both atherosclerosis and thrombosis are triggered by inflammation, and evidence suggests that several hemostatic factors other than the glycoprotein fibrinogen not only have an important role in thrombotic events but are also recognized as potentially important CHD risk factors.

Inflammation and Oxidative Damage

Many diseases that have an inflammatory basis such as cancer, sepsis, and chronic inflammatory diseases such as rheumatoid arthritis (RA) have symptoms mediated by pro-inflammatory mediators named cytokines. These mediators, which include interleukins (IL) 1–8, tumor necrosis factors (TNF), and interferons, are essential for protection from invading bodies. They act by producing a situation in which immune cells are attracted to the inflammatory site and are activated. An inflammatory stimulus, such as tissue damage incurred by trauma or invasion of tissue by bacteria or viruses, induces production of IL-1, IL-6, and TNF from a range of immune cells, including phagocytic leucocytes and T and B lymphocytes. Once induced, IL-6, IL-1, and TNF further induce each other's production, leading to a cascade of cytokines, which are capable of producing metabolic and immune effects. Inflammatory stimuli also bring about the activation of neutrophils to release free radicals, which enhance the production of TNF and other cytokines. Overproduction of these pro-inflammatory mediators may, therefore, allow excessive release of reactive oxygen species (ROS) into extracellular fluid to damage its macromolecular components.

Oxidative damage

Free radicals are any species capable of an independent existence that contain one or more unpaired electrons. ROS is a collective term, referring not only to oxygen-centered radicals such as superoxide

$(O_2^{\cdot})$ and the hydroxy radical $(^{\cdot}OH)$, but also to hydrogen peroxide (H_2O_2), ozone (O_3), and singlet oxygen $(^1O_2)$. These are produced as the by-products of normal metabolism and, as such, are highly reactive in chemical terms. In order to become more stable chemically, the free radical reacts with other molecules by either donating or taking an electron, in either case leaving behind another unstable molecule, and hence this becomes a chain reaction. So, although oxygen is essential for life, in certain circumstances it may also be toxic. Damage caused by ROS to cellular target sites includes oxidative damage to proteins, membranes (lipid and proteins), and DNA. PUFA are particularly vulnerable to ROS attack because they have unstable double bonds in their structure. This process is termed 'lipid peroxidation'; because PUFA are an essential part of the phospholipid fraction of cell membranes, uncontrolled lipid peroxidation can lead to considerable cellular damage. The balance of MUFA in cell membranes is also critical to cell function, but, as already noted, MUFA are far less vulnerable to lipid peroxidation.

MUFA and inflammation

Oxidative damage by ROS to DNA and lipids contributes significantly to the etiology of cancer and atherosclerosis. A decrease in production of pro-inflammatory mediators would, therefore, be beneficial by decreasing the release of ROS. Diminishing the production of cytokines is also believed to improve the symptoms of RA. It has been suggested that olive oil may have anti-inflammatory properties as it can reduce the production of these proinflammatory mediators. Although few studies have been carried out on the benefits of olive oil on symptoms of inflammation, it is possible that olive oil produces a similar effect to fish oil. Fish oils and butter have both been shown to reverse the proinflammatory effects of one cytokine, TNF. Further research, where $C_{18:1}$ was added to a diet containing coconut oil, resulted in responses to TNF that were similar to those seen in animals fed butter. It was assumed that, as the anti-inflammatory effects of butter appeared to be due to its oleic acid content, olive oil should be more anti-inflammatory. This was put to the test, and, while both butter and olive oil reduced the extent of a number of symptoms of inflammation, olive oil showed a greater potency than butter. From this, it can be concluded that dietary factors such as olive oil may play a significant protective role in the development severity of RA.

Carcinogenesis

Cancer is second only to CHD as a cause of death in Western countries. Cancer in humans is a multistep disease process in which a single cell can develop from an otherwise normal tissue into a malignancy that can eventually destroy the organism. Carcinogenesis is believed to proceed through three distinct stages. Initiation is brought about when carcinogens mutate a single cell. This mutation provides a growth advantage, and cells rapidly proliferate during the second stage, promotion. Tumor promotion produces relatively benign growths, which can be converted into cancer in the third stage, malignant conversion. While the causes of cancer are not known with certainty, both initiation and conversion require some form of genetic alteration, and ROS and other free radicals have long been known to be mutagenic (**Figure 4**).

Oxidation and cancer

Although PUFA are the most reactive of substrates for ROS attack leading to lipid peroxidation, interest is centering on the detection of oxidized nucleic acids as an indicator of pro-oxidant conditions. It has been indicated that significant oxidative damage occurs *in vitro* and contributes to the etiology of cancer. It has become apparent that many genotoxic agents act through the common mechanism of oxidative damage to DNA. Oxidative processes may be responsible for initiating carcinogenic

changes via DNA oxidative damage and may also act as tumor promoters, modulating the expression of genes that regulate cell differentiation and growth and act synergistically with the initiators. Animal studies have indicated diets containing high levels of $C_{18:2}$ as strong promoters of tumors, and this may be as a result of increased oxidative stress. The fact that MUFA are much less readily oxidized may therefore confer a protective effect against carcinogenesis.

Immune function and cancer

The diet is believed to play an important role in the onset of carcinogenesis, and there are a number of carcinogens present in food, including mycotoxins, polycyclic hydrocarbons, and pesticides. Associations have been made between dietary fat intake and morbidity and mortality from breast and colon cancer. Another possible mechanism for the proposed protective effects against cancer of olive oil compared with sunflower oil involves diet-induced alterations in host immune responses. Both the type and concentration of dietary fats have been reported to influence immune status in several animal models. The PUFA $C_{18:2}$ is necessary for T-cell-mediated immunity, but high intakes will suppress immune function and may therefore increase the risk of cancer. Furthermore, comparisons between the effects of diets rich in $C_{18:2}$ and those rich in $C_{18:1}$ on varying indicators of immune function in mice have shown that, while dietary $C_{18:2}$ predisposed

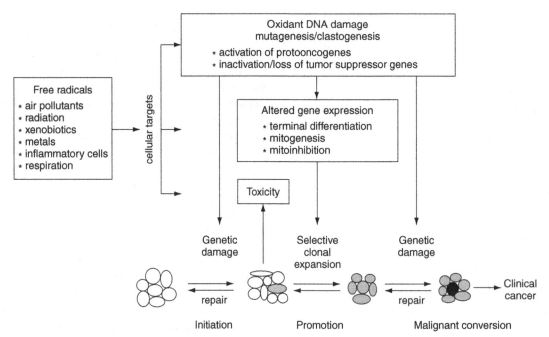

Figure 4 The role of oxidants in multistage carcinogenesis. Reproduced with permission from Guyton KZ and Kensler TW (1993) Oxidative mechanisms in carcinogenesis. *British Medical Bulletin* **49**: 523–544.

animals to suppression of certain T-cell-mediated reactions, diets rich in $C_{18:1}$ did not. MUFA may therefore have a significant effect in humans against cancer, by lowering the risk of suppression of T-cell activity.

Other Physiological Effects

Because many, sometimes competing, mechanisms appear to mediate the relation between intake of MUFA and CHD incidence, no single surrogate biochemical or physiological response can predict with confidence the effect of a particular dietary pattern. For this reason examinations of the relation between specific dietary factors and CHD incidence itself are particularly valuable because such studies integrate the effects of all known and unknown mechanisms. The extremely low rate of CHD in countries with high consumption of olive oil, for instance, suggests the benefits of substituting this fat for other fats. This kind of analysis has been expanded further by noting that MUFA intake is inversely associated with total mortality as well as with CHD. Some effects may well be because of the amount of antioxidant vitamins olive oil contains. Vegetable oils are the most important source of α-tocopherol in most diets, and olive oil contains about 12 mg per 100 g. Evidence indicates that α-tocopherol functions as a free-radical scavenger to protect cellular membranes from oxidative destruction. Oxidative stress has been linked to an increased risk of many chronic diseases, including atherosclerosis, cancer, and inflammatory disorders. Other injuries such as cataract and reperfusion injury are also associated with an increase in oxidative stress and a decrease in antioxidant activity.

A large body of evidence suggests a beneficial effect of MUFA in the diet. Although much remains to be learned about the mechanisms by which $C_{18:1}$ acts, it is believed to lower risks of CHD, several common cancers, cataracts, and other inflammatory disorders. It is suggested, therefore, that consuming MUFA, for instance in the form of olive oil as used widely in the Mediterranean diet, is likely to enhance long-term health.

See also: **Antioxidants**: Diet and Antioxidant Defense. **Coronary Heart Disease**: Lipid Theory; Prevention. **Fatty Acids**: Metabolism; Monounsaturated; Omega-3 Polyunsaturated; Omega-6 Polyunsaturated; Saturated; *Trans* Fatty Acids.

Further Reading

Ashwell M (1993) *Diet and Heart Disease – A Round Table of Factors*. London: British Nutrition Foundation.

Barter P (1994) Cholesterol and cardiovascular disease: basic science. *Australia and New Zealand Journal of Medicine* 24: 83–88.

Besler HT and Grimble RF (1993) Modulation of the response of rats to endotoxin by butter and olive and corn oil. *Proceedings of the Nutrition Society* 52: 68A.

Cerutti PA (1985) Prooxidant states and tumor promotion. *Science* 227: 375–381.

Daae LW, Kierulf P, Landass S, and Urdal P (1993) Cardiovascular risk factors: interactive effects of lipid, coagulation, and fibrinolysis. *Scandinavian Journal of Clinical Laboratory Investigation* 532: 19–27.

Dunnigan MG (1993) The problem with cholesterol. No light at the end of the tunnel. *British Medical Journal* 306: 1355–1356.

Ernst E (1993) The role of fibrinogen as a cardiovascular risk factor. *Atherosclerosis* 100: 1–12.

Guyton KZ and Kensler TW (1993) Oxidative mechanisms in carcinogenesis. *British Medical Bulletin* 49: 523–544.

Halliwell B (1989) Tell me about free radicals, doctor: a review. *Journal of the Royal Society of Medicine* 82: 747–752.

Hannigan BM (1994) Diet and immune function. *British Journal of Biomedical Science* 51: 252–259.

Hoff HF and O'Neil J (1991) Lesion-derived low density lipoprotein and oxidized low density lipoprotein share a lability for aggregation, leading to enhanced macrophage degradation. *Arteriosclerosis and Thrombosis* 11: 1209–1222.

Linos A, Kaklamanis E, and Kontomerkos A (1991) The effect of olive oil and fish consumption on rheumatoid arthritis – a case control study. *Scandinavian Journal of Rheumatology* 20: 419–426.

Mensink RP and Katan MB (1989) An epidemiological and an experimental study on the effect of olive oil on total serum and HDL cholesterol in healthy volunteers. *European Journal of Clinical Nutrition* 43(supplement 2): 43–48.

Morel DW, Dicorleto PE, and Chisolm GM (1984) Endothelial and smooth muscle cells alter low density lipoprotein *in vitro* by free radical oxidation. *Arteriosclerosis* 4: 357–364.

National Dairy Council (1992) *Coronary Heart Disease*. Fact File No. 8. London: NDC.

Visioli F and Galli C (1995) Natural antioxidants and prevention of coronary heart disease: the potential role of olive oil and its minor constituents. *Nutrition Metabolism and Cardiovascular Disease* 5: 306–314.

Omega-3 Polyunsaturated

A P Simopoulos, The Center for Genetics, Nutrition and Health, Washington, DC, USA

Introduction

Over the past 20 years many studies and clinical investigations have been carried out on the metabolism of polyunsaturated fatty acids (PUFAs) in general and on n-3 fatty acids in particular. Today we know that n-3 fatty acids are essential for normal growth and development. Research has been carried out in animal models, tissue cultures, and human beings. The original observational studies have given way to controlled clinical intervention trials. Great progress has taken place in our knowledge of the physiologic and molecular mechanisms of the n-3 fatty acids in health and disease. Specifically, their beneficial effects have been shown in the prevention and management of coronary heart disease, hypertension, type 2 diabetes, renal disease, rheumatoid arthritis, ulcerative colitis, Crohn's disease, and chronic obstructive pulmonary disease. This chapter focuses on the sources, desaturation and elongation of n-6 and n-3 fatty acids; evolutionary aspects of diet relative to n-3 fatty acids and the n-6:n-3 balance; eicosanoid metabolism and biological effects of n-6 and n-3 fatty acids; nutrigenetics – interaction between the n-6:n-3 fatty acids and the genome; effects of dietary α-linolenic acid compared with long-chain n-3 fatty acid derivatives on physiologic indexes; human studies in growth and development; coronary heart disease; inflammation – a common

base for the development of coronary heart disease, diabetes, arthritis, mental health and cancer; the need to return the n-3 fatty acids into the food supply for normal homeostasis; and future considerations.

n-6 and n-3 Fatty Acids: Sources, Desaturation and Elongation

Unsaturated fatty acids consist of monounsaturates and polyunsaturates. There are two classes of PUFA: n-6 and n-3. The distinction between n-6 and n-3 fatty acids is based on the location of the first double bond, counting from the methyl end of the fatty acid molecule. In the n-6 fatty acids, the first double bond is between the 6th and 7th carbon atoms and in the n-3 fatty acids the first double bond is between the 3rd and 4th carbon atoms. Monounsaturates are represented by oleic acid an n-9 fatty acid, which can be synthesized by all mammals including humans. Its double bond is between the 9th and 10th carbon atoms (**Figure 1**).

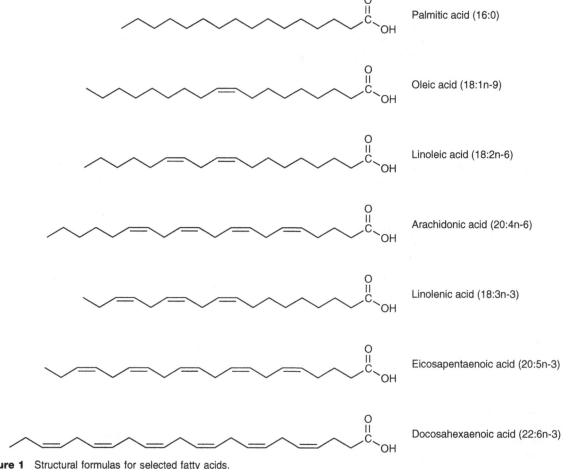

Figure 1 Structural formulas for selected fatty acids.

Table 1 Polyunsaturated oils high in n-6 and n-3 fatty acids

n-6 oils	n-3 oils
Corn oil	Fish oil
Safflower oil	Chia oil
Sunflower seed oil	Perilla oil
Cottonseed oil	Flaxseed oil
Soybean oil	Canola oil
Peanut oil	Walnut oil
Sesame oil	Soybean oil[a]
Grapeseed oil	
Borage oil	
Primrose oil	

[a]note: soybean oil is higher in n-6 fatty acids than most n-3 oils, so it belongs in both categories.

n-6 and n-3 fatty acids are also known as essential fatty acids (EFAs) because humans, like all mammals, cannot make them and must obtain them in their diet. n-6 fatty acids are represented by linoleic acid (LA; 18:2n-6) and n-3 fatty acids by α-linolenic acid (ALA; 18:3n-3). LA is plentiful in nature and is found in the seeds of most plants except for coconut, cocoa, and palm. ALA, on the other hand, is found in the chloroplasts of green leafy vegetables and in the seeds of flax, rape, chia, perilla, and in walnuts (**Tables 1, 2,** and **3**). Both EFAs are metabolized to longer chain fatty acids of 20 and 22 carbon atoms. LA is metabolized to arachidonic acid (AA; 20:4n-6) and LNA to eicosapentaenoic acid (EPA; 20:5n-3) and docosahexaenoic acid (DHA; 22:6n-3),

increasing the chain length and degree of unsaturation by adding extra double bonds to the carboxyl end of the fatty acid molecule (**Figure 2**).

Humans and other mammals, except for carnivores such as lions, can convert LA to AA and ALA to EPA and DHA. This conversion was shown by using deuterated ALA. There is competition between n-6 and n-3 fatty acids for the desaturation enzymes. However, both Δ-4 and Δ-6 desaturases prefer n-3 to n-6 fatty acids. But a high LA intake interferes with the desaturation and elongation of ALA. *Trans*-fatty acids interfere with the desaturation and elongation of both LA and ALA. Δ-6 desaturase is the limiting enzyme and there is some evidence that it decreases with age. Premature infants, hypertensive individuals, and some diabetics are limited in their ability to make EPA and DHA from ALA. These findings are important and need to be considered when making dietary recommendations. EPA and DHA are found in the oils of fish, particularly fatty fish (**Table 4**). AA is found predominantly in the phospholipids of grain-fed animals and eggs.

LA, ALA, and their long-chain derivatives are important components of animal and plant cell membranes. In mammals and birds, the n-3 fatty acids are distributed selectively among lipid classes. ALA is found in triglycerides, in cholesteryl esters, and in very small amounts in phospholipids. EPA is found in cholesteryl esters, triglycerides, and phospholipids. DHA is found

Table 2 Comparison of dietary fats (fatty acid content normalized to 100%)

Dietary fat	Saturated fat	Polyunsaturated fat			Monounsaturated fat	Cholesterol
		LA	ALA	LA:ALA		
Flaxseed oil	10	16	53	(0.3)	20	0
Canola (rapeseed) oil	6	22	10	(2.2)	62	0
Walnut oil	12	58	12	(4.8)	18	0
Safflower oil	10	77	Trace	(77)	13	0
Sunflower oil	11	69	–	(69)	20	0
Corn oil	13	61	1	(61)	25	0
Olive oil	14	8	1	(8.0)	77	0
Soybean oil	15	54	7	(7.7)	24	0
Margarine	17	32	2	(16)	49	0
Peanut oil	18	33	–	(33)	49	0
Palm oil[a]	51	9	0.3	(30)	39	0
Coconut oil[a]	92	2	0	(2.0)	7	0
Chicken fat	31	21	1	(21)	47	11
Lard	41	11	1	(11)	47	12
Beef fat	52	3	1	(3.0)	44	14
Butter fat	66	2	2	(1.0)	30	33

[a]palm oil has arachidic of 0.2 and coconut oil has arachidic of 0.1.
Data on canola oil from data on file, Procter & Gamble. All other data from Reeves JB and Weihrauch JL (1979) *Composition of Foods, Agriculture Handbook No. 8-4*. Washington, DC: US Department of Agriculture.

Table 3 Terrestrial sources of n-3 (18:3n-3) fatty acids (grams per 100 g edible portion, raw)

Nuts and seeds

Butternuts, dried	8.7
Walnuts, English/Persian	6.8
Chia seeds, dried	3.9
Walnuts, black	3.3
Beechnuts, dried	1.7
Soya bean kernels, roasted and toasted	1.5
Hickory nuts, dried	1.0

Oils

Linseed oil	53.3
Rapeseed oil (canola)	11.1
Walnut oil	10.4
Wheat germ oil	6.9
Soya bean oil	6.8
Tomato seed oil	2.3
Rice bran oil	1.6

Vegetables

Soya beans, green, raw	3.2
Soya beans, mature seeds, sprouted, cooked	2.1
Seaweed, Spirulina, dried	0.8
Radish seeds, sprouted, raw	0.7
Beans, navy, sprouted, cooked	0.3
Beans, pinto, sprouted, cooked	0.3
Kale, raw	0.2
Leeks, freeze-dried	0.2
Broccoli, raw	0.1
Cauliflower, raw	0.1
Lettuce, butterhead	0.1
Spinach, raw	0.1

Fruits

Avocados, raw, California	0.1
Raspberries, raw	0.1
Strawberries	0.1

Legumes

Soya beans, dry	1.6
Beans, common, dry	0.6
Cowpeas, dry	0.3
Lima beans, dry	0.2
Peas, garden, dry	0.2
Chickpeas, dry	0.1
Lentils, dry	0.1

Grains

Oats, germ	1.4
Wheat, germ	0.7
Barley, bran	0.3
Corn, germ	0.3
Rice, bran	0.2
Wheat, bran	0.2
Wheat, hard red winter	0.1

Data from United States Department of Agriculture. Provisional table on the content of n-3 fatty acids and other fat components in selected foods from Simopoulos AP, Kifer RR, and Martin RE (eds.) (1986) *Health Effects of Polyunsaturated Fatty Acids in Seafoods*. Orlando, FL: Academic Press.

mostly in phospholipids. In mammals, including humans, the cerebral cortex, retina, and testis and sperm are particularly rich in DHA. DHA is one of the most abundant components of the brain's structural lipids. DHA, like EPA, can be derived only from direct ingestion or by synthesis from dietary EPA or ALA.

Evolutionary Aspects of Diet Relative to n-3 Fatty Acids and the n-6:n-3 Balance

On the basis of estimates from studies in Paleolithic nutrition and modern-day hunter-gatherer populations, it appears that human beings evolved consuming a diet that was much lower in saturated fatty acids than today's diet. Furthermore, the diet contained small and roughly equal amounts of n-6 and n-3 PUFAs (ratio of 1–2:1) and much lower amounts of *trans*-fatty acids than today's diet (**Figure 3**). The current Western diet is very high in n-6 fatty acids (the ratio of n-6 to n-3 fatty acids ranges between 10:1 and 30:1) because of the recommendation to substitute vegetable oils high in n-6 fatty acids for saturated fats to lower serum cholesterol concentrations. Furthermore, intake of n-3 fatty acids is much lower today because of the decrease in fish consumption and the industrial production of animal feeds rich in grains containing n-6 fatty acids, leading to production of meat rich in n-6 and poor in n-3 fatty acids. The same is true for cultured fish and eggs. Even cultivated vegetables contain fewer n-3 fatty acids than do plants in the wild. In summary, modern agriculture, with its emphasis on production, has decreased the n-3 fatty acid content in many foods: green leafy vegetables, animal meats, eggs, and even fish, while it has increased the amount of n-6 fatty acids in foods, leading to high n-6 intake for the first time in the history of human beings in many countries around the world (**Table 5**). The traditional diet of Crete (Greece) is consistent with the Paleolithic diet relative to the n-6:n-3 ratio. The Lyon Heart Study, which was based on a modified diet of Crete, had an n-6:n-3 ratio of 4:1 resulting in a 70% decrease in risk for cardiac death. As shown in **Table 6**, the higher the ratio of n-6 to n-3 fatty acids in platelet phospholipids, the higher the death rate from cardiovascular disease. As the ratio of n-6 PUFAs to n-3 PUFAs increases, the prevalence of type 2 diabetes also increases (**Figure 4**). As will be discussed below, a balance between the n-6 and n-3 fatty acids is a more physiologic state in terms of gene expression, eicosanoid metabolism, and cytokine production.

Further support for the need to balance the n-6:n-3 PUFAs comes from studies that clearly show the ability of both normal rat cardiomyocytes and human breast cancer cells in culture to

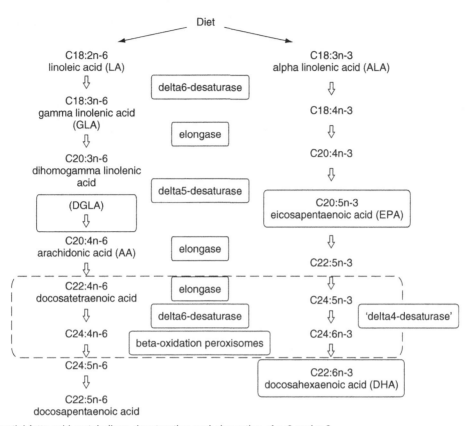

Figure 2 Essential fatty acid metabolism: desaturation and elongation of n-6 and n-3.

form all the n-3 fatty acids from n-6 fatty acids when fed the cDNA encoding n-3 fatty acid desaturase obtained from the roundworm *Caenorhabditis elegans*. The n-3 desaturase efficiently and quickly converted the n-6 fatty acids that were fed to the cardiomyocytes in culture to the corresponding n-3 fatty acids. Thus, n-6 LA was converted to n-3 ALA and AA was converted to EPA, so that at equilibrium, the ratio of n-6 to n-3 PUFAs was close to 1:1. Further studies demonstrated that the cancer cells expressing the n-3 desaturase underwent apoptotic death whereas the control cancer cells with a high n-6:n-3 ratio continued to proliferate.

Eicosanoid Metabolism and Biological Effects of n-6 and n-3 Fatty Acids

When humans ingest fish or fish oil, the ingested EPA and DHA partially replace the n-6 fatty acids (especially AA) in cell membranes, particularly those of platelets, erythrocytes, neutrophils, monocytes, and liver cells.

Because of the increased amounts of n-6 fatty acids in the Western diet, the eicosanoid metabolic products from AA, specifically prostaglandins,

thromboxanes, leukotrienes, hydroxy fatty acids, and lipoxins, are formed in larger quantities than those formed from n-3 fatty acids, specifically EPA. As a result (**Figure 5**), ingestion of EPA and DHA from fish or fish oil leads to: (1) decreased production of prostaglandin E2 metabolites; (2) decreased concentrations of thromboxane A2, a potent platelet aggregator and vasoconstrictor; (3) decreased formation of leukotriene B4, an inducer of inflammation and a powerful inducer of leukocyte chemotaxis and adherence; (4) increased concentrations of thromboxane A3, a weak platelet aggregator and vasoconstrictor; (5) increased concentrations of prostacyclin prostaglandin I3 (PGI3), leading to an overall increase in total prostacyclin by increasing PGI3 without decreasing PGI2 (both PGI2 and PGI3 are active vasodilators and inhibitors of platelet aggregation); and (6) increased concentrations of leukotriene B5, a weak inducer of inflammation and a chemotactic agent. The eicosanoids from AA are biologically active in small quantities and if they are formed in large amounts, they contribute to the formation of thrombi and atheromas; the development of allergic and inflammatory disorders, particularly in susceptible people; and cell proliferation. Thus, a

Table 4 Content of n-3 fatty acids and other fat components in selected fish (grams per 100 g edible portion, raw)

Fish	Total fat	Fatty acids (g/100 g)			18:3	20:5	22:6	Cholesterol (mg/100 g)
		Total saturated	Total monounsaturated	Total polyunsaturated				
Anchovy, European	4.8	1.3	1.2	1.6	–	0.5	0.9	–
Bass, striped	2.3	0.5	0.7	0.8	Tr	0.2	0.6	80
Bluefish	6.5	1.4	2.9	1.6	–	0.4	0.8	59
Carp	5.6	1.1	2.3	1.4	0.3	0.2	0.1	67
Catfish, brown Bullhead	2.7	0.6	1.0	0.8	0.1	0.2	0.2	75
Catfish, channel	4.3	1.0	1.6	1.0	Tr	0.1	0.2	58
Cod, Atlantic	0.7	0.1	0.1	0.3	Tr	0.1	0.2	43
Croaker, Atlantic	3.2	1.1	1.2	0.5	Tr	0.1	0.1	61
Flounder, unspecified	1.0	0.2	0.3	0.3	Tr	0.1	0.1	46
Grouper, red	0.8	0.2	0.1	0.2	–	Tr	0.2	–
Haddock	0.7	0.1	0.1	0.2	Tr	0.1	0.1	63
Halibut, Greenland	13.8	2.4	8.4	1.4	Tr	0.5	0.4	46
Halibut, Pacific	2.3	0.3	0.8	0.7	0.1	0.1	0.3	32
Herring, Pacific	13.9	3.3	6.9	2.4	0.1	1.0	0.7	77
Herring, round	4.4	1.3	0.8	1.5	0.1	0.4	0.8	28
Mackerel, king	13.0	2.5	5.9	3.2	–	1.0	1.2	53
Mullet, striped	3.7	1.2	1.1	1.1	0.1	0.3	0.2	49
Ocean perch	1.6	0.3	0.6	0.5	Tr	0.1	0.1	42
Plaice, European	1.5	0.3	0.5	0.4	Tr	0.1	0.1	70
Pollock	1.0	0.1	0.1	0.5	–	0.1	0.4	71
Pompano, Florida	9.5	3.5	2.6	1.1	–	0.2	0.4	50
Salmon, Chinook	10.4	2.5	4.5	2.1	0.1	0.8	0.6	–
Salmon, pink	3.4	0.6	0.9	1.4	Tr	0.4	0.6	–
Snapper, red	1.2	0.2	0.2	0.4	Tr	Tr	0.2	–
Sole, European	1.2	0.3	0.4	0.2	Tr	Tr	0.1	50
Swordfish	2.1	0.6	0.8	0.2	–	0.1	0.1	39
Trout, rainbow	3.4	0.6	1.0	1.2	0.1	0.1	0.4	57
Tuna, albacore	4.9	1.2	1.2	1.8	0.2	0.3	1.0	54
Tuna, unspecified	2.5	0.9	0.6	0.5	–	0.1	0.4	–

Dashes denote lack of reliable data for nutrient known to be present; Tr, trace (<0.05 g/100 g food). Adapted from the United States Department of Agriculture Provisional Table on the Content of Omega-3 Fatty Acids and Other Fat Components in Seafoods as presented by Simopoulos AP, Kifer RR, and Martin RE (eds.) (1986) *Health Effects of Polyunsaturated Fatty Acids in Seafoods*. Orlando, FL: Academic Press.

diet rich in n-6 fatty acids shifts the physiologic state to one that is prothrombotic and proaggregatory, with increases in blood viscosity, vasospasm, and vasoconstriction and decreases in bleeding time. Bleeding time is shorter in groups of patients with hypercholesterolemia, hyperlipoproteinemia, myocardial infarction, other forms of atherosclerotic disease, type 2 diabetes, obesity, and hypertriglyceridemia. Atherosclerosis is a major complication in type 2 diabetes patients. Bleeding time is longer in women than in men and in younger than in older persons. There are ethnic differences in bleeding time that appear to be related to diet. The hypolipidemic, antithrombotic, anti-inflammatory, and anti-arrhythmic effects of n-3 fatty acids have been studied extensively in animal models, tissue cultures, and cells (**Table 7**).

Nutrigenetics: Interaction between the n-6:n-3 Fatty Acids and the Genome

As expected, earlier studies focused on mechanisms that involve eicosanoid metabolites. More recently, however, the effects of fatty acids on gene expression have been investigated and this focus of interest has led to studies at the molecular level (**Tables 8, 9**). Previous studies have shown that fatty acids, whether released from membrane phospholipids by cellular phospholipases or made available to the cell from the diet or other aspects of the extracellular environment, are important cell signaling molecules. They can act as second messengers or substitute for the classic second messengers of the inositide phospholipid and cyclic AMP signal transduction pathways. They can also act as modulator molecules mediating responses of the cell to

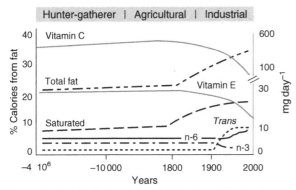

Figure 3 Hypothetical scheme of fat, fatty acid (n-6, n-3, *trans* and total) intake (as per cent of calories from fat) and intake of vitamins E and C (mg day^{-1}). Data were extrapolated from cross-sectional analyses of contemporary hunter-gatherer populations and from longitudinal observations and their putative changes during the preceding 100 years. *Trans*-fatty acids, the result of the hydrogenation process, have increased dramatically in the food supply during this century. (Reproduced with permission from Simopoulos AP (1999) Genetic variation and evolutionary aspects of diet. In: Papas A (ed.) *Antioxidants in Nutrition and Health*, pp. 65–88. Boca Raton: CRC Press.)

Table 5 n-6:n-3 ratios in various populations

Population	n-6:n-3
Paleolithic	0.79
Greece prior to 1960	1.00–2.00
Current Japan	4.00
Current India, rural	5–6.1
Current UK and northern Europe	15.00
Current US	16.74
Current India, urban	38–50

Reproduced with permission from Simopoulos AP (2003) Importance of the ratio of omega-6/omega-3 essential fatty acids: Evolutionary aspects. *World Review of Nutrition and Diet* **92**: 1–22.

Table 6 Ethnic differences in fatty acid concentrations in thrombocyte phospholipids and percentage of all deaths from cardiovascular disease

	Europe and US	Japan	Greenland Eskimos
Arachidonic acid (20:4n-6)	26%	21%	8.3%
Eicosapentaenoic acid (20:5n-3)	0.5%	1.6%	8.0%
Ratio of n-6:n-3	50%	12%	1%
Mortality from cardiovascular disease	45%	12%	7%

Modified from Weber PC (1989) Are we what we eat? Fatty acids in nutrition and in cell membranes: cell functions and disorders induced by dietary conditions. In: *Fish, Fats and your Health*, Report no. 4, pp. 9–18. Norway: Svanoybukt Foundation.

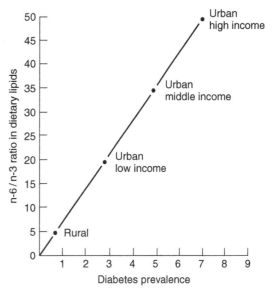

Figure 4 Relation between the ratio of n-6 to n-3 fatty acids in dietary lipids in the Indian diet and the prevalence of type 2 diabetes. (Reproduced with permission from Raheja BS, Sadikot SM, Phatak RB, and Rao MB (1993) Significance of the n-6/n-3 ratio for insulin action in diabetes. *Annals of the New York Academy of Science* **683**: 258–271.)

extracellular signals. It has been shown that fatty acids rapidly and directly alter the transcription of specific genes.

5-Lipoxygenase and Atherosclerosis: An Example of Nutrigenetics/Nutrigenomics

Leukotrienes are eicosanoids derived through the action of 5-lipoxygenase (5-LO). It has been recently shown that genetic variants of the 5-LO promoter, already known to be associated with variable sensitivity to anti-asthmatic medications, also influence atherosclerosis. Variant genotypes of the 5-LO gene were found in 6% of a cohort of 470 healthy middle-aged men and women. Carotid intima-media thickness (IMT), taken as a marker of the atherosclerotic burden, was significantly increased, by 80% in the variant group compared to carriers of the common allele, suggesting increased 5-LO promoter activity associated with the mutant (variant) allele. Furthermore, dietary AA intake significantly enhanced the proatherogenic effect of 5-LO gene variants, while intake of EPA and DHA decreased (blunted) the effect of 5-LO and was associated with less IMT. EPA and DHA decrease the formation of leukotrienes of the 4-series by competing with AA (**Figure 5**) as substrates for 5-LO and generate weaker leukotrienes of the 5-series. The results of this study suggest that person with genetic variants are at higher risk for atherosclerosis at higher AA

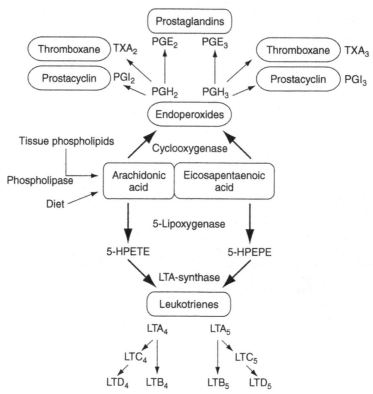

Figure 5 Oxidative metabolism of arachidonic acid and eicosapentaenoic acid by the cyclooxygenase and 5-lipoxygenase pathways. 5-HPETE denotes 5-hydroperoxyeicosatetranoic acid and 5-HPEPE denotes 5-hydroxyeicosapentaenoic acid.

intake. It also suggests that the effects of EPA and DHA may be stronger in individuals with genetic variants associated with increased 5-LO activity. Therefore, clinical trials in the future should be controlled for genetic variation.

Effects of Dietary ALA Compared with Long-Chain n-3 Fatty Acid Derivatives on Physiologic Indexes

Several clinical and epidemiologic studies have been conducted to determine the effects of long-chain n-3 PUFAs on various physiologic indexes. Whereas the earlier studies were conducted with large doses of fish or fish oil concentrates, more recent studies have used lower doses. ALA, the precursor of n-3 fatty acids, can be converted to long-chain n-3 PUFAs and can therefore be substituted for fish oils. The minimum intake of long-chain n-3 PUFAs needed for beneficial effects depends on the intake of other fatty acids. Dietary amounts of LA as well as the ratio of LA to ALA appear to be important for the metabolism of ALA to long-chain n-3 PUFAs. While keeping the amount of dietary LA constant (3.7 g) ALA appears to have biological effects similar to those of 0.3 g long-chain n-3

PUFAs with conversion of 11 g ALA to 1 g long-chain n-3 PUFAs. Thus, a ratio of 4 (15 g LA:3.7 g ALA) is appropriate for conversion. In human studies, the conversion of deuterated ALA to longer chain metabolites was reduced by $\cong$50% when dietary intake of LA was increased from 4.7% to 9.3% of energy as a result of the known competition between n-6 and n-3 fatty acids for desaturation. After ALA supplementation there is an increase in long-chain n-3 PUFAs in plasma and platelet phospholipids and a decrease in platelet aggregation. ALA supplementation does not alter triacylglycerol concentrations. Only long-chain n-3 PUFA have triacylglycerol-lowering effects. Supplementation with ALA to lower the n-6:n-3 ratio from 13:1 to 1:1 led to a 50% reduction in C-reactive protein (CRP), a risk factor for coronary heart disease.

In Australian studies, ventricular fibrillation in rats was reduced with canola oil as much or even more efficiently than with fish oil, an effect attributable to ALA. Further studies should be able to show whether this result is a direct effect of ALA per se or whether it occurs as a result of its desaturation and elongation to EPA and possibly DHA.

Table 7 Effects of n-3 fatty acids on factors involved in the pathophysiology of atherosclerosis and inflammation

Factor	Function	Effect of n-3 fatty acid
Arachidonic acid	Eicosanoid precursor; aggregates platelets; stimulates white blood cells	↓
Thromboxane A_2	Platelet aggregation; vasoconstriction; increase of intracellular Ca^{++}	↓
Prostacyclin ($PGI_{2/3}$)	Prevent platelet aggregation; vasodilation; increase cAMP	↑
Leukotriene (LTB_4)	Neutrophil chemoattractant; increase of intracellular Ca^{++}	↓
Fibrinogen	A member of the acute phase response; and a blood clotting factor	↓
Tissue plasminogen activator	Increase endogenous fibrinolysis	↑
Platelet activating factor (PAF)	Activates platelets and white blood cells	↓
Platelet-derived growth factor (PDGF)	Chemoattractant and mitogen for smooth muscles and macrophages	↓
Oxygen free radicals	Cellular damage; enhance LDL uptake via scavenger pathway; stimulate arachidonic acid metabolism	↓
Lipid hydroperoxides	Stimulate eicosanoid formation	↓
Interleukin 1 and tumor necrosis factor	Stimulate neutrophil O_2 free radical formation; stimulate lymphocyte proliferation; stimulate PAF; express intercellular adhesion molecule-1 on endothelial cells; inhibit plasminogen activator, thus, procoagulants	↓
Interleukin-6	Stimulates the synthesis of all phase proteins involved in the inflammatory response: C-reative protein; serum amyloid A; fibrinogen; α_1-chymotrypsin; and haptoglobin	↓
C-reactive protein (CRP)	An acute phase reactant and an independent risk factor for cardiovascular disease	↓
Endothelial-derived relaxation factor	Reduces arterial vasoconstrictor response	↑
Insulin sensitivity		↑
VLDL		↓
HDL	Decreases the risk for coronary heart disease	↑
Lp(a)	Lipoprotein(a) is a genetically determined protein that has atherogenic and thrombogenic properties	↓
Triglycerides and chylomicrons	Contribute to postprandial lipemia	↓

Source: Updated and modified from Weber PC, Leaf A. Cardiovascular effects of omega-3 fatty acids. Atherosclerosis risk factor modification by omega-3 fatty acids. World Rev Nutr Diet 1991, **66**: 218–32. With permission.

Table 8 Effects of polyunsaturated fatty acids on several genes encoding enzyme proteins involved in lipogenesis, glycolysis, and glucose transport

Function and gene	Linoleic acid	α-Linolenic acid	Arachidonic acid	Eicosapentaenoic acid	Docosahexaenoic acid
Hepatic cells					
Lipogenesis					
FAS	↓	↓	↓	↓	↓
S14	↓	↓	↓	↓	↓
SCD1	↓	↓	↓	↓	↓
SCD2	↓	↓	↓	↓	↓
ACC	↓	↓	↓	↓	↓
ME	↓	↓	↓	↓	↓
Glycolysis					
G6PD	↓				
GK	↓	↓	↓	↓	↓
PK	—	↓	↓	↓	↓
Mature adiposites					
Glucose transport					
GLUT4	—	—	↓	↓	—
GLUT1	—	—	↑	↑	—

↓ = Suppress or decrease; ↑ = induce or increase
Source: Modified from Simopoulos AP. The role of fatty acids in gene expression: Health implications. Ann Nutr Metab 1996, **40**: 303–311. With permission.

Table 9 Effects of polyunsaturated fatty acids on several genes encoding enzyme proteins involved in cell growth, early gene expression, adhesion molecules, inflammation, β-oxidation, and growth factors[a]

Function and gene	Linoleic acid	α-Linolenic acid	Arachidonic acid	Eicosapentaenoic acid	Docosahexaenoic acid
Cell growth and early gene expression					
c-fos	—	—	↑	↓	↓
Egr-1	—	—	↑	↓	↓
Adhesion molecules					
VCAM-1 mRNA[b]	—	—	↓	[c]	↓
Inflammation					
IL-1β	—	—	↑	↓	↓
β-oxidation					
Acyl-CoA oxidase[d]	↑	↑	↑	↑	↑↑
Growth factors					
PDGF	—	—	↑	↓	↓

[a]VCAM, vascular cell adhesion molecule; IL, interleukin: PDGF, platelet-derived growth factor. ↓ suppresses or decreases, ↑ induces or increases.
[b]Monounsaturated fatty acids (MONOs) also suppress VCAM1 mRNA, but to a lesser degree than does DHA. AA also suppresses to a lesser extent than DHA.
[c]Eicosapentachoic acid has no effect by itself but enhances the effect of docosahexachoic acid (DHA)
[d]MONOs also induce acyl-CoA oxidase mRNA
Source: Modified from Simopoulos AP. The role of fatty acids in gene expression: Health implications. Ann Nutr Metab 1996, **40**: 303–311. With permission.

The diets of Western countries have contained increasingly larger amounts of LA, which has been promoted for its cholesterol-lowering effect. It is now recognized that dietary LA favors oxidative modification of low-density lipoprotein (LDL) cholesterol, increases platelet response to aggregation, and suppresses the immune system. In contrast, ALA intake is associated with inhibitory effects on the clotting activity of platelets, on their response to thrombin, and on the regulation of AA metabolism. In clinical studies, ALA contributed to lowering of blood pressure. In a prospective study, ALA was inversely related to the risk of coronary heart disease in men.

ALA is not equivalent in its biological effects to the long-chain n-3 fatty acids found in fish oils. EPA and DHA are more rapidly incorporated into plasma and membrane lipids and produce more rapid effects than does ALA. Relatively large reserves of LA in body fat, as are found in vegans or in the diet of omnivores in Western societies, would tend to slow down the formation of long-chain n-3 fatty acids from ALA. Therefore, the role of ALA in human nutrition becomes important in terms of long-term dietary intake. One advantage of the consumption of ALA over n-3 fatty acids from fish is that the problem of insufficient vitamin E intake does not exist with a high intake of ALA from plant sources.

Human Studies in Growth and Development

Pregnancy and Fetal Growth

Since World War II, the role of maternal nutrition in fetal growth and development has been extensively studied in the context of protein-calorie malnutrition. The role of n-3 fatty acids has only recently come into focus, despite the evidence of its importance having been demonstrated in a series of studies between 1928 and 1930 involving rats and primates. Lipid nutrition during pregnancy and lactation is of special relevance to human development, because brain development in the human takes place during fetal life and in the first 2 years after birth. DHA is found in larger amounts in the gray matter of the brain and in the retinal membranes, where it accounts for 30% or more of the fatty acids in the ethanolamine and serine phospholipid. DHA accumulates in the neurons of the brain between weeks 26 and 40 of gestation in humans.

During the third trimester of human development, rapid synthesis of brain tissue occurs in association with increasing neuromotor activity. The increase in cell size, number, and type requires de novo synthesis of structural lipids, leading to accumulation of DHA in the brain of the human infant during the last trimester. The levels of ALA and LA are low in the brain, whereas marked accretion of long-chain desaturation products, specifically DHA and AA, occurs. More recent data indicate that the main developmental changes in the brain seem to be an increase in DHA at the end of gestation and a decrease in oleic acid (18:1n-9) and AA in phosphatidylethanolamine (PE). Similar changes occur in the liver. Therefore, a premature infant (prior to 37 weeks' gestation) has much lower amounts of DHA in the brain and liver and is at risk of becoming deficient in DHA unless it is supplied in the diet. In the full-term newborn, about half of the DHA accumulates in the brain before birth and the other half after birth.

There is epidemiologic evidence that the birth weights of newborns in the Faroe Islands (where fish intake is high) are higher than those in Denmark, as is the length of gestation: 40.3 ± 1.7 weeks for the Faroese versus 39.7 ± 1.8 weeks for the Danish pregnant women. The average birth weight of primiparas is 194 g higher for the Faroe Islands. The higher dietary n-3 fatty acid intake quite possibly influences endogenous prostaglandin metabolism. It is hypothesized that the dietary n-3 fatty acids inhibit the production of the dienoic prostaglandins, especially PGF_{2a} and PGE_2, because they are involved in the mediation of uterine contractions and the ripening of the cervix that lead to labor and delivery. These important observations need to be further investigated, as the prevention of prematurity is one of the most critical issues to be overcome in perinatal medicine.

Human Milk and Infant Feeding

A number of studies from around the world indicate that human milk contains both LNA and LA and their long-chain n-6 and n-3 fatty acids, whereas cow's milk does not. The long-chain fatty acid composition of red blood cell membrane phospholipids may reflect the composition of phospholipids in the brain. Therefore, determination of red blood cell membrane phospholipids has been carried out by many investigators to determine the long-chain PUFA content in breast-fed and bottle-fed infants. As expected, the fatty acids 22:5n-3 and 22:6n-3 were higher in the erythrocytes from breast-fed infants than those from bottle-fed babies and the 20:3n-9 was lower in the erythrocytes of the breast-fed infants.

Following birth, the amount of red blood cell DHA in premature infants decreases; therefore the amount of DHA available to the premature infant assumes critical importance. Preterm infants have a limited ability to convert LNA to DHA (**Figure 2**); therefore, a number of studies have been carried out on the DHA status of the premature infant. Premature babies have decreased amounts of DHA, but human milk contains enough DHA to support normal growth of the premature baby. The amount of n-3 fatty acids in human milk varies with the mother's diet; in particular, DHA is lower in vegetarians than in omnivores. One can increase the amount of DHA in human milk by giving fish oil rich in DHA to the mother.

The need to supplement infant formula with n-3 fatty acids and, particularly, DHA for the premature is now recognized and many countries have licensed infant formula enriched with n-3 fatty acids. DHA is essential for normal visual function and visual maturation, particularly of the premature infant. Studies are currently in progress comparing the growth and development of both the premature and full-term infant who are fed mother's milk with those who are receiving formula supplemented with n-3 fatty acids and those whose formula is not supplemented, to define precisely the effects of DHA on intelligence quotient (IQ) and overall neuromotor development. **Tables 10** and **11** show the EFA dietary recommendations for adults, pregnant women, and infants made by a scientific group at a workshop held at the National Institutes of Health in Bethesda, Maryland in 1999.

Aging

ALA deficiency has been found in patients on long-term gastric tube-feeding that included large amounts of skim milk without ALA supplementation. These patients, who were in nursing homes, developed skin lesions diagnosed as scaly dermatitis, which disappeared with ALA supplementation. A number of other patients were reported to have n-3 fatty acid deficiency, again patients on long-term gastric tube-feeding or prolonged total parenteral nutrition because of chronic illnesses. If a deficiency of total n-3 fatty acid intake is suspected, its concentration in plasma should be measured. A decrease in the concentration of 20:5n-3, 22:5n-3, and particularly 22:6n-3 in plasma or erythrocyte phospholipids indicates that the dietary intake of n-3 fatty acids has been low. The presence of clinical symptoms, along with the biochemical determinations, provides additional support for the diagnosis. To verify the diagnosis, it is essential that the clinical symptoms disappear upon supplementation of the deficient diet with n-3 fatty acids.

With the increase in the number of elderly persons in the population, and the proliferation of nursing homes, particular attention must be given to the nutritional requirements of the elderly, especially those who are fed enterally or parenterally.

Table 10 Adequate intake (AI) for adults

Fatty acid	Grams/day (2000 kcal diet)	% Energy
LA	4.44	2.0
(upper limit)[a]	6.67	3.0
ALA	2.22	1.0
DHA + EPA	0.65	0.3
DHA to be at least[b]	0.22	0.1
EPA to be at least	0.22	0.1
TRANS-FA		
(upper limit)[c]	2.00	1.0
SAT		
(upper limit)[d]	–	<8.0
MONOs[e]	–	–

[a]Although the recommendation is for AI, the Working Group felt that there is enough scientific evidence to also state an upper limit (UL) for LA of 6.67 g day^{-1} based on a 2000 kcal diet or of 3.0% of energy.
[b]For pregnant and lactating women, ensure 300 mg day^{-1} of DHA.
[c]Except for dairy products, other foods under natural conditions do not contain trans-FA. Therefore, the Working Group does not recommend trans-FA to be in the food supply as a result of hydrogenation of unsaturated fatty acids or high-temperature cooking (reused frying oils).
[d]Saturated fats should not comprise more than 8% of energy.
[e]The Working Group recommended that the majority of fatty acids are obtained from monounsaturates. The total amount of fat in the diet is determined by the culture and dietary habits of people around the world (total fat ranges from 15% to 40% of energy) but with special attention to the importance of weight control and reduction of obesity.
If sufficient scientific evidence is not available to calculate an estimated average requirement, a reference intake called an adequate intake is used instead of a recommended dietary allowance. The AI is a value based on experimentally derived intake levels or approximations of observed mean nutrient intakes by a group (or groups) of healthy people. The AI for children and adults is expected to meet or exceed the amount needed to maintain a defined nutritional state or criterion of adequacy in essentially all members of a specific healthy population.
LA, linoleic acid; ALA, α-linolenic acid; DHA, docosahexaenoic acid; EPA, eicosapentaenoic acid; TRANS-FA, trans-fatty acids; SAT, saturated fatty acids; MONOs, monounsaturated fatty acids.
Reproduced with permission from Simopoulos AP, Leaf A, and Salem N Jr (1999) Essentiality of and recommended dietary intakes for omega-6 and omega-3 fatty acids. *Annals of Nutrition and Metabolism* **43**: 127–130.

Table 11 Adequate intake (AI) for infant formula/diet

Fatty acid	Per cent of fatty acids
LA[a]	10.00
ALA	1.50
AA[b]	0.50
DHA	0.35
EPA[c]	
(upper limit)	<0.10

[a]The Working Group recognizes that in countries like Japan the breast milk content of LA is 6–10% of fatty acids and the DHA is higher, about 0.6%. The formula/diet composition described here is patterned on infant formula studies in Western countries.
[b]The Working Group endorsed the addition of the principal long-chain polyunsaturates, AA and DHA, to all infant formulas.
[c]EPA is a natural constituent of breast milk, but in amounts more than 0.1% in infant formula may antagonize AA and interfere with infant growth.
If sufficient scientific evidence is not available to calculate an estimated average requirement, a reference intake called an adequate intake is used instead of a recommended dietary allowance. The AI is a value based on experimentally derived intake levels or approximations of observed mean nutrient intakes by a group (or groups) of healthy people. The AI for children and adults is expected to meet or exceed the amount needed to maintain a defined nutritional state or criterion of adequacy in essentially all members of a specific healthy population.
LA, linoleic acid; ALA, α-linolenic acid; AA, arachidonic acid; DHA, docosahexaenoic acid; EPA, eicosapentaenoic acid; TRANS-FA, trans-fatty acids; SAT, saturated fatty acids; MONOs, monounsaturated fatty acids.
Reproduced with permission from Simopoulos AP, Leaf A, and Salem N Jr (1999) Essentiality of and recommended dietary intakes for omega-6 and omega-3 fatty acids. *Annals of Nutrition and Metabolism* **43**: 127–130.

Coronary Heart Disease

Most epidemiologic studies and clinical trials using n-3 fatty acids in the form of fish or fish oil have been carried out in patients with coronary heart disease. However, studies have also been carried out on the effects of ALA in normal subjects and in patients with myocardial infarction.

The hypolipidemic effects of n-3 fatty acids are similar to those of n-6 fatty acids, provided that they replace saturated fats in the diet. n-3 fatty acids

have the added benefit of not lowering high-density lipoprotein (HDL) and consistently lowering serum triacylglycerol concentrations, whereas the n-6 fatty acids do not and may even increase triglyceride levels.

Another important consideration is the finding that during chronic fish oil feeding postprandial triacylglycerol concentrations decrease. Furthermore, consumption of high amounts of fish oil blunted the expected rise in plasma cholesterol concentrations in humans. These findings are consistent with the low rate of coronary heart disease found in fish-eating populations. Studies in humans have shown that fish oils reduce the rate of hepatic secretion of very low-density lipoprotein (VLDL) triacylglycerol. In normolipidemic subjects, n-3 fatty acids prevent and rapidly reverse carbohydrate-induced hypertriglyceridemia. There is also evidence from kinetic studies that fish oil increases the fractional catabolic rate of VLDL (**Table 7**).

The effects of different doses of fish oil on thrombosis and bleeding time have been investigated. A dose of 1.8 g EPA day^{-1} did not result in any prolongation in bleeding time, but 4 g day^{-1} increased bleeding time and decreased platelet count with no adverse effects. In human studies, there has never been a case of clinical bleeding, even in patients undergoing angioplasty, while the patients were taking fish oil supplements. Clinical investigations indicate that n-3 fatty acids prevent sudden death. A series of intervention trials have clearly shown that the addition of n-3 fatty acids in the form of fish oil (EPA and DHA) decrease the death rate in the secondary prevention of coronary heart disease by preventing ventricular arrhythmias that lead to sudden death.

Antiarrhythmic Effects of n-3 Fatty Acids (ALA, EPA, and DHA)

Studies have shown that n-3 fatty acids, more so than n-6 PUFA, can prevent ischemia-induced fatal ventricular arrhythmias in experimental animals. n-3 fatty acids make the heart cells less excitable by modulating the conductance of the sodium and other ion channels. Clinical studies further support the role of n-3 fatty acids in the prevention of sudden death due to ventricular arrhythmias which, in the US, account for 50–60% of the mortality from acute myocardial infarction and cause 250 000 deaths a year. In the intervention trials, there was no change in lipid concentration, suggesting that the beneficial effects of n-3 fatty acids were due to their antithrombotic and antiarrhythmic effects.

The antiarrhythmic effects of n-3 fatty acids are supported by clinical intervention trials (Diet and Reinfarction Trial (DART), Lyon Heart Study, Gruppo Italiano per lo Studio della Sopravvivenza nell'Infarto miocardico (GISSI)-Prevenzione Trial, Indo-Mediterranean Diet Heart Study). Their results strongly support the role of fish or fish oil in decreasing total mortality and sudden death in patients with one episode of myocardial infarction. Therefore, the addition of 1 g/d of n-3 fatty acids is highly recommended for the primary and secondary prevention of coronary heart disease.

Inflammation: a Common Base for the Development of Coronary Heart Disease, Diabetes, Arthritis, Mental Health, Neurodegenerative Diseases and Cancer

Anti-inflammatory Aspects of n-3 Fatty Acids

Many experimental studies have provided evidence that incorporation of alternative fatty acids into tissues may modify inflammatory and immune reactions and that n-3 fatty acids in particular are potent therapeutic agents for inflammatory diseases. Supplementing the diet with n-3 fatty acids (3.2 g EPA and 2.2 g DHA) in normal subjects increased the EPA content in neutrophils and

monocytes more than sevenfold without changing the quantities of AA and DHA. The anti-inflammatory effects of fish oils are partly mediated by inhibiting the 5-lipoxygenase pathway in neutrophils and monocytes and inhibiting the leukotriene B_4 (LTB_4)-mediated function of LTB_5 (**Figure 5**). Studies show that n-3 fatty acids influence interleukin metabolism by decreasing IL-1β and IL-6. Inflammation plays an important role in both the initiation of atherosclerosis and the development of atherothrombotic events. An early step in the atherosclerotic process is the adhesion of monocytes to endothelial cells. Adhesion is mediated by leukocyte and vascular cell adhesion molecules (CAMs) such as selectins, integrins, vascular cell adhesion molecule 1 (VCAM-1), and intercellular adhesion molecule 1 (ICAM-1). The expression of E-selectin, ICAM-1, and VCAM-1, which is relatively low in normal vascular cells, is upregulated in the presence of various stimuli, including cytokines and oxidants. This increased expression promotes the adhesion of monocytes to the vessel wall. The monocytes subsequently migrate across the endothelium into the vascular intima, where they accumulate to form the initial lesions of atherosclerosis. Atherosclerosis plaques have been shown to have increased CAM expression in animal models and human studies.

Diabetes is a major risk factor for coronary heart disease. EPA and DHA increase sensitivity to insulin and decrease the risk of coronary heart disease. Rheumatoid arthritis has a strong inflammatory component characterized by an increase in interleukin (IL)-1β. n-3 fatty acids decrease IL-1β as well as the number of swollen and painful joints. Supplementation with EPA and DHA, changing the ratio of n-6:n-3 of the background diet by increasing the n-3 and decreasing the n-6 intake, is now standard treatment for patients with rheumatoid arthritis along with medication in a number of centers around the world. Similarly, changing the background diet in patients with asthma has led to decreases in the dose of nonsteroidal anti-inflammatory drugs.

These studies suggest the potential for complementarity between drug therapy and dietary choices and that increased intake of n-3 fatty acids and decreased intake of n-6 fatty acids may lead to drug sparing effects. Therefore, future studies need to address the fatty acid composition and the ratio of n-6:n-3 of the background diet, and the issue of concurrent drug use. A diet rich in n-3 fatty acids and low in n-6 fatty acids provides the appropriate background biochemical environment in which drugs function.

Psychologic stress in humans induces the production of proinflammatory cytokines such as interferon gamma (IFNγ), TNFα, IL-6, and IL-10. An imbalance of n-6 and n-3 PUFA in the peripheral blood causes an over-production of proinflammatory cytokines. There is evidence that changes in fatty acid composition are involved in the pathophysiology of major depression. Changes in serotonin (5-HT) receptor number and function caused by changes in PUFAs provide the theoretical rationale connecting fatty acids with the current receptor and neurotransmitter theories of depression. The increased 20:4n-6/20:5n-3 ratio and the imbalance in the n-6:n-3 PUFA ratio in major depression may be related to the increased production of proinflammatory cytokines and eicosanoids in that illness. Studies have shown that EPA and DHA prolong remission, that is, reduce the risk of relapse in patients with bipolar disorder. There are a number of studies evaluating the therapeutic effect of EPA and DHA in major depression.

Earlier studies in rodents showed that ALA intake improved learning, memory and cognition. In Zellweger's syndrome (a genetic neurodegenerative disease) high amounts of DHA early in life decreased somewhat the rate of progression of the disease. A number of studies have suggested that people who eat a diet rich in fish are less likely to develop Alzheimer's disease. Learning and memory depend on dendritic spine action assembly and DHA. High DHA consumption is associated with reduced risk for Alzheimer's disease, yet mechanisms and therapeutic potential remain elusive. In an Alzheimer's disease mouse model, reduction of dietaty n-3 fatty acid resulted in 80%-90% losses of the p85 alpha subunit of phosphoinositol 3-kinase and the postsynaptic action-regulating protein drebrin as in the brain of patients with Alzheimer's disease. The loss of postsynaptic proteins was associated with increased oxidation without concomitant neuron or presynaptic protein loss. Treatment of the n-3 fatty acid restricted mice with DHA protected against these effects and behavioral deficits. Since n-3 fatty acids are essential for p85-mediated central nervous system insulin signaling and selective protection of postsynaptic proteins, these findings have implications for neurodegenerative diseases, where synaptic loss is critical, especially in Alzheimer's disease. A few case control studies suggest that higher EPA and DHA intake is associated with lower risk of Alzheimer's disease and severity of the disease. Inflammation is a risk factor for Alzheimer's disease. It remains to be determined whether low n-3 fatty acids, especially low DHA status, in patients with Alzheimer's disease is a causal factor in the pathogenesis and progression of Alzheimer's disease and other neurodegenerative diseases.

Cancer is characterized by inflammation, cell proliferation, and elevated IL-6 levels. Since EPA and DHA suppress IL-6, fish oil supplementation suppresses rectal epithelial cell proliferation and PGE_2 biosynthesis. This was achieved with a dietary n-6:n-3 ratio of 2.5:1, but not with the same absolute level of fish oil intake and an n-6:n-3 ratio of 4:1. Case control studies in women with breast cancer support the hypothesis that the balance between n-6 and n-3 in breast adipose tissue plays an important role in breast cancer and in breast cancer metastasis.

Future Work, Conclusions, and Recommendations

n-3 fatty acids should be added to foods rather than be used solely as dietary supplements, which is a quasi-pharmaceutical approach. Furthermore, the development of a variety of n-3-rich foodstuffs would allow increased n-3 dietary intakes with little change of dietary habits. n-3 fatty acids maintain their preventative and therapeutic properties when packaged in foods other than fish. Efficient use of dietary n-3 fatty acids will require the simultaneous reduction in the food content of n-6 fatty acids and their substitution with monounsaturated oils. Dietary n-3 fats give rise to higher tissue levels of EPA when the 'background' diet is low in n-6 fats. Compared to n-6 fatty acids, olive oil increases the incorporation of n-3 fatty acids into tissues.

In the past, industry focused on improvements in food production and processing to increase shelf life of the products, whereas now and in the future the focus will be on nutritional quality in product development. This will necessitate the development of research for the nutritional evaluation of the various food products and educational programs for professionals and the public. The definition of food safety will have to expand in order to include nutrient structural changes and food composition. The dawn of the twenty-first century will enhance the scientific base for product development and expand collaboration among agricultural, nutritional, and medical scientists in government, academia, and industry. This should bring about a greater involvement of nutritionists and dieticians in industrial research and development to respond to an ever-increasing consumer interest in the health attributes of foods.

Today, more is known about the mechanisms and functions of n-3 fatty acids than other fatty acids. It is evident that Western diets are relatively deficient in n-3 fatty acids and that they contain much higher amounts of n-6 fatty acids than ever before in the evolution of human beings. Research has shown that DHA is essential for the development of the premature infant relative to visual acuity, visual function, and maturation. In the full-term infant, DHA may influence visual acuity and neural pathways associated with the developmental progression of language acquisition. These findings have led to the inclusion of DHA and AA in infant formulas in most countries around the world.

Most of the research on the role of n-3 fatty acids in chronic diseases has been carried out in patients with coronary heart disease. Intervention trials have clearly shown that n-3 fatty acids decrease sudden death and all cause mortality in the secondary prevention of coronary heart disease and in one study also in the primary prevention of coronary heart disease. The decrease in sudden death is most likely due to the anti-arrhythmic effects of n-3 fatty acids.

Most recent research suggests that the response to n-3 fatty acids may be genotype dependent, since certain individuals respond more than others. The time has come to take genetic variation into consideration when setting up clinical intervention trials. We need to move away from the long-term prospective studies and proceed with genotype-specific clinical intervention trials.

Inflammation and cell proliferation are at the base of many chronic diseases and conditions, especially atherosclerosis and cancer, but also diabetes, hypertension, arthritis, mental health, and various autoimmune diseases. Individuals carrying genetic variants for these conditions are much more prone to develop them because the high n-6:n-3 ratio leads to proinflammatory and prothrombotic states.

The time has come to return to high n-3 fatty acid levels in the diet and to decrease the n-6 intake. There is good scientific evidence from studies on the Paleolithic diet, the diet of Crete, other traditional diets (Okinawa), intervention studies, and finally studies at the molecular level using transgenic rodents that the physiologic n-6:n-3 ratio should be 1:1 or 2:1. Japan has already recommended a ratio of 2:1. Industry has moved in the direction of including n-3 fatty acids in various products starting with n-3 enriched eggs, which are based on the *Ampelistra* (Greek) egg as a model obtained under completely natural conditions and which has a ratio of n-6:n-3 of 1:1.

It is essential that Nutrition Science drives Food Science and the production of foods rather than Food Technology. This is of the utmost importance in the development of novel foods. The scientific evidence is strong for decreasing the n-6 and increasing the n-3 fatty acid intake to improve health throughout the life cycle. The scientific basis for the development of a public policy to develop dietary recommendations for EFA, including a balanced n-6:n-3 ratio, is robust. What is needed is a scientific consensus, education of professionals and the public,

the establishment of an agency on nutrition and food policy at the national level, and willingness of governments to institute changes. Education of the public is essential to demand changes in the food supply.

Abbreviations

ALA	α-linolenic acid
CAM	cell adhesion molecule
CRP	C-reactive protein
DHA	docosahexaenoic acid
EFA	essential fatty acid
EPA	eicosapentaenoic acid
FAS	fatty acid synthase
GK	glucokinase
GLUT	glucose transporter
ICAM	intercellular adhesion molecule
IFN	interferon
IL	interleukin
IMT	intima-media thickness
LA	linoleic acid
LO	lipoxygenase
ME	malic enzyme
PDGF	platelet-derived growth factor
PE	phosphatidylethanolamine
PG	prostaglandin
PK	pyruvate kinase
PUFA	polyunsaturated fatty acid
TNF	tumor necrosis factor
VCAM	vascular cell adhesion molecule

See also: **Coronary Heart Disease**: Lipid Theory; Prevention. **Fatty Acids**: Omega-6 Polyunsaturated.

Further Reading

Burr ML, Fehily AM, Gilbert JF, Rogers S, Holliday RM, Sweetnam PM, Elwood PC, and Deadman NM (1989) Effect of changes in fat fish and fibre intakes on death and myocardial reinfarction: diet and reinfarction trial (DART). *Lancet 2: 757–761.*

Calon F, Lim GP, Yang F, Morihara T, Teter B, Ubeda O, Rostaing P, Triller A, Salem N Jr, Ashe KH, Frautschy SA, and Cole GM (2004) Docosahexaenoic acid protects from dendritic pathology in an Alzheimer's disease mouse model. *Neuron* 43: 633–645.

de Lorgeril M, Renaud S, Mamelle N, Salen P, Martin JL, Monjaud I, Guidollet J, Touboul P, and Delaye J (1994) Mediterranean alpha-linolenic acid rich-diet in the secondary prevention of coronary heart disease. *Lancet* 343: 1454–1459.

Dwyer JH, Allayee H, Dwyer KM, Fan J, Wu H, Mar R, Lusis AJ, and Mehrabian M (2004) Arachidonate 5-lipoxygenase promoter genotype, dietary arachidonic acid, and atherosclerosis. *New England Journal of Medicine* 350: 29–37.

GISSI-Prevenzione Investigators (1999) Dietary supplementation with n-3 polyunsaturated fatty acids and vitamin E after myocardial infarction: results of the GISSI-Prevenzione trial. *Lancet* 354: 447–455.

Kang JX, Wang J, Wu L, and Kang ZB (2004) *Fat-1* mice convert n-6 to n-3 fatty acids. *Nature* 427: 504.

Maes M, Smith R, Christophe A, Cosyns P, Desynder R, and Meltzer H (1996) Fatty acid composition in major depression: decreased omega 3 fractions in cholesteryl esters and increased C20:4 omega 6/C20:5 omega 3 ratio in cholesteryl esters and phospholipids. *Journal of Affective Disorders* 38(1): 35–46.

Mechanisms of Action of LCPUFA (2003) Effects on infant growth and neurodevelopment. Proceedings of a conference held in Arlington, Virginia, May 14–15, 2002. *Journal of Pediatrics* 143(supplement 4): S1–S109.

Simopoulos AP (2001) N-3 fatty acids and human health: defining strategies for public policy. *Lipids* 36: S83–S89.

Simopoulos AP (2002) Omega-3 fatty acids in inflammation and autoimmune diseases. *Journal of American College of Nutrition* 21: 494–505.

Simopoulos AP and Cleland LG (eds.) (2003) *Omega-6/Omega-3 Essential Fatty Acid Ratio: The Scientific Evidence*. World Review of Nutrition and Dietetics, vol. 92 Basel: Karger.

Simopoulos AP, Leaf A, and Salem N Jr (1999) Essentiality of and recommended dietary intakes for omega-6 and omega-3 fatty acids. Annals of Nutrition and Metabolism 43: 127–130.

Simopoulos AP and Nestel PJ (eds.) (1997) *Genetic Variation and Dietary Response*. World Review of Nutrition and Dietetics, vol. 80, Basel: Karger.

Simopoulos AP and Robinson J (1999) In *The Omega Diet. The Lifesaving Nutritional Program Based on the Diet of the Island of Crete*. New York: Harper Collins.

Simopoulos AP and Visioli F (eds.) (2000) *Mediterranean Diets*. World Review of Nutrition and Dietetics, vol. 87. Basel: Karger.

Singh RB, Dubnov G, Niaz MA, Ghosh S, Singh R, Rastogi SS, Manor O, Pella D, and Berry EM (2002) Effect of an Indo-Mediterranean diet on progression of coronary artery disease in high risk patients (Indo-Mediterranean Diet Heart Study): a randomised single-blind trial. *Lancet* 360(9344): 1455–1461.

Yehuda S (2003) Omega-6/omega-3 ratio and brain-related functions. *World Review of Nutrition and Dietetics* 92: 37–56.

Omega-6 Polyunsaturated

J M Hodgson and T A Mori, University of Western Australia, Perth, WA, Australia
M L Wahlqvist, Monash University, Victoria, VIC, Australia

Structure, Function, and Nutritional Requirements

Omega-6 (n-6) fatty acids are a class of polyunsaturated fatty acids (PUFA). They have two or more *cis* double bonds, with the position of the first double bond six carbon atoms from the methyl end of the molecule. The general formula of n-6 fatty acids is $CH_3(CH_2)_4(CH=CHCH_2)_x(CH_2)_yCOOH$ [where $x = 2–5$]. Linoleic acid (*cis*-9, *cis*-12-octadecadienoic acid, 18:2n-6, LA) and α-linolenic acid (*cis*-9,

cis-12, *cis*-15-octadecatrienoic acid, 18:3n-3, ALA) are the precursor fatty acids of the n-6 and omega-3 (n-3) fatty acids, respectively. These two fatty acids cannot be made by mammals and are therefore termed essential fatty acids (EFA). In addition, mammals are unable to interconvert LA and ALA, or any of the n-6 and n-3 fatty acids, because mammalian tissues do not contain the necessary desaturase enzyme. Plant tissues and plant oils tend to be rich sources of LA. ALA is also present in plant sources such as green vegetables, flaxseed, canola, and some nuts. Once consumed in the diet, LA can be converted via chain elongation and desaturation to γ-linolenic acid (GLA, 18:3n-6), dihomo-γ-linolenic acid (DGLA, 20:3n-6), and arachidonic acid (AA, 20:4n-6) (**Figure 1**). The same enzymes involved in elongation and desaturation of the n-6 fatty acids are common to the n-3 series of fatty acids (**Figure 1**). Thus, ALA can be converted to eicosapentaenoic acid (EPA, 20:5n-3) and docosahexaenoic acid (DHA, 22:6n-3). EPA and DHA are found in relatively high proportions in marine oils.

The n-6 and n-3 fatty acids are metabolically and functionally distinct and often have important opposing physiological functions. Indeed, the balance of EFA is important for good health and normal development. Historically, human beings evolved on a diet in which the ratio of n-6 to n-3 fatty acids was about 1:1. In contrast, Western diets have a ratio of approximately 15:1. Evidence for this change in diet through history comes from studies on the evolutionary aspects of diet, modern-day hunter–gatherers, and traditional diets. Modern agriculture has led to a substantial increase in n-6 fatty acids at the expense of n-3 fatty acids, which has resulted in excessive consumption of n-6 fatty acids by humans.

The n-6 EFAs have two main functions. First, they act as structural components of membranes forming the basis of the phospholipid component of the lipid bilayer of plasma membranes in every cell in the body, thus providing a membrane impermeable to most water-soluble molecules. The length and degree of saturation of the fatty acids determine how the phospholipid molecules pack together and consequently affect membrane fluidity, signal transduction, and the expression of cellular receptors. The second role of n-6 fatty acids is as precursors to the eicosanoids (**Figure 1**). The eicosanoids are a family of 'hormone-like' compounds including prostaglandins (PGs), leukotrienes (LTs), and hydroxy- (HETEs), dihydroxy- (DiHETEs), and epoxy- (EETs) fatty acids. Eicosanoids, however, are distinct from most hormones in that they act locally, near their sites of synthesis, and they are catabolized extremely rapidly. Thus, they are considered to be locally acting

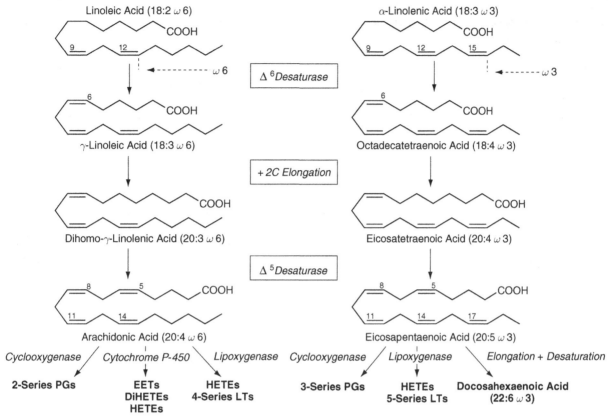

Figure 1 Essential fatty acid metabolism.

hormones. The eicosanoids modulate renal and pulmonary function, vascular tone, and inflammatory responses. The enzymes involved in AA metabolism include the cyclooxygenases and lipoxygenases, which yield the 2-series PGs and 4-series LTs, respectively. Lipoxygenase also utilizes AA for the formation of the HETEs. A third pathway for the utilization of AA involves the cytochrome P-450 enzymes found in the liver, kidney, lung, intestines, heart, small blood vessels, and white blood cells. AA metabolized via cytochrome P-450 yields EETs, DiHETEs, as well as HETEs. The cytochrome P-450 metabolites play an important role as paracrine factors and second messengers in the regulation of pulmonary, cardiac, renal, and vascular function and modulate inflammatory and growth responses.

Endothelial Function, Atherosclerosis, and Cardiovascular Disease

Differences in n-6 fatty acid intake have the potential to influence several chronic diseases and disorders. This article will focus on the effects of n-6 fatty acids on cardiovascular disease and atherosclerosis.

The vascular endothelium is the most important organ controlling vascular function and consists of a single layer of epithelial cells lining blood vessels. Its primary function is to regulate vascular tone, but it plays a critical role in modulating coagulation and fibrinolysis, inflammation, smooth muscle cell proliferation, and macrophage function. Many of these functions are regulated through the release of various mediators including eicosanoids. There is multiple and close interaction of the endothelial cells with circulating cells, smooth muscle cells, and macrophages. There is also evidence that endothelial dysfunction precedes clinically apparent atherosclerosis.

Atherosclerosis is an inflammatory disease involving multiple cellular and molecular responses that lead to an alteration in vascular function and structure, and the development and progression of cardiovascular disease. Atherosclerosis is characterized by degenerative changes, deposition of cholesterol, proliferation of smooth muscle cells, involvement of a range of circulating proinflammatory cell types, and fibrosis. Resulting atheromatous plaques cause narrowing of arteries and increase the likelihood of thrombosis and occlusion. When this process occurs in the coronary arteries, the outcome is myocardial infarction and with possible death.

Eicosanoids: Relevance to Endothelial Function, Thrombosis, Inflammation, and Atherosclerosis

In general, the eicosanoids derived from AA have potent prothrombotic and proinflammatory activity. In contrast, the eicosanoids derived from EPA have reduced biological activity and are less prothrombotic and proinflammatory. Eicosanoid production is generally tightly controlled through homeostatic mechanisms. However, eicosanoid production can be significantly altered in situations in which endothelial dysfunction, atherosclerosis and plaque rupture, or various thrombotic or inflammatory conditions are present.

Prostaglandins and Leukotrienes

Prostaglandins have a central role in the regulation of platelet aggregation and vascular tone. In this regard, two of the major prostaglandins derived from AA are thromboxane A_2, produced in platelets, and prostacyclin I_2, produced in endothelial cells. Thromboxane A_2 promotes platelet aggregation and blood vessel constriction, while prostacyclin I_2 has the opposite effects. An increase in availability of EPA can decrease platelet thromboxane A_2 and increase thromboxane A_3, the latter having considerably less physiological activity. EPA supplementation also stimulates formation of prostacyclin I_3, while prostacyclin I_2 is unaffected. Prostacyclin I_3 and prostacyclin I_2 are equipotent in their biological activity. The net result following intake of n-3 fatty acids is a shift in the thromboxane/prostacyclin balance toward a reduced prothrombotic state.

Leukotriene B_4 is a potent inflammatory mediator produced by neutrophils from 20:4n-6 at the site of injury. Leukotriene B_4 is also a powerful chemotactic factor responsible for attracting neutrophils to the site of injury. Leukotriene B_5, which is produced from EPA, has significantly lower biological activity. Therefore an increased availability of EPA has the potential to reduce inflammation.

Fatty Acid Intake and Eicosanoids

The proportional concentration of the eicosanoid precursor fatty acids both circulating and in tissues depends on dietary intake. DGLA and AA can be obtained from animal meat and fat, and by desaturation and chain elongation of LA. The major dietary source of EPA is fish. EPA can also be obtained indirectly from ALA, although desaturation and chain elongation of ALA appears to be a less important pathway in humans.

Only the free form of the fatty acid precursors of eicosanoids can be utilized by the enzymes for conversion to the biologically active metabolites. However, the amount of precursor free fatty acid in the cytoplasm and circulating is usually low and so too is basal eicosanoid formation. Furthermore, basal eicosanoid formation may depend on dietary and adipose tissue fatty acid composition. The amount of eicosanoid precursor free fatty acids is controlled to a large extent by incorporation and release from cellular phospholipids. Which eicosanoids are produced during stimulated synthesis may depend on membrane fatty acid composition as well as the cell type involved. Dietary fatty acid composition, therefore, has the potential to effect basal and stimulated synthesis of eicosanoids and influence endothelial function and thrombotic and inflammatory responses.

n-6 Fatty Acids and Risk of Cardiovascular Disease

Evidence that differences in n-6 fatty acid intake can influence cardiovascular disease risk derives from several sources. Population studies may provide useful data for establishing optimal intakes of n-6 fatty acids. However, valuable information on the potential mechanisms and effects of these fatty acids is derived from studies focusing on their impact on thrombosis, inflammation, endothelial function, and other cardiovascular risk factors.

Cardiovascular Disease: Population Studies

The incidence of cardiovascular disease within populations with either very high or very low intakes of n-6 fatty acids may provide some indication for optimal intakes of n-6 fatty acids. Within populations with low n-6 fatty acid intakes ($\leq 3\%$) there would appear to be a benefit of having a higher n-6 fatty acid intake on cardiovascular disease risk reduction. These observations suggest that very low n-6 fatty acid intakes increase the risk for cardiovascular disease. The presence of EFA deficiency in a significant proportion of such populations may explain the increased risk. Several populations, including the Israelis, Taiwanese, and !Kung bushmen in the African Kalahari desert, have high to very high intakes of n-6 fatty acids. The contribution of n-6 fatty acids to total energy intake is about 10% in the Israelis and Taiwanese and about 30% in the !Kung bushmen. Rates of cardiovascular disease are low in the Taiwanese, where dietary n-6 fatty acids are obtained mainly from soybean oil, and estimated to be very low in the

!Kung bushmen, where dietary n-6 fatty acids were obtained mainly from the monongo fruit and nut. In the Taiwanese, the soybean oil is refined but is accompanied by a diet rich in antioxidant polyphenols, notably from tea, fruits, and vegetables. In the !Kung bushmen the oil is unrefined and is therefore likely to contain a range of phytochemicals. There is, however, a high prevalence of cardiovascular disease in the Israeli population, where n-6 PUFAs are obtained largely from refined sources. These observations suggest that a high n-6 fatty acid intake can be compatible with low risk of cardiovascular disease, but the dietary context may be very important. Given that n-6 fatty acids are susceptible to lipid peroxidation, high n-6 fatty acid intake may increase risk for cardiovascular disease when consumed against a background diet low in antioxidants. The potential impact on eicosanoid metabolism remains uncertain.

Several factors may need to be considered in the interpretation of the results of population studies. First, the effect of LA on atherosclerosis and cardiovascular disease may depend on the background intake in the population being studied. Second, any relationships observed may be confounded by intake of other foods from which LA derives. Third, LA may have differential effects on aspects of the aetiology of cardiovascular disease, including endothelial function, thrombosis, arrhythmia, and atherosclerosis.

Thrombosis

Dietary fatty acids influence thrombosis by altering the activity and function of endothelial cells, platelets, and other circulating cells—effects that can be mediated, in part, by alterations in eicosanoid metabolism. Replacement of dietary saturated fatty acids with unsaturated fatty acids, including n-6 fatty acids, generally lowers the risk of thrombosis and cardiovascular disease. Furthermore, studies have shown that an increase in n-3 fatty acid intake can increase vasodilation, attenuate platelet aggregation, and alter circulating concentrations of factors involved in coagulation and fibrinolysis. The net effect of increasing n-3 fatty acid intake is a tendency toward reduced risk for thrombosis. These findings are supported by population studies demonstrating that n-3 fatty acids may reduce the risk of thrombosis. It remains uncertain whether the major factor influencing these functions is the absolute increase in n-3 fatty acids or the relative proportions of n-6 and n-3 fatty acids in the diet and cell membranes. There is evidence, however, that increased n-3 fatty acid intake may be more

beneficial in populations consuming relatively small quantities of fish, which includes many Western populations.

Much of the evidence for a potential impact of n-6 fatty acids on thrombosis derives from research on platelet function. The role of platelets in thrombosis is established and the influence of fatty acid intake on platelet function has been assessed in many studies. Platelets play a part in thrombosis by adhering to, and aggregating at, the site of injury. Platelet reactivity and increased platelet activation may increase the risk of thrombosis. In vitro and in vivo studies assessing effects of n-6 fatty acids on platelet aggregation are inconsistent. To date there is little evidence that a high n-6 fatty acid diet in humans decreases platelet aggregation and some studies are suggestive of increased aggregation with high n-6 fatty acid diets, primarily in the form of LA. The effects of AA on platelet aggregation are also not clear. One of the main difficulties in interpreting these studies is the unresolved issue as to how the in vitro aggregation test reflects platelet function in vivo.

Inflammation

Conditions of increased inflammation, such as inflammatory arthritis, dermatological conditions such as psoriasis and atopic dermatitis, chronic inflammatory bowel disease, autoimmune diseases, and bronchial asthma, appear to be beneficially influenced by n-3 fatty acids but not by n-6 fatty acids.

Whether or not increased intake of n-6 fatty acids can exacerbate inflammation via increased production of proinflammatory eicosanoids remains uncertain. Results of in vitro studies and intervention studies in humans are generally consistent with this theoretical potential of n-6 fatty acids to enhance inflammation, at least in comparison to n-3 fatty acids and probably n-9 monounsaturated fatty acids. The importance of absolute and relative intakes of n-6 fatty acids to inflammatory processes also remains unclear. The effects of changes in n-6 fatty acid intake on inflammatory processes may depend on the background dietary fatty acid intake, as well as proportional and absolute intake of n-3 fatty acids.

Cholesterol and Lipoproteins

The major classes of circulating lipoproteins in human plasma are chylomicrons, very low-density lipoproteins (VLDL), low-density lipoproteins (LDL), and high-density lipoproteins (HDL). High fasting plasma concentrations of LDL cholesterol and triglycerides—predominantly circulating as part of VLDL—and low plasma concentrations of HDL cholesterol are associated with increased risk of cardiovascular disease. Dietary fatty acids can influence lipoprotein metabolism and therefore have the potential to influence atherosclerosis and cardiovascular disease risk. Most studies examining the effects of n-6 PUFAs on cholesterol metabolism have focused on LA, the major dietary n-6 fatty acid.

It is now established that LDL cholesterol lowering reduces the risk of cardiovascular disease. In the fasting state LDL is the major cholesterol carrying lipoprotein in human plasma. The mechanisms through which raised plasma LDL cholesterol concentrations increase cardiovascular disease risk are not entirely understood but oxidative modification of LDL is thought to be involved. An increase in LA intake results in a lowering of plasma LDL cholesterol concentrations and therefore has the potential to reduce cardiovascular disease risk. These effects may not be linear over the entire range of LA intake and most of the benefits appear to be gained by moving from lower (<2% of energy) to moderate (~4–5% of energy) intakes. In addition, it is worthy of note that the effects of dietary n-6 PUFAs are less than half that of lowering dietary saturated fatty acids. Therefore, if total fat intake is maintained, the LDL cholesterol lowering effects of increasing n-6 PUFA intake are greatly enhanced if saturated fatty acid intake is decreased.

HDL cholesterol is inversely associated with cardiovascular disease risk. The mechanism by which HDL reduces cardiovascular disease risk may involve reverse cholesterol transport and reductions in cholesterol accumulation in the arterial wall. Intakes of LA within the normal ranges of intakes in most populations do not appear to alter HDL cholesterol concentrations. However, very high intakes—above 12% of energy—can lower HDL cholesterol concentrations.

Oxidative Stress

Several lines of evidence suggest that oxidatively modified LDL plays an important role in the development of atherosclerosis. Oxidative modification of LDL involves peroxidation of PUFAs. LDL particles enriched in PUFAs have been shown to be more susceptive to oxidative modification compared to LDL particles rich in monounsaturated fatty acids. Others have also suggested that a diet high in PUFAs may overwhelm the antioxidant defenses of cells. In particular, studies have shown that LA-enriched LDL is more prone to *in vitro* oxidation than oleic acid-enriched LDL. Concern also remains with

respect to the potential for increased lipid peroxidation following n-3 fatty acids. To date, however, the data *in vivo* are inconclusive, with observations of increased, unchanged, and decreased lipid peroxidation. The most plausible explanation relates to differences in the methodologies employed to assess lipid peroxidation. Much of the literature relating to PUFAs and lipid peroxidation is based on indirect and nonspecific assays, including measurement of LDL oxidative susceptibility, which relies on the isolation of LDL from plasma. In this regard, the recent discovery of F_2-isoprostanes, which are nonenzymatic prostaglandin-like products of free radical peroxidation of arachidonic acid, has allowed for the direct assessment of *in vivo* lipid peroxidation. There is now good evidence that quantitation of F_2-isoprostanes provides a reliable measure of *in vivo* oxidative stress. Using measurement of F_2-isoprostanes, recent data have demonstrated that n-3 fatty acids decrease oxidative stress. It has also been suggested that the concentration of PUFAs may be a more important factor affecting lipid peroxidation than the degree of unsaturation. Further research using better markers of lipid peroxidation is required before definitive statements can be made relating to the effect of n-6 fatty acids, and indeed PUFAs in general, on oxidative stress.

Blood Pressure

The possible effects of dietary fatty acids on blood pressure have been explored in population studies and dietary intervention trials. With the exception of studies comparing vegetarian and nonvegetarian populations, from which there is a suggestion of a blood pressure lowering effect of diets high in PUFAs, including LA, and lower in saturated fatty acids, the results of most within- and between-population studies have generally not found significant associations. The results of intervention studies suggest that n-6 fatty acids, LA in particular, may be responsible for a small blood pressure lowering effect. However, these studies are also inconsistent, with several failing to find a significant blood pressure lowering effect.

Conclusions

Diets low in n-6 fatty acids, principally LA, appear to be associated with an increased risk of cardiovascular disease. The results of studies examining the effects of LA on risk factors for atherosclerosis and cardiovascular disease are consistent with this observation. An increase in n-6 PUFA intake from a low to a moderate intake level, in conjunction with decreases in total and saturated fat intake, may beneficially influence lipoprotein metabolism, lower blood pressure, and reduce cardiovascular disease risk. Observations in populations with high n-6 PUFA intake indicate that high intakes of n-6 fatty acids (>10%) can occur together with low rates of cardiovascular disease and possibly also cancer. However, where antioxidant composition of the diet is low, there is the potential for increased risk of cardiovascular disease. An increased susceptibility of PUFAs to oxidative damage, particularly in the presence of low concentrations of protective antioxidants, may be an important factor involved. The source of n-6 PUFAs in the diet, refined versus unrefined, and the composition of the background diet may therefore be important determinants of whether high n-6 fatty acid intake increases or decreases risk of cardiovascular disease. In addition, the proportion of n-6 to n-3 fatty acids in the diet may also play an important role in determining cardiovascular risk.

The available evidence suggests that n-6 fatty acid-derived eicosanoids are generally proinflammatory and prothrombotic. In contrast, eicosanoids derived from n-3 fatty acids have attenuated biological activity on cardiovascular risk factors. The effects of altering n-6 PUFA intake, in conjunction with changes in other polyunsaturated fatty acids, as well as other classes of fatty acids, on endothelial function, thrombosis, and inflammation are not understood. The relative proportion of all the classes of fatty acids in the diet may well be more important and relevant to cardiovascular risk reduction than any single class of fatty acids. Clearly such research warrants further investigation.

See also: **Coronary Heart Disease**: Lipid Theory. **Fatty Acids**: Metabolism; Monounsaturated; Omega-3 Polyunsaturated; Saturated; *Trans* Fatty Acids. **Fish**.

Further Reading

Grundy SM (1996) Dietary fat. In: Ziegler EE and Filer LJ Jr. (eds.) *Present knowledge in Nutrition*, 7th edn., pp. 44–57. Washington, DC: ILSI Press.

Hodgson JM, Wahlqvist ML, Boxall JA, and Balazs NDH (1993) Can linoleic acid contribute to coronary artery disease? *American Journal of Clinical Nutrition* 58: 228–234.

Hodgson JM, Wahlqvist ML, and Hsu-Hage B (1995) Diet, hyperlipidaemia and cardiovascular disease. *Asia Pacific Journal of Clinical Nutrition* 4: 304–313.

Hornsrtra G, Barth CA, Galli C *et al.* (1998) Functional food science and the cardiovascular system. *British Journal of Nutrition* 80(supplement 1): S113–S146.

Horrobin DF (ed.) (1990) *Omega-6 Essential Fatty Acids: Pathophysiology and Roles in Clinical Medicine*. New York: Wiley-Liss.

Jones GP (1997) Fats. In: Wahlqvist ML (ed.) *Food and Nutrition, Australia, Asia and the Pacific*, pp. 205–214. Sydney: Allen & Unwin.

Jones PJH and Kubow S (1999) Lipids, sterols and their metabolism. In: Shils ME, Olson JA, Shike M, and Ross AC (eds.) *Modern Nutrition in Health and Disease*, 9th edn., pp. 67–94. Baltimore: Williams & Wilkins.

Knapp HR (1997) Dietary fatty acids in human thrombosis and hemostasis. *American Journal of Clinical Nutrition* 65(supplement 5): 1687S–1698S.

Lyu LC, Shieh MJ, Posner BM *et al.* (1994) Relationship between dietary intake, lipoproteins and apolipoproteins in Taipei and Framingham. *American Journal of Clinical Nutrition* 60: 765–774.

Mensink R and Connor W (eds.) (1996) *Nutrition. Current Opinion in Lipidology* 7: 1–53.

National Health and Medical Research Council (1992) *The role of polyunsaturated fats in the Australian diet: Report of the NHMRC working party*. Canberra: Australian Government Publishing Service.

Salem N, Simopoulos AP, Galli, Lagarde M, and Knapp HR (eds.) (1996) Fatty acids and lipids from cell biology to human disease: Proceedings of the 2nd International Congress of the International Society for the Study of Fatty Acids and Lipids. *Lipids* 31 (supplement).

Truswell AS (1977) Diet and nutrition of hunter gatherers. *Ciba Foundation Symposium*, 213–221.

Yam D, Eliraz A, and Berry EM (1996) Diet and disease—The Israeli paradox: Possible dangers of a high omega-6 polyunsaturated fatty acid diet. *Israeli Journal of Medical Sciences* 32: 1134–1143.

Saturated

R P Mensink, Maastricht University, Maastricht, The Netherlands
E H M Temme, University of Leuven, Leuven, Belgium

Fats and oils always consist of a mixture of fatty acids, although one or two fatty acids are usually predominant. **Table 1** shows the fatty acid composition of some edible fats rich in saturated fatty acids. In the Western diet, palmitic acid ($C_{16:0}$) is the major saturated fatty acid. A smaller proportion comes from stearic acid ($C_{18:0}$), followed by myristic acid ($C_{14:0}$), lauric acid ($C_{12:0}$), and short-chain and medium-chain fatty acids (MCFA) ($C_{10:0}$ or less).

When discussing the health effects of the total saturated fat content of diets, this class of fatty acids has to be compared with some other component of the diet that provides a similar amount of energy (isoenergetic). Otherwise, two variables are being introduced: changes in total dietary energy

Table 1 Composition of fats rich in satured fatty acids

| | Weight per 100 g of total fatty acids (g) | | | | | | | | |
	$\leq C_{10:0}$	$C_{12:0}$	$C_{14:0}$	$C_{16:0}$	$C_{18:0}$	$C_{18:1}$	$C_{18:2}$	$C_{18:3}$	Other
Butterfat	9	3	17	25	13	27	3	1	2
Palm kernel fat	8	50	16	8	2	14	2		
Coconut fat	15	48	17	8	3	7	2		
Palm oil		1	45	5	39	9			1
Beef fat		3	26	22	38	2	1		8
Pork fat (lard)		2	25	12	44	10	1		6
Cocoa butter			26	35	35	3			1

intake and, as a consequence, changes in body weight. Normally, an isoenergetic amount from carbohydrates is used for comparisons.

Cholesterol Metabolism

Lipoproteins and their associated apoproteins are strong predictors of the risk of coronary heart disease (CHD). Concentrations of total cholesterol, low-density lipoproteins (LDL), and apoprotein B are positively correlated with CHD risk; high-density lipoprotein (HDL) and apoprotein AI concentrations are negatively correlated. Controlled dietary trials have now demonstrated that the total saturated fat content and the type of saturated fatty acid in the diet affect serum lipid and lipoprotein levels.

Total Saturated Fat Content of Diets

Using statistical techniques, results from independent experiments have been combined to develop equations that estimate the mean change in serum lipoprotein levels for a group of subjects when carbohydrates are replaced by an isoenergetic amount of a mixture of saturated fatty acids. The predicted changes for total LDL and HDL cholesterol and triacylglycerols are shown in **Figure 1**. Each bar represents the predicted change in the concentration of that particular lipid or lipoprotein when a particular fatty acid class replaces 10% of the daily energy intake from carbohydrates. For a group of adults with an energy intake of 10 MJ daily, 10% of energy is provided by about 60 g of carbohydrates or 27 g of fatty acids.

A mixture of saturated fatty acids strongly elevates serum total cholesterol levels. It was predicted that when 10% of dietary energy provided by carbohydrates was exchanged for a mixture of saturated fatty acids, serum total cholesterol concentrations would increase by 0.36 mmol l^{-1}. This increase in total cholesterol will result from a

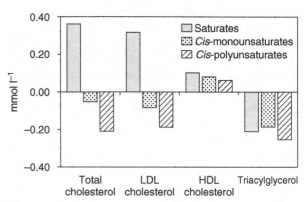

Figure 1 Predicted changes in serum lipids and lipoproteins when 10% of energy from dietary carbohydrates is replaced by an isoenergetic amount of saturated fatty acids. From Mensink *et al.* (2003) *American Journal of Clinical Nutrition* **77**: 1146–1155. Reproduced with permission by the *American Journal of Clinical Nutrition*. © Am J Clin Nutr. American Society for Clinical Nutrition.

rise in both LDL and HDL cholesterol concentrations. Saturated fatty acids will also lower fasting triacylglycerol concentrations compared with carbohydrates. Besides affecting LDL and HDL cholesterol concentrations, a mixture of saturated fatty acids also changes the concentrations of their associated apoproteins. In general, strong associations are observed between changes in LDL cholesterol and changes in apo-B and between changes in HDL cholesterol and apo-AI.

Figure 1 also shows that total and LDL cholesterol concentrations decrease when saturated fatty acids are replaced by unsaturated fatty acids. In addition, slight decreases of HDL cholesterol concentrations are then predicted.

Effects of Specific Saturated Fatty Acids

Cocoa butter raises total cholesterol concentrations to a lesser extent than palm oil. This difference in the serum cholesterol-raising potency of two fats high in saturated fatty acids (see **Table 1**) showed that not all saturated fatty acids have equal effects

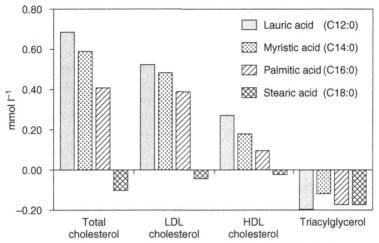

Figure 2 Overview of the effects of particular fatty acids on serum total, LDL, and HDL cholesterol concentration when 10% of energy from dietary carbohydrates is replaced by an isoenergetic amount of a particular saturated fatty acid. From Mensink *et al.* (2003) *American Journal of Clinical Nutrition* **77**: 1146–1155. Reproduced with permission by the *American Journal of Clinical Nutrition.* © Am J Clin Nutr. American Society for Clinical Nutrition.

on cholesterol concentrations. **Figure 2** illustrates the effects of lauric, myristic, palmitic, and stearic acids on LDL and HDL cholesterol concentrations. Compared with other saturated fatty acids, lauric and myristic acids have the strongest potency to increase serum total and LDL cholesterol concentrations and also HDL cholesterol concentrations. Effects of lauric acid on HDL are stronger than those of myristic acid.

Scientists are not unanimous about the cholesterol-raising properties of palmitic acid, the major dietary saturated fatty acid. Many studies have indicated that, compared with carbohydrates, palmitic acid raises serum total and LDL cholesterol levels but has less effect on HDL cholesterol (**Figure 2**). However, a few studies indicated that palmitic acid might not raise total and LDL cholesterol concentrations compared with carbohydrates. It has been proposed that this negative finding is only present when the linoleic acid content of the diet is adequate (6–7% of energy). It is hypothesized that the increased hepatic apo-B100 production caused by palmitic acid, and the consequent elevation of concentrations of serum very low density lipoproteins (VLDL) and LDL particles, is counteracted by an increased uptake of LDL particles by the LDL receptor which is upregulated by linoleic acid. To explain the discrepancy with other studies, it has been suggested that in some situations, such as hypercholesterolaemia or obesity, linoleic acid is unable to increase LDL receptor activity sufficiently to neutralize the cholesterol-raising effects of palmitic acid. This theory, however, awaits confirmation, and for now it seems justified to classify palmitic acid as a cholesterol-raising saturated fatty acid.

Stearic acid, a major fatty acid in cocoa butter, does not raise total, LDL, and HDL cholesterol levels compared with carbohydrates. Also, MCFA have been reported not to raise LDL and HDL cholesterol concentrations compared with carbohydrates, but data are limited. Like carbohydrates, diets containing large amounts of MCFA increase fasting triacylglycerol concentrations compared with the other saturated fatty acids. However, such diets are the sole energy source only in parenteral or enteral nutrition or in sports drinks. Other saturated fatty acids have not been reported to raise triacylglycerol concentrations compared with each other, but lower triacylglycerol concentrations compared with carbohydrates.

Platelet Aggregation

Increased platelet aggregation may be an important risk marker for the occurrence of cardiovascular disease, and different types of fatty acids can modify platelet aggregation *in vitro*. However, reports of research on this topic are confusing. All measurements have their limitations, and it is not known whether measurement *in vitro* of platelet aggregation reflects the reality of platelet reactivity *in vivo*.

Many methods are available to measure platelet aggregation *in vitro*. First, the blood sample is treated with an anticoagulant to avoid clotting of the blood in the test tube or in the aggregometer; many different anticoagulants are used, which all differ in their mechanism of action. Second, platelet aggregation can be measured in whole blood, in platelet-rich plasma, or (to remove the influence of the plasma constituents) in a washed platelet sample. Finally, the platelet aggregation reaction in the aggregometer can be initiated with many different compounds, such as collagen, ADP, arachidonic acid, and thrombin. Platelet aggregation can also be studied by measuring the stable metabolites of the proaggregatory thromboxane A_2 (TxA_2), thromboxane B_2 (TxB_2), the stable metabolite of the antiaggregatory prostaglandin (prostacyclin: PGI_2), or 6-keto-$PGF1\alpha$.

Total Saturated Fat Content of Diets

Platelet aggregation and clotting activity of plasma were studied in British and French farmers, who were classified according to their intake of saturated fatty acids. A positive correlation was observed between thrombin-induced aggregation of platelet-rich plasma and the intake of saturated fatty acids. Aggregation induced by ADP or collagen, however, did not correlate with dietary saturated fat intake. In a follow-up study, a group of farmers consuming high-fat diets were asked to replace dairy fat in their diets with a special margarine rich in polyunsaturated fatty acids. Besides lowering the intake of saturated fatty acids, this intervention also resulted in a lower intake of total fat. A control group of farmers did not change their diets. After this intervention the thrombin-induced aggregation of platelet-rich plasma decreased when saturated fat intake decreased. Aggregation induced by ADP, however, increased in the intervention group. From these studies, it is not clear whether the fatty acid composition of the diets or the total fatty acid content is responsible for the changes in platelet aggregation. Furthermore, it is not clear if one should favor increased or decreased platelet aggregation after decreasing the saturated fat content of diets as effects did depend on the agonist used to induce platelet aggregation. Saturated fatty acids from milk fat have also been compared with unsaturated fatty acids from sunflower and rapeseed oils. Aggregation induced by ADP or collagen in platelet-rich plasma was lower with the milk fat diet than with either oil.

One of the mechanisms affecting platelet aggregation is alteration of the proportion of arachidonic acid in the platelet phospholipids. Arachidonic acid is a substrate for the production of the proaggregatory TxA_2 and the antiaggregatory PGI_2, and the balance between these two eicosanoids affects the degree of platelet activation. The proportion of arachidonic acid in membranes can be modified through changes in dietary fatty acid composition. Diets rich in saturated fatty acids increase the arachidonic acid content of the platelet phospholipids, but this is also dependent on the particular saturated fatty acid consumed (see below).

Diets rich in saturated fatty acids have also been associated with a lower ratio of cholesterol to phospholipids in platelet membranes, which may affect receptor activity and platelet aggregation. However, these mechanisms have been described from studies in vitro and on animals and have not adequately been confirmed in human studies.

Effects of Specific Saturated Fatty Acids

Diets rich in coconut fat have been reported to raise TxB_2 and lower 6-keto-$PGF_{1\alpha}$ concentrations in collagen-activated plasma compared with diets rich in palm or olive oils, indicating a less favourable eicosanoid profile. The main saturated fatty acids of coconut fat — lauric and myristic acids — did not, however, change collagen-induced aggregation in whole-blood samples compared with a diet rich in oleic acid. Also, diets rich in MCFA or palmitic acid did not change collagen-induced aggregation in whole-blood samples. Compared with a diet rich in a mixture of saturated fatty acids, a stearic acid diet increased collagen-induced aggregation in platelet-rich plasma. In addition, a decreased proportion of arachidonic acid in platelet phospholipids was demonstrated after a cocoa butter diet compared with a diet rich in butterfat. Changes in eicosanoid metabolite concentrations in urine, however, were not observed after either diet. These results are conflicting and it is debatable whether measurement in vitro of platelet aggregation truly reflects the situation in vivo.

Coagulation and Fibrinolysis

Processes involved in thrombus formation include not only those required for the formation of a stable thrombus (platelet aggregation and blood clotting) but also a mechanism to dissolve the thrombus (fibrinolysis). Long-term prospective epidemiological studies have reported that in healthy men factor VII coagulant activity (factor VIIc) and fibrinogen concentrations were higher in subjects who developed cardiovascular diseases at a later stage of the study. Factor VIIc in particular was associated with an increased risk of dying from cardiovascular disease. A high concentration of plasminogen activator inhibitor type 1 (PAI-1) indicates impaired fibrinolytic capacity of the plasma and is associated with increased risk of occurrence of coronary events.

Saturated fatty acids can affect the plasma activity of some of these coagulation and fibrinolytic factors and thus the prethrombotic state of the blood. However, the effects of saturated fatty acids on coagulation and fibrinolytic factors in humans, unlike effects on cholesterol concentrations, have received little attention, and few well-controlled human studies have been reported. Also, regression equations derived from a meta-analysis, which predict the effects on coagulation and fibrinolytic factors of different fatty acid classes compared with those of carbohydrates, do not exist. Therefore, the reference fatty acid is dependent on the experiment discussed. In the epidemiological studies that have found associations between CHD risk and factors involved in thrombogenesis or atherogenesis, subjects were mostly fasted. Also, the effects of saturated fatty acids on cholesterol metabolism, platelet aggregation, and coagulation and fibrinolysis have been studied mainly in fasted subjects. It should be noted, however, that concentrations of some coagulation factors (e.g., factor VIIc) and fibrinolytic factors change after a meal.

Total Saturated Fat Content of Diets

Coagulation Results of studies on the effects of low-fat diets compared with high-fat diets provide some insight into the effects of decreasing the saturated fat content of diets. However, in these studies multiple changes are introduced which makes interpretation of results difficult.

Figure 3 demonstrates that decreased factor VIIc levels were observed in subjects on low-fat diets compared with those on high-saturated fat diets. In many of these studies, the low-fat diet provided smaller quantities of both saturated and unsaturated fatty acids and more fiber than the high-saturated fat diets. The combined results, however, suggest

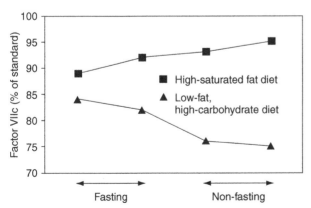

Figure 3 Effects of a high-saturated fat diet on fasting and postprandial factor VIIc activity From Miller (1998) *American Journal of Clinical Nutrition* **67**(supplement): 542S–545S. Reproduced with permission by the *American Journal of Clinical Nutrition*. © Am J Clin Nutr. American Society for Clinical Nutrition.

that, apart from a possible effect of dietary fiber, saturates increase factor VII levels compared with carbohydrates. Effects on other clotting factors are less clear. Measurements of markers of *in vivo* coagulation (e.g., prothrombin fragment $1+2$) might have provided more information on the effect of saturates on blood coagulation but were unfortunately not measured in most experiments.

Fibrinolysis Effects of low-fat and high-fat diets on the fibrinolytic capacity of the blood have also been studied. A similar problem, as stated before, is that multiple changes were introduced within a single experiment. Results of longer term and shorter term studies with dietary changes of total fat (decrease of saturated and unsaturated fatty acids contents) and increased fiber content indicate beneficially increased euglobulin fibrinolytic capacity of the blood. However, when the saturated fatty acid and fiber content of two diets were almost identical and only the unsaturated fatty acid content was changed, no significant differences in fibrinolytic capacity were observed.

Little is known about the relative effects on fibrinolytic capacity of saturated fatty acids compared with unsaturated fatty acids. It has been reported, however, that diets rich in butterfat decreased PAI-1 activity compared with a diet rich in partially hydrogenated soybean oil, but whether this is because of changes in the saturated acid or the *trans* fatty acid content is not clear from this study.

As for coagulation factors, the findings on the fibrinolytic effects of saturates are still inconclusive and need to be examined by more specific assays, measuring the activities of the separate fibrinolytic factors such as tPA and PAI-1.

Effects of Specific Saturated Fatty Acids

Coagulation The interest in the effects of particular fatty acids on coagulation and fibrinolytic factors has increased since the observation that different saturated fatty acids raise serum lipids and lipoproteins in different ways (see section on cholesterol metabolism). Although results are conflicting, some studies indicate that the most potent cholesterol-raising saturated fatty acids also increase factor VII activity.

Diets rich in lauric plus myristic acids compared with a diet rich in stearic acid also increase concentrations of other vitamin K-dependent coagulation proteins. In addition, this mixture of saturated fatty acids raised $F1+2$ concentrations, indicating increased *in vivo* turnover of prothrombin to thrombin. This agreed with a study in rabbits where increased $F1+2$ concentrations were associated with increased hepatic synthesis of vitamin K-dependent clotting factors.

Diets rich in certain saturated fatty acids (lauric acid and palmitic acid) and also diets rich in butterfat have been reported to raise fibrinogen concentrations, but increases were small.

Postprandially, increased factor VIIc concentrations have been demonstrated after consumption of diets rich in fat compared with fat-free meals (**Figure 3**). The response is stronger when more fat is consumed, but this occurs regardless of whether the fat is high in saturated or unsaturated fatty acids. Only meals with unrealistically high amounts of MCFA have been reported not to change factor VIIc levels in comparison with a meal providing a similar amount of olive oil.

Fibrinolysis Increased PAI-1 activity of a palmitic acid-rich diet has been observed compared with diets enriched with oleic acid, indicating impaired fibrinolytic capacity of the plasma. However, this was not confirmed by other experiments on the effects of particular saturated fatty acids (including palmitic acid), which did not indicate changes in fibrinolytic capacity of the blood, measured as tPA, PAI-1 activity, or antigen concentrations of tPA and PAI-1.

Conclusion

Saturated fatty acids as a group affect factors involved in cholesterol metabolism. Relative to the carbohydrate content of the diet, a decrease in saturated fat content induces a favorable decrease in serum total and LDL cholesterol concentrations but unfavorably reduces HDL cholesterol concentrations. Both increasing and decreasing effects of saturates on platelet aggregation have been observed, as well as the absence of effect, so results are inconsistent and difficult to interpret. Whether the beneficial effect of a diet low in saturated fat on the prethrombotic state of blood depends on the dietary fiber content is still unclear.

Of the saturated fatty acids, lauric and myristic acids have the strongest potency to raise total and LDL cholesterol concentrations. In addition, both of these saturated fatty acids raise HDL cholesterol levels. Palmitic acid raises total and LDL cholesterol levels compared with carbohydrates but is less potent than lauric and myristic acids. Stearic acid does not raise LDL and HDL cholesterol concentrations compared with carbohydrates. Lauric, myristic, and palmitic acids increase factor VII activity in a similar way, whereas the effects of MCFA and stearic acid seem limited.

See also: **Coronary Heart Disease**: Lipid Theory; Prevention. **Fatty Acids**: Metabolism.

Further Reading

Hornstra G and Kester ADM (1997) Effect of the dietary fat type on arterial thrombosis tendency: Systematic studies with a rat model. *Atherosclerosis* 131: 25–33.

Khosla P and Sundram K (1996) Effects of dietary fatty acid composition on plasma cholesterol. *Progress in Lipid Research* 35: 93–132.

Kris-Etherton PM, Kris-Etherton PM, Binkoski AE *et al.* (2002) Dietary fat: Assessing the evidence in support of a moderate-fat diet; The benchmark based on lipoprotein metabolism. *Proceedings of the Nutrition Society* 61: 287–298.

Masson LF, McNeill G, and Avenell A (2003) Genetic variation and the lipid response to dietary intervention: A systematic review. *American Journal of Clinical Nutrition* 77: 1098–1111.

Mensink RP, Zock PL, Kester AD, and Katan MB (2003) Effects of dietary fatty acids and carbohydrates on the ratio of serum total to HDL cholesterol and on serum lipids and apolipoproteins: A meta-analysis of 60 controlled trials. *American Journal of Clinical Nutrition* 77: 1146–1155.

Miller GJ (1998) Effects of diet composition on coagulation pathways. *American Journal of Clinical Nutrition* 67(supplement): 542S–545S.

Mutanen M and Freese R (1996) Polyunsaturated fatty acids and platelet aggregation. *Current Opinion in Lipidology* 7: 14–19.

Mutanen M and Freese R (2001) Fats, lipids and blood coagulation. *Current Opinion in Lipidology* 12: 25–29.

Sacks FM and Katan M (2002) Randomized clinical trials on the effects of dietary fat and carbohydrate on plasma lipoproteins and cardiovascular disease. *American Journal of Medicine* 113(Supplement 9B): 13S–24S.

Temme EHM, Mensink RP, and Hornstra G (1998) Saturated fatty acids and effects on whole blood aggregation in vitro. *European Journal of Clinical Nutrition* 52: 697–702.

Temme EHM, Mensink RP, and Hornstra G (1999) Effects of diets enriched in lauric, palmitic or oleic acids on blood coagulation and fibrinolysis. *Thrombosis and Haemostasis* 81: 259–263.

Tholstrup T, Miller GJ, Bysted A, and Sandström B (2003) Effect of individual dietary fatty acids on postprandial activation of blood coagulation factor VII and fibrinolysis in healthy young men. *American Journal of Clinical Nutrition* 77: 1125–1132.

Trans Fatty Acids

M J Sadler, MJSR Associates, Ashford, UK

This article is reproduced from the previous edition, pp. 769–776, © 1998, Elsevier Ltd.

Chemistry

The *trans* fatty acids are unsaturated fatty acids that contain one or more ethylenic double bonds in the *trans* geometrical configuration, i.e., on opposite sides of the carbon chain (**Figure 1**). The *trans*

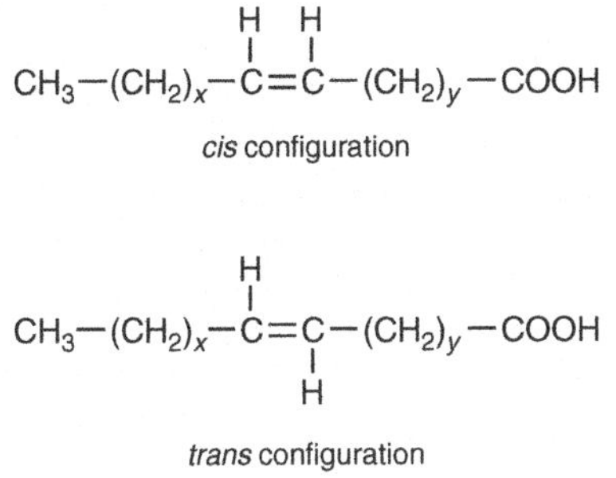

$$CH_3-(CH_2)_x-\overset{\overset{H}{|}}{C}=\overset{\overset{H}{|}}{C}-(CH_2)_y-COOH$$

cis configuration

$$CH_3-(CH_2)_x-\overset{\overset{H}{|}}{C}=\underset{\underset{H}{|}}{C}-(CH_2)_y-COOH$$

trans configuration

Figure 1 The *trans* and *cis* configurations of unsaturated bonds. Reproduced with kind permission of the British Nutrition Foundation.

bond is more thermodynamically stable than the *cis* bond and is therefore less chemically reactive.

Trans bonds have minimal effect on the conformation of the carbon chain such that their physical properties more closely resemble those of saturated fatty acids than of *cis* unsaturated fatty acids. The conformation remains linear, compared with *cis* fatty acids, which are kinked (**Figure 2**). Hence, *trans* isomers can pack together more closely than their *cis* counterparts.

Trans fatty acids have higher melting points than their *cis* counterparts, while saturated fatty acids have higher melting points than both *trans* and *cis* fatty acids. For example, the melting points of C_{18} fatty acids are $69.6\,°C$ for stearic acid (18:0), $44.8\,°C$ for elaidic acid (*trans*-18:1), and $13.2\,°C$ for oleic acid (*cis*-18:1). The relative proportion of these different types of fatty acids influences the physical properties of cooking fats and their suitability for different uses in the food processing industry.

In addition to geometrical isomerism (*cis* and *trans*), unsaturated fatty acids also exhibit positional isomerism, where the double bonds can occur in different positions along the chain in fatty acids which have identical chemical formulae. As with *cis* fatty acids, *trans* fatty acids also occur as mixtures of positional isomers.

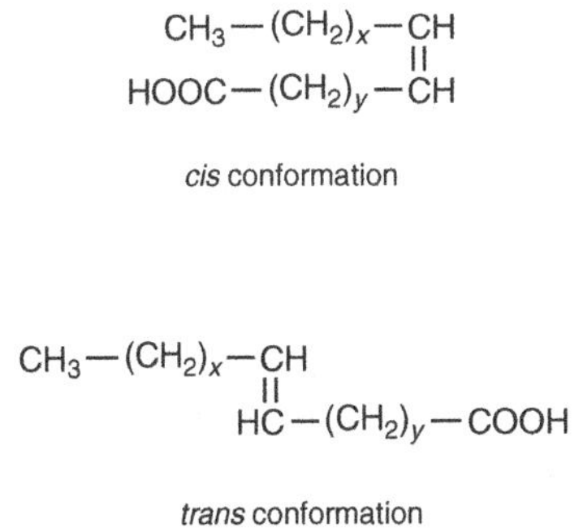

$$CH_3-(CH_2)_x-CH$$
$$HOOC-(CH_2)_y-\overset{\overset{||}{}}{CH}$$

cis conformation

$$CH_3-(CH_2)_x-CH$$
$$HC-(CH_2)_y-COOH$$

trans conformation

Figure 2 Conformation of the carbon chain with *trans* and *cis* bonds. Reproduced with kind permission of the British Nutrition Foundation.

Occurrence

Trans fatty acids present in the diet arise from two origins. The first is from bacterial biohydrogenation in the forestomach of ruminants, which is the source of *trans* fatty acids present in mutton and beef fats. These are present at a concentration of 2–9% of bovine fat. *Trans*-11-octadecenoic acid is the main isomer produced although *trans*-9- and *trans*-10-octadecenoic acid are also produced. Thus, *trans* fatty acids occur in nature and cannot be considered to be foreign substances.

The second origin is from the industrial catalytic hydrogenation of liquid oils (mainly of vegetable origin, but also of fish oils). This produces solid fats and partially hydrogenated oils and is undertaken to increase the thermal stability of liquid oils and to alter their physical properties. The margarines, spreads, shortenings, and frying oils produced are thus more useful in the food processing industry than liquid oils. Chemically, a range of *trans* isomers is produced that, for vegetable oils containing predominantly C_{18} unsaturated fatty acids, is qualitatively similar to those produced by biohydrogenation, although the relative proportions of the isomers may differ. Use of fish oils containing a high proportion of very long-chain (C_{20} and C_{22}) fatty acids with up to six double bonds produces more complex mixtures of *trans, cis,* and positional isomers. However, the use of hydrogenated fish oils in food processing is declining, owing to a general fall in edible oil prices and to consumer preference for products based on vegetable oils.

Analysis

Methods available for the estimation of total *trans* unsaturation and to determine individual *trans* fatty acids are outlined in **Table 1**. At present there is no one simple and accurate method suitable for both research applications and for use in the food industry. In dietary studies data for *trans* fatty acid intake are generally expressed as the sum of the fatty acids containing *trans* double bonds, and there is generally no differentiation between the different isomers.

A report from the British Nutrition Foundation (BNF) in 1995 highlighted concerns over the variations in estimations of *trans* fatty acid concentrations in some food products provided by different analytical techniques. A thorough review of the available analytical techniques was called for.

Table 1 Analytical methods for *trans* fatty acids

General method	Determines	Advantages	Disadvantages
Infrared (IR) absorption spectrometry	Total *trans* unsaturation	Inexpensive; reliable results provided concentrations of *trans* isomers exceed 5%; can analyze intact lipids	Unreliable results if concentrations of *trans* isomers less than 5%; interpretive difficulties—need to apply correction factors
Fourier transform IR spectroscopy	Total *trans* unsaturation	Reliable results if concentrations of *trans* isomers less than 2%	Does not distinguish between two esters each with one *trans* bond or between one ester with two *trans* bonds and one with none
Gas–liquid chromatography (GLC)	Individual *trans* fatty acids		Presence of unidentified compounds can give false estimates of *trans* fatty content
Argentation—GLC	Individual *trans* fatty acids	Saturated, monounsaturated, and diunsaturated fatty acids can be resolved	Method is time-consuming
Capillary column GLC	Individual *trans* fatty acids which can be summated to give total *trans* unsaturation	Accurate resolution of fatty acid esters including *cis* and *trans* isomers	Great skill required for preparing columns and interpretation of chromatograms
High-performance liquid chromatography	Individual *trans* fatty acids	*cis,cis*- and *trans,trans*-dienoic fatty acids can be separated	
Nuclear magnetic resonance (NMR)	Individual *trans* fatty acids	Intact lipids can be analyzed; can identify *trans*-diene isomers by use of proton (^{1}H) NMR	Equipment is costly; more use as a research tool than for general analysis

Sources and Intakes

The main sources of *trans* fatty acids in the UK diet are cereal-based products (providing 27% of total *trans* fatty acid intake), margarines, spreads, and frying oils (22%), meat and meat products (18%), and milk, butter, and cheese (16%). In the USA, the main sources of intake are baked goods (28%), fried foods (25%), margarine, spreads, and shortenings (25%), savory snacks (10%), and milk and butter (9%).

Typical ranges of *trans* fatty acids in foods are shown in **Table 2**. *Trans* isomers of $C_{18:1}$ (elaidic acid) are the most common *trans* fatty acids, accounting for 65% of the total *trans* fatty acids in the UK diet.

Intakes of *trans* fatty acids are difficult to assess because of:

- analytical inaccuracies;
- difficulties of obtaining reliable information about food intake.

A number of countries have attempted to assess intakes of *trans* fatty acids (**Table 3**). Reliable intake data are available for the UK, based on a 7-day weighed intake of foods eaten both inside and outside the home, for 2000 adults aged 16–64 years (**Table 3**). Data from the UK National Food Survey, which does not include food eaten outside the home,

show a steady decline in intake of *trans* fatty acids from 5.6 g per person per day in 1980 to 4.8 g in 1992. In the UK *trans* fatty acids account for approximately 6% of dietary fat, and in the USA for approximately 7–8% of dietary fat. Estimates of *trans* fatty acid intake are likely to show a downward trend because of:

- improved analytical techniques which give lower but more accurate values for the *trans* fatty acid content of foods;
- the availability of values for *trans* fatty acids in a wider range of foods which allows more accurate estimation of intakes;
- the reformulation of some products which has led to a reduction in the concentration of *trans* fatty acids in recent years.

Advances in food technology that are enabling a gradual reduction in the *trans* fatty acid content include:

1. refinements in hydrogenation processing conditions which will enable the reduction and in the future, the elimination of *trans* fatty acids;
2. the interesterification (rearrangement of fatty acids within and between triacylglycerols) of liquid oils with solid fats;
3. the future genetic modification of oils.

Table 2 Typical content of *trans* fatty acids in a range of foods

Food	Content of trans fatty acids per 100 g product (g)
Butter	3.6
Soft margarine, not high in PUFA	9.1
Soft margarine, high in PUFA	5.2
Hard margarine	12.4
Low-fat spread, not high in PUFA	4.5
Low-fat spread, high in PUFA	2.5
Blended vegetable oil	1.1
Vegetable oil (sunflower, safflower, soya, sesame)	0
Commercial blended oil	6.7
Potato crisps	0.2
Whole wheat crisps	0.2
Low-fat crisps	0.3
Beefburger, 100% beef frozen, fried, or grilled	0.8
Sausage, pork, fried	0.1
Sausage roll, flaky pastry	6.3
Hamburger in bun with cheese, take-away	0.5
Biscuits, cheese-flavored	0.2
Biscuits, chocolate, full coated	3.4
Chocolate cake and butter icing	7.1
Chips, old potatoes, fresh, fried in commercial blended oil	0.7
Chips, frozen, fine cut, fried in commercial blended oil	0.7

PUFA, polyunsaturated fatty acids. *Trans* fatty acid methyl esters were determined by capillary gas chromatography.
Reproduced with kind permission of the British Nutrition Foundation.

Table 3 Estimated intakes of *trans* fatty acids in various countries

Country	Estimated daily intake of total trans fatty acids (g)	Year published and basis for estimation
UK	5.6 (men) 4.0 (women)	1990: 7-day weighed intake undertaken in 1986–87 including food eaten outside the home
USA	8.1	1991: availability data
	3.8	1994: food frequency questionnaire
Denmark	5.0	1995: availability data
Finland	1.9	1992: duplicate diets
Spain	2.0–3.0	1993: calculated from food consumption data
Norway	8.0	1993: food frequency questionnaire

Physiology of *trans* Fatty Acids

Extensive reviews of the health effects of *trans* fatty acids conducted in the 1980s found no evidence for any adverse effects of *trans* fatty acids on growth, longevity, reproduction, or the occurrence of disease, including cancer, from studies conducted in experimental animals.

Digestion, Absorption, and Metabolism

Trans fatty acids are present in the diet in esterified form, mainly in triacylglycerols but those from ruminant sources may also be present in phospholipids. Before absorption into the body, triacylglycerols must be digested by pancreatic lipase in the upper small intestine. There is no evidence of differences in the hydrolysis and absorption of *trans* fatty acids, in comparison with that of *cis* fatty acids. *Trans* fatty acids are transported from the intestine mainly in chylomicrons, but some are also incorporated into cholesteryl esters and phospholipids.

Trans fatty acids are incorporated into the lipids of most tissues of the body and are present in all the major classes of complex lipids. The positional distribution of *trans* fatty acids tends to show more similarity to that of saturated fatty acids than to that of the corresponding *cis* fatty acids. Some selectivity between tissues results in an uneven distribution of *trans* fatty acids throughout the body.

Trans fatty acids occur mainly in positions 1 and 3 of triacylglycerols, the predominant lipids in adipose tissue. The concentration of *trans* fatty acids in adipose tissue is approximately proportional to long-term dietary intake, and determination of the concentrations in storage fat is one method used to estimate *trans* fatty acid intake. However, this is not entirely straightforward as variation has been reported in the composition of adipose tissue obtained from different sites and depths, and factors that influence adipose tissue turnover rates such as dieting and exercise are also complicating factors. *Trans*-18:1 isomers account for approximately 70% of the *trans* fatty acids found in adipose tissue, and *trans*-18:2 isomers (*trans,trans*, *trans,cis*, and *cis,trans*) account for about 20%.

In heart, liver, and brain, *trans* fatty acids occur mainly in membrane phospholipids. The position of the double bond as well as the conformation of the carbon chain may determine the pattern of *trans* fatty acid esterification in phospholipids, but there is evidence that *trans*-18:1 fatty acids are preferentially incorporated into position 1 of the phospho-acylgly-cerols, as are saturated fatty acids; in contrast, oleic acid is randomly distributed.

The turnover of *trans* fatty acids parallels that of other types of fatty acids in the body, and *trans* fatty acids are readily removed from the tissues for oxidation. Studies in which human subjects were fed labelled carbon-13 isotope have demonstrated that the whole-body oxidation rate for *trans*-18:1 is similar to that for *cis*-18:1. *Trans* fatty acids are a minor component of tissue lipids, and their concentrations in tissues are much lower than their concentrations in the diet. However, research has focused on C_{18} *trans* fatty acids, and more studies are needed to investigate the effects of very long-chain *trans* fatty acids derived from the hydrogenation of fish oils.

Interactions with Metabolism of Essential Fatty Acids

From experiments mainly with laboratory animals, it has been demonstrated that relatively high intakes of *trans* fatty acids in the diet in conjunction with marginal intakes of essential fatty acids (less than 2% dietary energy from linoleic acid) can lead to the presence of Mead acid (*cis*-5,8,11–20:3) in tissue lipids and an increase in the ratio of 20:3 n-9 to 20:4 n-6. This has been interpreted to suggest early signs of essential fatty acid deficiency, with potentially increased requirements for essential fatty acids. Mead acid can accumulate in the presence of linoleic acid, if large amounts of nonessential fatty acids are also present. Two mechanisms have been suggested to explain these observations in relation to intake of *trans* fatty acids:

- that *trans* fatty acids may compete with linoleic acid in metabolic pathways;
- that *trans* fatty acids may inhibit enzymes involved in elongation and further desaturation of linoleic acid.

The consensus is that the significance of Mead acid production in humans has not been established, and further research is needed in this area. It is unlikely that a competitive effect between polyunsaturated fatty acids (PUFA) and *trans* fatty acids would arise, because of the relatively high intakes of linoleic acid in people freely selecting their own diets. Also, as there is a large body pool of linoleic acid available for conversion to long-chain PUFA, it is unlikely that the *trans* fatty acids in the body would interfere even at relatively low ratios of dietary linoleic acid to *trans* fatty acids. The appearance of Mead acid is not specifically induced by *trans* fatty acids, and experiments in animals have not demonstrated any adverse health effects of its production.

Effect of *trans* Fatty Acids on Plasma Lipoproteins

Raised plasma concentrations of low-density lipoprotein (LDL) are considered to be a risk factor for coronary heart disease (CHD); in contrast, reduced concentrations of high-density lipoprotein (HDL) are

considered to increase risk. It therefore follows that to help protect against CHD, diets should ideally help to maintain plasma concentrations of HDL cholesterol and to lower those of LDL cholesterol. Dietary factors that raise LDL and lower HDL concentrations would be considered to be undesirable in this context.

Several trials have evaluated the effects of C_{18} *trans* monounsaturated fatty acids on plasma lipoproteins (**Figure 3**). The results have been relatively consistent, and the following general conclusions have been drawn from these studies:

- C_{18} monounsaturated *trans* fatty acids raise LDL cholesterol concentration; the cholesterol-raising effect is similar in magnitude to that of the cholesterol-raising saturated fatty acids, i.e., myristic (14:0) and palmitic (16:0) acids.
- C_{18} monounsaturated *trans* fatty acids decrease HDL cholesterol concentration; this is in contrast to saturated fatty acids which produce a small rise in HDL levels.
- In comparison with the effects of oleic and linoleic fatty acids, C_{18} monounsaturated *trans* fatty acids raise LDL cholesterol and lower HDL cholesterol levels.

It has been calculated that 'theoretically', each 1% increase in energy from *trans* fatty acids (18:1) in place of oleic acid (*cis*-18:1) would raise plasma LDL concentration by $0.040 \, \text{mmol} \, l^{-1}$ (an approximately 1% increase based on average UK plasma cholesterol concentration); HDL would be decreased by $0.013 \, \text{mmol} \, l^{-1}$ (a 1% decrease).

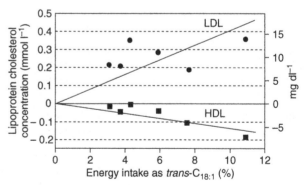

Figure 3 Effects of monounsaturated C_{18} *trans* fatty acids on lipoprotein cholesterol concentrations relative to oleic acid (*cis*-$C_{18:1}$). Data are derived from six dietary comparisons between *trans* and *cis* monounsaturated fatty acids; differences between diets in fatty acids other than *trans* and *cis* monounsaturated fatty acids were adjusted for by using regression coefficients from a meta-analysis of 27 controlled trials. The regression lines were forced through the origin because a zero change in intake will produce a zero change in lipoprotein concentrations. From Zock *et al.* (1995), reproduced with kind permission of the *American Journal of Clinical Nutrition*.

The 1995 BNF Task Force calculated that, in the UK, replacing 2% energy from *trans* fatty acids with 2% energy from oleic acid would reduce mean plasma LDL cholesterol concentration by 0.08 mmol l^{-1}; plasma HDL concentration would rise by 0.026 mmol l^{-1}, and the HDL ratio would fall from 3.92 to 3.77. From estimates of the effect of changes in LDL and HDL concentrations on CHD risk, this was predicted to reduce the risk of CHD by 5–15%. In comparison, replacing *trans* fatty acids with either saturated fatty acids or carbohydrate would decrease risk by up to 8%.

The influence of *trans* fatty acids on plasma lipoproteins in relation to CHD risk would thus appear to be more unfavorable than that of saturated fatty acids, as determined by the effect on the ratio of LDL to HDL cholesterol. However, the overall magnitude of the effect would be dependent on the relative intakes of *trans* fatty acids and saturated fatty acids. In the UK *trans* fatty acids contribute about 2% of dietary energy, in contrast to saturated fatty acids which contribute about 15% dietary energy, and this needs to be considered when formulating dietary advice. The Task Force also estimated, on the same basis, that a reduction of 6% in energy from saturated fatty acids would decrease risk by 37%.

However, these conclusions of the adverse effect of *trans* fatty acid on plasma lipoprotein concentrations are not universally accepted. It has been commented that some trials used an inappropriate basis for comparison of the different diets and did not always control for other fatty acids that are known to influence blood cholesterol levels.

Several studies have suggested that *trans* fatty acids raise the plasma concentration of lipoprotein(a), particularly in individuals with already raised levels. Lipoprotein(a) has been suggested to be an independent risk marker for CHD, although this is not universally accepted.

Atherosclerosis and Hemostasis

Despite the reported effects of *trans* fatty acids on blood lipoproteins, experiments with laboratory animals have not provided evidence that dietary *trans* fatty acids are associated with the development of experimental atherosclerosis, provided that the diet contains adequate levels of linoleic acid. Similarly, there is no evidence that *trans* fatty acids raise blood pressure or affect the blood coagulation system. However, there has been no thorough evaluation of the effect of *trans* fatty acids on the coagulation system, and this is an area worthy of investigation.

The Role of *trans* Fatty Acids in Coronary Heart Disease

A number of epidemiological studies have suggested an association between *trans* fatty acids and CHD.

Case–Control Studies

A study by Ascherio in 1994 demonstrated that in subjects who had suffered acute myocardial infarction (AMI), past intake of *trans* fatty acids, assessed from a food frequency questionnaire, was associated with increased risk. *Trans* fatty acid intake per day in the top quintile was 6.5 g compared with 1.7 g in the lowest quintile. After adjusting for age, energy intake, and sex, relative risk of a first AMI for the highest compared with the lowest quintile was 2.44 (95% confidence interval, 1.42–4.10). However, there was not a clear dose–response relationship.

A case–control study of sudden cardiac death found that higher concentrations of *trans* isomers of linoleic acid in adipose tissue, compared with lower concentrations, were associated with increased risk of sudden death. After controlling for smoking and making an allowance for social class, this relationship became insignificant.

A multicenter study in eight European countries plus Israel found that the risk of AMI was not significantly different across quartiles of the concentration of *trans*-18:1 fatty acids in adipose tissue, the multivariate odds ratio being 0.97 (95% confidence interval, 0.56–1.67) for the highest compared with the lowest quartiles. However, there were significant differences within countries. In Norway and Finland, relative risk was significantly increased in the highest compared with the lowest quartiles, but in Russia and Spain relative risk was significantly decreased in these groups. Exclusion from the multicenter analysis of the Spanish centers, which had particularly low intakes of *trans* fatty acids, resulted in a tendency to increased risk of AMI in the highest quartiles of *trans*-18:1 concentration. However, the trend was not statistically significant, and adjustment for confounding factors had no effect on the results.

A Prospective Study

The relationship between *trans* fatty acid intake and subsequent CHD events was investigated in approximately 85 000 US nurses (the Nurses Health Study). *Trans* fatty acid intake was calculated from food frequency questionnaires for women who had been diagnosed free from CHD, stroke, diabetes, and hypercholesterolemia. The subjects were followed up for 8 years and CHD events were recorded. The relative risk of CHD in the highest compared with the lowest quintile was 1.5 (95% confidence interval, 1.12–2.0), after adjustment for age, energy intake, social class, and smoking. However, there was no clear dose–response relationship between the highest and the lowest intake groups. The intake of *trans* fatty acids in the top quintile was 3.2% dietary energy compared with 1.3% in the lowest quintile.

It has been commented on that the benefit predicted by the authors, that individuals in the top quintile of intake could halve their risk of myocardial infarction by reducing their intake of *trans* fatty acids to that of the lowest quintile, seems a large effect in view of the small difference in intakes between these groups (3.3 g). The changes in plasma lipoprotein cholesterol concentrations that would be predicted to occur as a result of lowering *trans* fatty acid intake would not explain all of the observed increase in risk. Also, the study was carried out in a selected population of women and it is unclear that the findings are applicable to the whole population or to other population groups.

Cancer

Although there is much evidence concerning the effect of different intakes of different types of fats on experimental carcinogenesis, data for *trans* fatty acids are limited and are hampered by confounding due to the lack of a suitable control diet.

Studies using different tumor models in mice and rats have shown no effect of *trans* fatty acids on tumor development. Increasing the intake of *trans* fatty acids, in place of *cis* fatty acids, has not demonstrated an adverse outcome with regard to cancer risk. In humans, there is little to suggest that *trans* fatty acids are adversely related to cancer risk at any of the major cancer sites. Early studies did not generally find that *trans* fatty acids were an important risk factor for malignant or benign breast disease. One study did report an association between the incidence of cancer of the colon, breast, and prostate and the use of industrially hydrogenated vegetable fats in the USA; however, other known risk factors were not allowed for.

Cancer of the Breast

Some epidemiological evidence suggests that total fat intake may be related to increased risk of cancer of the breast, although this is by no means conclusive. There is no strong evidence that intake of *trans* fatty acids *per se* is related to increased risk of breast cancer and many studies have not reported examining this relationship. A study in which adipose tissue concentrations of *trans*-18:1 fatty acids were assessed in 380 women with breast cancer at various stages and in controls revealed no consistent pattern of association. A similar, smaller study suggested an increased risk with higher body stores of *trans* fatty acids, but it was concluded that any such association may be modified by adipose tissue concentrations of polyunsaturated fatty acids.

Cancer of the colon

Epidemiological data from the Nurses Health Study suggested a link between intake of meat and meat products and colon cancer. The data indicated that high intakes of total, animal, saturated, and monounsaturated fat were associated with increased risk. Consuming beef, pork, or lamb as a main dish was positively associated with risk; though beef and lamb contain *trans* fatty acids, there was no evidence that high intakes of *trans* fatty acids increased risk. The Health Professionals Follow-up Study (a prospective study in male health professionals of parallel design to the Nurses Health Study) found similar dietary associations for colon cancer risk, with no suggestion of any link with intake of *trans* fatty acids.

Prostate Cancer

Dietary associations with risk of prostate cancer were also assessed from the Health Professionals Follow-up Study. High intakes of total, saturated, and monounsaturated fatty acids and of α-linolenic acid were associated with increased risk, whereas high intakes of saturated fatty acids and linoleic acid were found to be protective. Intake of *trans* fatty acids was not found to be associated with risk of prostate cancer.

Dietary Guidelines

The details of population dietary guidelines for the quality and quantity of fat intake differ between countries. However, in consideration of prevention of CHD, dietary guidelines generally reflect advice to reduce average total fat intakes to 30–35% dietary energy and to lower saturated fat intakes to approximately 10% of dietary energy. Though the effect of *trans* fatty acids on the plasma LDL/HDL ratio is less favorable than that of saturated fatty acids, dietary advice needs to reflect the relative intakes of these two types of fatty acids. Since the contribution of saturated fat intake to dietary energy is approximately 5–7 times higher than that of *trans* fatty acids, advice on *trans* fatty acids should not assume more importance than advice to lower saturated fatty acids. However, because of the unfavorable effect of *trans* fatty acids on plasma lipoprotein concentrations, the 1995 BNF Task Force report concluded that the average intake of *trans* fatty acids in the UK diet (2% of energy) should not rise, and that dietary advice should continue to focus on reducing intake of saturated fatty acids as a priority.

Extreme consumers of *trans* fatty acids may be at greater risk, and individuals with high intakes may benefit from advice to lower their intake. It has been calculated that lowering total fat and increasing carbohydrate intake (which reduces plasma HDL cholesterol) will have minimal effect on risk of CHD. Substituting *cis* unsaturated fatty acids for saturated and *trans* fatty acids would be predicted to have a greater impact. For individuals at risk of CHD, high intakes of *trans* fatty acids would appear to be undesirable. Most dietary guidelines call for a reduction in *trans* fatty acids "as much as possible" recognizing that small amounts of *trans* fats are naturally present in the food chain. The food industry in general has reduced or eliminated *trans* in many products by improving manufacturing techniques and reducing *trans* fats generated during the hydrogenation process. Additionally, several countries now have regulations requiring that *trans* fatty acid be listed on products' labels. In some cases, like in the US, *trans* must be added to the saturated fat content reported on the Nutrition Facts label, based on their similar adverse effects on health. Although listing both fats together may not be correct in chemical terms, it is a practical way to allow consumers to quickly assess the content of unhealthy fat in a product.

Conclusions

Several lines of evidence indicate that *trans* fats have an adverse effect on the lipoprotein profile and likely on risk of cardiovascular disease. Although reducing intake of *trans* fats is a desirable goal, public health policy should keep as a central recommendation the reduction of saturated fats, which constitute four to six times more percent calories in the diet than *trans* fats. Since the largest proportion of *trans* fats is generated during food processing, industry bears the main responsibility for reducing the *trans* content of its products, thus helping the general public to lower their intake of this type of fat.

See also: **Coronary Heart Disease**: Lipid Theory.

Further Reading

AIN/ASCN (1996) Position paper on *trans* fatty acids. *American Journal of Clinical Nutrition* 63: 663–670.

Aro AV, Kardinal AFM, Salminen I *et al.* (1995) Adipose tissue isomeric *trans* fatty acids and the risk of myocardial infarction in different countries: the EURAMIC study. *Lancet* 345: 273–278.

Ascherio A, Hennekens CH, Buring JE *et al.* (1994) *Trans* fatty acids intake and risk of myocardial infarction. *Circulation* 89: 94–101.

Berger KG (1996) In *Lipids and Nutrition: Current Hot Topics*. Bridgwater: PJ Barnes.

British Nutrition Foundation (1995) *Trans Fatty Acids*. Report of the British Nutrition Foundation Task Force. London: BNF.

Giovannucci E, Rimm E, Colditz GA *et al.* (1993) A prospective study of dietary fat and risk of prostate cancer. *Journal of the National Cancer Institute* 85: 1571–1579.

Giovannucci E, Rimm EB, Stampfer MJ *et al.* (1994) Intake of fat, meat and fiber in relation to risk of colon cancer in men. *Cancer Research* 54: 2390–2397.

Gurr MI (1996) Dietary fatty acids with *trans* unsaturation. *Nutrition Research Reviews* 9: 259–279.

International Life Sciences Institute (1995) *Trans* fatty acids and coronary heart disease risk. Report of the expert panel on *trans* fatty acids and coronary heart disease. *American Journal of Clinical Nutrition* 62: 655S–707S.

Ip C and Marshall JR (1996) *Trans* fatty acids and cancer. *Nutrition Reviews* 54: 138–145.

Mensink RP and Katan MB (1990) Effect of dietary fatty acids on high density and low density lipoprotein levels in healthy subjects. *New England Journal of Medicine* 323: 439–444.

Willett WC, Stampfer MJ, Manson JE *et al.* (1993) Intake of *trans* fatty acids and risk of coronary heart disease among women. *Lancet* 341: 581–585.

Zock PL, Katan MB, and Mensink RP (1995) Dietary *trans* fatty acids and lipoprotein cholesterol. *American Journal of Clinical Nutrition* 61: 617.

FISH

A Ariño, J A Beltrán, A Herrera and P Roncalés,
University of Zaragoza, Zaragoza, Spain

Introduction

In discussing the food uses of fishes, the term 'fish' refers to edible species of finfish, molluscs, and crustacea coming from the marine or freshwater bodies of the world, either by capture fisheries or by aquaculture. Accordingly, "fishery products" means any human food product in which fish is a characterizing ingredient, such as dried, salted, and smoked fish, marinated fish, canned seafood, minced fish flesh such as surimi, and miscellaneous products.

Fish is a source of high-quality animal protein, supplying approximately 6% of the world's protein requirements and 16.4% of the total animal protein. According to Food and Agriculture Organization figures, the contribution of fish to the total animal-protein intake is 26.2% in Asia, 17.4% in Africa, 9.2% in Europe, 9% in the former USSR, 8.8% in Oceania, 7.4% in North and Central America, 7.2% in South America, and 21.8% in the low-income food-deficit countries (including China). There are wide differences among countries in fish consumption measured as the average yearly intake per person, ranging from countries with less than 1.0 kg per person to countries with over 100 kg per person.

Edible fish muscle contains 18–20% protein and 1–2% ash; the percentage of lipids varies from less than 1% to more than 20% (in high-fat finfish), and fish has the added advantage of being low in saturated fat. In general, lean fish is not an important source of calories, which are mostly obtained from the staple carbohydrates in the diet. Fatty fish, however, is a significant energy source in many fish-consuming communities in both the developed and the developing worlds. Today it is recognized that fish is probably more important as a source of micronutrients, minerals, and particularly essential fatty acids than for its energy or protein value. The essential micronutrients and minerals in fish include vitamins A and D, calcium, phosphorus, magnesium, iron, zinc, selenium, fluorine, and iodine (in marine fishes).

The protective effect of a small amount of fish against mortality from coronary heart disease (CHD) has been established by numerous epidemiological studies. A diet including two or three servings of fish per week has been recommended on this basis, and researchers have reported a 50% reduction in CHD mortality after 20 years with intakes of as little as 400 g of fish per week.

It has been suggested that the long-chain omega-3 (n-3) polyunsaturated fatty acids (PUFAs) (eicosapentanoic acid (EPA; C20:5) and docosahexanoic acid (DHA; C22:6)) in fish offer this protection against CHD. Several recent studies have shown that a large intake of omega-3 fatty acids is beneficial in lowering blood pressure, reducing triacylglycerols, decreasing the risk of arrhythmia, and lowering the tendency of blood platelets to aggregate.

As fish become more popular, the reports of foodborne diseases attributed to fish have increased. Food-borne diseases linked with exposure to fish can result from the fish itself (i.e., toxic species, allergies) or from bacterial (i.e., *Clostridium botulinum*, *Listeria monocytogenes*, *Salmonella*, *Vibrio*, and *Staphylococcus*), viral (i.e., hepatitis, Norwalk gastroenteritis), or parasitic (i.e., *Anisakis* and related worms) contamination. Also, naturally occurring seafood toxins (i.e., scombrotoxin, ciguatoxins, shellfish poisoning from toxic algae) or the presence of additives and chemical residues due to environmental contamination can cause food-borne illnesses. In recent years, reports of contamination of some fish with methylmercury have raised concerns about the healthfulness of certain fish for some populations.

General Characteristics of Finfish

A very large number of species of finfish are used for food by the world's population. The dressing percentage of finfish (60–70%) is similar to that of beef, pork, or poultry. The percentage of edible tissue in the dressed carcasses of finfish (without head, skin, and viscera) is higher than that of other food animals, because fishes contain less bone, adipose tissue, and connective tissue. There are three main categories of finfish that are widely used as foods. The bony fishes (teleosts) provide two compositional categories: white fishes (or lean fishes) and fatty fish. The third category is the cartilaginous elasmobranch fishes.

White fishes

The flesh of these fishes is very low in fat and consists primarily of muscle and thin layers of connective tissue. The concentrations of most of the B vitamins are similar to those in mammalian lean meats, although fish may contain higher amounts of vitamins B_6 and B_{12}. The mineral levels are also similar, although the very fine bones that are eaten with the fish flesh can raise the calcium content; fish is also a significant source of iodine. These fishes accumulate oils only in their livers, which are a rich source of vitamin A (retinol), vitamin D, and long-chain PUFAs in their triacylglycerols (TAGs).

Fatty Fishes

These fishes have fat in their flesh, which is usually much darker than that of white fishes, with similar blocks of muscle and connective tissue. The amount of fat is related to the breeding cycle of the fish, so that the fat content falls considerably after breeding. The flesh of fatty fishes is generally richer in the B vitamins than that of white fishes, and significant amounts of vitamins A and D are present. The mineral concentrations are not very different, but fatty fish is a better source of iron. The oil of these fishes is particularly rich in very-long-chain PUFA, especially those of the omega-3 (n-3) series such as EPA and DHA. These fishes accumulate oils in their muscles, belly flap, and skin (subdermal fat).

Cartilaginous Fishes

The cartilaginous fishes include the sharks and rays, whose flesh is rich in connective tissue and relatively low in fat, although they do accumulate oils in their livers. The concentrations of vitamins and minerals are very similar to those in white fish. These fishes contain urea in relatively large amounts, and so protein values based on total nitrogen are overestimated. The ammonia smell of cooked sharks and rays is not an indication that the fish is spoiled but rather is the result of enzymatic degradation of urea.

General Characteristics of Shellfish

The term 'shellfish' includes any aquatic invertebrate, such as molluscs or crustaceans, that has a shell or shell-like exoskeleton. The cephalopods have an internal shell (as in squids) or no shell (as in octopods). Owing to the presence of the tough exoskeleton, the edible portion in shellfish (around 40%) is less than that in finfish, with the exception of cephalopods, whose dressing percentage is 70–75%. The lipid content of the edible parts of most shellfish is low, as bivalves store their energy surplus as glycogen and not as depot fat, while crustaceans and cephalopods store their fat in their digestive glands (hepatopancreas). In many fish-eating communities, these foods are very highly valued gastronomically.

Molluscs

A wide range of molluscs are eaten by man, including bivalves (such as mussels, oysters, and scallops), gastropods (such as winkles and whelks), and cephalopods (such as squids and octopuses). The flesh is muscular with low levels of fat, although the fat is more saturated and richer in cholesterol than that of finfish. The mineral levels in shellfish are usually somewhat higher than those in finfish, and the vitamin concentrations are low. Bivalves and gastropods are often eaten whole after boiling or sometimes raw; usually, only the muscular mantles of cephalopods are eaten. In some cultures, only selected parts are eaten; for example, only the white adductor muscle of the scallop is eaten in North America.

Crustaceans

Crustaceans include a range of species, both freshwater (such as crayfish) and marine (such as crabs, shrimps, prawns, and lobsters). These animals have a segmented body, a chitinous exoskeleton, and paired jointed limbs. The portions eaten are the muscular parts of the abdomen and the muscles of the claws of crabs and lobsters. The flesh is characteristically low in fat and high in minerals, with vitamin levels similar to those found in finfish.

Nutritional Value of Fish and Shellfish: Introductory Remarks

Fish and shellfish are excellent sources of protein. A 100 g cooked serving of most types of fish and shellfish provides about 18–20 g of protein, or about a third of the average daily recommended protein intake. The fish protein is of high quality, containing an abundance of essential amino-acids, and is very digestible by people of all ages. Seafood is also loaded with minerals such as iron, zinc, and calcium.

The caloric value of fish is related to the fat content and varies with species, size, diet, and season. Seafood is generally lower in fat and calories than beef, poultry, or pork. Most lean or low-fat species of fish, such as cod, hake, flounder, and sole, contain less than 100 kcal (418 kJ) per 100 g portion, and even fatty fish, such as mackerel, herring, and salmon, contain approximately 250 kcal (1045 kJ) or less in a 100 g serving. Most crustaceans contain less than 1% fat in the tail muscle because depot fat is stored in the hepatopancreas, which is in the head region.

Interest in the health benefits of fish and shellfish began decades ago when researchers noted that certain groups of people – including the Inuit and the Japanese, who rely on fish as a dietary staple – have a low rate of ischemic diseases (i.e., heart attack or stroke). Fish, particularly fatty fish, is a good source of the omega-3 fatty acids EPA and DHA. These fats help to lower serum triacylglycerols and cholesterol, help prevent the blood clots that form in heart attacks, and lower the chance of having an irregular heartbeat. In fact, one study found that women who ate fish at least once a week were 30% less likely to die of heart disease than women who ate fish less than once a month. Similar benefits have been found for men. Fish consumption is also related to slower growth of atherosclerotic plaque and lower blood pressure. Especially good sources of omega-3 fats are salmon, tuna, herring, mackerel, and canned tuna and sardines.

When included in the diet of pregnant and breast-feeding women, DHA is thought to be beneficial to infant brain (learning ability) and eye (visual acuity) development. Scientists have found that women who ate fatty fish while pregnant gave birth to children with better visual development. Babies of mothers who had significant levels of DHA in their diet while breastfeeding experienced faster-than-normal eyesight development. Preliminary research also suggests that a diet rich in omega-3 fatty acids – and in DHA in particular – may help to decrease the chance of preterm birth, thus allowing the baby more time for growth and development.

Recent research found that eating just one serving a week of fish decreased the risk of developing dementia by 30%. Eating fatty fish several times a week may also lower the risk of developing prostate cancer by as much as half. A Swedish study of 3500 postmenopausal women eating two servings of fatty fish a week found that they were 40% less likely to develop endometrial cancer than those eating less than one-fourth of a serving a week.

Eating a variety of fish and seafood, rather than concentrating on one species, is highly recommended for both safety and nutrition. It is recommended that pregnant women should avoid certain species of fish and limit their consumption of other fish to an average of 400 g of cooked fish per week. The reason for this recommendation is that, whereas nearly all fish contain trace amounts of methylmercury (an environmental contaminant), large predatory fish, such as swordfish, shark, tilefish, and king mackerel, contain the most. Excess exposure to methylmercury from these species of fish can harm an unborn child's developing nervous system. It is also suggested that nursing mothers and young children should not eat these particular species of fish.

Fish Lipids

In fish, depot fat is liquid at room temperature (oil) and is seldom visible to the consumer; an exception is the belly flaps of salmon steaks. Many species of finfish and almost all shellfish contain less than 2.5% total fat, and less than 20% of the total calories come from fat. Almost all fish has less than 10% total fat, and even the fattiest fish, such as herring, mackerel, and salmon, contains no more than 20% fat (**Table 1**). In order to obtain a good general idea of the fat contents of most finfish species, flesh color might be considered. The leanest species, such as cod and flounder, have a white or lighter color, while fattier fishes, such as salmon, herring, and mackerel, have a much darker color.

The triacylglycerol depot fat in edible fish muscle is subject to seasonal variation in all marine and freshwater fishes from all over the world. Fat levels tend to be higher during times of the year when fishes are feeding heavily (usually during the warmer

Table 1 Fat levels in marine and freshwater fish and shellfish commonly found in the marketplace

Low (<2.5% fat) less than 20% of total calories from fat	Medium (2.5–5% fat) between 20% and 35% of total calories from fat	High (>5% fat) between 35% and 50% of total calories from fat
Saltwater fish		
Cod	Anchovy	Dogfish
Grouper	Bluefish	Herring[a]
Haddock	Sea bass	Mackerel[a]
Hake	Swordfish	Salmon[a]
Most flatfishes (flounder, sole, plaice)	Tuna (yellowfin)	Sardine
Pollock		Tuna (bluefin)
Shark		
Skate		
Snapper		
Whiting		
Most crustaceans		
Most molluscs		
Freshwater fish		
Pike	Bream	Catfish (farmed)
Perch, bass	Carp	Eel[a]
Tilapia	Trout (various)	Whitefish

[a]More than 10% fat.
Reproduced with permission from Ariño A, Beltran JA, and Roncalés P (2003) Dietary importance of fish and shellfish. In: Caballero B, Trugo L, and Finglas P (eds.) *Encyclopedia of Food Sciences and Nutrition*, 2nd edn. Oxford: Elsevier Science Ltd. pp. 2471–2478.

months) and in older and healthier individual fishes. Fat levels tend to be lower during spawning or reproduction. When comparing fat contents between farmed and wild-caught food fish, it should be remembered that farmed species have a tendency to show a higher proportion of muscle fat than their wild counterparts. Also, the fatty-acid composition of farmed fish depends on the type of dietary fat used in raising the fish. Cholesterol is independent of fat content and is similar in wild and cultivated fishes.

Most protein-rich foods, including red meat and poultry as well as fish, contain cholesterol. However, almost all types of fish and shellfish contain well under 100 mg of cholesterol per 100 g, and many of the leaner types of fish typically have 40–60 mg of cholesterol in each 100 g of edible muscle. It is known that most shellfish also contain less than 100 mg of cholesterol per 100 g. Shrimp contain somewhat higher amounts of cholesterol, over 150 mg per 100 g, and squid is the only fish product with a significantly elevated cholesterol content, which averages 300 mg per 100 g portion. Fish roe, caviar, internal organs of fishes (such as livers), the tomalley of lobsters, and the hepatopancreas of crabs can contain high amounts of cholesterol.

Omega-3 PUFA in Fish and Shellfish

The PUFA of many fish lipids are dominated by two members of the omega-3 (n-3) family, C20:5 n-3 (EPA) and C22:6 n-3 (DHA). They are so named because the first of several double bonds occurs three carbon atoms away from the terminal end of the carbon chain.

All fish and shellfish contain some omega-3, but the amount can vary, as their relative concentrations are species specific (**Table 2**). Generally, the fattier fishes contain more omega-3 fatty acids than the leaner fishes. The amount of omega-3 fatty acids in farm-raised products can also vary greatly, depending on the diet of the fishes or shellfish. Many companies now recognize this fact and provide a source of omega-3 fatty acids in their fish diets. Omega-3 fatty acids can be destroyed by heat, air, and light, so the less processing, heat, air exposure, and storage time the better for preserving omega-3 in fish. Freezing and normal cooking cause minimal omega-3 losses, whereas deep frying and conditions leading to oxidation (rancidity) can destroy some omega-3 fatty acids.

The beneficial effects of eating fish for human health have been well documented. Research has shown that EPA and DHA are beneficial in protecting against cardiovascular and other diseases (**Table 3**). Studies examining the effects of fish

Table 2 Selected fish and shellfish grouped by their omega-3 fatty-acid content

Low-level group (<0.5 g per 100 g)	Medium-level group (0.5–1 g per 100 g)	High-level group (>1 g per 100 g)
Finfish		
Carp	Bass	Anchovy
Catfish	Bluefish	Herring
Cod, Haddock, Pollock	Halibut	Mackerel
Grouper	Pike	Sablefish
Most flatfishes	Red Snapper	Salmon (most species)
Perch	Swordfish	Tuna (bluefin)
Snapper	Trout	Whitefish
Tilapia	Whiting	
Shellfish		
Most crustaceans	Clams	
Most molluscs	Oysters	

Reproduced with permission from Ariño A, Beltran JA, and Roncalés P (2003) Dietary importance of fish and shellfish. In: Caballero B, Trugo L, and Finglas P (eds.) *Encyclopedia of Food Sciences and Nutrition*, 2nd edn. Oxford: Elsevier Science Ltd. pp. 2471–2478.

consumption on serum lipids indicate a reduction in triacylglycerol and VLDL-cholesterol levels, a factor that may be protective for some individuals. Research also indicates that EPA in particular reduces platelet aggregation, which may help vessels injured by plaque formation. Fish oils also appear to help stabilize the heart rhythm, a factor that may be important in people recovering from heart attacks.

The major PUFA in the adult mammalian brain is DHA. It is among the materials required for development of the fetal brain and central nervous system and for retinal growth in late pregnancy. Brain growth uses 70% of the fetal energy, and 80–90% of cognitive function is determined before birth. However, the placenta depletes the mother of DHA, a situation that is exacerbated by multiple pregnancies. Dietary enhancement or fortification with marine products before and during pregnancy, rather than after the child is born, would be of great benefit to the child and mother. Furthermore, the food sources that are rich in DHA are also rich in zinc, iodine, and vitamin A, so it may be possible to provide several dietary supplements at one time. Deficiencies of the latter micronutrients are established causes of mental retardation and blindness.

The typical Western diet has a ratio of omega-6 to omega-3 essential fatty acids of between 15:1 and 20:1. Several sources of information suggest that a very high omega-6 to omega-3 ratio may promote many diseases, including cardiovascular disease, cancer, and inflammatory and autoimmune diseases. Fish

Table 3 Summary of the beneficial effects of eating fish for cardiovascular and other diseases

Cardiovascular disease	Other diseases
Protects against heart disease	Protects against age-related macular degeneration
Prolongs the lives of people after a heart attack	Alleviates autoimmune diseases such as rheumatoid arthritis
Protects against sudden cardiac arrest caused by arrhythmia	Protects against certain types of cancer
Protects against stroke (thrombosis)	Mitigates inflammation reactions and asthma
Lowers blood lipids such as triacylglycerols and VLDL-cholesterol	
Lowers blood pressure	

VLDL, very low-density lipoprotein.
Reproduced with permission from Ariño A, Beltran JA, and Roncalés P (2003) Dietary importance of fish and shellfish. In: Caballero B, Trugo L, and Finglas P (eds.) *Encyclopedia of Food Sciences and Nutrition*, 2nd edn. Oxford: Elsevier Science Ltd. pp. 2471–2478.

provides an adequate intake of these omega-3 fats, thus improving the omega-6 to omega-3 fatty-acid ratio. Most experts do not advise the routine use of fish-oil supplements: they favor eating fish and shellfish regularly in the context of a healthy diet and a regular pattern of physical activity. Whereas some research shows benefits of fish-oil supplements, research has also shown that people with weakened immune systems should avoid large doses of fish oil. The final conclusion as to whether it is possible to substitute fish consumption with fish oils or omega-3 fatty-acid supplements, and gain the same reduction in mortality from CHD, awaits more studies. However, the protective role of fish consumption is unquestioned.

Fish Proteins

Both finfish and shellfish are highly valuable sources of proteins in human nutrition. The protein content of fish flesh, in contrast to the fat content, is highly constant, independent of seasonal variations caused by the feeding and reproductive cycles, and shows only small differences among species. Table 4 summarizes the approximate protein contents of the

Table 4 Protein content of the different groups of fish and shellfish

Fish group	g per 100 g
White finfish	16–19
Fatty finfish	18–21
Crustaceans	18–22
Bivalves	10–12
Cephalopods	16–18

Reproduced with permission from Ariño A, Beltran JA, and Roncalés P (2003) Dietary importance of fish and shellfish. In: Caballero B, Trugo L, and Finglas P (eds.) *Encyclopedia of Food Sciences and Nutrition*, 2nd edn. Oxford: Elsevier Science Ltd. pp. 2471–2478.

various finfish and shellfish groups. Fatty finfish and crustaceans have slightly higher than average protein concentrations. Bivalves have the lowest values if the whole body mass is considered (most of them are usually eaten whole), whereas values are roughly average if specific muscular parts alone are consumed; this is the case with the scallop, in which only the adductor muscle is usually eaten.

The essential amino-acid compositions of fish and shellfish are given in **Table 5**. Fish proteins, with only slight differences among groups, possess a high nutritive value, similar to that of meat proteins and slightly lower than that of egg. It is worth pointing out the elevated supply, relative to meat, of essential amino-acids such as lysine, methionine, and threonine. In addition, owing in part to the low collagen content, fish proteins are easily digestible, giving rise to a digestibility coefficient of nearly 100.

The recommended dietary allowances (RDA) or dietary reference intakes (DRI) of protein for human male and female adults are in the range of 45–65 g per day. In accordance with this, an intake of 100 g of fish would contribute 15–25% of the total daily protein requirement of healthy adults and 70% of that of children. A look at the dietary importance of the Mediterranean diet is convenient: one of its characteristics is the high consumption of all kinds of fish, chiefly fatty fish. In many Mediterranean countries, fish intake averages over 50 g per day (edible flesh); thus, fish protein contributes over 10% of the total daily protein requirements steadily over the whole year in those countries.

Less well known is the fact that the consumption of fish protein, independently of the effect exerted by fish fat, has been related to a decrease in the risk of atherogenic vascular diseases. In fact, it has been demonstrated that diets in which fish is the only source of protein increase the blood levels of high-density lipoprotein relative to those resulting from diets based on milk or soy proteins.

Table 5 Content of essential amino-acids in fish and shellfish (g per 100 g of protein)

Fish group	Isoleucine	Leucine	Lysine	Methionine	Phenylalanine	Threonine	Tryptophan	Valine
Finfish	5.3	8.5	9.8	2.9	4.2	4.8	1.1	5.8
Crustaceans	4.6	8.6	7.8	2.9	4.0	4.6	1.1	4.8
Molluscs	4.8	7.7	8.0	2.7	4.2	4.6	1.3	6.2

Reproduced with permission from Ariño A, Beltran JA, and Roncalés P (2003) Dietary importance of fish and shellfish. In: Caballero B, Trugo L, and Finglas P (eds.) *Encyclopedia of Food Sciences and Nutrition*, 2nd edn. Oxford: Elsevier Science Ltd. pp. 2471–2478.

Nonprotein Nitrogen Compounds in Fish

Nonprotein nitrogen (NPN) compounds are found mostly in the fiber sarcoplasm and include free amino-acids, peptides, amines, amine oxides, guanidine compounds, quaternary ammonium molecules, nucleotides, and urea (**Table 6**). NPN compounds account for a relatively high percentage of the total nitrogen in the muscles of some aquatic animals, 10–20% in teleosts, about 20% in crustaceans and molluscs, and 30–40% (and in special cases up to 50%) in elasmobranchs. In contrast, NPN compounds in land animals usually represent no more than 10% of total nitrogen.

Most marine fishes contain trimethylamine oxide (TMAO); this colorless, odorless, and flavorless compound is degraded to trimethylamine, which gives a 'fishy' odor and causes consumer rejection. This compound is not present in land animals and freshwater species (except for Nile perch and tilapia from Lake Victoria). TMAO reductase catalyzes the reaction and is found in several fish species (in the red muscle of scombroid fishes and in the white and red muscle of gadoids) and in certain microorganisms (*Enterobacteriaceae, Shewanella putrefaciens*).

Creatine is quantitatively the main component of the NPN fraction. This molecule plays an important role in fish muscle metabolism in its phosphorylated form; it is absent in crustaceans and molluscs.

Endogenous and microbial proteases yield some free amino-acids; taurine, alanine, glycine, and imidazole-containing amino-acids seem to be the most frequent. Glycine and taurine contribute to the sweet flavor of some crustaceans. Migratory marine species such as tuna, characterized by a high proportion of red muscle, have a high content (about 1%) of free histidine. A noticeable amount of this amino-acid has been reported in freshwater carp. The presence of free histidine is relevant in several fish species because it can be microbiologically decarboxylated to histamine. Cooking the fish may kill the bacteria and destroy the enzymes, but histamine is not affected by heat, thus becoming a hazard to consumers. The symptoms of the resulting illness (scombroid poisoning) are itching, redness, allergic symptoms, headache, diarrhea, and peppery taste. Scombroid poisoning is most common after ingesting mahi-mahi, tuna, bluefish, mackerel, and skipjack.

Nucleotides and related compounds generally play an important role as coenzymes. They participate actively in muscle metabolism and supply

Table 6 Nonprotein nitrogen compounds in several commercially important fish species and mammalian muscle (mg per 100 g wet weight)

Compounds	Cod	Herring	Shark species	Lobster	Mammal
Total NPN	1200	1200	3000	5500	3500
Total free amino-acids:	75	300	100	3000	350
Arginine	<10	<10	<10	750	<10
Glycine	20	20	20	100–1000	<10
Glutamic acid	<10	<10	<10	270	36
Histidine	<1.0	86	<1.0	—	<10
Proline	<1.0	<1.0	<1.0	750	<1.0
Creatine	400	400	300	0	550
Betaine	0	0	150	100	—
Trimethylamine oxide	350	250	500–1000	100	0
Anserine	150	0	0	0	150
Carnosine	0	0	0	0	200
Urea	0	0	2000	—	35

NPN, nonprotein nitrogen.
Reproduced with permission from Ariño A, Beltran JA, and Roncalés P (2003) Dietary importance of fish and shellfish. In: Caballero B, Trugo L, and Finglas P (eds.) *Encyclopedia of Food Sciences and Nutrition*, 2nd edn. Oxford: Elsevier Science Ltd. pp. 2471–2478.

energy to physiological processes. They have a noticeable participation in flavor; moreover, some of them may be used as freshness indices. Adenosine triphosphate (ATP) is degraded to adenosine diphosphate (ADP), adenosine monophosphate (AMP), inosine monophosphate (IMP), inosine, and hypoxanthine. This pattern of degradation takes place in finfish, whereas AMP is degraded to adenosine and thereafter to inosine in shellfish. The degradation chain to IMP and AMP in finfish and shellfish, respectively, is very fast. IMP degradation to inosine is generally slow, except in scombroids and flat fishes. Inosine degradation to hypoxanthine is slower. IMP is a flavor potentiator, whereas hypoxanthine imparts a sour taste and it is toxic at high levels. ATP, ADP, and AMP decompose quickly leading to a build-up of inosine and hypoxanthine. As this corresponds well to a decline in freshness, the ratio of the quantity of inosine and hypoxanthine to the total quantity of ATP and related substances is called the *K*-value and used as a freshness index of fish meat.

Guanosine is an insoluble compound that gives fish eyes and skin their characteristic brightness. It is degraded to guanine, which does not have this property; therefore, brightness decreases until it completely disappears.

The NPN fraction contains other interesting compounds, such as small peptides. Most of them contribute to flavor; besides this, they have a powerful antioxidant activity. Betaines are a special group of compounds that contribute to the specific flavors of different aquatic organisms: homarine in lobster and glycine-betaine, butiro-betaine, and arsenic-betaine in crustaceans. Arsenic-betaine has the property of fixing arsenic into the structure, giving a useful method for studying water contamination.

Fish Vitamins

The vitamin content of fish and shellfish is rich and varied in composition, although somewhat variable in concentration. In fact, significant differences are neatly evident among groups, especially regarding fat-soluble vitamins. Furthermore, vitamin content shows large differences among species as a function of feeding regimes.

The approximate vitamin concentration ranges of the various finfish and shellfish groups are summarized in **Table 7**. The RDA for adults is also given, together with the percentage supplied by 100 g of fish. Of the fat-soluble vitamins, vitamin E (tocopherol) is distributed most equally, showing relatively high concentrations in all fish groups, higher than those of meat.

However, only a part of the vitamin E content is available as active tocopherol on consumption of fish, since it is oxidized in protecting fatty acids from oxidation. The presence of vitamins A (retinol) and D is closely related to the fat content, and so they are almost absent in most low-fat groups. Appreciable but low concentrations of vitamin A are found in fatty finfish and bivalve molluscs, whereas vitamin D is very abundant in fatty fish. In fact, 100 g of most fatty species supply over 100% of the RDA of this vitamin.

Water-soluble vitamins are well represented in all kinds of fish, with the sole exception of vitamin C (ascorbic acid), which is almost absent in all of them. The concentrations of the rest are highly variable; however, with few exceptions, they constitute a medium-to-good source of such vitamins, comparable with, or even better than, meat. The contents of vitamins B_2 (riboflavin), B_6 (pyridoxine), niacin, biotin, and B_{12} (cobalamin) are relatively high. Indeed, 100 g of fish can contribute up to 38%, 60%, 50%, 33%, and 100%, respectively, of the total daily requirements of those vitamins. Fatty fish also provides a higher supply of many of the water-soluble vitamins (namely pyridoxine, niacin, pantothenic acid, and cobalamin) than does white fish or shellfish. Crustaceans also possess a relatively higher content of pantothenic acid, whereas bivalve molluscs have much higher concentrations of folate and cobalamin.

A Mediterranean diet rich in fish – and especially in fatty finfish – contributes steadily over the year to an overall balanced vitamin supply. The last row of **Table 7** illustrates this; the supply of vitamins D, B_2, B_6, B_{12}, and niacin from this particular diet is more than 15% of the daily requirements; all other vitamins, except ascorbic acid, are supplied to a lesser, but significant, extent.

Fish Minerals

The approximate amounts of selected minerals contained in fish are given in **Table 8**. The first point to note is that all kinds of finfish and shellfish present a well-balanced content of most minerals, either macroelements or oligoelements, with only a few exceptions. Sodium content is low, as in other muscle and animal origin foods. However, it must be remembered that sodium is usually added to fish in most cooking practices in the form of common salt; also, surimi-based and other manufactured foods contain high amounts of added sodium. Potassium and calcium levels are also relatively low, though the latter are higher in fish than in meat; in addition, small fish bones are frequently eaten with fish flesh, thus increasing the calcium intake. Fish is a good source of magnesium and phosphorus, at least as good as meat. These elements

Table 7 Vitamin content of the different groups of fish and shellfish (mg or μg per 100 g)

	A (μg)	D (μg)	E (mg)	B_1 (mg)	B_2 (mg)	B_6 (mg)	Niacin (mg)	Biotin (μg)	Pantothenic acid (mg)	Folate (μg)	B_{12} (μg)	C (mg)
White finfish	Tr	Tr	0.3–1.0	0.02–0.2	0.05–0.5	0.15–0.5	1.0–5.0	1.0–10	0.1–0.5	5.0–15	1.0–5.0	Tr
Fatty finfish	20–60	5–20	0.2–3.0	0.01–0.1	0.1–0.5	0.2–0.8	3.0–8.0	1.0–10	0.4–1.0	5.0–15	5.0–20	Tr
Crustaceans	Tr	Tr	0.5–2.0	0.01–0.1	0.02–0.3	0.1–0.3	0.5–3.0	1.0–10	0.5–1.0	1.0–10	1.0–10	Tr
Molluscs	10–100	Tr	0.5–1.0	0.03–0.1	0.05–0.3	0.05–0.2	0.2–2.0	1.0–10	0.1–0.5	20–50	2.0–30	Tr
Cephalopods	Tr	Tr	0.2–1.0	0.02–0.1	0.05–0.5	0.3–0.1	1.0–5.0	1.0–10	0.5–1.0	10–20	1.0–5.0	Tr
RDA	900	5	15	1.2	1.3	1.3	16	30	5.0	400	2.4	90
% RDA/100 g	0–11	0–100	2–20	1–20	2–38	5–60	1–50	3–33	2–20	0.3–12	40–100	0
% RDA/Md	2	50	7	5	15	25	18	5	8	2	100	0

Tr, trace; RDA, recommended dietary allowance; Md, Mediterranean diet.
Reproduced with permission from Ariño A, Beltran JA, and Roncalés P (2003) Dietary importance of fish and shellfish. In: Caballero B, Trugo L, and Finglas P (eds.) *Encyclopedia of Food Sciences and Nutrition*, 2nd edn. Oxford: Elsevier Science Ltd. pp. 2471–2478.

Table 8 Selected mineral content of the different groups of fish and shellfish (mg per 100 g)

	Na	K	Ca	Mg	P	Fe	Zn	Mn	Cu	Se	Cr	Mo	I
White finfish	50–150	200–500	10–50	15–30	100–300	0.2–0.6	0.2–1.0	0.01–0.05	0.01–0.05	0.02–0.1	0.005–0.02	0.005–0.02	0.01–0.5
Fatty finfish	50–200	200–500	10–200	20–50	200–500	1.0–5.0	0.2–1.0	0.01–0.05	0.01–0.05	0.02–0.1	0.005–0.02	0.005–0.02	0.01–0.5
Crustaceans	100–500	100–500	20–200	20–200	100–700	0.2–2.0	1.0–5.0	0.02–0.2	0.1–2.0	0.05–0.1	0.005–0.02	0.01–0.05	0.01–0.2
Molluscs	50–300	100–500	50–200	20–200	100–300	0.5–10	2.0–10	0.02–0.2	0.02–10	0.05–0.1	0.005–0.02	0.01–0.2	0.05–0.5
Cephalopods	100–200	200–300	10–100	20–100	100–300	0.2–1.0	1.0–5.0	0.01–0.1	0.02–0.1	0.02–0.1	0.005–0.02	0.01–0.2	0.01–0.1
RDA			1000	420	700	8	11	2.3	0.9	0.055	0.035	0.045	0.15
% RDA/100 g			1–20	4–50	15–100	2–50	1–90	0–10	1–100	25–100	15–60	10–100	8–100
% RDA/Md			6	5	30	18	2		2	100			100

RDA, recommended dietary allowance; Md, Mediterranean diet.

Reproduced with permission from Ariño A, Beltran JA, and Roncalés P (2003) Dietary importance of fish and shellfish. In: Caballero B, Trugo L, and Finglas P (eds.) *Encyclopedia of Food Sciences and Nutrition*, 2nd edn. Oxford: Elsevier Science Ltd. pp. 2471–2478.

are particularly abundant in crustaceans; fatty finfish show elevated levels of phosphorus, and bivalve molluscs have high amounts of magnesium.

Fish is a highly valuable source of most oligoelements. Fatty fish provides a notable contribution to iron supply, similar to that of meat, whereas shellfish have higher concentrations of most dietary minerals. In particular, crustaceans and bivalve molluscs supply zinc, manganese, and copper concentrations well above those of finfish. Worth mentioning is the extraordinary dietary supply of iodine in all kinds of finfish and shellfish; however, this depends on the concentration present in feed, particularly in planktonic organisms.

In summary, 100 g of fish affords low levels of sodium and medium-to-high levels of all the remaining dietary minerals. In fact, it can contribute 50–100% of the total daily requirements of magnesium, phosphorus, iron, copper, selenium, and iodine. A Mediterranean diet, rich in fatty fish and all kinds of shellfish, can lead to an overall balanced mineral supply, which may well reach over 20% of daily requirements of phosphorus, iron, selenium, and iodine.

See also: **Coronary Heart Disease**: Prevention. **Fatty Acids**: Omega-3 Polyunsaturated. **Iodine**: Physiology, Dietary Sources and Requirements. **Supplementation**: Dietary Supplements.

Further Reading

Ackman RG (1995) Composition and nutritive value of fish and shellfish lipids. In: Ruiter A (ed.) *Fish and Fishery Products: Composition, Nutritive Properties and Stability*, pp. 117–156. Wallingford: CAB International.

Ariño A, Beltran JA, and Roncalés P (2003) Dietary importance of fish and shellfish. In: Caballero B, Trugo L, and Finglas P (eds.) *Encyclopedia of Food Sciences and Nutrition*, 2nd edn., pp. 2471–2478. Oxford: Elsevier Science Ltd.

Exler J (1987, updated 1992) *Composition of Foods: Finfish and Shellfish Products, Human Nutrition Information Service Agriculture Handbook 8-15* Washington DC: US Department of Agriculture.

Food and Agriculture Organization of the United Nations (1989) *Yield and Nutritional Value of the Commercially More Important Species. FAO Fisheries Technical Paper 309. Rome: Food and Agriculture Organization.*

Food and Drug Administration (1989) *The Fish List, FDA Guide to Acceptable Market Names for Food Fish Sold in Interstate Commerce 1988.* Washington DC: US Government Printing Office.

Haard NF (1995) Composition and nutritive value of fish proteins and other nitrogen compounds. In: Ruiter A (ed.) *Fish and Fishery Products: Composition, Nutritive Properties and Stability*, pp. 77–115. Wallingford: CAB International.

Holland B, Brown J, and Buss DH (1993) Fish and fish products. In: *Supplement to the 5th Edition of McCance and Widdowson's The Composition of Foods*. London: The Royal Society of Chemistry and Ministry of Agriculture, Fisheries and Food.

Huss HH (1995) *Quality and Quality Changes in Fresh Fish*, FAO Fisheries Technical Paper 348. Rome: Food and Agriculture Organization.

Lands WEM (1988) *Fish and Human Health* Orlando, FL: Academic Press.

Lovell RT (1989) *Nutrition and Feeding of Fish* New York: Van Nostrand Reinhold.

National Fisheries Institute. http://www.nfi.org.

Nettleton JA (1993) *Omega-3 Fatty Acids and Health* New York: Chapman & Hall.

Southgate DAT (2000) Meat, fish, eggs and novel protein. In: Garrow JS, James WPT, and Ralph A (eds.) *Human Nutrition and Dietetics*, 10th edn. Edinburgh: Churchill Livingstone.

United States Department of Agriculture. Composition of foods. http://www.nal.usda.gov/fnic/foodcomp.

Valdimarsson G and James D (2001) World fisheries – utilisation of catches. *Ocean and Coastal Management* 44: 619–633.

FOLIC ACID

J McPartlin, Trinity College, Dublin, Ireland

Introduction

Folic acid was initially distinguished from vitamin B_{12} as a dietary anti-anemia factor by Wills in the 1930s. The subsequent chemical isolation of folic acid and the identification of its role as a cofactor in one-carbon metabolism led to the elucidation of deficiency diseases at the molecular level. The term 'folate' encompasses the entire group of folate vitamin forms, comprising the naturally occurring folylpolyglutamates found in food and folic acid (pteroylglutamic acid), the synthetic form of the vitamin added as a dietary supplement to foodstuffs. 'Folate' is thus the general term used for any form of the vitamin irrespective of the state of reduction, type of substitution, or degree of polyglutamylation.

Folate functions metabolically as an enzyme cofactor in the synthesis of nucleic acids and amino-acids. Deficiency of the vitamin leads to impaired cell replication and other metabolic alterations, particularly related to methionine synthesis. The similar clinical manifestations of cobalamin deficiency and folate deficiency underline the metabolic interrelationship between the two vitamins. Folate deficiency, manifested clinically as megaloblastic anemia, is the most common vitamin deficiency in developed countries. Much attention has focused recently on a number of diseases for which the risks are inversely related to folate status even within the range of blood indicators previously considered 'normal.' Food-fortification programs introduced to prevent neural-tube defects (NTD) have proved effective in increasing folate intakes in populations and may be shown potentially to reduce the risk of cardiovascular disease.

Physiology and Biochemistry

Chemistry and Biochemical Functions

Folic acid (**Figure 1**) consists of a pterin moiety linked via a methylene group to a para-aminobenzoylglutamate moiety. Folic acid is the synthetic form of the vitamin; its metabolic activity requires reduction to the tetrahydrofolic acid (THF) derivative, addition of a chain of glutamate residues in γ-peptide linkage, and acquisition of one-carbon units.

One-carbon units at various levels of oxidation are generated metabolically and are reactive only as moieties attached to the N5 and/or N10 positions of the folate molecule (**Table 1**).

The range of oxidation states for folate one-carbon units extends from methanol to formate as methyl, methylene, methenyl, formyl, or formimino moieties. When one-carbon units are incorporated into folate derivatives, they may be converted from one oxidation state to another by the gain or loss of electrons.

The source of one-carbon units for folate   One-carbon units at the oxidation level of formate can enter

Table 1 Structure and nomenclature of folate compounds (see **Figure 1**)

Compound	R	Oxidation state
5-formylTHF	—CHO	Formate
10-formylTHF	—CHO	Formate
5-formiminoTHF	—CH=NH	Formate
5,10-methenylTHF	—CH=	Formate
5,10-methyleneTHF	—CH$_2$—	Formaldehyde
5-methylTHF	—CH$_3$	Methanol

directly into the folate pool as formic acid in a reaction catalyzed by 10-formylTHF synthase (**Figure 2**). Entry at the formate level of oxidation can also take place via a catabolic product of histidine, formaminoglutamic acid. The third mode of entry at the formate level of oxidation involves the formation of 5-formylTHF from 5,10-methenylTHF by the enzyme serine hydroxymethyl transferase (SHMT). The 5-formylTHF may be rapidly converted to other forms of folate.

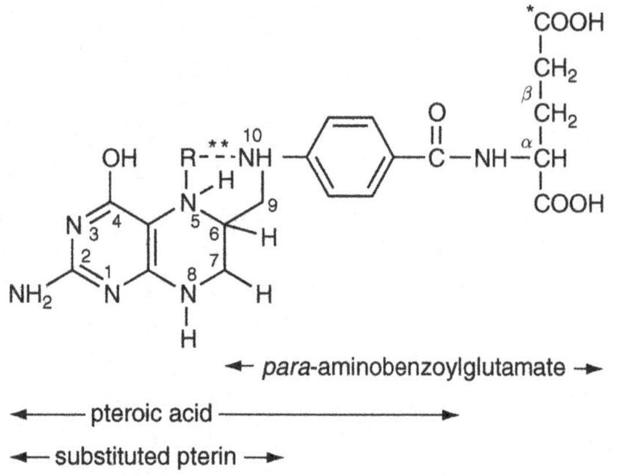

The enzyme SHMT is involved in the entry of one-carbon units at the formaldehyde level of oxidation by catalyzing the transfer of the β-carbon of serine to form glycine and 5,10-methyleneTHF. Other sources of one-carbon entry at this level of oxidation include the glycine cleavage system and the choline-dependent pathway; both enzyme systems generate 5,10-methylene in the mitochondria of the cell.

The removal and use of one-carbon units from folate   Single-carbon units are removed from folate by a number of reactions. The enzyme 10-formylTHF dehydrogenase provides a mechanism for disposing of excess one-carbon units as carbon dioxide. (Folate administration to animals enhances the conversion of ingested methanol and formate to carbon dioxide, diminishing methanol toxicity.) Additionally, single-carbon units from 10-formylTHF are used for the biosynthesis of purines (**Figure 2**).

The one-carbon unit of 5,10-methyleneTHF is transferred in two ways. Reversal of the SHMT reaction produces serine from glycine, but since serine is also produced from glycolysis via phosphoglycerate this reaction is unlikely to be important. However, one-carbon transfer from 5,10-methyleneTHF to deoxyuridylate to form thymidylic acid, a precursor of DNA, is of crucial importance to the cell. While the source of the one-carbon unit, namely 5,10-methyleneTHF, is at the formaldehyde level of oxidation, the one-carbon unit transferred to form thymidylic acid appears at the methanol level of oxidation. Electrons for this reduction come from THF itself to generate dihydrofolate as a product. The dihydrofolate must in turn be reduced back to THF in order to accept further one-carbon units.

Figure 1 Structural formula of tetrahydrofolate (THF) compounds. In tetrahydrofolic acid R = H; other substituents are listed in **Table 1**. The asterisk indicates the site of attachment of extra glutamate residues; the hatched line and double asterisk indicates the N5 and/or N10 site of attachment of one-carbon units.

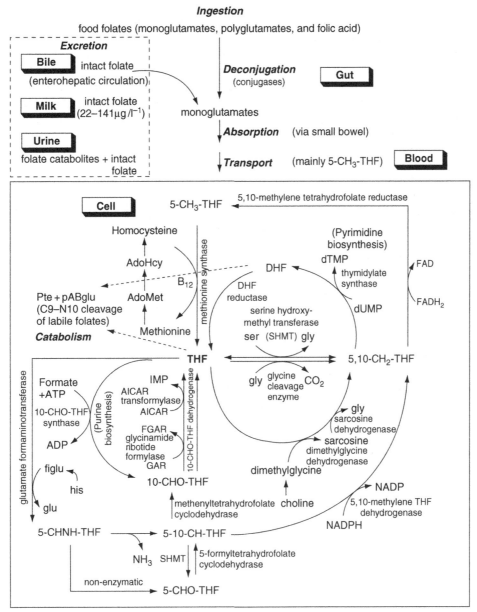

Figure 2 Physiology and metabolism of folate. GAR, glycinamide ribonucleotide; FGAR, formylglycinamide ribonucleotide; AICAR: aminoimidazolecarboxamide ribonucleotide; figlu, formiminoglutamic acid; IMP, inosine monophosphate.

A solitary transfer of one-carbon units takes place at the methanol level of oxidation. It involves the transfer of the methyl group from 5-methylTHF to homocysteine to form methionine and THF. This reaction is catalyzed by the enzyme methionine synthase and requires vitamin B_{12} as a cofactor. The substance 5-methylTHF is the dominant folate in the body, and it remains metabolically inactive until it is demethylated to THF, whereupon polyglutamylation takes place to allow subsequent folate-dependent reactions to proceed efficiently.

Clinical implications of methionine synthase inhibition The inhibition of methionine synthase due to vitamin B_{12} deficiency induces megaloblastic anemia that is clinically indistinguishable from that caused by folate deficiency. The hematological effect in both cases results in levels of 5,10-methyleneTHF that are inadequate to sustain thymidylate biosynthesis. Clinically, it is essential to ascertain whether the anemia is the result of folate deficiency or vitamin B_{12} deficiency by differential diagnostic techniques. Vitamin B_{12} is essential for the synthesis of myelin in nerve tissue, a function probably related to methionine production from the methionine synthase reaction and the subsequent formation of S-adenosyl-methionine. Hence, vitamin B_{12} deficiency probably leads to nervous disorders in addition to the hematological effects. While the latter respond to treatment with folic acid, the neurological effects do not. Thus, inappropriate administration of folic acid in patients with vitamin B_{12} deficiency may treat the anemia but mask the progression of the neurological defects. Where possible, vitamin B_{12} and folate statuses should be checked before giving folate supplements to treat megaloblastic anemia. The main objection to fortifying food with folate is the potential to mask vitamin B_{12} deficiency in the elderly, who are most prone to it.

In summary, the biochemical function of folate coenzymes is to transfer and use these one-carbon units in a variety of essential reactions (**Figure 2**), including *de novo* purine biosynthesis (formylation of glycinamide ribonucleotide and 5-amino-4-imidazole carboxamide ribonucleotide), pyrimidine nucleotide biosynthesis (methylation of deoxyuridylic acid to thymidylic acid), amino-acid interconversions (the interconversion of serine to glycine, catabolism of histidine to glutamic acid, and conversion of homocysteine to methionine (which also requires vitamin B_{12})), and the generation and use of formate.

Many of the enzymes involved in these reactions are multifunctional and are capable of channelling substrates and one-carbon units from reaction to reaction within a protein matrix. Another feature of intracellular folate metabolism is the compartmentation of folate coenzymes between the cytosol and the mitochondria. For instance, 5-methylTHF is associated with the cytosolic fraction of the cell, whereas most of 10-formylTHF is located in the mitochondria. Similarly, some folate-dependent enzymes are associated with one or other compartment, though some are found in both. Metabolic products of folate-dependent reactions, such as serine and glycine, are readily transported between the two locations, but the folate coenzymes are not.

Folate Deficiency and Hyperhomocysteinemia An important consequence of folate deficiency is the inability to remethylate homocysteine (**Figure 2**). Indeed, there is an inverse correlation between the levels of folate and those of homocysteine in the blood of humans. Many clinical studies, beginning with the observations of children with homocysteinuria presenting with vascular abnormalities and thromboembolism, have demonstrated an association between hyperhomocysteinemia and an increased risk of premature atherosclerosis in the coronary, carotid, and peripheral vasculatures. Even mild hyperhomocysteinemia is recognized to be an independent risk factor for cardiovascular disease. The risk of heart disease was found to increase proportionately in most, but not all, studies, throughout the full of range of blood homocysteine concentrations. An increase in plasma homocysteine of $5\,\mu mol\,l^{-1}$ is associated with a combined odds ratio of 1.3 for cardiovascular disease. Plasma homocysteine is usually shown to be a greater risk factor for cardiovascular disease in prospective studies than in retrospective studies, probably because the populations in the former studies are older. Metabolically, homocysteine may be disposed of by the methionine synthase reaction (dependent on folate and vitamin B_{12}), the transsulfuration pathway (dependent on vitamin B_6), and the choline degradation pathway. Marginal deficiencies of these three vitamins are associated with hyperhomocysteinemia. Of the three vitamins, however, folic acid has been shown to be the most effective in lowering levels of homocysteine in the blood. Convincing evidence of the potential role of folate intake in the prevention of vascular disease has come from a significant inverse relationship between serum folate levels and fatal coronary heart disease. While most studies have focused on the homocysteine-lowering effects of folate, other benefits have also been reported. Potential mechanisms include antioxidant actions and interactions with the enzyme endothelial nitric oxide synthase.

Absorption of Folates

Food folates mainly consist of reduced polyglutamates, which are hydrolyzed to monoglutamates in the gut prior to absorption across the intestinal mucosa. The conjugase enzyme that hydrolyzes dietary folates has been found on the luminal brush border membrane in the human jejunum and has equal affinity for polyglutamates of various chain lengths. Transport is facilitated by a saturable carrier-mediated uptake system, although changes in luminal pH and the presence of conjugase inhibitors, folate binders, or other food components can adversely affect the rate of hydrolysis and intestinal absorption. Such factors account for the wide variation in the bioavailability of the vitamin from foods of plant and animal origins. Some metabolism of the resultant monoglutamate, mainly to 5-methylTHF, appears to occur during the absorption process, though this may not be necessary for transport across the basolateral membrane of the intestinal mucosa into the portal circulation. The degree of metabolic conversion of dietary folic acid depends on the dose; pharmacological amounts are transported unaltered into the circulation.

Transport in the Circulation, Cellular Uptake, and Turnover

Folate circulates in the blood predominantly as 5-methylTHF. A variable proportion circulates freely or bound either to low-affinity protein binders such as albumin, which accounts for about 50% of bound folate, or to a high-affinity folate binder in serum, which carries less than 5% of circulating folate. The physiological importance of serum binders is unclear, but they may control folate distribution and excretion during deficiency.

Though most folate is initially taken up by the liver following absorption, it is delivered to a wide variety of tissues in which many types of folate transporters have been described. Because these transporters have affinities for folate in the micromolar range, they would not be saturated by normal ambient concentrations of folate. Therefore, folate uptake into tissues should be responsive to any increases in serum folate levels arising from folate supplementation. An important determinant of folate uptake into cells is their mitotic activity, as would be expected given the dependence of DNA biosynthesis on folate coenzyme function. Folate accumulation is more rapid in actively dividing cells than in quiescent cells, a factor that is probably related to the induction and activity of folylpoly-γ-glutamate synthase. This enzyme catalyzes the addition of glutamate by γ-peptide linkage to the initial glutamate moiety of the folate molecule. Although polyglutamate derivatization may be considered a storage strategem, this elongation is the most efficient coenzyme form for normal one-carbon metabolism. The activity of folylpoly-γ-glutamate synthase is highest in the liver, the folate stores of which account for half of the estimated 5–10 mg adult complement. Retention within the cell is facilitated by the high proportion of folate associated with proteins, and this is likely to be increased in folate deficiency.

The mobilization of liver and other stores in the body is not well understood, particularly in deficiency states, though some accounts describe poor turnover rates in folate-depleted rats. Transport across cell membranes during redistribution requires deconjugation of the large negatively charged polyglutamates. Mammalian γ-glutamylhydrolases that hydrolyze glutamate moieties residue by residue and transpeptidases that can hydrolyze folylpolyglutamates directly to mono- or di-glutamate forms of the vitamin have been described for a number of tissues. Thus, mammalian cells possess two types of enzyme that can play a key role in folate homeostasis and regulation of one-carbon metabolism: the folylpolyglutamate synthetase that catalyzes the synthesis of retentive and active folate, and a number of deconjugating enzymes that promote the release of folate from the cell. Polyglutamate forms released into the circulation either through cell death or by a possible exocytotic mechanism would be hydrolyzed rapidly by plasma γ-glutamyl-hydrolase to the monoglutamate form.

Catabolism and Excretion

Folate is concentrated in bile, and enterohepatic recirculation from the intestine accounts for considerable re-absorption and reuse of folate (about $100\,\mu g\,day^{-1}$). Fecal folates mostly arise through biosynthesis of the vitamin by the gut microflora, with only a small contribution from unabsorbed dietary folate. Urinary excretion of intact folates accounts for only a small fraction of ingested folate under normal physiological conditions. The greater amount of excretion in urine is accounted for by products that arise from cleavage of the folate molecule at the C9–N10 bond, consisting of one or more pteridines and p-acetamido-benzoylglutamate. The rate of scission of the folate molecule increases during rapid-mitotic conditions such as pregnancy and rapid growth. Scission of folate is perhaps the major mechanism of folate turnover in the body.

Human Folate Requirements

The folate requirement is the minimum amount necessary to prevent deficiency. Dietary recommendations for populations, however, must allow a margin of safety to cover the needs of the vast majority of the population. As is the case with most nutrients, the margin of safety for folate requirement corresponds to two standard deviations above the mean requirement for a population and should therefore meet the needs of 97.5% of the population. Thus, international dietary recommendations contain allowances for individual variability, the bioavailability of folate from different foodstuffs, and periods of low intake and increased use. Current international folate recommendations for FAO/WHO, USA/Canada, and the European Union are listed in **Table 2**.

Table 2 Recommended dietary folate allowances for various population groups (μg day^{-1})

Category	Age	FAO/WHO (1998)	USA/Canada RDA (1998)	EU (1993)
Infants	Up to 6 months	80	65	100
	6 months–1 year	80	80	100
	1–3 years	160	150	100
Children	4–6 years	200	200	130
	7–10 years	300 (age 9–13 years)	300	150
Males	11–14 years	400	300	180
	15–18 years	400	400	200
	19–24 years	400	400	200
	25–50 years	400	400	200
	Over 50 years	400	400	200
Females	11–14 years	400	300	180
	15–18 years	400	400	200
	19–24 years	400	400	200
	25–50 years	400	400	200
	Over 50 years	400	400	200
Pregnant women		600	600	400
Lactating women		500	500	350

The 1998 recommendations for folate are expressed using a term called the dietary folate equivalent (DFE). The DFE was developed to help account for the difference in bioavailability between naturally occurring dietary folate and synthetic folic acid. The Food and Nutrition Board of the US National Academy of Sciences reasoned that, since folic acid in supplements or in fortified food is 85% bioavailable, but food folate is only about 50% bioavailable, folic acid taken as supplements or in fortified food is 85/50 (i.e., 1.7) times more available. Thus, the calculation of the DFE for a mixture of synthetic folic acid and food is μg of DFE = μg food folate + (1.7 × μg synthetic folate).

International recommendation tables are constantly subject to review, particularly in view of the relationship between folate status and the risk of NTD and specific chronic diseases including coronary artery disease and colorectal cancer.

Pregnancy

The crucial role of folate in the biosynthesis of precursors for DNA suggests that folate requirements may vary with age, though folate use is most obviously increased during pregnancy and lactation. Maintaining adequate folate status in women in their child-bearing years is particularly important since a large proportion of pregnancies are unplanned and many women are likely to be unaware of their pregnancy during the first crucial weeks of fetal development. Pregnancy requires an increase in folate supply that is large enough to fulfil considerable mitotic requirements related to fetal growth, uterine expansion, placental maturation, and expanded blood volume. The highest prevalence of poor folate status in pregnant women occurs among the lowest socioeconomic groups and is often exacerbated by the higher parity rate of these women. Indeed, the megaloblastic anemia commonly found amongst the malnourished poor during pregnancy probably reflects the depletion of maternal stores to the advantage of the fetal–placental unit, as indicated by the several-fold higher serum folate levels in the newborn compared with the mother. Considerable evidence indicates that maternal folate deficiency leads to fetal growth retardation and low birth weight. The higher incidence of low-birth-weight infants among teenage mothers compared with their adult counterparts is probably related to the additional burden that adolescent growth places on folate resources.

The lack of hard evidence about the extent of supplementation required in pregnancy prompted the development of a laboratory-based assessment of metabolic turnover, which involved the assay of total daily folate catabolites (along with intact folate) in the urine of pregnant women. The rationale of the procedure was that this catabolic product represents an ineluctable daily loss of folate, the replacement of which should constitute the daily requirement. Correcting for individual variation in catabolite excretion and the bioavailability of dietary folate, the recommended allowances based on this mode of assessment are in close agreement with the latest recommendations of the USA/Canada and FAO/WHO. The data produced by the catabolite-excretion method may provide a useful adjunct to current methods based on intakes, clinical examination, and blood folate measurements to provide a more accurate assessment of requirement.

Folate and Neural-Tube Defects

Much attention has focused over the past 15 years on a number of diseases for which the risks are inversely related to folate status even within the range of serum folate levels previously considered 'normal.' Foremost among these is NTD, a malformation in the developing embryo that is related to a failure of the neural tube to close properly during the fourth week of embryonic life. Incomplete closure of the spinal cord results in spina bifida, while incomplete closure of the cranium results in anencephaly. The risk of NTD was found to be 10-fold higher (6 affected pregnancies per 1000) in people with poor folate status (i.e., less than 150 µg red cell folate per litre) than in those with good folate status (400 µg l^{-1}). International agencies have published folic acid recommendations for the prevention of NTD. To prevent recurrence, 5 mg of folic acid daily in tablet form is recommended, while 400 µg daily is recommended for the prevention of occurrence, to be commenced prior to conception and continued until the 12th week of pregnancy. Given the high proportion of unplanned pregnancies, the latter recommendations are applicable to all fertile women. This amount, however, could not be introduced through fortification because high intakes of folic acid by people consuming fortified flour products would risk preventing the diagnosis of pernicious anemia in the general population and of vitamin B$_{12}$ deficiency in the elderly.

The introduction of 140 µg of folic acid per 100 g of flour in the USA, calculated to increase individual consumption of folic acid by 100 µg day^{-1}, has reduced the incidence of abnormally low plasma folate from 21% to less than 2%, the incidence of mild hyperhomocysteinemia from 21% to 10%, and, most importantly, the incidence of NTD by about 20% over the first years of universal fortification. Because 30% of the population takes vitamin supplements and presumably would not be expected to derive significant benefit from fortification, the actual effect may be closer to a 30% decrease due to fortification. Recent calculations suggest that, for a variety of reasons, the overall fortification amount was about twice the mandatory amount.

On balance, the introduction of food fortification with folate is regarded as beneficial not only in preventing NTD but also in reducing the incidences of hyperhomocysteinemia (mentioned earlier), colorectal cancer, and a number of neurological and neuropsychiatric diseases in which folate is postulated to play a protective role.

Lactation

Unlike during pregnancy, in which the bulk of folate expenditure arises through catabolism, during lactation the increased requirement is chiefly due to milk secretion. Several observations indicate that mammary tissue takes precedence over other maternal tissues for folate resources. For instance, maternal folate status deteriorates in both early and late lactation, but milk folate concentration is maintained or increased. Moreover, supplemental folate appears to be taken up by mammary epithelial cells preferentially over hematopoietic cells in lactating women with folate deficiency, indicating that maternal reserves are depleted to maintain milk folate content in lactating women. Recommendations are based on the maintenance requirement of nonpregnant nonlactating women and the estimated folate intake required to replace the quantity lost in milk. This increment of between 60 µg and 100 µg daily is based on a milk secretion rate of 40–60 µg l^{-1} and an absorption rate from dietary sources of between 50% and 70%. The official recommendations might be underestimated, however. On the one hand, a less efficient absorption rate of 50% from a mixed diet is more likely, and, on the other hand, the most recent estimations of milk folate secretion are as high as 100 µg daily. Therefore, an additional 200 µg of folate daily or a total of 500 µg daily seems a more realistic recommended amount for lactating women.

Infants and Children

The high concentration of circulating folate in newborn infants coincides with the rapid rate of cell division in the first few months of life and is reflected in the higher folate requirement for infants on a weight basis than for adults. Though the recommendation standards (see **Table 2**) may underestimate the quantities consumed by many breastfed infants, intake is generally sufficiently above the recommendations that folate deficiency is unlikely.

Data on requirements for older children are sparse, so recommendations for up to adolescence are based on interpolations between the values for very young children and those for adults. Daily recommended levels are above 3.6 µg per kg of body weight, an amount associated with no overt folate deficiency in children and shown to maintain plasma folate concentrations at a low but acceptable level.

Adolescents and Adults

Folate recommendations for adolescents are set at a similar level to that for adults, the smaller weights of adolescents being compensated for by higher rates of growth.

The Elderly

Although folate deficiency occurs more frequently in the elderly than in young adults, recommendations are set at the same level for both groups. Reference recommendations apply to healthy subjects. However, a significant proportion of the elderly are likely to suffer from clinical conditions and to be exposed to a range of factors such as chronic smoking, alcohol, and prescription drugs that may have a detrimental effect on folate status.

Food Sources of Folate

Folate is synthesized by microorganisms and higher plants but not by mammals, for which it is an essential vitamin. The most concentrated food folate sources include liver, yeast extract, green leafy vegetables, legumes, certain fruits, and fortified breakfast cereals. Folate content is likely to depend on the maturity and variety of particular sources. Foods that contain a high concentration of folate are not necessarily those that contribute most to the overall intakes of the vitamin in a population. For example, liver is a particularly concentrated source, providing 320 µg of folate per 100 g, but it is not eaten by a sufficient proportion of the population to make any major contribution to total dietary folate intakes. The potato, on the other hand, although not particularly rich in folate, is considered a major contributor to folate in the UK diet, accounting for 14% of total folate intake because of its high consumption. Prolonged exposure to heat, air, or ultraviolet light is known to inactivate the vitamin; thus, food preparation and cooking can make a difference to the amount of folate ingested; boiling in particular results in substantial food losses. The major source of folate loss from vegetables during boiling may be leaching as opposed to folate degradation. Broccoli and spinach are particularly susceptible to loss through leaching during boiling compared with potatoes because of their larger surface areas. The retention of folate during cooking depends on the food in question as well as the method of cooking. Folates of animal origin are stable during cooking by frying or grilling. In addition to highlighting good food

Table 3 Contributions of the main food groups to the average daily intake of folate in British and US adults (%)

Food group	USA (1994)	UK (1998)
Dairy products	8.1	9.8
Meat, poultry, fish	8.5	6.5
Grain products	21.2[a]	31.8
Fruit, fruit juices	10.2	6.9
Vegetables	26.4	31.8
Legumes, nuts, soy	18.5	—
Eggs	5.1	2.4
Tea	—	4.1
Other food	2.1	5.7

[a]Prior to mandatory fortification of flour-based products.

sources, public-health measures promoting higher folate intake should include practical advice on cooking. For example, steaming in preference to boiling is likely to double the amount of folate consumed from green vegetables.

While cultural differences and local eating habits determine the contribution of different foodstuffs to folate intake (**Table 3**), as with other nutrients, globalization and the integration of the international food industry may lead to more predictable 'Westernized' diets in the developed and developing world. Internationally, much of the dietary folate in the 'Western' diet currently comes from fortified breakfast cereals, though this foodstuff is likely to be joined shortly in this regard by fortified flour products in the light of the experience of the US food fortification program. In the main, though, adherence to dietary recommendations to increase the consumption of folate-rich foods is likely to enhance the intake not only of folate but also of other nutrients essential to health.

See also: **Amino Acids**: Specific Functions.

Further Reading

Bailey LB (ed.) (1995) *Folate in Health and Disease*. New York: Marcel Dekker.

Blakley R (1969) The biochemistry of folic acid and related pteridines. In: Newbergen H and Taton EL (eds.) *North Holland Research Monographs Frontiers of Biology*, vol. 13, Amsterdam: North Holland Publishing Company.

Boushey CJ, Beresford SA, Omenn GS, and Motulsky AG (1995) A quantitative assessment of plasma homocysteine as a risk factor for vascular disease. *JAMA* 274: 1049–1057.

Chanarin I (1979) *The Megaloblastic Anaemias*, 2nd edn. Oxford: Blackwell Scientific Publications.

Duthie SJ (1999) Folic acid deficiency and cancer: mechanisms of DNA instability. *British Medical Bulletin* 55: 578–592.

Homocysteine Lowering Trialists' Collaboration (1998) Lowering blood homocysteine with folic acid based supplements: meta-analysis of randomised trials. *BMJ* **316**: 894–898.

National Academy of Sciences (1998) *Dietary Reference Intakes: Folate, other B Vitamins and Choline.* Wasington, DC: National Academy Press.

Refsum H, Ueland PM, Bygard MD, and Vollset SE (1998) Homocysteine and cardiovascular disease. *Annual Review of Medicine* **49**: 31–62.

Reynolds EH (2002) Folic acid, ageing, depression, and dementia. *BMJ* **324**: 1512–1515.

Scott JM and Weir DG (1994) Folate/vitamin B$_{12}$ interrelationships. *Essays in Biochemistry* **28**: 63–72.

UK Department of Health (2000) *Folic Acid and the Prevention of Disease. Report of the Committee on Medical Aspects of Food and Nutritional Policy.* Norwich: Her Majesty's Stationary Office.

FUNCTIONAL FOODS

Health Effects and Clinical Applications

L Galland, Applied Nutrition Inc., New York, NY, USA

Introduction

Functional foods are foods with health benefits that exceed those attributable to the nutritional value of the food. The term is usually applied to foods that have been modified or combined in order to enhance the health benefits but may include any food that naturally possesses components with demonstrable pharmacologic activity. Functional foods are most often selected because they contain ingredients with immune-modulating, antioxidant, anti-inflammatory, antitoxic, or ergogenic effects. The most widely studied functional ingredients are plant-derived phenolic chemicals, probiotic bacteria, and fiber or other poorly digested carbohydrates, but colostrum, egg yolk, and other nonplant foods may also serve as functional food sources. Although pharmacologic activity of most of these substances is well established *in vitro* or in small mammals, establishing clinical effects in humans poses a challenge for functional food research.

Concept and Definition

The concept of functional foods derives from the observation that certain foods and beverages exert beneficial effects on human health that are not explained by their nutritional content (i.e., macronutrients, vitamins, and minerals). The definition of functional foods varies among countries for reasons that are historical, cultural, and regulatory. In its broadest use, functional foods are food-derived products that, in addition to their nutritional value, enhance normal physiological or cognitive functions or prevent the abnormal function that underlies disease. A hierarchy of restrictions narrows the definition. In most countries, a functional food must take the form of a food or beverage, not a medication, and should be consumed the way a conventional food or beverage is consumed. If the ingredients are incorporated into pills, sachets, or other dosage forms they are considered dietary supplements or nutraceuticals, not functional foods. In Japan and Australia, the functional food appellation has been applied only to food that is modified for the purpose of enhancing its health benefits; in China, Europe, and North America, any natural or preserved food that enhances physiological function or prevents disease might be considered a functional food. If food is modified, there is lack of international consensus as to whether a vitamin or mineral-enriched food (e.g., folate-fortified flour or calcium-fortified orange juice) should be considered a functional food, or whether functional foods are described by the presence of their nonnutritive components (e.g., fiber or polyphenols). Future development of functional foods is likely to be driven by scientific research rather than government regulation, so it is likely that the concept (if not the definition) of functional foods will remain fluid and flexible.

History

If the broadest, least restrictive definition is employed, the use of functional foods for promoting health and relieving symptoms is as old as the practice of medicine. Specific dietary recommendations for treating or preventing various types of illness have been documented in Hippocratic and Vedic texts and the canons of traditional Chinese medicine. Traditional Chinese remedies frequently contain recipes for combining specific foods with culinary and nonculinary herbs to produce healing mixtures. Folk medicine, East and West, has always depended upon functional foods. Peppermint (*Mentha piperita*) tea has a long history of use for digestive complaints. Peppermint oil contains spasmolytic components that block calcium channels in smooth muscle. Cranberry (*Vaccinium macrocarpon*) juice contains proanthocyanidins that inhibit the attachment of *E.coli* to the epithelium of the urinary bladder, explaining its efficacy in prevention of bacterial cystitis and its traditional use for treatment of urinary infection.

Herbs and spices are added to food to enhance flavor and initially were used to inhibit spoilage. Many of these have documented medicinal uses that render them functional foods, broadly defined. Thyme (*Lamiaceae* spp.) was used to treat worms in ancient Egypt. Thyme oils possess potent antimicrobial properties. Ginger (*Zingiber officinale* root), cinnamon (*Cinnamomum* spp. bark), and licorice (*Glycyrrhiza glabra* root) are common ingredients in Chinese herbal tonics and have been widely used in Western folk medicine for treating digestive disorders. Ginger contains over four hundred biologically active constituents. Some have antimicrobial, anti-inflammatory, or anti-platelet effects; others enhance intestinal motility, protect the intestinal mucosa against ulceration and dilate or constrict blood vessels. Cinnamon oil contains cinnamaldehyde and various phenols and terpenes with antifungal, antidiarrheal, vasoactive, and analgesic effects. Recent research has identified phenolic polymers in cinnamon with actions that increase the sensitivity of cells to insulin, leading to the recognition that regular consumption of cinnamon may help to prevent type 2 diabetes. The most studied component of licorice, glycyrrhizin, inhibits the enzyme11 beta-hydroxysteroid dehydrogenase type 2, potentiating the biological activity of endogenous cortisol. Glycyrrhizin also inhibits the growth of *Helicobacter pylori*. Glycyrrhizin and its derivatives may account for the anti-inflammatory and anti-ulcerogenic effects of licorice.

Fermentation is a form of food modification initially developed for preservation. The health-enhancing effects of fermented foods have a place in folk medicine. Several fermented foods have health benefits that exceed those of their parent foods and can be considered functional foods, broadly defined. These include red wine, yogurt, and tempeh. Red wine is a whole fruit alcohol extract that concentrates polyphenols found primarily in the seed and skin of the grape. Its consumption is associated with protection against heart disease, perhaps because red

wine polyphenols inhibit the production of free radicals and lipid peroxides that result from the simultaneous ingestion of cooked meat. Fresh yogurt contains live cultures of lactic acid-producing bacteria that can prevent the development of traveler's diarrhea, antibiotic-induced diarrhea, rotavirus infection, and vaginal yeast infection, decrease the incidence of postoperative wound infection following abdominal surgery and restore the integrity of the intestinal mucosa of patients who have received radiation therapy. Tempeh is made from dehulled, cooked soy beans fermented by the fungus *Rhizopus oligosporus*. Not only is its protein content higher than the parent soy bean, but it also has antibiotic activity *in vitro* and the ability to shorten childhood diarrhea *in vivo*.

Modification of a food to make it less harmful by removing potential toxins or allergens may create a functional food. Using this criterion, infant formula, protein hydrolysates, low-sodium salt substitutes, low-fat dairy products, and low-erucic-acid rapeseed oil (canola oil) might be considered functional foods.

If the most restrictive definition of functional foods is employed, the functional food movement began in Japan during the 1980s, when the Japanese government launched three major research initiatives designed to identify health-enhancing foods to control the rising cost of medical care. In 1991, a regulatory framework, Foods for Special Health Uses (FOSHU), was implemented, identifying those ingredients expected to have specific health benefits when added to common foods, or identifying foods from which allergens had been removed. FOSHU products were to be in the form of ordinary food (not pills or sachets) and consumed regularly as part of the diet. Initially, 11 categories of ingredients were identified for which sufficient scientific evidence indicated beneficial health effects. The Japanese Ministry of Health recognized foods containing these ingredients as functional foods. They were intended to improve intestinal function, reduce blood lipids and blood pressure, enhance calcium or iron absorption, or serve as noncariogenic sweeteners (see **Table 1**). In addition, low-phosphorus milk was approved for people with renal insufficiency and protein-modified rice for people with rice allergy.

Interest in the development of functional foods quickly spread to North America and Europe, where the concept was expanded to include any food or food component providing health benefits in addition to its nutritive value. In Europe, functional food proponents distinguished functional foods from dietetic foods, which are defined by

Table 1 Some ingredients conferring FOSHU status on Japanese functional foods

Ingredient	Physiological function
Dietary fiber	Improve gastrointestinal function
Psyllium seed husk	
Wheat bran	
Hydrolyzed guar gum	
Oligosaccharides	Improve gastrointestinal function
Xylo-, fructo-, isomalto-	and mineral absorption
Soy-derived	
Polydextrose	
Bacterial cultures	Improve gastrointestinal function
Lactobacilli	
Bifidobacteria	
Soy protein isolates	Reduce cholesterol levels
Diacylglycerols	Reduce triglyceride levels
Sugar alcohols	Prevent dental caries
Maltitol	
Palatinose	
Erythritol	
Green tea polyphenols	Prevent dental caries
Absorbable calcium	Improve bone health
Calcium citrate malate	
Casein	
phosphopeptide	
Heme iron	Correct iron deficiency
Eucommiacea (tochu)	Reduce blood pressure
leaf glycosides	
Lactosucrose, lactulose,	Improve gastrointestinal function
indigestible dextrin	

law. European dietetic foods are intended to satisfy special nutritional requirements of specific groups rather than to enhance physiologic function or prevent disease through nonnutritive influences. They include infant formula, processed baby foods (weanling foods), low-calorie foods for weight reduction, high-calorie foods for weight gain, ergogenic foods for athletes, and foods for special medical purposes like the treatment of diabetes or hypertension. In the US, functional food proponents have distinguished functional foods from medical foods, defined by law as special foods designed to be used under medical supervision to meet nutritional requirements in specific medical conditions. In both domains, functional foods have been viewed as whole foods or food components with the potential for preventing cancer, osteoporosis, or cardiovascular disease; improving immunity, detoxification, physical performance, weight loss, cognitive function, and the ability to cope with stress; inhibiting inflammation, free-radical pathology and the ravages of aging; and modulating the effects of hormones. Researchers have sought to validate biomarkers that demonstrate functional improvement in response to dietary intervention, identify the chemical components of functional foods responsible for those effects, and elucidate the mechanism of action of those components. The scientific substantiation of claims is a major objective.

In China, functional foods (referred to as health foods) have been viewed as part of an unbroken medical tradition that does not separate medicinal herbs from foods. Over 3000 varieties of health foods are available to Chinese consumers, most derived from compound herbal formulas for which the active ingredients and their mechanism of action are unknown, all claiming multiple effects on various body systems, with little experimental evidence for safety and efficacy but widespread acceptance due to their history of use.

Edible Plants and Phytochemicals

Because their consumption is known to enhance health, vegetables, fruits, cereal grains, nuts, and seeds are the most widely researched functional foods. The health benefits of a plant-based diet are usually attributed to the content of fiber and of a variety of plant-derived substances (phytonutrients and phytochemicals) with antioxidant, enzyme-inducing, and enzyme-inhibiting effects. Some phytochemicals may also exert their health effects by modifying gene expression. Carotenoids, for example, enhance expression of the gene responsible for production of Connexin 43, a protein that regulates intercellular communication. The protective effect of carotenoid consumption against the development of cancer is more strongly related to the ability of individual carotenoids to upregulate Connexin 43 expression than their antioxidant effects or conversion to retinol. Dietary supplementation with betacarotene reduces the blood levels of other carotenoids, some of which are more potent inducers of Connexin 43 than is beta-carotene. The unexpected and highly publicized increase in incidence of lung cancer among smokers taking beta-carotene supplements may be explained by this mechanism.

Phytochemicals associated with health promotion and disease prevention are described in **Table 2**. The most studied food sources of these phytonutrients are soy beans (*Glycine max*) and tea (*Camellia sinensis* leaves), but tomatoes (*Lycopersicon esculentum*), broccoli (*Brassica oleracea*), garlic (*Allium sativum*), turmeric (*Curcuma longa*), tart cherries (*Prunus cerasus*), and various types of berries are also receiving considerable attention as functional food candidates. An overview of the research on soy and tea illustrates some of the clinical issues encountered in the development of functional foods from edible plants.

Soy protein extracts have been found to lower cholesterol in humans, an effect that appears to be

Table 2 Phytochemicals associated with health promotion and disease prevention

Group	Typical components	Biological activities	Food sources
Carotenoids	Alpha- and beta-carotene cryptoxanthin, lutein, lycopene, zeaxanthin	Quench singlet and triplet oxygen, increase cell–cell communication	Red, orange and yellow fruits and vegetables, egg yolk, butter fat, margarine
Glucosinolates, isothiocyanates	Indole-3-carbinol sulphoraphane	Increase xenobiotic metabolism, alter estrogen metabolism	Cruciferous vegetables, horseradish
Inositol phosphates	Inositol hexaphosphate (phytate)	Stimulate natural killer cell function, chelate divalent cations	Bran, soy foods
Isoflavones	Genistein, daidzein	Estrogen agonist and antagonist, induce apoptosis	Soy foods, kudzu
Lignans	Enterolactone, enterolactone	Estrogen agonists and antagonists, inhibit tyrosine kinase	Flax seed, rye
Phenolic acids	Gallic, ellagic, ferulic, chlorogenic, coumaric	Antioxidant, enhance xenobiotic metabolism	Diverse fruits, vegetables
Phytoallexins	Resveratrol	Antioxidant, platelet inhibition, induce apoptosis	Red wine, grape seed
Polyphenols	Flavonoids, chalcones, catechins, anthocyanins, proanthocyanidins	Antioxidant, enhance xenobiotic metabolism, inhibit numerous enzymes	Diverse fruits, vegetables, red wine, tea
Saponins	Glycyrrhizin, ginsenosides	Antimicrobial, immune boosting, cytotoxic to cancer cells	Legumes, nuts, herbs
Sterols	Beta-sistosterol, campestrol	Bind cholesterol, decrease colonic cell proliferation, stimulate T-helper-1 cells	Nuts, seeds, legumes, cereal grains
Sulfides	Diallyl sulfides	Antimicrobial, antioxidant	Garlic, onions

related to amino acid composition. Soy protein extracts frequently contain nonprotein isoflavones, which have received considerable attention because of their structural similarity to estrogen. Soy isoflavones are weak estrogen agonists and partial estrogen antagonists. Epidemiologic and experimental data indicate that isoflavone exposure during adolescence may diminish the incidence of adult breast cancer. *In vitro* studies show conflicting effects. On the one hand, soy isoflavones induce apoptosis of many types of cancer cells; on the other hand, estrogen receptor-bearing human breast cancer cells proliferate in tissue culture when exposed to isoflavones. Although the widespread use of soy in Asia is cited in support of the safety of soy foods, the intake of isoflavones among Asian women consuming soy regularly is in the range of 15–40 mg day^{-1}, significantly less than the isoflavone content of a serving of soymilk as consumed in the US. In clinical trials, soy isoflavones have not been effective in relieving hot flashes of menopausal women but do diminish the increased bone resorption that causes postmenopausal bone loss. In premenopausal women, soy isoflavones may cause menstrual irregularities. The successful development of soy derivatives as functional foods will require that these complex and diverse effects of different soy components in different clinical settings be better understood.

Regular consumption of tea, green or black, is associated with a decreased risk of heart disease and several kinds of cancer. These benefits are attributed to tea's high content of catechin polymers, especially epigallocatechin gallate (ECGC), which has potent antioxidant and anti-inflammatory effects, that may lower cholesterol in hyperlipidemic individuals and alter the activity of several enzymes involved in carcinogenesis. Catechin content is highest in young leaves. Aging and the fermentation used to produce black tea oxidize tea catechins, which polymerize further to form the tannins, theaflavin and thearubigen. Although ECGC is a more potent antioxidant than theaflavin, theaflavin is far more potent an antioxidant than most of the commonly used antioxidants, like glutathione, vitamin E, vitamin C, and butylated hydroxytoluene (BHT). Both ECGC and theaflavin are partially absorbed after oral consumption, but a clear dose–response relationship has not been established. Tea-derived catechins and polymers are being intensively studied as components of functional foods, because the results of epidemiologic, *in vitro*, and animal research indicate little toxicity and great potential benefit in preventing cancer or treating inflammation-associated disorders. Clinical trials have shown a mild cholesterol-lowering effect and perhaps some benefit for enhancing weight loss.

Probiotics and Prebiotics

Probiotics are live microbes that exert health benefits when ingested in sufficient quantities. Species of lactobacilli and bifidobacteria, sometimes combined with *Streptococcus thermophilus*, are the main bacteria used as probiotics in fermented dairy products. Most probiotic research has been done with nutraceutical preparations, but yogurt has been shown to alleviate lactose intolerance, prevent vaginal candidosis in women with recurrent vaginitis, and reduce the incidence or severity of gastrointestinal infections.

Prebiotics are nondigestible food ingredients that stimulate the growth or modify the metabolic activity of intestinal bacterial species that have the potential to improve the health of their human host. Criteria associated with the notion that a food ingredient should be classified as a prebiotic are that it remains undigested and unabsorbed as it passes through the upper part of the gastrointestinal tract and is a selective substrate for the growth of specific strains of beneficial bacteria (usually lactobacilli or bifidobacteria), rather than for all colonic bacteria, inducing intestinal or systemic effects through bacterial fermentation products that are beneficial to host health. Prebiotic food ingredients include bran, psyllium husk, resistant (high amylose) starch, inulin (a polymer of fructofuranose), lactulose, and various natural or synthetic oligosaccharides, which consist of short-chain complexes of sucrose, fructose, galactose, glucose, maltose, or xylose. The best-known effect of prebiotics is to increase fecal water content, relieving constipation. Bacterial fermentation of prebiotics yields short-chain fatty acids (SCFAs) that nourish and encourage differentiation of colonic epithelial cells. Absorbed SCFAs decrease hepatic cholesterol synthesis. Fructooligosaccharides (FOSs) have been shown to alter fecal biomarkers (pH and the concentration of bacterial enzymes like nitroreductase and beta-glucuronidase) in a direction that may convey protection against the development of colon cancer.

Several prebiotics have documented effects that are probably independent of their effects on gastrointestinal flora. Whereas the high phytic acid content of bran inhibits the absorption of minerals, FOSs have been shown to increase absorption of calcium and magnesium. Short-chain FOSs are sweet enough to be used as sugar substitutes. Because they are not hydrolyzed in the mouth or upper gastrointestinal tract, they are noncariogenic and noninsulogenic. Bran contains immunostimulating polysaccharides, especially beta-glucans and inositol phosphates, which have been shown to stimulate macrophage

and natural killer cell activity *in vitro* and in rodent experiments. The poor solubility and absorption of beta-glucans and inositol phosphates are significant barriers to clinical effects in humans.

Immune Modulators

Several substances produced by animals and fungi have been investigated for immune-modulating effects. Fish oils are the most studied. As a source of *n*-3 fatty acids, fish oil consumption by humans has been shown to influence the synthesis of inflammatory signaling molecules like prostaglandins, leukotrienes, and cytokines. In addition to direct effects on prostanoid synthesis, *n*-3 fats have also been shown to directly alter the intracellular availability of free calcium ions, the function of ion channels, and the activity of protein kinases. Generally administered as nutraceuticals rather than as functional foods, fish oil supplements have demonstrated anti-inflammatory and immune suppressive effects in human adults. A high intake of the *n*-3 fatty acids eicosapentaenoic (20:5*n*-3) and docosahexaenoic (22:6*n*-3) acid (DHA) from seafood or fish oil supplements has also been associated with prevention of several types of cancer, myocardial infarction, ventricular arrhythmias, migraine headaches, and premature births, and with improved control of type 2 diabetes mellitus, inflammatory bowel disease, rheumatoid arthritis, cystic fibrosis, multiple sclerosis, bipolar disorder, and schizophrenia. 20:5*n*-3 but not 22:6*n*-3 is effective for schizophrenia and depression; 22:6*n*-3 but not 20:5*n*-3 improves control of blood sugar in diabetics. The benefits of fish oil supplements have prompted efforts at increasing the *n*-3 fatty acid content of common foods by adding fish oil or flax oil extracts. Consumption of these has been associated with decreased levels of some inflammatory biomarkers, including thromboxane B2, prostaglandin E2, and interleukin 1-beta.

Feeding flax seed meal or fish meal to hens enriches the *n*-3 fatty acid content of the yolks of the eggs they lay. Consumption of these eggs increases the *n*-3 fatty acid content of plasma and cellular phospholipids and produces an improved blood lipid profile when compared with consumption of standard eggs. Egg yolk is not only a source of fatty acids, but also of carotenoids and immunoglobulins. The xanthophyll carotenoids zeaxanthin and its stereoisomer lutein are readily absorbed from egg yolk. Their consumption is associated with a decreased incidence of macular degeneration and cataract. Immunizing hens to specific pathogens and extracting the antibodies present in their egg yolks yields a functional food that has been shown to prevent enteric bacterial or viral infection in experimental animals.

Bovine colostrum, the milk produced by cows during the first few days postpartum, has a long history of use as a functional food. Compared to mature milk, colostrum contains higher amounts of immunoglobulins, growth factors, cytokines, and various antimicrobial and immune-regulating factors. Consumption of bovine colostrum has been shown to reduce the incidence of diarrheal disease in infants and the symptoms of respiratory infection in adults. Specific hyperimmune bovine colostrums, produced by immunizing cows to pathogenic organisms like *Cryptosporidium parvum*, *Helicobacter pylori*, rotavirus, and *Shigella* spp., may prevent or treat infection by these organisms.

Human studies have also shown that consumption of bovine colostrum can improve anaerobic athletic performance and prevent the enteropathy induced by use of nonsteroidal anti-inflammatory drugs.

Mushrooms play a major role in traditional Chinese medicine and as components of contemporary Chinese health foods. Many *Basidiomycetes* mushrooms contain biologically active polysaccharides in fruiting bodies, cultured mycelium, or culture broth. Most belong to the group of beta-glucans that have both beta-$(1\rightarrow3)$ and beta-$(1\rightarrow6)$ linkages. Although they stimulate macrophages and natural killer cells, the anticancer effect of mushroom polysaccharide extracts appears to be mediated by thymus-derived lymphocytes. In experimental animals, mushroom polysaccharides prevent oncogenesis, show direct antitumor activity against various cancers, and prevent tumor metastasis. Clinical trials in humans have shown improvement in clinical outcome when chemotherapy was combined with the use of commercial mushroom polysaccharides like lentinan (from *Lentinus edodes* or shiitake), krestin (from *Coriolus versicolor*), or schizophyllan (from *Schizophyllum commune*). Mushroom extracts may fulfill their potential more as medicines than as functional foods.

Designer Foods

An important direction in the development of functional foods is the combination of numerous ingredients to achieve a specific set of goals, rather than efforts to uncover the potential benefits of a single food source. Infant formula was probably the first area for designer foods of this type, because of the profound influence of nutrients on the developing brain and immune system. The addition of DHA to infant formula for enhancing brain and visual development, the alteration of allergenic components in food, and the possible use of probiotics and nucleotides to enhance immune response are important developments in this area.

Sports nutrition is another established arena for designer foods. Specific nutritional measures and dietary interventions have been devised to support athletic performance and recuperation. Oral rehydration products for athletes were one of the first categories of functional foods for which scientific evidence of benefit was obtained. Oral rehydration solutions must permit rapid gastric emptying and enteral absorption, improved fluid retention, and thermal regulation, to enhance physical performance and delay fatigue. Carbohydrates with relatively high glycemic index combined with whey protein concentrates or other sources of branched chain amino acids have been shown to enhance recovery of athletes. Caffeine, creatine, ribose, citrulline, L-carnitine, and branched chain amino acids have each been shown to improve exercise performance or diminish postexercise fatigue. Whether combinations of these ingredients, blended into foods or beverages, will perform better than the individual ingredients will help to determine the design of future sports foods.

Optimal cardiovascular health involves prevention of excessive levels of oxidant stress, circulating homocysteine, cholesterol, triglycerides and fibrinogen, and protection of the vascular endothelium. A mix of ingredients supplying all of these effects could consist of soy protein powder, oat beta-glucan, plant sterols and stanols, folic acid, L-arginine, 22:6n-3, magnesium, and red wine or green tea polyphenols. Evidence suggests that addressing multiple nutritional influences on cardiovascular health will be more beneficial than addressing only one influence, but more definitive studies are needed. Genetic factors may need to be incorporated for designer foods to achieve their full potential. Polyunsaturated fatty acids, for example, raise the serum concentration of HDL-cholesterol among individuals who carry the Apo A1-75A gene polymorphism, but reduce HDL-cholesterol levels of individuals who carry the more common Apo A1-75G polymorphism.

See also: **Carotenoids**: Chemistry, Sources and Physiology; Epidemiology of Health Effects. **Dietary Fiber**: Physiological Effects and Effects on Absorption. **Fatty Acids**: Omega-3 Polyunsaturated. **Microbiota of the Intestine**: Probiotics. **Phytochemicals**: Classification and Occurrence; Epidemiological Factors. **Sports Nutrition**.

Further Reading

Ashwell M (2001) Functional foods: a simple scheme for establishing the scientific basis for all claims. *Public Health Nutrition* 4(3): 859–862.

Bellisle F, Diplock AT, Hornstra G *et al.* (eds.) (1998) Functional food science in Europe. *British Journal of Nutrition* 80(supplement 1): S1–S193.

Clydesdale FM and Chan SH (eds.) (1995) First International Conference on East–West Perspectives on Functional Foods. *Nutrition Reviews* 54(11, part II): S1–S202.

Constantinou AI and Singletary KW (eds.) (2002) Controversies in functional foods. *Pharmaceutical Biology* 40(supplement): 5–74.

Diplock AT, Aggett PJ, Ashwell M *et al.* (eds.) (1999) Scientific Concepts of Functional Foods in Europe: Consensus Document. *British Journal of Nutrition* 81(supplement): S1–S27.

Farnworth ER (2003) *Handbook of Fermented Functional Foods.* USA: CRC Press.

Goldberg I (ed.) (1994) *Functional Foods, Designer Food, Pharmafoods, Nutraceuticals.* New York: Chapman and Hall.

ILSI North America Technical Committee on Food Components for Health Promotion (1999). *Food Component Report.* Washington, DC: ILSI Press.

Knorr D (1999) Technology aspects related to microorganisms in functional food. *Trends in Food Science and Technology.* 9(8–9, Special Issue): 295–306.

Langseth L (1995) *Oxidants, Antioxidants and Disease Prevention: ILSI Europe Concise Monograph Series.* Washington, DC: ILSI Press.

Langseth L (1996) *Nutritional Epidemiology: Possibilities and Limitations: ILSI Europe Concise Monograph Series.* Washington, DC: ILSI Press.

Langseth L (1999) *Nutrition and Immunity in Man: ILSI Europe Concise Monograph Series.* Washington, DC: ILSI Press.

Meskin MS, Biidlack BI, Davies AJ, and Omaye ST (eds.) (2002) *Phytochemicals in Nutrition and Health.* USA: CRC Press.

Roberfroid MB (2000) Defining functional foods. In: Gibson G and Williams C (eds.) *Functional Foods.* Cambridge: Woodhead Publishing Ltd.

Truswell AS (1995) *Dietary Fat: Some Aspects of Nutrition and Health and Product Development: ILSI Europe Concise Monograph Series.* Washington, DC: ILSI Press.

IODINE

Contents
Deficiency Disorders
Physiology, Dietary Sources and Requirements

Deficiency Disorders

B S Hetzel, Women's and Children's Hospital, North Adelaide, SA, Australia

Iodine deficiency is discussed as a risk factor for the growth and development of up to 2.2 million people living in iodine-deficient environments in 130 countries throughout the world. The effects of iodine deficiency on growth and development, called the iodine deficiency disorders (IDD), comprise goiter (enlarged thyroid gland), stillbirths and miscarriages, neonatal and juvenile thyroid deficiency, dwarfism, mental defects, deaf mutism, and spastic weakness and paralysis, as well as lesser degrees of loss of physical and mental function.

Iodine deficiency is now accepted by the World Health Organization as the most common preventable cause of brain damage in the world today.

Since 1990, a major international health program to eliminate iodine deficiency has developed that uses iodized salt. The progress of this program and the continuing challenge are discussed as a great opportunity for the elimination of a noninfectious disease, which is quantitatively a greater scourge than the infectious diseases of smallpox and polio.

History

The first records of goiter and cretinism date back to ancient civilizations, the Chinese and Hindu cultures and then to Greece and Rome. In the Middle Ages, goitrous cretins appeared in the pictorial art, often as angels or demons. The first detailed descriptions of these subjects occurred in the Renaissance. The paintings of the madonnas in Italy so commonly showed goiter that the condition must have been regarded as virtually normal. In the seventeenth and eighteenth centuries, scientific studies multiplied and the first recorded mention of the word 'cretin' appeared in Diderot's *Encyclopédie* in 1754. The nineteenth century marked the beginning of serious attempts to control the problem; however, not until the latter half of the twentieth century was the necessary knowledge for effective prevention acquired.

Mass prophylaxis of goiter with iodized salt was first introduced in Switzerland and in Michigan in the United States. In Switzerland, the widespread occurrence of a severe form of mental deficiency and deaf mutism (endemic cretinism) was a heavy charge on public funds. However, following the introduction of iodized salt, goiter incidence declined rapidly and cretins were no longer born. Goiter also disappeared from army recruits.

A further major development was the administration of injections of iodized oil to correct iodine deficiency in Papua New Guinea for people living in inaccessible mountain villages. These long-lasting injections corrected iodine deficiency and prevented goiter for 3–5 years, depending on the dosage.

Subsequently, the prevention of cretinism and stillbirths was demonstrated by the administration of iodized oil before pregnancy in a controlled trial in the Highlands of Papua New Guinea. This proved the causal role of iodine deficiency.

To further establish the relation between iodine deficiency and fetal brain development, an animal model was developed in the pregnant sheep given an iodine-deficient diet. Subsequently, similar models were developed in the primate marmoset monkey and in the rat.

Studies with animal models confirmed the effect of iodine deficiency on fetal brain development (as already indicated by the results of the field trial with iodized oil in Papua New Guinea). The combination of the controlled human trials and the results of the studies in animal models clearly indicated that prevention was possible by correction of the iodine deficiency before pregnancy.

This work led Hetzel to propose the concept of the IDD resulting from all the effects of iodine deficiency on growth and development, particularly brain development, in an exposed population that can be prevented by correction of the iodine deficiency. Iodine deficiency is now recognized by the World Health Organization (WHO) as the most common form of preventable mental defect.

Although the major prevalence of iodine deficiency is in developing countries, the problem continues to be very significant in many European countries (France, Italy, Germany, Greece, Poland, Romania, Spain, and Turkey) because of the threat to brain development in the fetus and young infant.

Ecology of Iodine Deficiency

There is a cycle of iodine in nature. Most of the iodine resides in the ocean. It was present during the primordial development of the earth, but large amounts were leached from the surface soil by glaciation, snow, or rain and were carried by wind, rivers, and floods into the sea. Iodine occurs in the deeper layers of the soil and is found in oil well and natural gas effluents, which are now a major source for the production of iodine.

The better known areas that are leached are the mountainous areas of the world. The most severely deficient soils are those of the European Alps, the Himalayas, the Andes, and the vast mountains of China. However, iodine deficiency is likely to occur to some extent in all elevated regions subject to glaciation and higher rainfall, with runoff into rivers. It has become clear that iodine deficiency also occurs in flooded river valleys, such as the Ganges in India, the Mekong in Vietnam, and the great river valleys of China.

Iodine occurs in soil and the sea as iodide. Iodide ions are oxidized by sunlight to elemental iodine, which is volatile so that every year approximately 400,000 tons of iodine escapes from the surface of the sea. The concentration of iodide in the seawater is approximately $50–60\,\mu g/l$, and in the air it is approximately $0.7\,\mu g/m^3$. The iodine in the atmosphere is returned to the soil by rain, which has a concentration of $1.8–8.5\,\mu g/l$. In this way, the cycle is completed (**Figure 1**).

However, the return of iodine is slow and the amount is small compared to the original loss of iodine, and subsequent repeated flooding ensures the

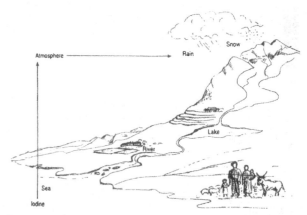

Figure 1 The iodine cycle in nature. The atmosphere absorbs iodine from the sea, which then returns through rain and snow to mountainous regions. It is then carried by rivers to the lower hills and plains, eventually returning to the sea. High rainfall, snow, and flooding increase the loss of soil iodine, which has often been already denuded by past glaciation. This causes the low iodine content of food for man and animals. (Reproduced from Hetzel BS (1989) *The Story of Iodine Deficiency: An international Challenge in Nutrition.* Oxford: Oxford University Press.)

continuity of iodine deficiency in the soil. Hence, no natural correction can take place and iodine deficiency persists in the soil indefinitely. All crops grown in these soils will be iodine deficient. The iodine content of plants grown in iodine-deficient soils may be as low as $10\,\mu g/kg$ compared to $1\,mg/kg$ dry weight in plants in a non-iodine-deficient soil.

As a result, human and animal populations that are totally dependent on food grown in such soil become iodine deficient. This accounts for the occurrence of severe iodine deficiency in vast populations in Asia that live within systems of subsistence agriculture in flooded river valleys (India, Bangladesh, Burma, Vietnam, and China).

Iodine Deficiency Disorders

The effects of iodine deficiency on the growth and development of a population that can be prevented by correction of iodine deficiency, denoted by the term IDD, are evident at all stages, including particularly the fetus, the neonate, and in infancy, which are periods of rapid brain growth. The term goiter has been used for many years to describe the enlarged thyroid gland caused by iodine deficiency (**Figure 2**). Goiter is indeed the obvious and familiar feature of iodine deficiency, but knowledge of the effects of iodine deficiency on brain development has greatly expanded in the past 30 years so that the term IDD was introduced to refer to all the effects of iodine deficiency on growth and development, particularly brain development, in a

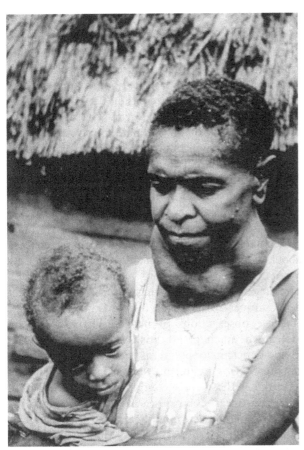

Figure 2 A mother and child from a New Guinea village who are severely iodine deficient. The mother has a large goiter and the child is also affected. The larger the goiter, the more likely it is that she will have a cretin child. This can be prevented by eliminating the iodine deficiency before the onset of pregnancy. (Reproduced from Hetzel BS and Pandav CS (eds.) (1996) *SOS for a Billion: The Conquest of Iodine Deficiency Disorders*, 2nd edn. Oxford: Oxford University Press.)

Table 1 Spectrum of Iodine Deficiency Disorders

Fetus	Abortions
	Stillbirths
	Congenital anomalies
	Neurological cretinism
	Mental deficiency, deaf mutism, spastic diplegia, squint
	Hypothyroid cretinism
	Mental deficiency, dwarfism, hypothyroidism
	Psychomotor defects
Neonate	Increased perinatal mortality
	Neonatal hypothyroidism
	Retarded mental and physical development
Child and adolescent	Increased infant mortality
	Retarded mental and physical development
Adult	Goiter with its complications
	Iodine-induced hyperthyroidism
All ages	Goiter
	Hypothyroidism
	Impaired mental function
	Increased susceptibility to nuclear radiation

Reproduced with permission from Oxford University Press and the World Health Organization, WHO/UNICEF/ICCIDD (2001).

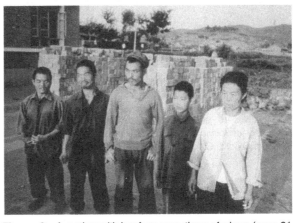

Figure 3 A mother with her four sons, three of whom (ages 31, 29, and 28 years) are cretins born before iodized salt was introduced, and the fourth is normal (age 14 years), born after iodized salt became available in Chengde, China. (Reproduced from Hetzel BS and Pandav CS (eds.) (1996) *SOS for a Billion: The Conquest of Iodine Deficiency Disorders*, 2nd edn. Oxford: Oxford University Press.)

population that can be prevented by correction of the deficiency (**Table 1**).

The following sections discuss in detail the IDD at various stages of life: the fetus, the neonate, the child and adolescent, and the adult (**Table 1**).

The Fetus

Iodine deficiency of the fetus is the result of iodine deficiency in the mother (**Figure 2**). The condition is associated with a greater incidence of stillbirths, abortions, and congenital abnormalities, which can be prevented by iodization.

Another major effect of fetal iodine deficiency is the condition of endemic cretinism, which is quite distinct from the condition of sporadic cretinism or congenital hypothyroidism due to a small or absent thyroid gland.

Endemic cretinism-associated with an iodine intake of less than 25 μg per day, in contrast to a normal intake of 100–150 μg per day, has been widely prevalent, affecting up to 10% of populations living in severely iodine-deficient regions in India, Indonesia, and China. In its most common form, it is characterized by mental deficiency, deaf mutism, and spastic diplegia (**Figure 3**). This form of cretinism is referred to as the nervous or

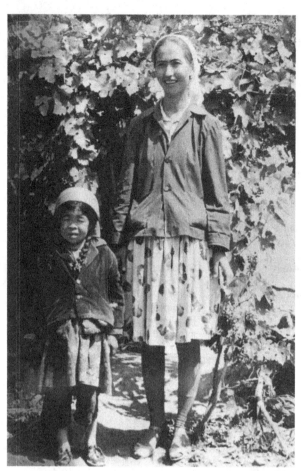

Figure 4 A hypothyroid cretin from Sinjiang, China, who is also deaf mute. This condition is completely preventable. (Right) The barefoot doctor of her village. Both are approximately 35 years old. (Reproduced from Hetzel BS (1989) *The Story of Iodine Deficiency: An international Challenge in Nutrition.* Oxford: Oxford University Press.)

neurological type, in contrast to the less common hypothyroid or myxedematous type characterized by hypothyroidism with dwarfism (**Figure 4**).

In addition to Asia, cretinism also occurs in Africa, (Zaire, now the Republic of the Congo), South America in the Andean region (Ecuador, Peru, Bolivia, and Argentina), and the more remote areas of Europe. In all these areas, with the exception of the Congo, neurological features are predominant. In the Congo, the hypothyroid form is more common, probably due to the high intake of the root vegetable cassava, which contains substances inhibiting the function of the thyroid gland.

However, there is considerable variation in the clinical manifestations of neurological cretinism, which include isolated deaf mutism and mental defect of varying degrees. In China, the term cretinoid is used to describe these individuals, who may number 5–10 times those with overt cretinism.

The Neonate

Apart from the question of mortality, the importance of the state of thyroid function in the neonate relates to the fact that at birth the brain of the human infant has only reached approximately one-third of its full size and continues to grow rapidly until the end of the second year. The thyroid hormone, dependent on an adequate supply of iodine, is essential for normal brain development, as has been confirmed by animal studies.

Data on iodine nutrition and neonatal thyroid function in Europe confirm the continuing presence of severe iodine deficiency. This affects neonatal thyroid function and hence represents a threat to early brain development. These data have raised great concern about iodine deficiency, which is also heightened by awareness of the hazard of nuclear radiation with carcinogenic effects following the Chernobyl disaster in the former Soviet Union (**Table 1**).

These observations of neonatal hypothyroidism indicate a much greater risk of mental defects in iodine-deficient populations than is indicated by the presence of cretinism. Apart from the developing world, there has been a continuing major problem in many European countries, such as Italy, Germany, France, and Greece, and Romania, Bulgaria, and Albania still have very severe iodine deficiency with overt cretinism.

The Child

Iodine deficiency in children is characteristically associated with goiter. The goiter rate increases with age and reaches a maximum at adolescence. Girls have a higher prevalence than boys. Goiter rates in schoolchildren over the years provide a useful indication of the presence of iodine deficiency in a community.

In a review of 18 studies, a comparison was made between IQ scores in iodine-deficient children and carefully selected control groups. The iodine-deficient group had a mean IQ that was 13.5 points lower than that of the non-iodine-deficient control group. Detailed individual studies demonstrating these defects in Italian and Spanish schoolchildren as well as those from Africa, China, Indonesia, and Papua New Guinea have been published. There is a serious problem in Europe as well as in many developing countries.

The Adult

Long-standing large goiter may require surgery to reduce pressure in the neck. Long-standing goiter may also be associated with iodine-induced hyperthyroidism (IIH) due to an increase in iodine intake. IIH is associated with nervousness, sweating, and tremor, with loss of weight due to excessive levels of circulating thyroid hormone. This condition no longer occurs following correction of iodine deficiency and therefore is within the spectrum of IDD.

In northern India, a high degree of apathy has been noted in whole populations living in iodine-deficient areas. This may even affect domestic animals such as dogs. It is apparent that reduced mental function is widely prevalent in iodine-deficient communities, with effects on their capacity for initiative and decision making. This is due to the effect of hypothyroidism on brain function. This condition can be readily reversed by correction of the iodine deficiency, unlike the effects on the fetus and in infancy, so that villages can come to life.

Thus, iodine deficiency is a major block to the human and social development of communities living in an iodine-deficient environment. Correction of the iodine deficiency is indicated as a major contribution to economic development. An increase in physical and mental energy leads to improved work output, improved learning by children, and improved quality of life. Improved livestock productivity (chickens, cattle, and sheep) is also a major economic benefit.

Magnitude of the Problem

The number of cases of IDD throughout the world was estimated by WHO in 1990 to be 1.6 billion, including more than 200 million cases with goiter and more than 20 million cases with some degree of brain damage due to the effects of iodine deficiency in pregnancy. Recent estimates of the population at risk have been increased to 2.2 billion, with the recognition that even mild iodine deficiency in the mother has effects on the fetus. There are now estimated to be 130 IDD-affected countries, including the most populous: Bangladesh, Brazil, China, India, Indonesia, and Nigeria. Therefore, there is a global scourge of great magnitude, which provides one of the major challenges in international health today.

Correction of Iodine Deficiency

Iodized Salt

Since the successful introduction of iodized salt in Switzerland and the United States in the 1920s, successful programs have been reported from a number of countries, including those in Central and South America (e.g., Guatemala and Colombia) and Finland and Taiwan. However, there has been great difficulty in sustaining these programs in Central and South America mainly due to political instability. Following the breakup of the Soviet Union, iodine deficiency recurred in the Central Asian republics.

The difficulties in the production and quality maintenance of iodized salt for the millions who are iodine deficient, especially in Asia, were vividly demonstrated in India, where there was a breakdown in supply. These difficulties led to the adoption of universal salt iodization (USI) for India and subsequently for many other countries. This policy includes legislation to provide for compulsory iodization of all salt for human and animal consumption, and this legislation makes it illegal for noniodized salt to be available for human or animal consumption.

In Asia, the cost of iodized salt production and distribution is on the order of 3–5 cents per person per year. This must be considered cheap in relation to the social benefits that have already been described.

However, there is still the problem of the iodine in the salt actually reaching the iodine-deficient subject. There may be a problem with distribution or preservation of the iodine content: It may be left uncovered or exposed to heat. Thus, it should be added after cooking to reduce the loss of iodine.

Potassium iodate is the preferred vehicle compared to potassium iodide because of its greater stability in the tropical environment. A dose of 20–40 mg iodine as potassium iodate per kilo is recommended to cover losses to ensure an adequate household level. This assumes a salt intake of 10 g per day; if the level is below this, then an appropriate correction can readily be made by increasing the concentration of potassium iodate.

Iodized Oil

Iodized oil by injection or by mouth is singularly appropriate for isolated communities characteristic of mountainous endemic goiter areas. The striking regression of goiter following iodized oil administration, with improved well-being from correction of hypothyroidism, ensures general acceptance of the measure (**Figure 5**).

Iodized oil is more expensive than iodized salt but is used especially for severe iodine deficiency in remote areas. It provides instant correction of the deficiency and the consequent prevention of brain damage.

In a suitable area, the oil (1 ml contains 480 mg iodine) should be administered to all females up to the age of 40 years and all males up to the age of 20 years. A dose of 480 mg will provide coverage for 1 year by mouth and for 2 years by injection.

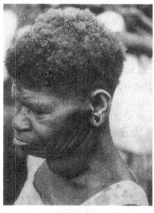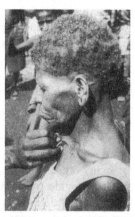

Figure 5 Subsidence of goiter in a New Guinea woman 3 months after the injection of iodized oil. This is accompanied by a feeling of well-being due to a rise in the level of the thyroid hormone in the blood. This makes the injections very popular. (Reproduced from Hetzel BS (1989) *The Story of Iodine Deficiency: An international Challenge in Nutrition.* Oxford: Oxford University Press.)

Iodized Milk

This is particularly important for infants receiving formula milk as an alternative to breast-feeding. An increase in levels from 5 to 10 µg/dl has been recommended for full-term infants and 20 µg/dl for premature infants. However, breast-fed infants will be iodine deficient if the mother is iodine deficient.

Iodized milk has been available in the United States, the United Kingdom and Northern Europe, Australia, and New Zealand as a result of the addition of iodophors as disinfectants by the dairy industry. This has been a major factor in the elimination of iodine deficiency in these countries. However, in most countries of Southern Europe and Eastern Europe, this has not occurred and the risk of iodine deficiency continues. Recently, the use of iodophors has been phased out, with a substantial decrease in the level of urine iodine excretion. Recurrence of iodine deficiency has been confirmed in Australia and New Zealand.

The Role of the United Nations

In 1990 the United Nations Sub-Committee on Nutrition recognized IDD as a major international public health problem and adopted a global plan for the elimination of IDD by the year 2000 proposed by the International Council for Control of Iodine Deficiency Disorders (ICCIDD) working in close collaboration with UNICEF and WHO.

The ICCIDD, founded in 1986, is an independent multidisciplinary expert group of more than 700 professionals in public health, medical, and nutritional science, technologists, and planners from more than 90 countries.

In 1990, the World Health Assembly and the World Summit for Children both accepted the goal of elimination of IDD as a public health problem by the year 2000. These major meetings included government representatives, including heads of state at the World Summit for Children, from 71 countries, and an additional 88 countries signed the plan of action for elimination of IDD as well as other major problems in nutrition and health.

Since 1989, a series of joint WHO/UNICEF/ICCIDD regional meetings have been held to assist countries with their national programs for the elimination of IDD. The impact of these meetings has been that governments now better realize the importance of iodine deficiency to the future potential of their people.

A dramatic example is provided by the government of the People's Republic of China. As is well-known, China has a one child per family policy, which means that an avoidable hazard such as iodine deficiency should be eliminated. In China, iodine deficiency is a threat to 40% of the population due to the highly mountainous terrain and flooded river valleys—in excess of 400 million people at risk. In recognition of this massive threat to the Chinese people, in 1993 the government held a national advocacy meeting in the Great Hall of the People sponsored by the Chinese Premier, Li Peng. The commitment of the government to the elimination of iodine deficiency was emphasized by Vice Premier Zhu Rongyi to the assembly of provincial delegations led by the provincial governors and the representatives of international agencies.

In 1998, an international workshop was held in Beijing by the Ministry of Health of China with the ICCIDD. Dramatic progress was reported, as indicated by a reduction in mean goiter rate (from 20 to 10%) with normal urine iodine levels. Severe iodine deficiency has persisted in Tibet due to difficulty in the implementation of salt iodization. In other provinces, excess iodine intake was noted in 10% of the population. The need for continuation of monitoring with urine iodine was emphasized at the meeting. Tibet is now receiving special assistance with a program supported by WHO, UNICEF, and the Australian Aid Program (AusAID).

Elimination of Iodine Deficiency Disorders at the Country Level

It is now recognized that an effective national program for the elimination of IDD requires a multisectoral approach as shown in **Figure 6**, which provides a model in the form of a wheel.

Wheel model for IDD Elimination Program

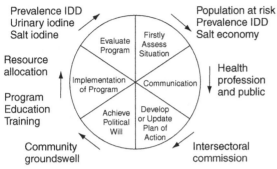

Figure 6 Wheel model for the iodine deficiency disorders (IDD) elimination program. The model shows the social process involved in a national IDD control program. The successful achievement of this process requires the establishment of a national IDD control commission, with full political and legislative authority to carry out the program. (Reproduced from Hetzel BS (1989) *The Story of Iodine Deficiency: An international Challenge in Nutrition.* Oxford: Oxford University Press.)

This wheel model represents the continuous feedback process involved in the national IDD control (elimination) program. All actors in the program need to understand the whole social process. The wheel must keep turning to maintain an effective program.

The wheel model also shows the social process involved in a national IDD control program. The successful achievement of this process requires the establishment of a national IDD control commission, with full political and legislative authority to carry out the program.

The program consists of the following components:

1. Assessment of the situation requires baseline IDD prevalence surveys, including measurement of urinary iodine levels and an analysis of the salt economy.
2. Dissemination of findings implies communication to health professionals and the public so that there is complete understanding of the IDD problem and the potential benefits of elimination of the most common preventable cause of brain damage.
3. Development of a plan of action includes the establishment of an intersectoral task force on IDD and the formulation of a strategy document on achieving the elimination of IDD.
4. Achieving political will requires intensive education and lobbying of politicians and other opinion leaders.
5. Implementation requires the complete involvement of the salt industry. Special measures, such as negotiations for monitoring and quality control of imported iodized salt, will be required. It will also be necessary to ensure that iodized salt delivery systems reach all affected populations,

including the neediest. In addition, the establishment of cooperatives for small producers, or restructuring to larger units of production, may be needed. Implementation will require training in management, salt technology, laboratory methods, and communication at all levels.

In addition, a community education campaign is required to educate all age groups about the effects of iodine deficiency, with particular emphasis on the brain.
6. Monitoring and evaluation require the establishment of an efficient system for the collection of relevant scientific data on salt iodine content and urinary iodine levels. This includes suitable laboratory facilities.

Striking progress with USI has occurred, as indicated by the WHO/UNICEF/ICCIDD report to the 1999 World Health Assembly. Data show that of 5 billion people living in countries with IDD, 68% now have access to iodized salt. Of the 130 IDD-affected countries, it was reported that 105 (81%) had an intersectoral coordinating body and 98 (75%) had legislation in place.

Criteria for tracking progress toward the goal of elimination of IDD have been agreed on by ICCIDD, WHO, and UNICEF. These include salt iodine (90% effectively iodized) and urine iodine in the normal range (median excretion, 100–200 µg/l).

The major challenge is not only the achievement but also the sustainability of effective salt iodization. In the past, a number of countries have achieved effective salt iodization, but in the absence of monitoring the program lapsed with recurrence of IDD. To this end, ICCIDD, WHO, and UNICEF offer help to governments with partnership evaluation to assess progress toward the goal and also provide help to overcome any bottlenecks obstructing progress.

The Global Partnership

Since 1990, a remarkable informal global partnership has come together composed of the people and countries with an IDD problem, international agencies (particularly UNICEF, WHO, and ICCIDD), bilateral aid agencies (Australia (AusAID) and Canada (CIDA)), the salt industry (including the private sector), and Kiwanis International. Kiwanis International is a world service club with 500,000 members throughout the world that has achieved a fundraising target of $75 million toward the elimination of IDD through UNICEF.

This partnership exists to support countries and governments in their elimination of IDD.

A more recent development is the establishment of the Global Network for the Sustainable Elimination of Iodine Deficiency, in collaboration with the salt industry.

The achievement of the global elimination of iodine deficiency will be a great triumph in international health in the field of noninfectious disease, ranking with the eradication of the infectious diseases smallpox and polio.

However, the goal of elimination is a continuing challenge. Sustained political will at both the people and the government level is necessary to bring the benefits to the many millions who suffer the effects of iodine deficiency.

Nomenclature

Endemic Occurrence of a disease confined to a community

Endemic Cretinism A state resulting from the loss of function of the maternal thyroid gland due to iodine deficiency during pregnancy characterised by mental defect, deaf-mutism and spastic paralysis in its fully developed form

Goiter An enlarged thyroid gland most commonly due to iodine deficiency in the diet

Hypothyroidism The result of a lowered level of circulating thyroid hormone causing loss of mental and physical energy

Hyperthyroidism The result of excessive circulating thyroid hormone with nervousness, sweating, tremor, with a rapid heart rate and loss of weight

ICCIDD International Council for Control of Iodine Deficiency Disorders-an international non-government organization made up of a network of 700 health professionals from more than 90 countries available to assist IDD elimination programs in affected countries

IDD Iodine Deficiency Disorders referring to all the effects of iodine deficiency in a population that can be prevented by correction of the iodine deficiency

IIH Iodine Induced Hyperthyroidism-due to increase in iodine intake following long standing iodine deficiency. The condition is transient and no longer occurs following correction of iodine deficiency

Iodization The general term covering fortification programs using various agents (iodide, iodate) or various vehicles (salt, oil, bread and water)

Iodized Oil Iodine in poppy seed oil-lipiodol is extensively used in radiology as a radio-contrast medium to demonstrate holes (cavities) in the lung. Available both by injection (lipiodol) and by mouth (oriodol) for the instant correction of iodine deficiency

Iodized Salt Salt to which potassium iodate or potassium iodide has been added at a recommended level of 20–40 milligrams of iodine per kilogram of salt

Kiwanis International A World Service Group including more than 10,000 clubs and over 500,000 members based in the USA

Thyroid size Measured by ultrasound-a much more sensitive and reproducible measurement than is possible by palpation of the thyroid

Thyroxine Thyroid Hormone (T_4) an amino acid which includes four iodine atoms

Triiodothyronine A more rapidly active thyroid hormone (T_3) which includes 3 iodine atoms on the amino acid molecule

UNICEF United Nations Children's Fund

USI Universal Salt Iodization-iodization of all salt for human and animal consumption which requires legislation and has been adopted by a number of countries

WHO World Health Organization-the expert group on health within the UN System

See also: **Iodine**: Physiology, Dietary Sources and Requirements. **Supplementation**: Role of Micronutrient Supplementation.

Further Reading

Buttfield IH and Hetzel BS (1967) Endemic goiter in Eastern New Guinea with special reference to the use of iodized oil in prophylaxis and treatment. *Bulletin of the World Health Organization* 36: 243–262.

Delange F, Dunn JT, and Glinoer D (eds.) (1993) *Iodine Deficiency in Europe: A Continuing Concern*, NATO ASI Series A: Life Sciences vol. 241. New York: Plenum.

Hetzel BS (1983) Iodine deficiency disorders (IDD) and their eradication. *Lancet* 2: 1126–1129.

Hetzel BS (1989) *The Story of Iodine Deficiency: An International Challenge in Nutrition*. Oxford: Oxford University Press.

Hetzel BS and Pandav CS (eds.) (1996) *SOS for a Billion: The Conquest of Iodine Deficiency Disorders*, 2nd edn. Oxford: Oxford University Press.

Hetzel BS, Pandav CS, Dunn JT, Ling J, and Delange F (2004) *The Global Program for the Elimination of Brain Damage Due to Iodine Deficiency*. Oxford: Oxford University Press.

Ma T, Lu T, Tan U et al. (1982) The present status of endemic goiter and endemic cretinism in China. *Food and Nutrition Bulletin* 4: 13–19.

Pharoah POD, Buttfield IH, and Hetzel BS (1971) Neurological damage to the fetus resulting from severe iodine deficiency during pregnancy. *Lancet* 1: 308–310.

Stanbury JB (ed.) (1994) *The Damaged Brain of Iodine Deficiency*. New York: Cognizant Communication Corporation.

Stanbury JB and Hetzel BS (eds.) (1980) *Endemic Goiter and Endemic Cretinism*. New York: John Wiley.

World Health Organization (1990) *Report to the 43rd World Health Assembly*. Geneva: World Health Organization.

World Health Organization (1996) *Recommended Iodine Levels in Salt and Guidelines for Monitoring Their Adequacy and Effectiveness*, WHO/NUT/96.13. Geneva: WHO/UNICEF/ICCIDD.

World Health Organization (1999) *Progress towards the Elimination of Iodine Deficiency Disorders (IDD)*, WHO/NHD/99.4. Geneva: World Health Organization.

WHO/UNICEF/ICCIDD (2001) Assessment of Iodine Deficiency Disorders and their Elimination: A guide for Program Managers WHO/NHD/01.1.

Physiology, Dietary Sources and Requirements

R Houston, Emory University, Atlanta, GA, USA

This article is reproduced from the previous edition, pp. 1138–1145, © 1998, Elsevier Ltd.

A relevant thing, though small, is of the highest importance

MK Gandhi

Iodine is classified as a nonmetallic solid in the halogen family of the Periodic Table of the elements and therefore is related to fluorine, chlorine, and bromine. The halogen family lies between the oxygen family and the rare gases. Iodine sublimates at room temperature to form a violet gas; its name is derived from the Greek *iodes*, meaning 'violet-colored.' Iodine was discovered by Bernard Courtois in Paris in 1811, the second halogen (after chlorine) to be discovered. It took nearly 100 years to understand its critical importance in human physiology. In 1896, Baumann determined the association of iodine with the thyroid gland, and in 1914 Kendall, with revisions by Harrington in 1926, described the hormone complexes synthesized by the thyroid gland using iodine that are so integral to human growth and development.

As the biochemistry of iodine and the thyroid was being established, the scarcity of the element in the natural environment became evident and the link between deficiency and human disease was revealed. Enlargement of the thyroid, or goitre, is seen in ancient stone carvings and Renaissance paintings, but it was not until years later that the link with lack of iodine was firmly established. Even with this knowledge, many years passed before preventive measures were established. From 1910 to 1920 in Switzerland and the USA work was done on the use of salt fortified with iodine to eliminate iodine deficiency, with classic work being done by Dr David Marine in Michigan. Recently the linkage of iodine deficiency with intellectual impairment has brought iodine into the international spotlight.

Recent work has demonstrated that the halogens, including iodine, are involved through the halo-peroxidases in enzymatic activity and production of numerous active metabolites in the human body. While the importance of iodine for the thyroid has been known for some time, recent research on halogen compounds in living organisms suggests additional more complex roles including antibiotic and anticancer activity. Yet it is the critical importance of iodine in the formation of the thyroid hormones thyroxine (T_4) and triiodothyronine (T_3) that makes any discussion of this element and human physiology of necessity bound up with a review of thyroid function.

Existence of Iodine in the Natural Environment

The marine hydrosphere has high concentrations of halogens, with iodine being the least common and chlorine the most. Halogens, including iodine, are concentrated by various species of marine organisms such as macroalgae and certain seaweeds. Release from these organisms makes a major contribution to the atmospheric concentration of the halogens. Iodine is present as the least abundant halogen in the Earth's crust. It is likely that in primordial times the concentration in surface soils was higher, but today the iodine content of soils varies and most has been leached out in areas of high rainfall or by previous glaciation. Environmental degradation caused by massive deforestation and soil erosion is accelerating this process. This variability in soil and water iodine concentration is quite marked, with some valleys in China having relatively high iodine concentrations in water, and other parts of China with negligible amounts in soil and water. **Table 1** shows the relative abundance of various halogens in the natural environment, while **Figure 1** illustrates the cycle of iodine in nature.

Commercial production of iodine occurs almost exclusively in Japan and Chile, with iodine extracted from concentrated salt brine from underground wells, seaweed, or from Chilean saltpetre deposits.

Absorption, Transport, and Storage

Iodine is usually ingested as an iodide or iodate compound and is rapidly absorbed in the intestine. Iodine entering the circulation is actively trapped by the thyroid gland. This remarkable capacity to concentrate iodine is a reflection of the fact that the most

Table 1 Relative abundance of halogens in the natural environment

Element	Abundance in oceans (ppm)	Abundance in Earth's crust (ppm)	Abundance in human body (mol)
Fluorine	1.3	625	0.13
Chlorine	19400	130	2.7
Bromine	67	2.5	0.0033
Iodine	0.06	0.05	0.00013

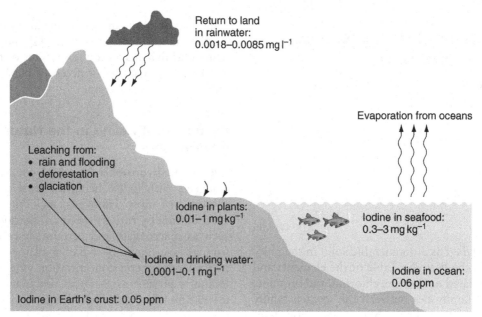

Figure 1 Cycle of iodine in nature.

critical physiological role for iodine is the normal functioning of the thyroid gland. Circulating iodide enters the capillaries within the thyroid and is rapidly transported into follicular cells and on into the lumen of the follicle. This active transport is likely to be based on cotransport of sodium and iodine, allowing iodine to move against its electrochemical gradient. Several anions, such as thiocyanate, perchlorate, and pertechnetate, inhibit this active transport. There is evidence that the active transport clearly demonstrated in the thyroid gland is also true for extrathyroidal tissues, including the salivary glands, mammary glands, and gastric mucosa.

In addition to trapping iodine, follicular cells also synthesize the glycoprotein, thyroglobulin (Tg), from carbohydrates and amino acids (including tyrosine) obtained from the circulation. Thyroglobulin moves into the lumen of the follicle where it becomes available for hormone production. Thyroid peroxidase (TPO), a membrane-bound hem-containing glycoprotein, catalyzes the oxidation of the iodide to its active form, I_2, and the binding of this active form to the tyrosine in thyroglobulin to form mono- or diiodotyrosine (MIT or DIT). These in turn combine to form the thyroid hormones triiodothyronine (T_3) and thyroxine (T_4). Thyroglobulin is very concentrated in the follicles through a process of compaction, making the concentration of iodine in the thyroid gland very high. Only a very small proportion of the iodine remains as inorganic iodide, although even for this unbound iodide the concentration in the thyroid remains much

greater than that in the circulation. This remarkable ability of the thyroid to concentrate and store iodine allows the gland to be very rapidly responsive to metabolic needs for thyroid hormones. **Figure 2** shows the structures of the molecules tyrosine and thyroxine.

Formation of thyroid hormones is not restricted to humans. Marine algae have an 'iodine pump' that facilitates concentration; invertebrates and all vertebrates demonstrate similar mechanisms to concentrate iodine and form iodotyrosines of various types. Although the function of these hormones in invertebrates is not clear, in vertebrates these iodine-containing substances are important for a variety of functions, such as metamorphosis in amphibians, spawning changes in fish, and general translation of genetic messages for protein synthesis.

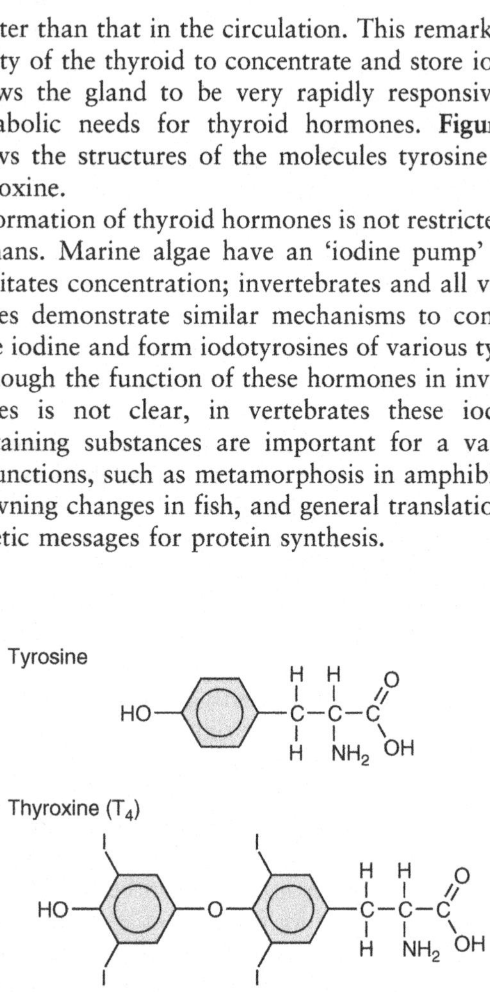

Tyrosine

Thyroxine (T_4)

Figure 2 Structures of tyrosine and thyroxine (T_4).

Metabolism and Excretion

Once iodine is 'captured' by the thyroid and thyroid hormones formed in the lumen of the follicles, stimulation of the gland causes release of the hormones into the circulation for uptake by peripheral tissues. Both production and release of the hormones are regulated in two ways. Stimulation is hormonally controlled by the hypothalamus of the brain through thyroid releasing hormone (TRH) which stimulates the pituitary gland to secrete thyroid stimulating hormone (TSH), which in turn stimulates the thyroid to release T_3 and T_4. In addition to the regulation of thyroid hormones by TSH, iodine itself plays a major role in autoregulation. The rate of uptake of iodine into the follicle, the ratio of T_3 to T_4, and the release of these into the circulation, among other things, are affected by the concentration of iodine in the gland. Thus, an increase in iodine intake causes a decrease in organification of iodine in the follicles and does not necessarily result in a corresponding increase in hormone release. Recent research suggests that this autoregulation is not entirely independent of TSH activity and that several other factors may contribute. However, regardless of the mechanism, these regulatory mechanisms allow for stability in hormone secretion in spite of wide variations in iodine intake.

When stimulated to release thyroid hormones, thyroglobulin is degraded through the activity of lysosomes and T_3 and T_4 are released and rapidly enter the circulation. Iodide freed in this reaction is for the most part recycled and the iodinated tyrosine reused for hormone production. Nearly all of the released hormones are rapidly bound to transport hormones, with 70% bound to thyroxine binding globulin (TBG). Other proteins, such as transthyretin (TTR), albumin, and lipoproteins, bind most of the remainder; with significant differences in the strengths of the affinity for the hormones, these proteins transport the hormones to different sites.

This remarkable ability of the thyroid to actively trap and store the iodine required creates a relatively steady state, with daily intake used to ensure full stores. T_4, with a longer half-life, serves as a reservoir for conversion to the more active hormone, T_3, with a much shorter half-life of 1 day. Target organs for thyroid hormone activity all play a role in the complex interplay between conversion of T_4 to T_3 deiodination, and metabolism of various other proteins involved with thyroid function. The liver, which is estimated to contain 30% of the extrathyroidal T_4, is responsible, through the activity of the liver cell enzyme, deiodinase, for ensuring adequate supply of T_3 to peripheral tissues and degradation of metabolic by-products. The kidney demonstrates a strong ability to take up the iodothyronines. Iodine is ultimately excreted in the urine, with average daily excretion rates of approximately $100\,\mu g$ per day. This accounts for the vast majority of iodine excretion, with negligible amounts excreted in feces. **Figure 3** illustrates a thyroid follicle and summarizes iodine transport.

Metabolic Functions

Separating the role of iodine from the complex and pervasive function of the thyroid gland is difficult since iodine is a critical component of the hormones that mediate these functions, and whatever other roles iodine may have are poorly understood. Thyroid hormones affect a wide range of physiological functions, from liver and kidney to heart and brain. Earlier work supported a role for thyroid hormones in affecting the energy generating capacity of cells through biochemical changes in mitochondria. More recent work has shown, however, that these hormones act on specific genetic receptors in cell nuclei, and perhaps through other extranuclear mechanisms. The nuclear receptors belong to a large family of receptors that bind other extranuclear molecules including vitamins A and D and steroids. Through this interaction, along with a number of other proteins, thyroid hormones modify genetic expression. A great deal of research currently focuses on these thyroid hormone receptors, and the effect primarily of T_3 on the physiological function of the target organ through genetic transcription. These receptors are present in pituitary, liver, heart, kidney, and brain cells.

In the pituitary gland, thyroid hormones, along with many cofactors, regulate the synthesis and secretion of growth hormone by increasing gene transcription. Similarly, as part of the feedback loop for hormone regulation and release, thyroid hormones affect transcription of TSH in the pituitary. In cardiac and skeletal muscle, thyroid hormones affect production of the muscle tissue myosin in a variety of ways, depending on the stage of life and specific muscle tissue affected. In addition, the hormones affect muscle contraction through genetic alteration of calcium uptake within the cell. Carbohydrate metabolism and formation of certain fats (lipogenesis) are affected through hormone-induced changes in gene transcription in liver cells.

In the adult brain, receptors have been identified, but the specific genes affected by thyroid hormones have not yet been located. However, in the developing brain of the fetus and neonate, the effects of

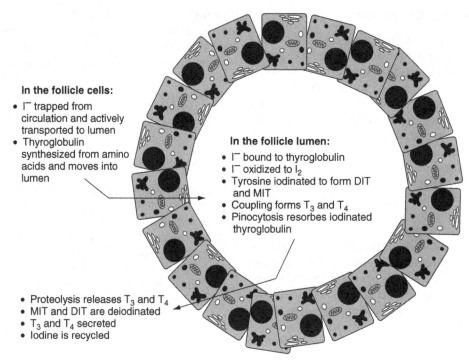

In the follicle cells:
- I^- trapped from circulation and actively transported to lumen
- Thyroglobulin synthesized from amino acids and moves into lumen

In the follicle lumen:
- I^- bound to thyroglobulin
- I^- oxidized to I_2
- Tyrosine iodinated to form DIT and MIT
- Coupling forms T_3 and T_4
- Pinocytosis resorbes iodinated thyroglobulin

- Proteolysis releases T_3 and T_4
- MIT and DIT are deiodinated
- T_3 and T_4 secreted
- Iodine is recycled

Figure 3 Thyroid follicle (courtesy of Kiely Houston).

thyroid hormones are significant even though the exact mechanisms are still not fully understood. The effects of thyroid hormones on brain development are suggested by failure in development of the nerve elements, failure of differentiation of cerebellar cells, and reduced development of other brain cells, in hypothyroid states. It is this early effect that has recently elevated the status of iodine from an element whose deficiency caused goitre to one whose deficiency is the leading cause of mental impairment worldwide.

In addition to these nuclear mechanisms, several alternative pathways have been suggested, some based on earlier historical studies. The thermogenic effects of thyroid hormones were originally felt to be a direct action on mitochondria, though this has recently been questioned. Thyroid hormones stimulate glucose transport, and again though originally attributed to a direct action on the plasma membrane, recent evidence suggests a genetic mechanism. There may also be a direct effect of thyroid hormones on brain enzymatic activity.

The overall effect of these cellular and systemic actions is to stimulate respiratory and other enzyme synthesis, which results in increased oxygen consumption and resultant increased basal metabolic rate. This affects heart rate, respiratory rate, mobilization of carbohydrates, cholesterol metabolism, and a wide variety of other physiological activities. In addition, thyroid hormones stimulate growth and development and, as noted earlier, are critical for the normal proliferation, growth, and development of brain cells. **Table 2** shows the estimated iodine concentration in selected organs.

Iodine Deficiency and Excess

Iodine Deficiency

Iodine deficiency is the most common cause of preventable mental retardation in the world. This fact, along with the recognition that iodine deficiency is not limited to remote rural populations, has stimulated agencies and governments to

Table 2 Estimated iodine concentrations in selected organs

Total body	Thyroid gland	Brain	Liver	Blood
15–20 mg	8–12 mg (for a 15–25 g gland)	0.02 μg g^{-1} (wet weight)	0.2 μg g^{-1} (wet weight)	0.08–0.60 μg dl^{-1} (plasma inorganic iodide)

mobilize resources to eliminate this problem. This global effort, focusing primarily on iodization of salt for human and animal consumption, is slowly succeeding in eliminating a hidden set of disorders that have plagued mankind for centuries.

Unlike many nutritional deficiencies that are more directly related to socioeconomic status, insufficient intake of iodine is a geographical disease, related to lack of iodine in the environment. Iodine originally present in soil was subjected to leaching by snow and rain, and while a portion of the iodine in the oceans evaporates and is returned to the soil in rainwater, this amount is small. Thus, many areas have insufficient iodine in the environment, and this is reflected in plants grown in that environment. The diets in many developing countries are limited in variability and contain few processed foods. This places large populations at risk of iodine deficiency. The World Health Organization (WHO) estimates that at least 1572 million people are at risk in 118 countries, with 43 million affected by 'some degree of mental impairment.'

In the most simplistic physiological model, inadequate intake of iodine results in a reduction in thyroid hormone production, which stimulates increased TSH production. TSH acts directly on thyroid cells, and without the ability to increase hormone production, the gland becomes hyperplastic. In addition, iodine trapping becomes more efficient, as demonstrated by increased radioactive iodine uptake in deficient individuals. However, this simplistic model is complicated by complex adaptive mechanisms which vary depending on the age of the individual affected. In adults with mild deficiency, reduced intake causes a decrease in extrathyroidal iodine and reduced clearance, demonstrated by decreased urinary iodine excretion, but iodine concentration in the gland may remain within normal limits. With further reduction in intake, this adaptive mechanism is overwhelmed, and the iodine content of the thyroid decreases with alterations in iodination of thyroglobulin, in the ratio of DIT to MIT, and reduction in efficient thyroid hormone production. The ability to adapt appears to decrease with decreasing age, and in children the iodine pool in the thyroid is smaller, and the dynamics of iodine metabolism and peripheral use more rapid. In neonates, the effects of iodine deficiency are more directly reflected in increased TSH. Diminished thyroid iodine content and increased turnover make neonates the most vulnerable to the effects of iodine deficiency and decreased hormone production, even with mild deficiency.

A number of other factors influence iodine balance. Active transport of iodide is competitively inhibited by several compounds, including complex ions such as perchlorate, and by thiocyanate, a metabolic product of several foods. Other compounds, such as propylthiouracil, affect coupling reactions and iodination, doing so regardless of iodine intake, e.g., without blocking iodide transport. Several pharmaceuticals affect peripheral hormone action. Dietary goitrogens, as these compounds have been called, include cassava, lima beans, sweet potatoes, cabbage, and broccoli; these contain cyanide compounds that are detoxified to thiocyanate, which may inhibit iodide transport. Cabbage and turnips, and other plants of the genus *Brassica*, also contain thionamide compounds which block iodination. Certain industrial waste products, such as resorcinol from coal processing, contain phenols that cause irreversible inhibition of TPO and block iodination. In some countries the staple diet includes such goitrogens, and iodine deficiency may be exacerbated, as has been well documented for cassava. While this may be a significant problem in some geographical areas, in most instances adequate dietary iodine can reverse the goitrogenic effect.

The most important clinical effect of deficiency relates to the fact that thyroid hormone is required for the normal development of the brain in both humans and other animals. Numerous studies have demonstrated reduced psychomotor skills and intellectual development in the presence of iodine deficiency, and most experts now believe that there is a continuum of deficits, from mild impairment in IQ to severe mental retardation. Studies in China demonstrated shifts in IQ point distributions in rural communities that were deficient, suggesting an impact of deficiency of 10–15 IQ points. In Europe, where mild deficiency still exists, studies have demonstrated decreased psychomotor, perceptual integrative motor ability as well as lower verbal IQ scores in schoolchildren. Studies in Iran showed similar findings. A recent meta-analysis of 18 studies demonstrated a strong relationship, with an overall 13.5 IQ point difference between deficient and non deficient populations. These findings, coupled with the high prevalence of deficiency in many countries, have major implications for development.

The most severe effect of iodine deficiency is cretinism, which is rare in areas of mildly endemic deficiency but may have reached 5–10% or more in areas with severe deficiency. There are general classifications of cretinism, the symptoms of which frequently overlap. Neurological cretinism presents as extreme mental retardation, deaf-mutism, and impaired motor function including spastic gait.

Myxoedematous cretinism presents as disturbances of growth and development including short stature, coarse facial features, retarded sexual development, mental retardation, and other signs of hypothyroidism. It appears likely that severe deficiency resulting in decreased maternal T_4 may be responsible for the impaired neurological development of the fetus occurring early in pregnancy. The effect of deficiency on the fetus after 20 weeks' gestation may result in hyperstimulation of the developing fetal thyroid, with the extreme manifestation being thyroid failure causing myxoedematous cretinism. Other factors may affect thyroid hormone metabolism. Selenium deficiency, when present with iodine deficiency, may alter the clinical manifestations. Selenium deficiency decreases the activity of the enzyme, glutathione peroxidase (GPX), which, along with thyroid hormone synthesis, reduces hydrogen peroxide (H_2O_2). Combined with iodine deficiency and reduced hormone synthesis, it has been speculated that selenium deficiency may contribute to accumulation of H_2O_2 which may in turn lead to cell damage and contribute to thyroid failure. Selenium is also essential for the deiodinase enzyme activity affecting thyroid hormone catabolism, and deficiency may actually increase serum thyroxine. The balance between these two effects is still not fully understood. The study of cretinism has been critical to the evolution of our understanding of the critical role of iodine for normal mental development.

Iodine deficiency has a number of other effects, including development of goitre, clinical or subclinical hypothyroidism, decreased fertility rates, increased stillbirth and spontaneous abortion rates, and increased perinatal and infant mortality. This spectrum of clinical effects, collectively called 'iodine deficiency disorders,' underlines the importance of iodine in human health.

The most effective method to eliminate iodine deficiency in populations is through iodization of salt. The most classic success of salt iodization was demonstrated in Switzerland. Salt is universally consumed, and in most countries the amount consumed is relatively constant between 5 and 10 g per person per day. Iodine is usually added as iodide or iodate (which is more stable) to achieve 25–50 ppm iodine at consumption. This provides about 150–250 μg of iodine per person per day.

The challenge for national iodine deficiency elimination programs is to mobilize the various sectors that must be involved in a sustainable national program, including education, industry, health, and the political arena. There must be an appropriate regulatory environment, effective demand creation, adequate production to make iodized salt available, and quality assurance of both the product and all program elements to ensure that the program is sustained forever. Success in these efforts has the potential to have a greater impact on development than any public health program to date.

Iodine Excess

Iodine is used in many medications, food preservatives, and antiseptics with minimal adverse effects on populations. Pure iodine crystals are toxic, and ingestion can cause severe stomach irritation. Iodine is allergenic, and acute reactions to radiographic contrast media are not rare. Yet because of the thyroid's unique ability to regulate the body's iodine pool, quite a wide range in intake is tolerated without serious effects, particularly when the exposure is of limited duration.

When ingestion of iodine is in excess of the daily requirement of approximately 150 μg per day, changes in thyroid hormones can occur. A variety of clinical problems can occur, and these differ depending on the dose, the presence of thyroid disease, and whether the individual has been deficient in the past. In iodine-replete individuals without thyroid disease, goitre can result, and rarely, hypothyroidism, although the latter is more common in individuals with other illnesses such as lung disease or cystic fibrosis. The relationship of iodine excess to other diseases such as Hashimoto's thyroiditis remains controversial. In the US iodine levels were quite high from 1960 to 1980, with estimates for adult males as high as 827 μg per day. There was no immediate evidence of an impact on thyroid disease, although longer term longitudinal data are lacking. Effects usually remain subtle and transient, even with ingestion of up to 1500–4500 μg per day.

In the presence of thyroid disease, and in areas with endemic iodine deficiency, suddenly raising daily iodine intake may precipitate hyperthyroidism, and this has been the subject of some concern as salt iodization efforts proceed with fledgling quality assurance. This effect is felt to be related in part to autonomous nodules in the gland that synthesize and release excess thyroid hormone. The exact prevalence of iodine-induced hyperthyroidism in deficient areas is not clear. Many countries initiating salt iodization programs have reported increases in the incidence of toxic nodular goitre and iodine-induced thyrotoxicosis, usually in older people. While this may be a significant clinical problem, the risk is estimated to be between 0.01 and 0.06% and must be considered in the light of the benefit from correction of deficiency.

Assessment of Iodine Status

A standard set of indicators of iodine status has been established by the WHO in response to the need to determine prevalence in countries with endemic deficiency. These indicators reflect iodine status as mediated through the response of the thyroid gland to fluctuations in iodine intake. There are several additional indicators that are used to assess thyroid function, such as T_4 and T_3, but these are less accurate in reflecting iodine status since conversion of T_4 to T_3 and cellular uptake is so responsive to peripheral need.

Urinary iodine reflects iodine sufficiency, and output decreases with diminished intake. Since this indicator reflects the amount of iodine per unit volume of urine, its accuracy is impaired by variable fluid intake and factors affecting the concentration of the urine. Therefore, as a measure of iodine status in an individual, it is less accurate than as a measure of iodine status of a population. Median urinary iodine values are used extensively to assess population prevalence of iodine deficiency.

Thyroid size, either estimated by palpation or using ultrasound volume determination, reflects iodine status since deficiency results in thyroid enlargement, or goitre. Due to the relative ease of palpation, that measure has been a traditional standard to assess populations for iodine deficiency and has been particularly useful in schoolchildren. In adults, where long-standing thyroid enlargement from iodine deficiency may be minimally responsive to corrected iodine intake, palpation may be misleading and could overestimate the current level of iodine sufficiency. In children, palpation becomes increasingly difficult and significantly less accurate when deficiency is mild. Ultrasound volume determination provides a more accurate estimate of thyroid size. For any measure of thyroid size, other factors besides iodine deficiency can cause enlargement, including iodine excess, carcinoma, and infection. In areas of the world where deficiency is a problem, the prevalence of these other diseases compared with goitre from iodine deficiency is negligible.

TSH is produced in response to decreased iodine intake and diminished thyroid hormone production and is used as a measure of iodine status. TSH is best measured in neonates—in the developed world for surveillance against congenital hypothyroidism, and in endemic countries to estimate the magnitude of iodine deficiency. Neonatal TSH has been a useful advocacy tool to demonstrate to policy makers that iodine deficiency is not limited to rural remote populations but affects children born in big city hospitals. However, with the complexity of the interactions between TSH and other hormones, TSH has not been shown to be as useful in older children or adults in estimating prevalence of iodine deficiency. Also, use of iodine containing antiseptics affects TSH distributions in neonates.

Uptake of radioactive iodine isotopes can be used to scan the gland, and determine the affinity of the gland to introduced iodine, and is a measure of deficiency. The most common isotope used is ^{123}I because of its relatively short 13-h half-life and γ photon emission. Uptake is increased in iodine deficiency. Isotopes can also be used to examine the organification of iodine in the formation of thyroid hormones. This is an impractical method for surveying populations. Table 3 provides the WHO criteria for defining iodine deficiency as a public health problem.

Requirements and Dietary Sources

The daily requirement for iodine in humans has been estimated based on daily losses, iodine balance, and turnover, with most studies ranging from 40 to 200 µg per day, depending on age and metabolic needs, as shown in Table 4.

Table 3 WHO criteria for iodine deficiency as a public health problem in populations

Indicator	Population assessed	Mild deficiency (%)	Severe deficiency (%)
Goitre by palpation	Schoolchildren	5–19.9	≥30
Thyroid volume by ultrasound (>97th percentile)	Schoolchildren	5–19.9	≥30
Median urinary iodine (µg l^{-1})	Schoolchildren	50–99	<20
TSH (>5 mU l^{-1} whole blood)	Neonates	3–19.9	≥40

Table 4 Recommended dietary intake

Age	WHO recommended intake (µg per day)	US RDA 1989 (µg per day)
0–6 months	40	40
6–12 months	50	60 (at age 1 year)
1–10 years	70–120	60–120
11 years–adult	120–150	150
Pregnancy	175	175
Lactation	200	200

Table 5 Sample iodine content for various sources

Water	Cabbage	Eggs	Seafood	Sugar	Iodized salt
0.1–2 μg l^{-1} in endemic area	0–0.95 μg g^{-1}	4–10 μg egg^{-1}	300–3000 μg kg^{-1}	<1 μg kg^{-1} in refined sugar	20–50 ppm (at household level, depending on climate, and currently subject to review)
2–15 μg l^{-1} in nonendemic area				30 μg kg^{-1} in unrefined brown sugar	

Table 6 Iodine intake from average US and British diets

Country	Milk (μg per day)	Grains (μg per day)	Meat, fish, and poultry (μg per day)
US	534	152	103
Britain	92	31	36

Natural sources of iodine include seafood, seaweeds, and smaller amounts from crops grown on soil with sufficient iodine, or from meat where livestock has grazed on such soil. The contribution of the latter two is small, and in most countries other sources are required. Iodine added to salt, as noted above, is the primary source for many populations. **Table 5** shows sample iodine content for various sources.

In the US and Britain, as well as in other developed countries, most dietary iodine comes from food processing. Intake can vary, as illustrated in **Table 6**. Iodophors used as antiseptics in the dairy and baking industries provide residual iodine in milk and processed foods. In addition, iodine is present in several vitamin and pharmaceutical preparations.

Iodine as a trace element in low concentrations in most environments plays a critical role in the normal growth and development of many species. In humans, iodine is critical for brain development and correction of global deficiencies is an unparalleled opportunity to improve the well-being of our global community.

See also: **Iodine**: Deficiency Disorders.

Further Reading

Braverman LE and Utiger RD (eds.) (1996) *Werner and Ingbar's The Thyroid, A Fundamental and Clinical Text.* Philadelphia: Lippincott-Raven.

Burgi H, Supersaxo Z, and Selz B (1990) Iodine deficiency diseases in Switzerland one hundred years after Theodor Kocher's survey: A historical review with some new goitre prevalence data. *Acta Endocrinologica (Copenhagen)* **123**: 577–590.

Gaitan E (1990) Goitrogens in food and water. *Annual Review of Nutrition* **10**: 21–39.

Hall R and Kobberling J (1985) *Thyroid Disorders Associated with Iodine Deficiency and Excess.* New York: Raven Press.

Hetzel BS (1994) Iodine deficiency and fetal brain damage. *New England Journal of Medicine* **331**(26): 1770–1771.

Hetzel BS (1989) In *The Story of Iodine Deficiency: An International Challenge in Nutrition.* Oxford: Oxford University Press.

Hetzel BS and Pandav CS (eds.) (1994) *SOS for a Billion—The Conquest of Iodine Deficiency Disorders.* Delhi: Oxford University Press.

Mertz W (1986) *Trace Elements in Human and Animal Nutrition,* 5th edn. New York: Academic Press.

Patai S and Rappoport Z (eds.) (1995) *The Chemistry of Halides, Pseudo-halides and Azides,* Supplement D2: part 2. New York: John Wiley & Sons.

Stanbury JB (ed.) (1994) *The Damaged Brain of Iodine Deficiency.* New York: Cognizant Communication Corporation, The Franklin Institute.

Sullivan KM, Houston RM, Gorstein J, and Cervinskas J (1995) *Monitoring Universal Salt Iodization Programmes* Ottowa: UNICEF, MI, ICCIDD, WHO publication.

Thorpe-Beeston JG and Nicolaides KH (1996) *Maternal and Fetal Thyroid Function in Pregnancy* New York: The Parthenon Publishing Group.

Todd CH, Allain T, Gomo ZAR *et al.* (1995) Increase in thyrotoxicosis associated with iodine supplements in Zimbabwe. *Lancet* **346**: 1563–1564.

Troncone L, Shapiro B, Satta MA, and Monaco F (1994) *Thyroid Diseases: Basic Science Pathology, Clinical and Laboratory Diagnosis.* Boca Raton: CRC Press.

WHO, UNICEF, and ICCIDD (1994) *Indicators for Assessing Iodine Deficiency Disorders and Their Control through Salt Iodization,* (limited publication). Geneva: WHO, UNICEF, ICCID.

Wilson JD and Foster DW (eds.) (1992) *Williams Textbook of Endocrinology.* Philadelphia: WB Saunders.

LYCOPENES AND RELATED COMPOUNDS

C J Bates, MRC Human Nutrition Research,
Cambridge, UK

Introduction

Lycopene, the most abundant pigment in ripe red tomatoes and in a few other fruits, is one of the major carotenoid pigments that is widely present in the diet of the human population in the world today. **Figure 1** illustrates the chemical formula of selected carotenoids that occur widely both in human diets and in the noncellular fraction of human blood in most regions of the world. Carotenoids are yellow-to-red in color, with lycopene being nearer the red end of the carotenoid series. However, unlike the carotenes and cryptoxanthins, it does not possess a beta-ionone ring structure at either end of the molecule, and this precludes it from becoming a precursor of vitamin A in humans and animals. Nevertheless, it is readily transformed from the all-*trans* form that is characteristic of most plants and plant foods for animals and humans, to a range of mono- and di-*cis* forms within the animal's body. In addition, oxidation to epoxides and hydroxylated derivatives occurs, although the control of these oxidation pathways and the nature of their products are not yet well understood or characterized.

In plant tissues, where it is synthesized, lycopene is thought to help protect vulnerable photosynthetic tissues from light- and oxygen-catalyzed damage. Its role in humans and other animals, which can only obtain the pigment from their diet, is less well understood. Indeed it remains unproven that there is an essential role for lycopene in animal tissues. Nevertheless, considerable research effort is currently being undertaken to test hypotheses that are attempting to link human dietary and tissue lycopene levels to the risk of degenerative diseases, such as vascular diseases, cancers, etc., especially in older people. As discussed in more detail below, this research is being performed in a wide range of tissue culture and animal model systems and human epidemiological studies.

In this article, some key aspects of the chemical and physical properties, the dietary sources, biochemical status indices, and biological significance of lycopene will be described.

Chemical and Physical Properties of Lycopene; its Food Sources and Enteral Absorption

Lycopene is the most commonly encountered of that subgroup of the naturally occurring carotenoids that have a straight-chain poly-isoprenoid molecule without any terminal β-ionone ring structures (**Figure 1**). The chain length and number of conjugated double bonds determine the absorption spectrum, which peaks at 472 nm with a molar extinction coefficient, $\varepsilon^{1\%}$ of 3450. It is one of the most nonpolar members of the carotenoids, and in organic solution it is also one of the most easily oxidized and thus is easily destroyed, which necessitates the use of rigorous precautions against its oxidative destruction during its extraction and analysis from plants, foods, animal tissues, and body fluids. Currently, such analytical determination is usually based on high-performance liquid chromatography (HPLC), using either its characteristic light absorption property, or its natural fluorescence, or its redox character, for detection and quantitation by absorbance or fluorometric or electrochemical detection. Another characteristic that greatly affects its stability and the problems of its storage and analysis is the phenomenon of *cis-trans* isomerization. Naturally occurring lycopene in tomatoes, the major human food source of this carotenoid, is nearly 100% all-*trans* (**Figure 1**), but during the processing of food, and then during the processes of absorption and accumulation in animal tissues, there is a progressive increase in the proportion of a variety of *cis*-forms. Most of these *cis*-forms contain a single *cis*-bond (mono-*cis*-lycopene), and the 5-, 9-, 13- and 15- mono-

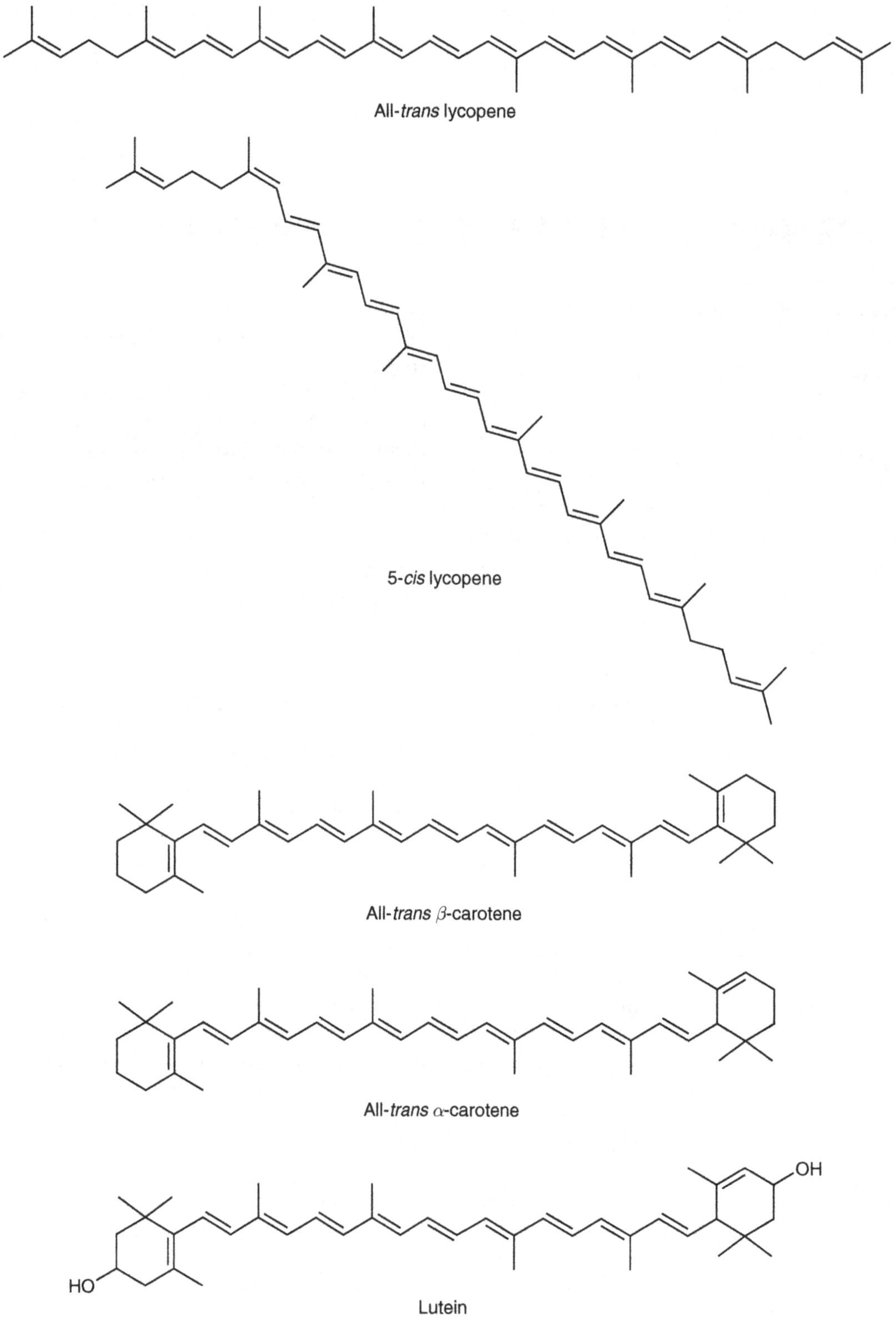

Figure 1 Structures of lycopene and certain other carotenoids found in human blood and tissues.

cis-lycopenes account for more than 50% of the total lycopene in human serum. Smaller quantities of di-cis-lycopenes are normally also present. Curiously, another food source of lycopene, red palm oil, has a much higher natural proportion of the cis-forms of the pigment. Isomerization is catalyzed by low pH; therefore, stomach acid is believed to be a major factor in the conversion of the all-trans-lycopene ingested from tomatoes and their products to a mixture of *cis*-forms in the digestive tract. There is also evidence that further isomerization occurs between the digestive tract and the portal lymphatic lipid micelles. The *cis*-isomers differ from the all-*trans* form in their absorption and intertissue transportation properties, and also in their functional characteristics; for instance, they are more soluble in lipophilic solvents and structures and are less likely to aggregate into crystalline forms. However, these physicochemical differences and their biological consequences have yet to be adequately explored and described.

Of all the most common naturally occurring carotenoids, lycopene is by far the most efficient in reacting with and quenching singlet oxygen, $^1O_2$, which is a non-free-radical excited and reactive form of oxygen. This form of oxygen reacts rapidly with lycopene to yield nonexcited triplet oxygen and excited triplet lycopene. The latter then dissipates its extra energy by solvent interactions, thus regenerating nonexcited lycopene and preserving its original structure by recycling. However, another of its chemical interactions with molecular oxygen appears to result in irreversible oxidation to yield one or more cyclic epoxides, which then probably undergo ring-opening. Nevertheless, there are many unresolved questions about the nature and importance of the many degradation and catabolic pathways that are believed to result in the irreversible destruction of lycopene both *in vitro* and *in vivo*.

Lycopene is an essential intermediate in the pathway for synthesis of the β-ionone ring-containing carotenoids such as β-carotene in plant tissues, and in most plant tissues it is present in only minor amounts. However, in a few, including tomato fruit, watermelon, and red grapefruit, this conversion to the β-ionone ring products by the enzyme lycopene cyclase is hindered, so that the intermediate carotenoid forms, lycopene, phytoene and phytofluene, accumulate instead.

In the US, tomato products provide more than 85% of the total quantity of lycopene consumed by the human population. Mean lycopene intakes in the US are considerably greater than they are in the UK, where the mean daily intake is thought to be less than one-third that in the US, while lycopene intakes in Far Eastern countries such as China and Thailand appear to be much lower still. Wild tomatoes originated in Central America and were introduced into Europe following the opening up of the New World, and were later introduced back into North America from Europe. Because tomatoes are the major source of dietary lycopene in many human populations, some epidemiological studies have been designed on the simplistic assumption that tomato consumption can be used as a general proxy for lycopene consumption, and that any disease associations with tomato consumption can be attributed to the biological effects of lycopene. However, tomatoes also contain significant amounts of other carotenoids, vitamin C, bioflavonoids such as naringenin, and phenolic acids such as chlorogenic acid. Much of the existing epidemiological evidence for possible beneficial effects of lycopene (see below) cannot distinguish unequivocally between the biological effects of lycopene and those of the many other bioactive constituents present in tomatoes.

The bioavailability of lycopene from raw tomatoes is low, but it is greatly increased by cooking or by commercial processing such as conversion to soup, sauce, ketchup, etc., and its availability is also increased by increasing the fat content of the food. Interactions with other carotenoids are complex and have only partly been studied, for instance β-carotene in the same dish seems to increase the absorption of lycopene, but large doses of β-carotene given separately seem to decrease the lycopene content of serum lipoproteins. The contribution of several categories of tomato product to intakes in a recent survey of older people in Britain is shown in **Table 2**. The strength of the correlation between dietary lycopene intake and blood (serum or plasma) lycopene concentration varies greatly among studies and clearly depends on many factors, one of which is the degree of sophistication of the food table values, since subtle differences in food sources and meal composition affect its bioavailability very considerably.

Table 1 Lycopene content of selected foods

Food category	Content as summarized by Clinton (1998) (mg per 100 g wet weight)
Fresh tomatoes	0.9–4.2
Canned tomatoes	
Tomato sauce	6.2
Tomato paste	5–150
Tomato juice	5–12
Tomato ketchup	10–13
Tomato soup	
Grapefruit	3.4
Guava	5.4
Papaya	2–5.3
Watermelon	2.3–7.2

Source: Clinton SK (1998) Lycopene: Chemistry, biology and implication for human health and disease. *Nutrition Reviews* **56**: 35–51.

Table 2 Tomato products consumed by people aged 65 years and over in Britain

Categories of tomatoes and tomato products	Percentage of each category consumed
Raw tomatoes	36.2
Processed tomatoes	
Soups	8.8
Canned tomatoes	7.0
Grilled	5.4
Fried	3.2
Ketchup	0.4
Tomato-based products	
Canned food	29.5
Pizza	2.3
Other	7.1
Total	99.9

Source: Re R, Mishra GD, Thane CW, and Bates CJ (2003) Tomato consumption and plasma lycopene concentration in people aged 65 years and over in a British National Survey. *European Journal of Clinical Nutrition* **57**: 1545–1554. Reproduced with permission from Nature Publishing Group.

Tissue Contents and Kinetics of Lycopene Turnover

Once absorbed, passively from lipid micelles by the enterocyte, lycopene enters the portal lymphatics and thence the liver, from which it enters the peripheral bloodstream, mainly in association with the β-lipoproteins, in which it is transported to the peripheral tissues. Its half-life in plasma is of the order of 12–33 days; longer than that of β-carotene, which is less than 12 days. Clearly, many of these factors are interdependent, and there is a need for further clarification of the key independent determinants of lycopene status, and whether plasma levels can provide an adequate picture of tissue and whole body status.

Patients with alcoholic cirrhosis of the liver have greatly reduced hepatic lycopene concentrations; indeed, hepatic lycopene seems to offer a sensitive index of hepatic health. Studies of organ concentrations (**Table 3**), suggest a gradient from circulating levels in plasma to different ones in specific tissues. The different carotenoid ratios between organs (not shown) also indicate selective transport and accumulation. However, the mechanisms involved are poorly understood. No lycopene is detectable in the retina or lens of the eye, where lutein and zeaxanthin are found; however, lycopene is present in the ciliary body.

Table 3 Concentrations of lycopene reported in human tissues

Tissue	Range of mean or median lycopene concentrations (nmol per g wet weight)
Adrenal	1.9–21.6
Testis	4.3–21.4
Liver	0.6–5.7
Brain	2.5
Lung	0.2–0.6
Kidney	0.1–0.6
Stomach, colon	0.2–0.3
Breast, cervix	0.2–0.8
Skin	0.4
Adipose tissue	0.2–1.3
Prostate	0.1–0.6
Plasma	0.2–1.1

Values were gathered from 11 publications, all based on HPLC analyses.

Functional Properties and Tissue Health

The capacity for quenching of singlet oxygen has been mentioned above; the exceptionally high rate constant, $K = 3.1 \times 10^{10}\,\mathrm{mol}^{-1}\,\mathrm{s}^{-1}$, renders it one of the most efficient of known quenchers of this powerful oxidant. In the plant, it probably protects chlorophyll, which produces singlet oxygen as a by-product of photosynthesis. In experiments with lymphoid cells, lycopene provided better protection against singlet oxygen damage than several other carotenoids tested. In skin exposed to UV light, lycopene disappears much more rapidly than β-carotene. Lycopene is also able, in model systems, to inhibit the peroxidation of polyunsaturated lipids and the oxidation of DNA bases to products such as 8-hydroxydeoxyguanosine (8-OHdG). It can react directly with hydrogen peroxide and nitrogen dioxide.

Several studies in cell culture have shown a reduction in the formation of oxidation damage products such as malondialdehyde, and have found less injury to cells exposed to oxidants such as carbon tetrachloride, if lycopene (or other carotenoids) are present.

Another characteristic of lycopene and other carotenoids that may be relevant to inhibition of cancer cell growth is the modulation of gap junction cell–cell communication processes. In particular, carotenoids including lycopene have been shown to enhance the efficacy of the protein, connexin43, which helps to ensure the maintenance of the differentiated state of cells and to reduce the probability of unregulated cell division, and which is deficient in many tumors. They may also interact with and enhance the synthesis of binding proteins that downregulate the receptor for the growth-promoting hormone insulin-like growth factor-1 (IGF-1).

In certain circumstances, lycopene can reduce LDL-cholesterol levels, possibly by inhibiting hydroxymethylglutaryl CoA reductase (HMGCoA reductase), the rate-limiting enzyme for cholesterol synthesis (see below). Lycopene was shown to have modest hypocholesterolemic properties in one small clinical trial.

Health, Research Models and Epidemiological Evidence

Table 4 summarizes the various types of evidence that have been used to test the hypothesis that lycopene may have health-promoting or protective properties in man. The ultimate proof of efficacy, which would be long-term controlled intervention studies with clinical diseases and or mortality as the end points, are extremely difficult, expensive, and time-consuming to obtain, and

cannot address all possible benefits in a single intervention trial.

The two disease categories that have so far received most attention for possible long-term benefits of lycopene have been the amelioration of cancers and of heart disease. Both benefits are plausible in view of the physicochemical and biological properties of lycopene outlined above, because both categories of disease are characterized by tissue damage, which is thought to be induced or exacerbated by reactive oxygen species in the environment or those generated within the body.

Evidence for Possible Anticancer Protection by Lycopene

Most of the indications with respect to cancer comes from human studies linking tomato intake, total estimated lycopene intake, and serum or plasma lycopene concentrations to the subsequent development of cancers (Table 5). There is a small amount of evidence from experimental animal studies, for instance, rat and mouse dimethylbenzanthracene-

Table 4 Types of evidence being sought, that a nutrient such as lycopene may protect against oxidation-induced or other disease processes

1. Model *in vitro* systems, e.g., oxygen-derived free-radical trapping in pure chemical mixtures.
2. Tissue (cell and organ) cultures, e.g., reduction of optical opacity development in cultured eye lenses; reduced growth rates or apoptosis in tumor cell cultures.
3. Animal studies demonstrating a reduction of oxidation-induced damage or disease with lycopene supplements or with lycopene-rich foods such as tomatoes or tomato products.
4. Human observation studies using intermediate biochemical markers: e.g., inverse relationships between lycopene intakes or its blood levels and biochemical markers, such as lipid or DNA oxidation products.
5. Studies using pathology-related intermediate markers, e.g., arterial thickening or reduced arterial elasticity; precancerous polyposis, etc.
6. Relationships (without intervention) between tomato intakes or estimated lycopene intakes or lycopene contents of serum, plasma, or tissues (e.g., fat biopsies) and actual disease prevalence or incidence in human cross-sectional, case-control, or prospective epidemiological studies.
7. Intervention studies: lycopene supplements producing a reduction in biochemical markers of oxidation damage or in functional markers, or, eventually, in actual human disease incidence or progression.

Table 5 Summary evidence for possible lycopene protection against prostate cancer

No. of studies	Locations	Total no. of participants	Types of trial	Outcome conclusion
2	Greece, Canada	937	Case–control (intake of tomato or lycopene, or blood level)	Significant association
7	USA, UK, Canada, New Zealand	3824	As above	No significant association
3	USA	954	Prospective studies based on dietary estimates	Significant association
1	Netherlands		As above	No association
3	USA	723	Prospective studies based on serum or plasma lycopene	Inconclusive; one study found a marginal ($P = 0.05$) benefit vs. aggressive cancer

induced mammary tumor studies have supported the hypothesis, as has a model of spontaneous mammary tumor formation in one strain of mice, but many of the animal models of tumor promotion have been criticized as being too dissimilar from the likely processes of spontaneous tumorigenesis in humans.

Partly for historical reasons, there has been a particular interest in prostate cancer (**Table 5**). A large and early trial in the US (US Health Professionals Follow-up Study) reported an impressive difference between groups with high and low intakes of tomatoes and hence of lycopene for subsequent prostate cancer development, which was not shared with other carotenoids. Plausibility was enhanced by the fact that although human prostate lycopene concentrations are not especially high on an absolute basis (**Table 3**), they are higher than those of other carotenoids in this tissue. Subsequent studies have had variable outcomes. A small pilot study reported that tomato oleoresin supplements given for a short period to prostate cancer sufferers who were due for radical prostatectomy resulted in smaller tumor size and other apparent benefits, but this trial now needs to be repeated on a larger scale.

Several studies have provided evidence for protection of certain regions of the digestive tract against tumor occurrence or growth. Two studies, one in Iran and another in Italy, found an inverse relationship between esophageal cancer and tomato consumption. Two Italian and one Japanese study reported evidence for protection against gastric cancer, and two studies claimed a reduction in pancreatic cancer. Results with others cancer have been mixed and inconclusive.

Lycopene and Cardiovascular Disease

Table 6 summarizes the evidence. The European Multicentre Euramic Study, which reported that risk of developing myocardial infarct was inversely related to lycopene intake, after appropriate adjustment for other cardiovascular risk factors. Some Scandinavian studies have subsequently supported this claim; moreover, lycopene is capable of reducing LDL-cholesterol levels, possibly by inhibiting hydroxymethylglutaryl CoA reductase (HMGCoA reductase), the rate-limiting enzyme for cholesterol synthesis.

Other Disease-Related Investigations

In an organ culture model, some evidence for protection of rat lenses against induction of cataractogenesis has been reported. There is good reason to believe that carotenoids in general may play a role in the protection of ocular tissues against the damaging effects of UV light and of reactive oxygen substances, whose exposure to light carries some analogy with the known

Table 6 Summary evidence of association of relatively high serum or plasma lycopene with lowered risk of cardiovascular disease (CVD)

Study	Location	Sex (total participants)	Types of trial and outcome measures	Outcome conclusion
Euramic	Europe, multicenter	M (1379)	C-C, MI	Significant association with protection[a]
ARIC	USA	M + F (462)	C-C, IMT	NS
Street	USA	M + F (369)	NC-C, MI in smokers	NS
Rotterdam	Netherlands	M + F (216)	C-C, PC	Significant association with protection
Bruneck	Italy	M + F (392)	CS + PFU, PC	NS
Linkoping –Vinus	Sweden and Lithuania	M (210)	CS, mortality from heart disease	NS
Kuopio (KHID)	Finland	M (725)	PFU, acute coronary event or stroke	Significant association with protection
Kuopio (ASP)	Finland	M + F (520)	IMT	Males significant; females not significant.

[a]No association with plasma β-carotene in this study.

C-C, case–control study; NC-C, nested case–control study; CS, cross-sectional study; PFU, prospective follow-up study; MI, myocardial infarct; IMT, intima-media thickness estimate; PC, plaque count. NS, no significant evidence for protection.Significance generally after appropriate adjustment for other known CVD risk factors.

functions of carotenoids in plant tissues. A possible protective role in the ciliary body and iris has been proposed, but not yet tested.

Conclusions

Clearly lycopene possesses chemical and biological properties, which make it a very attractive candidate for tissue protection and reduction of disease, especially degenerative diseases. Lycopene probably interacts more efficiently with one particular reactive oxygen species, singlet oxygen, than any other commonly occurring nutrient. It appears to share with several other carotenoids the capacity to reduce lipid peroxidation and DNA oxidative damage, and to enhance cell–cell gap junction communication and to protect normal IGF-1 function. It may reduce cholesterol formation and its tissue accumulation in some circumstances. Studies related to cancers and cardiovascular disease are ongoing and are attracting increased research interest.

See also: **Antioxidants**: Diet and Antioxidant Defense; Observational Studies; Intervention Studies. **Ascorbic Acid**: Physiology, Dietary Sources and Requirements. **Carotenoids**: Chemistry, Sources and Physiology; Epidemiology of Health Effects. **Vitamin A**: Biochemistry and Physiological Role; Deficiency and Interventions.

Further Reading

Arab L and Steck S (2000) Lycopene and cardiovascular disease. *American Journal of Clinical Nutrition* **71**(supplement): 1691S–1695S.

Arab L, Steck-Scott S, and Bowen P (2001) Participation of lycopene and beta-carotene in carcinogenesis: Defenders, aggressors or passive bystanders? *Epidemiologic Reviews* **23**: 211–230.

Britton G (1995) Structure and properties of carotenoids in relation to function. *FASEB J* **9**: 1551–1558.

Clinton SK (1998) Lycopene: chemistry, biology, and implications for human health and disease. *Nutrition Reviews* **56**: 35–51.

Gerster H (1997) The potential of lycopene for human health. *Journal of the American College of Nutrition* **16**: 109–126.

Giovanucci E (1999) Tomatoes, tomato-based products, lycopene, and cancer: review of the epidemiologic literature. *Journal of the National Cancer Institute* **91**: 317–331.

International Symposium on the Role of Tomato Products and Carotenoids in Disease Prevention (2002) 14 review articles by different authors, plus 17 symposium abstracts. *Experimental Biology and Medicine* **227**: 843–937.

Nguyen ML and Schwartz SJ (1999) Lycopene: chemical and biological properties. *Food Technology* **53**: 38–45.

Rao AV and Agarwal S (1999) Role of lycopene as antioxidant carotenoid in the prevention of chronic diseases: A review. *Nutrition Research* **19**: 305–323.

Stahl W and Sies H (1996) Lycopene: a biologically important carotenoid for humans? *Archives of Biochemistry and Biophysics* **336**: 1–9.

Weisburger J (1998) International symposium on lycopene and tomato products in disease prevention. *Proceedings of the Society for Experimental Biology and Medicine* **218**: 93–143.

MAGNESIUM

C Feillet-Coudray and Y Rayssiguier, National Institute for Agricultural Research, Clermont-Ferrand, France

Magnesium (Mg), the second intracellular cation after sodium, is a essential mineral. It is a critical cofactor in more than 300 enzymatic reactions. It may be required for substrate formation (Mg-ATP) and enzyme activation. It is critical for a great number of cellular functions, including oxidative phosphorylation, glycolysis, DNA transcription, and protein synthesis. It is involved in ion currents and membrane stabilization. Mg deficiency may be implicated in various metabolic disorders, including cardiovascular diseases, immune dysfunction and free radical damage.

Magnesium Metabolism

Distribution of Mg within the Body

The normal adult body contains approximately 25 g of Mg, with more than 60% in bone tissue (**Table 1**). Only a fraction of bone Mg (at the surface of the bone crystal) is exchangeable with extracellular Mg. The muscle contains 25% of total body Mg, and extracellular Mg accounts for only 1%. Plasma Mg is approximately 0.8 mmol/l, half of which is ionised and active in physiological reactions half bound to proteins or complexed to anions. In cells, Mg is associated with various structures, such as the nucleus and intracellular organelles, and free Mg accounts for 1–5% of total cellular Mg. Intracellular free Mg is maintained at a relatively constant level, even if extracellular Mg level varies. This phenomenon is due to the limited permeability of the plasma membrane to Mg and the existence of specific Mg transport systems that regulate the rates at which Mg is taken up by cells or extruded from cells. Mechanisms by which Mg is taken up by cells have not been completely elucidated, and Mg efflux particularly requires the antiport Na^+/Mg^{2+}. Various hormonal and pharmacological factors influence Mg transport, and it can be assumed that recent developments in molecular genetics will lead to the identification of proteins implicated in Mg transport.

Intestinal Absorption

Net Mg absorption results from dietary Mg absorption and Mg secretion into the intestinal tract via bile and gastric and pancreatic juice. In healthy adults, 30–50% of dietary Mg is absorbed. The secreted Mg is efficiently reabsorbed and endogenous fecal losses are only 20–50 mg/day. Mg absorption occurs along the entire intestinal tract, but the distal small intestine (jejunum and ileum) is the primary site. It is essentially a passive intercellular process by electrochemical gradient and solvent drag. The active transport occurs only for extremely low dietary Mg intake and its regulation is unknown. Mg uptake in the brush border may be mediated by a Mg/anion complex, and Mg efflux across the basolateral membrane may involve Na^+/Mg^{2+} antiport systems. A gene implicated in Mg deficit in humans has been identified. It is expressed in intestine and kidney and appears to encode for a protein that combines Ca- and Mg-permeable channel properties with protein kinase activity. This gene may be implicated in Mg absorption. Because of the importance of the passive process, the quantity of Mg in the digestive tract is the major factor controlling the amount of Mg absorbed.

The possibility of an adaptative increase in the fraction of Mg absorbed as Mg intake is lowered is controversial. In fact, experimental studies indicate that fractional intestinal absorption of Mg is directly proportional to dietary Mg intake. Because only soluble Mg is absorbed, all the factors increasing Mg solubility increase its absorption while formation of insoluble complexes in the intestine may decrease Mg absorption. Most well-controlled studies indicate that high calcium intake does not affect intestinal Mg absorption in humans. In contrast, dietary phytate in excess impairs Mg

Table 1 Magnesium in human tissues

	% distribution	Concentration
Bone	60–65	0.5% of bone ash
Muscle	27	6–10 mmol/kg wet weight
Other cells	6–7	6–10 mmol/kg wet weight
Extracellular	<1	
Erythrocytes		2.5 mmol/l
Serum		0.7–1.1 mol/l
Free	55	
Complexed	13	
Bound	32	
Mononuclear blood cells		2.3–3.5 fmol/cell
Cerebrospinal fluid		1.25 mmol/l
Free	55	
Complexed	45	
Sweat		0.3 mmol/l (in hot environment)
Secretions		0.3–0.7 mmol/l

From *Molecular Aspects of Medicine*, vol. 24, Vormann J: Magnesium: nutrition and metabolism, pp. 27–37, Copyright 2003, with permission from Elsevier.

absorption by formation of insoluble complexes in the intestinal tract. Negative effects of a high intake of dietary fiber have often been reported, but these actions have certainly been overestimated. In fact, only the impact of purified fiber was considered, but fiber-rich diets are a major source of Mg and roles of the intestinal fermentation and the large bowel in mineral absorption were neglected. It was demonstrated in animal models that fermentable carbohydrates (oligosaccharides and resistant starch) enhance Mg absorption in the large bowel and that a similar effect exists in humans. Other nutrients may influence Mg absorption but these effects are important only at low dietary Mg intake.

Urinary Excretion

Magnesium homeostasis is essentially regulated by a process of filtration–reabsorption in the kidney. Urinary Mg excretion increases when Mg intake is in excess, whereas the kidney conserves Mg in the case of Mg deprivation. Usually, 1000 mmol/24 h of Mg is filtered and only 3 mmol/24 h is excreted in urine.

A total of 10–15% of the filtered Mg is reabsorbed in the proximal tubule by a passive process. The majority of filtered Mg (65%) is reabsorbed in the thick ascending loop of Henle. The reabsorption in this segment is mediated by a paracellular mechanism involving paracellin-1. It is also related to sodium transport by a dependence on the transepithelial potential generated by NaCl absorption. Thus, factors that impair NaCl reabsorption in the thick

ascending loop of Henle, such as osmotic diuretics, loop diuretics, and extracellular fluid volume expansion, increase Mg excretion. At least 10–15% of the filtered Mg is reabsorbed in the distal tubule. The reabsorption occurs via an active transcellular mechanism and is under the control of special divalent cation-sensing receptors. Thus, elevated plasma Mg concentrations inhibit reabsorption of Mg from the distal tubule, leading to an increased magnesuria. Other active transport may also exist since some hormones (parathyroid hormone, glucagon, calcitonin, and insulin) may increase Mg reabsorption. Other factors may also influence Mg reabsorption, such as hypercalciuria or hypophosphatemia, which inhibit the tubular reabsorption of Mg. Metabolic alkalosis leads to renal Mg conservation, whereas metabolic acidosis is associated with urinary Mg wasting. Thus, the chronic low-grade metabolic acidosis in humans eating Western diets may contribute to decreased Mg status.

Dietary Sources of Magnesium

Mg is present in all foods, but the Mg content varies substantially (**Table 2**). Cereals and nuts have high Mg content. Vegetables are moderately rich in Mg, and meat, eggs, and milk are poor in Mg. A substantial amount of Mg may be lost during food processing, and refined foods generally have a low Mg content. In addition to Mg content, it is important to consider the Mg density of food (i.e., the quantity of Mg per unit of energy). Vegetables, legumes, and cereals thus contribute efficiently to daily Mg intake, whereas fat- and/or sugar-rich products have a minor contribution. Some water can also be a substantial source of Mg, but it depends on the area from which the water derives.

Table 2 Mg density of foods

Food	Magnesium density (mg/MJ)
Vegetables (lettuce, broccoli)	211
Legumes (bean)	113
Whole cereal (wheat)	104
Nuts (almond)	105
Fruits (apple)	30
Fish (cod)	75
Meat (roast beef)	40
Whole milk	38
Cheese (camembert)	15
Eggs	18
Dessert	
Biscuit	10
Chocolate	52

From Répertoire Général des Aliments (1996).

Requirements

Assessment of Mg Status

Several potential markers for estimating daily Mg requirement have been suggested. Plasma Mg concentration is the most commonly used marker to assess Mg status. In healthy populations, the plasma Mg value is 0.86 mmol/l and the reference value is 0.75–0.96 mmol/l. A low plasma Mg value reflects Mg depletion, but a normal plasma Mg level may coexist with low intracellular Mg. Thus, despite its interest, plasma Mg is not a good marker of Mg status.

Ion-specific electrodes have become available for determining ionized Mg in plasma, and this measurement may be a better marker of Mg status than total plasma Mg. However, further investigation is necessary to achieve a standardized procedure and to validate its use as an appropriate marker of Mg status.

Erythrocyte Mg level is also commonly used to assess Mg status, and the normal value is 2.06–2.54 mmol/l. However, erythrocyte Mg level is under genetic control, and numerous studies have shown no correlation between erythrocyte Mg and other tissue Mg.

The total Mg content of white blood cells has been proposed to be an index of Mg status. However, lymphocytes, polymorphonuclear blood cells, and platelets may have protective mechanisms against intracellular Mg deficiency, and the determination of total Mg content in leukocytes and platelets to assess Mg status is of questionable usefulness.

Mg excretion determination is helpful for the diagnosis of Mg deficit when there is an hypomagnesemia. In healthy populations, the urinary Mg value is 4.32 mmol/day and the reference value is 1.3–8.2 mmol/day. In the presence of hypomagnesemia, normal or high urinary Mg excretion is suggestive of renal wasting. On the contrary, Mg urinary excretion lower than normal values is convincing evidence of Mg deficiency.

The parenteral loading test is probably the best available marker for the diagnosis of Mg deficiency. The Mg retention after parenteral administration of Mg seems to reflect the general intracellular Mg content, and a Mg retention more than 20% of the administered Mg suggests Mg deficiency. However, this test is not valid in the case of abnormal urinary Mg excretion and is contraindicated in renal failure.

Determination of exchangeable Mg pools using Mg stable isotopes is an interesting approach to evaluate Mg status. In fact, Mg exchangeable pool sizes vary with dietary Mg in animals. However, more studies are necessary to better appreciate the relationship between Mg status and exchangeable Mg pool size in humans.

Magnesium Deficit

Two types of Mg deficit must be differentiated. Dietary Mg deficiency results from an insufficient intake of Mg. Secondary Mg deficiency is related to dysregulation of the control mechanisms of Mg metabolism.

Dietary Mg Deficiency

Severe Mg deficiency is very rare, whereas marginal Mg deficiency is common in industrialized countries. Low dietary Mg intake may result from a low energy intake (reduction of energy output necessary for physical activity and thermoregulation, and thus of energy input) and/or from low Mg density of the diet (i.e., refined and/or processed foods). Moreover, in industrialized countries, diets are rich in animal source foods and low in vegetable foods. This leads to a dietary net acid load and thus a negative effect on Mg balance. In fact, animal source foods provide predominantly acid precursors (sulphur-containing amino acids), whereas fruits and vegetables have substantial amounts of base precursor (organic acids plus potassium salts). Acidosis increases Mg urinary excretion by decreasing Mg reabsorption in the loop of Henle and the distal tubule, and potassium depletion impairs Mg reabsorption. Mg deficiency treatment simply requires oral nutritional physiological Mg supplementation.

Secondary Mg Deficiency

Failure of the mechanisms that ensure Mg homeostasis, or endogenous or iatrogenic perturbing factors of Mg status, leads to secondary Mg deficit. Secondary Mg deficiency requires a more or less specific correction of its causal dysregulation.

Intestinal Mg absorption decreases in the case of malabsorption syndromes, such as chronic diarrhoea, inflammatory enteropathy, intestinal resection, and biliary and intestinal fistulas.

Hypermagnesuria is encountered in the case of metabolic and iatrogenic disorders, such as primary and secondary hyperaldosteronism (extracellular volume expansion), hypercalcemia (competition Ca/Mg at the thick ascending loop of Henle), hyperparathyroidism, and phosphate or potassium depletion. Hypermagnesuria may also result from tubulopathy, as the selective defect of the Mg tubular reabsorption (chromosome 11q23), Bartter's syndrome (thick ascending loop of Henle), or Gitelman's syndrome (distal convoluted tubule).

Administration of medications can be a causal factor in the development of secondary Mg deficiency. Administration of diuretics is the main cause of iatrogenic deficit because it decreases NaCl reabsorption in the thick ascending loop of Henle and thus increases the fractional excretion of Mg.

Causes of Mg Deficit

Complex relations exist between Mg and carbohydrate metabolism. Diabetes is frequently associated with Mg deficit and insulin may play an important role in the regulation of intracellular Mg content by stimulating cellular Mg uptake. Hypomagnesemia is the most common ionic abnormality in alcoholism because of poor nutritional status and Mg malabsorption, alcoholic ketoacidosis, hypophosphatemia, and hyperaldosteronism secondary to liver disease.

Stress can contribute to Mg deficit by stimulating the production of hormones and thus increasing urinary Mg excretion and by impairing neurohormonal mechanisms that spare Mg.

Consequences of Mg Deficit and Implications in Various Metabolic Diseases

Mg deficit causes neuromuscular manifestations, including positive Chvostek and Trousseau signs, muscular fasciculations, tremor, tetany, nausea, and vomiting. The pathogenesis of the neuromuscular irritability is complex, and it implicates the central and peripheral nervous system, the neuromuscular junction, and muscle cells.

Mg deficit perturbs Ca homeostasis and hypocalcemia is a common manifestation of severe Mg deficit. Impaired release of parathyroid hormone (PTH) and skeletal end organ resistance to PTH appear to be the major factors implicated, probably by a decrease in adenylcyclase activity.

Perturbations in the action and/or metabolism of vitamin D may also occur in Mg deficit. Because Mg plays a key role in skeletal metabolism, Mg deficit may be a possible risk factor for osteoporosis. However, epidemiologic studies relating Mg intake to bone mass or rate of bone loss have been conflicting, and further investigation is necessary to clarify the role of Mg in bone metabolism and osteoporosis.

Hypokalemia is frequently encountered in Mg deficit. This is due to an inhibition of Na,K-ATPase activity that impairs K and Na transport in and out of the cell and to stimulation of renin and aldosterone secretion that increases K urinary excretion.

There is increasing evidence that Mg deficiency may be involved in the development of various pathologies. Mg deficit is frequent in diabetes and can be a factor in insulin resistance. It can modify insulin sensitivity, probably by influencing intracellular signaling and processing. Mg deficit has also been implicated in the development or progression of micro- and macroangiopathy and neuropathy.

Mg deficit appears to act as a cardiovascular risk factor. Experimental, clinical, and epidemiological evidence points to an important role of Mg in blood pressure regulation. Mg deficit can lead to cardiac arrhythmias and to increased sensitivity to cardiac glucosides. Mg deficit may also play a role in the development of atherosclerosis. In experimental animal models, dietary Mg deficiency results in dyslipidemia, increased sensitivity to oxidative stress, and a marked proinflammatory effect, thus accelerating atherogenosis. Macrophages and polynuclear neutrophils are activated and synthesize a variety of biological substances, some of which are powerful inducers of inflammatory events (cytokines, free radicals, and eicosanoids). The effect of Mg depletion or Mg supplementation may result in the ability of Mg to modulate intracellular calcium. Pharmacological doses of Mg may reduce morbidity and mortality in the period following infarction. The beneficial effect of Mg may result from calcium-antagonist action, decreased platelet aggregation, and decreased free radical damage.

Magnesium Excess

Magnesium overload can occur in individuals with impaired renal function or during massive intravenous administration of Mg. It is most often iatrogenic. Clinical symptoms such as drowsiness and hyporeflexia develop when plasma Mg is 2- or 3-fold higher than the normal value.

Recommended Dietary Allowances

The Estimated Average Requirement (EAR) is the nutrient intake value that is estimated to meet the requirement of 50% of individuals in a life stage and a gender group. Balance studies and data on stable isotopes suggest an EAR of 5 mg/kg/day for males and females. This value is greater during growth in adolescents and is estimated to be 5.3 mg/kg/day. The Mg requirement is also higher during pregnancy because of Mg transfer to the fetus in the last 3 months; therefore, an additional 35 mg/day is recommended.

In infants, the determination of the Adequate Intake (AI) is based on the Mg content of mother's milk and the progressive consumption of solid food.

Table 3 Recommended dietary allowances of Mg

Age	RDA (mg/day)		AI (mg/day)	
	Male	Female	Male	Female
0–6 months			30	30
6–12 months			75	75
1–3 years	80	80		
4–8 years	130	130		
9–13 years	240	240		
14–18 years	410	360		
19–30 years	400	310		
31–50 years	420	320		
51–70 years	420	320		
<70 years	420	320		
Pregnancy		+40		
Lactation		+0		

From the Institute of Medicine (1997).

Thus, the AI is 30 mg/day during the first 6 months of life and 75 mg/day the second 6 months of life.

The Recommended Dietary Allowance (RDA) is the average daily dietary intake that is sufficient to meet the nutrient requirement of 97.5% of individuals and is set at 20% above the EAR +2 CVs where the CV is 10%. During recent years, dietary reference intakes have been revised by the US Institute of Medicine. The recommended intakes of Mg are given in **Table 3**. It is not known whether decreased urinary Mg and increased maternal bone resorption provide sufficient amounts of Mg to meet increased needs during lactation. Thus, the French Society for Nutrition suggests adding 30 mg/day to intake for lactation.

The intake of Mg has been determined in various populations. Evidence suggests that the occidental diet is relatively deficient in Mg, whereas the vegetarian diet is rich in Mg. For instance, the mean Mg intake of the subjects in the French Supplementation with Antioxidant Vitamins and Minerals Study was estimated to be 369 mg/day in men and 280 mg/day in women. Thus, 77% of women and 72% of men had dietary Mg intakes lower than the RDA, and 23% of women and 18% of men consumed less than two-thirds of the RDA.

Conclusion

Based on evidence of low Mg intake in industrialized countries, intervention studies to improve Mg status and to assess its impact on specific health outcomes are required.

See also: **Calcium. Vitamin D**: Rickets and Osteomalacia.

Further Reading

Coudray C, Demigné C, and Rayssiguier Y (2003) Effects of dietary fibers on magnesium absorption in animals and humans. *Journal of Nutrition* 133: 1–4.

Durlach J (1988) *Magnesium in Clinical Practice* London: John Libbey.

Elin RJ (1989) Assessment of magnesium status. In: Itokawa Y and Durlach I (eds.) *Magnesium in Health and Disease*, pp. 137–146. London: John Libbey.

Feillet-Coudray C, Coudray C, Gueux E, Mazur A, and Rayssiguier Y (2002) A new approach to evaluate magnesium status: Determination of exchangeable Mg pool masses using Mg stable isotope. *Magnesium Research* 15: 191–198.

Galan P, Preziosi P, Durlach V *et al.* (1997) Dietary magnesium intake in a French adult population. *Magnesium Research* 10: 321–328.

Institute of Medicine (1997) *Dietary Reference Intakes for Calcium, Phosphorus, Magnesium, Vitamin D and Fluoride.* Washington, DC: National Academy Press.

Rayssiguier Y, Mazur A, and Durlach J (2001) *Advances in Magnesium Research, Nutrition and Health* London: John Libbey.

Répertoire général des aliments (1996) *Table de Composition Minérale.* Paris: Tec & Doc, Lavoisier.

Rude RK (1998) Magnesium deficiency: A cause of heterogeneous disease in humans. *Journal of Bone Mineral Research* 13(4): 749–758.

Shils ME (1994) Magnesium. In: Shils ME, Olson JA, and Shike M (eds.) *Modern Nutrition in Health and Disease*, 8th ed, pp. 164–184. Philadelphia, PA: Lea & Febiger.

Vormann J (2003) Magnesium: Nutrition and metabolism. *Molecular Aspects of Medicine* 24: 27–37.

Wilkinson SR, Welch RM, Mayland HF, and Grunes DL (1990) Magnesium in plants: Uptake, distribution, function and utilization by man and animals. In: Sigel H and Sigel A (eds.) *Compendium of Magnesium and Its Role in Biology, Nutrition and Physiology*, pp. 33–56. New York: Marcel Dekker.

MANGANESE

**C L Keen, J L Ensunsa, B Lönnerdal and
S Zidenberg-Cherr**, University of California at Davis,
Davis, CA, USA

The essentiality of manganese was established in 1931, when it was demonstrated that a deficit of it resulted in poor growth and impaired reproduction in rodents. Manganese deficiency can be a practical problem in the swine and poultry industries, and it may be a problem in some human populations. Conversely, manganese toxicity can be a significant human health concern. Here, literature related to manganese nutrition, metabolism, and metabolic function is reviewed.

Chemical and Physical Properties

Manganese is the 12th most abundant element in the Earth's crust and constitutes approximately 0.1% of it. Chemical forms of manganese in their natural deposits include oxides, sulfides, carbonates, and silicates. Anthropogenic sources of manganese are predominantly from the manufacturing of steel, alloys, and iron products. Manganese is widely used as an oxidizing agent, as a component of fertilizers and fungicides, and in dry cell batteries. Methylcyclopentadienyl manganese tricarbonyl (MMT) improves combustion in boilers and motors and can substitute for lead in gasoline as an antiknock agent. Concentrations of manganese in groundwater normally range between 1 and $100\,\mu g\,l^{-1}$, with most values being below $10\,\mu g\,l^{-1}$. Typical airborne levels of manganese (in the absence of excessive pollution) range from 10 to $70\,ng\,m^{-3}$.

Manganese is a transition element located in group VIIA of the periodic table. It occurs in 11 oxidation states ranging from -3 to $+7$, with the physiologically most important valences being $+2$ and $+3$. The $+2$ valence is the predominant form in biological systems and is the form that is thought to be maximally absorbed. The $+3$ valence is the form in which manganese is primarily transported in biological systems.

The solution chemistry of manganese is relatively simple. The aquo-ion is resistant to oxidation in acidic or neutral solutions. It does not begin to hydrolyze until pH 10, and therefore free Mn^{2+} can be present in neutral solutions at relatively high concentrations. Divalent manganese is a $3d^5$ ion and typically forms high-spin complexes lacking crystal field stabilization energies. The previous properties, as well as a large ionic radius and small charge-to-radius ratio, result in manganese tending to form weak complexes compared with other first-row divalent ions, such as Ni^{2+} and Cu^{2+}. Free Mn^{2+} has a strong isotropic electron paramagnetic resonance (EPR) signal that can be used to determine its concentration in the low micromolar range. Mn^{3+} is also critical in biological systems. For example, Mn^{3+} is the oxidative state of manganese in superoxide dismutase, is the form in which transferrin binds manganese, and is probably the form of manganese that interacts with Fe^{3+}. Given its smaller ionic radius, the chelation of Mn^{3+} in biological systems would be predicted to be more avid than that of Mn^{2+}. Cycling between Mn^{3+} and Mn^{2+} has been suggested to be deleterious to biological systems because it can generate free radicals. However, at low concentrations Mn^{2+} can provide protection against free radicals, and it appears to be associated with their clearance rather than their production.

Dietary Sources

Manganese concentrations in typical food products range from $0.4\,\mu g\,g^{-1}$ (meat, poultry, and fish) to $20\,\mu g\,g^{-1}$ (nuts, cereals, and dried fruit). Breast milk is exceptionally low in manganese, containing only $0.004\,\mu g\,g^{-1}$, whereas infant formula can contain up to $0.4\,\mu g\,g^{-1}$. Teas can be particularly rich in manganese, containing up to $900\,\mu g\,g^{-1}$ of the element. An important consideration with respect to food sources of manganese is the extent to which the manganese is available for absorption. For example, although tea contains high amounts of the element, the tannin in tea can bind a significant amount of manganese, reducing its absorption from the gastrointestinal tract. Similarly, the high content of phytates and fiber constituents in cereal grains may limit the absorption of manganese. Conversely, although meat products contain low concentrations of manganese, absorption and retention of manganese from them is relatively high. Based on studies utilizing whole body retention curves after dosing with ^{54}Mn, the estimated percentage absorption of 1 mg of manganese from a test meal was 1.35%, whereas that from green leafy vegetables (lettuce and spinach) was closer to 5%. Absorption from wheat and sunflower seed kernels was somewhat lower than that from the leafy greens at 1 or 2%, presumably due to a higher fiber content or to higher amounts of phytates and similar compounds in the wheat and sunflower seeds. The dephytinization of soy formula increased manganese absorption 2.3-fold from 0.7 to 1.6%.

Analysis

Although manganese is widely distributed in the biosphere, it occurs in only trace amounts in animal tissues. Serum concentrations can be as low as 20 nM and typical tissue concentrations are less than $4 \mu mol g^{-1}$ wet weight; tissue concentrations of $4–8 \mu mol g^{-1}$ wet weight are considered high. Because of the high environmental levels of manganese relative to its concentration in animal tissues, considerable effort must be made to minimize contamination of samples during their collection and handling.

The most common analytical methods that can sensitively measure manganese include neutron activation analysis, X-ray fluorescence, proton-induced X-ray emission, inductively coupled plasma emission, EPR, and flameless atomic absorption spectrophotometry (AAS). Currently, the most common method employed is flameless AAS. All of these methods, with the exception of EPR, measure the total concentration of manganese in the samples. EPR allows selective measurement of bound versus free manganese.

Physiological Role

Tissue Concentrations

The average human body contains between 200 and 400 μmol of manganese, which is fairly uniform in distribution throughout the body. There is relatively little variation among species with regard to tissue manganese concentrations. Manganese tends to be highest in tissues rich in mitochondria; its concentration in mitochondria is higher than in cytoplasm or other cell organelles. Hair can accumulate high concentrations of manganese, and it has been suggested that hair manganese concentrations may reflect manganese status. High concentrations of manganese are normally found in pigmented structures, such as retina, dark skin, and melanin granules. Bone, liver, pancreas, and kidney tend to have higher concentrations of manganese ($20–50 nmol g^{-1}$) than do other tissues. Concentrations of manganese in brain, heart, lung, and muscle are typically $<20 nmol g^{-1}$; blood and serum concentrations are approximately 200 and $20 nmol l^{-1}$, respectively. Typical concentrations in cow milk are on the order of $800 nmol l^{-1}$, whereas human milk contains $80 nmol l^{-1}$. Bone can account

for up to 25% of total body manganese because of its mass. Bone manganese concentrations can be raised or lowered by substantially varying dietary manganese intake over long periods of time, but bone manganese is not thought to be a readily mobilizable pool. The fetus does not accumulate liver manganese before birth, and fetal concentrations are significantly less than adult concentrations. This lack of fetal storage can be attributed to the apparent lack of storage proteins and the low prenatal expression of most manganese enzymes.

Absorption, Transport, and Storage

Absorption of manganese is thought to occur throughout the small intestine. Manganese absorption is not thought to be under homeostatic control. For adult humans, manganese absorption has been reported to range from 2 to 15% when [54]Mn-labeled test meals are used and to be 25% when balance studies are conducted; given the technical problems associated with balance studies, the [54]Mn data are probably more reflective of true absorption values. Data from balance studies indicate that manganese retention is very high during infancy, suggesting that neonates may be particularly susceptible to manganese toxicosis.

The higher retention of manganese in young animals relative to adults in part reflects an immaturity of manganese excretory pathways, particularly that of bile secretion, which is very limited in early life. The avid retention of the small amount of manganese from milk and the postnatal changes in its excretory pattern underscore the considerable changes in manganese metabolism that occur during the neonatal period.

In experimental animals, high amounts of dietary calcium, phosphorus, fiber, and phytate increase the requirements for manganese; such interactions presumably occur via the formation of insoluble manganese complexes in the intestinal tract with a concomitant decrease in the soluble fraction available for absorption. The significance of these dietary factors with regard to human manganese requirements remains to be clarified. Studies in avian species have demonstrated that high dietary phosphorus intakes decrease manganese deposition in bone by approximately 50%. Given that the diet of many individuals may be marginal in manganese ($\leq 2 mg$ per day intake) while high in phosphorus ($\geq 2000 mg$ per day intake), this antagonism may have important implications for human health. For example, the low fractional absorption of manganese from soy formula has been related to its relatively high phytate content. The mechanism underlying this effect of soy protein on manganese absorption/retention has not been fully delineated. However, dephytinization of soy formula with microbial phytase can markedly enhance manganese absorption.

An interaction between iron and manganese has been demonstrated in experimental animals and humans. Manganese absorption increases under conditions of iron deficiency, whereas high amounts of dietary iron can accelerate the development of manganese deficiency. The chronic consumption of high levels of iron supplements ($>60\,mg$ Fe per day) can have a negative effect on manganese balance in adult women. The mechanisms underlying the interactions between iron and manganese have not been fully elucidated; however, they likely involve competition for either a transport site or a ligand. Both iron and manganese can utilize divalent metal transporter 1 (DMT1); however, the expression of DMT1 is regulated by iron status via the IRE/IRP system. Thus, during iron deficiency, DMT1 is upregulated causing an increase in manganese absorption. Rats fed iron-deficient diets accumulate manganese in several brain regions compared to rats fed control diets; the involvement of DMT1 in this accumulation of manganese is an area of active study. It should be noted that the interaction between manganese and iron can also affect the functions of some enzymes. For example, manganese can replace iron in the iron–sulfur center of cytosolic aconitase (IRP-1), resulting in an inhibition of the enzyme and an increase in iron regulatory protein (IRP) binding activity. Given the central role of IRPs in cellular iron metabolism, elevated cellular manganese concentration could in theory disrupt numerous translational events dependent on IRPs. That this in fact occurs is illustrated by the observation that following the addition of manganese to cells in culture, there can be sharp reductions in ferritin protein abundance, whereas there are increases in transferrin receptor abundance. This results in changes in intracellular iron metabolism, as reflected by decreases in mitochondrial aconitase (m-aconitase) abundance.

Manganese entering the portal blood from the gastrointestinal tract may remain free or become associated with α_2-macroglobulin, which is subsequently taken up by the liver. A small fraction enters the systemic circulation, where it may become oxidized to Mn^{3+} and bound to transferrin. Studies *in vivo* suggest that the Mn^{3+} complex forms very quickly in blood, in contrast to the slow oxidation of the Mn^{2+}–transferrin complex *in vitro*. Manganese uptake by the liver has been reported to occur by a unidirectional, saturable process with the properties of passive mediated transport. After entering

the liver, manganese enters one of at least five metabolic pools. One pool represents manganese taken up by the lysosomes, from which it is transferred subsequently to the bile canaliculus. The regulation of manganese is maintained in part through biliary excretion of the element; up to 50% of manganese injected intravenously can be recovered in the feces within 24 h. A second pool of manganese is associated with the mitochondria. Mitochondria have a large capacity for manganese uptake, and the mitochondrial uptake and release of manganese and calcium are thought to be related. A third pool of manganese is found in the nuclear fraction of the cell; the roles of nuclear manganese have not been fully delineated, but one function may be to contribute to the stability of nucleosome structure. A fourth manganese pool is incorporated into newly synthesized manganese proteins; biological half-lives for these proteins have not been agreed upon. The fifth identified intracellular pool of manganese is free Mn^{2+}. Fluctuations in the free manganese pool may be an important regulator of cellular metabolic control in a manner analogous to those for free Ca^{2+} and Mg^{2+}. Consistent with this concept, in pancreatic islets manganese blocks glucose-induced insulin release by altering cellular calcium fluxes, and manganese directly augments contractions in smooth muscle by a mechanism comparable to that of calcium.

The mechanisms by which manganese is transported to, and taken up by, extrahepatic tissues have not been identified. Transferrin is the major manganese binding protein in plasma; however, it is not known to what extent transferrin facilitates the uptake of manganese by extrahepatic tissue. The concentration of manganese citrate in blood can be fairly high, and this complex may be important for manganese movement across the blood–brain barrier. DMT1 may be involved in manganese transport because it is expressed in discrete areas of the brain. Manganese uptake by extrahepatic tissue does not seem to be increased under conditions of manganese deficiency, suggesting that manganese, in marked contrast to iron, does not play a role in the induction (or suppression) of manganese transport proteins.

There is limited information concerning the hormonal regulation of manganese metabolism. Fluxes in the concentrations of adrenal, pancreatic, and pituitary–gonadal axis hormones affect tissue manganese concentrations; however, it is not clear to what extent hormone-induced changes in tissue manganese concentrations are due to alterations in cellular uptake of manganese-activated enzymes or metalloenzymes.

Metabolic Function and Essentiality

Manganese functions as a constituent of metallo-enzymes and as an enzyme activator. Manganese-containing enzymes include arginase (EC 3.5.3.1), pyruvate carboxylase (EC 6.4.1.1), and manganese–superoxide dismutase (MnSOD) (EC 1.15.1.1). Arginase, the cytosolic enzyme responsible for urea formation, contains $4\,mol\,Mn^{2+}$ per mole of enzyme. Reductions in arginase activity resulting from manganese deficiency result in elevated plasma concentrations of ammonia and lowered plasma concentrations of urea. Reductions in arginase activity due to manganese deficiency may affect flux of arginine through the nitric oxide synthase (NOS) pathway, resulting in alterations in NO production. It has been suggested that arginase plays a regulatory role in NO production by competing with NOS for the same substrate, arginine. Rats fed manganese-deficient diets have shown effects indicative of increased NO production, such as increases in plasma and urinary nitrates plus nitrites and decreased blood pressure; however, neither NOS activity nor NO production have been measured directly. In addition, manganese binding by arginase is critical for the pH-sensing function of this enzyme in the ornithine cycle, suggesting that manganese plays a role in the regulation of body pH. With experimental diabetes, liver and kidney manganese concentrations and arginase activity can be markedly elevated. This manganese effect on arginase has been suggested to be due to an effect of Mn^{2+} on the conformational properties of the enzyme with a resultant modification of arginase activity. Whether this finding implies an increased manganese requirement for people with diabetes has not been determined.

Pyruvate carboxylase, the enzyme that catalyses the first step of carbohydrate synthesis from pyruvate, also contains $4\,mol\,Mn^{2+}$ per mole enzyme. Although the activity of this enzyme can be lower in manganese-deficient animals than in controls, gluconeogenesis has not been shown to be markedly inhibited in manganese-deficient animals.

MnSOD catalyzes the disproportionation of O_2^- to H_2O_2 and O_2. The essential role of MnSOD in the normal biological function of tissues has been clearly demonstrated by the homozygous inactivation of the *SOD2* gene for MnSOD in mice. Mice with this phenotype die within the first 10 days of life with a dilated cardiomyopathy, accumulation of lipid in liver and skeletal muscle, and metabolic acidosis. The activity of MnSOD in tissues of manganese-deficient rats can be significantly lower than in controls due to downregulation of MnSOD at the (pre)transcriptional level. That this reduction is functionally significant is suggested by the observation of higher than normal levels of hepatic mitochondrial lipid peroxidation in manganese-deficient rats. Tissue MnSOD activity can be increased by several diverse stressors, including alcohol, ozone, irradiation, interleukin-1, and tumor necrosis factor-α, presumably as a consequence of stressor-associated increases in cellular free radical (or oxidized target(s)) concentrations. Stressor-induced increases in MnSOD activity can be attenuated in manganese-deficient animals, potentially increasing their sensitivity to these insults. Transgenic mice have also been produced that overexpress MnSOD; a decreased severity of reperfusion injury has been noted in these animals, further supporting its physiological significance.

Considerable research is focused on the introduction of the human MnSOD gene into research animals utilizing viral vectors or plasmid/liposome delivery. This gene therapy has been shown to decrease radiation-induced injury, extend pancreatic islet transplant function, and slow the growth of malignant tumors in animal models via overexpression of the MnSOD protein. Another field of research that is rapidly advancing utilizes MnSOD mimetics for treatment of a variety of diseases in which the native SOD enzyme has been found to be effective. These mimetics are small manganese-containing synthetic molecules that have catalytic activity equivalent or superior to the native enzyme. They possess the additional beneficial properties of being nonimmunogenic because they are nonpeptides, able to penetrate cells, selective for superoxide (they do not interact with biologically important molecules), stable *in vivo*, and not deactivated by the destructive free radical peroxynitrite, which is capable of deactivating native MnSOD via nitration of tyrosine. These mimetic compounds have been found to be protective in animal models of acute and chronic inflammation, reperfusion injury, shock, and radiation-induced injury. Both of these therapies, MnSOD gene delivery and MnSOD mimetics, hold promise for future treatments in human chronic and acute conditions.

Finally, further evidence for the biological and research relevance of MnSOD is that experiments have been undertaken on the International Space Station to improve three-dimensional growth of MnSOD crystals in order to develop a better understanding of the role of structure in the reaction mechanism of this enzyme.

In contrast to the relatively few manganese metalloenzymes, there are a large number of manganese-activated enzymes, including hydrolases, kinases, decarboxylases, and transferases.

Manganese activation of these enzymes can occur as a direct consequence of the metal binding to the protein, causing a subsequent conformation change, or by binding to the substrate, such as ATP. Many of these metal activations are nonspecific in that other metal ions, particularly Mg^{2+}, can replace Mn^{2+}. An exception is the manganese-specific activation of glycosyltransferases. Several manganese deficiency-induced pathologies have been attributed to a low activity of this enzyme class. A second example of an enzyme that may be specifically activated by manganese is phosphoenolpyruvate carboxykinase (PEPCK; EC 4.1.1.49), the enzyme that catalyzes the conversion of oxaloacetate to phosphoenolpyruvate, GDP, and CO_2. Although low activities of PEPCK can occur in manganese-deficient animals, the functional significance of this reduction is not clear.

A third example of a manganese-activated enzyme is glutamine synthetase (EC 6.3.1.2). This enzyme, found in high concentrations in the brain, catalyzes the reaction $NH_3 + glutamate + ATP \rightarrow glutamine + ADP + P_i$. Brain glutamine synthetase activity can be normal even in severely manganese-deficient animals, suggesting that the enzyme either has a high priority for this element or magnesium can act as a substitute when manganese is lacking. It should be noted that this enzyme can be inactivated by oxygen radicals; therefore, a manganese deficiency-induced reduction in MnSOD activity theoretically could act to depress further the activity of glutamine synthetase.

Manganese Deficiency

Manganese deficiency has been demonstrated in several species, including rats, mice, pigs, and cattle. Signs of manganese deficiency include impaired growth, skeletal abnormalities, impaired reproductive performance, ataxia, and defects in lipid and carbohydrate metabolism.

The effects of manganese deficiency on bone development have been studied extensively. In most species, manganese deficiency can result in shortened and thickened limbs, curvature of the spine, and swollen and enlarged joints. The basic biochemical defect underlying the development of these bone defects is a reduction in the activities of glycosyltransferases; these enzymes are necessary for the synthesis of the chondroitin sulfate side chains of proteoglycan molecules. In addition, manganese deficiency in adult rats can result in an inhibition of both osteoblast and osteoclast activity. This observation is particularly noteworthy, given the reports that women with osteoporosis tend to have low blood manganese concentrations and that

the provision of manganese supplements might be associated with an improvement in bone health in postmenopausal women.

One of the most striking effects of manganese deficiency occurs during pregnancy. When pregnant animals (rats, mice, guinea pigs, and mink) are deficient in manganese, their offspring exhibit a congenital, irreversible ataxia characterized by incoordination, lack of equilibrium, and retraction of the head. This condition is the result of impaired development of the otoliths, the calcified structures in the inner ear responsible for normal body-righting reflexes. The block in otolith development is secondary to depressed proteoglycan synthesis due to low activity of manganese-requiring glycosyltransferases.

Defects in carbohydrate metabolism, in addition to those described previously, have been shown in manganese-deficient rats and guinea pigs. In the guinea pig, perinatal manganese deficiency results in pancreatic pathology, with animals exhibiting aplasia or marked hypoplasia of all cellular components. Manganese-deficient guinea pigs and rats given a glucose challenge often respond with a diabetic-type glucose tolerance curve. In addition to its effect on pancreatic tissue integrity, manganese deficiency can directly impair pancreatic insulin synthesis and secretion as well as enhance intracellular insulin degradation. The mechanism(s) underlying the effects of manganese deficiency on pancreatic insulin metabolism have not been fully delineated, but they are thought to be multifactorial. For example, the flux of islet cell manganese from the cell surface to an intracellular pool may be a critical signal for insulin release. It is also known that insulin mRNA levels are reduced in manganese-deficient animals, which is consistent with their depressed insulin synthesis. In addition, insulin sensitivity of adipose tissue is reduced in manganese-deficient rats, a phenomenon that may be related to fewer insulin receptors per adipose cell. Manganese deficiency may also affect glucose metabolism by means of a reduction in the number of glucose transporters in adipose tissue by an unidentified mechanism. Finally, the effect of manganese deficiency on insulin production may also be due to the destruction of pancreatic J3 cells. It is worth noting that constitutive pancreatic MnSOD activity is lower than in most tissues; this, coupled with the observation that most diabetogenic agents function via the production of free radicals with subsequent tissue damage, suggests that an additional mechanism underlying pancreatic dysfunction in manganese-deficient animals may be free radical mediated.

In addition to its effect on endocrine function, manganese deficiency can affect pancreatic exocrine function. For example, manganese-deficient rats can be characterized by an increase in pancreatic amylase content. The mechanism underlying this effect of manganese deficiency has not been delineated; however, it is thought to involve a shift in amylase synthesis or degradation because secretagogue-stimulated acinar secretion is comparable in control and manganese-deficient rats.

Although the majority of studies concerning the influence of manganese deficiency on carbohydrate metabolism have been conducted with experimental animals, there is one report in the literature of an insulin-resistant diabetic patient who responded to oral doses of manganese (doses ranged from 5 to 10 mg) with decreasing blood glucose concentrations. Although this is an intriguing case report, others have reported a lack of an effect of oral manganese supplements (up to 30 mg) in diabetic subjects, and low blood manganese concentrations have not been found to be a characteristic of diabetics.

Abnormal lipid metabolism is also characteristic of manganese deficiency: Specifically, a lipotrophic effect of manganese has been suggested in the literature. Severely manganese-deficient animals can be characterized by high liver fat, hypocholesterolemia, and low high-density lipoprotein (HDL) concentrations. Deficient animals can also be characterized by a shift to smaller plasma HDL particles, lower HDL apolipoprotein (apoE) concentrations, and higher apoC concentrations. As stated previously, tissue lipid peroxidation rates can be increased in manganese-deficient animals, possibly as a result of low tissue MnSOD activity.

There is considerable debate as to the extent to which manganese deficiency affects humans under free-living conditions. Manganese deficiency can be induced in humans under highly controlled experimental conditions. In one study, manganese deficiency was induced in adult male subjects by feeding a manganese-deficient diet (0.1 mg Mn per day) for 39 days. The subjects developed temporary dermatitis, as well as increased serum calcium and phosphorus concentrations and increased alkaline phosphatase activity, suggestive of bone resorption. Since the late 1980s, several diseases have been reported to be characterized, in part, by low blood manganese concentrations. These diseases include epilepsy, Mseleni disease, maple syrup urine disease and phenylketonuria, Down's syndrome, osteoporosis, and Perthes' disease. The finding of low blood manganese levels in subsets of individuals with the previously mentioned diseases is significant since blood manganese levels can reflect soft tissue manganese concentrations. The reports of low blood manganese concentrations in individuals with

epilepsy are particularly intriguing, given the observations that manganese-deficient animals can show an increased susceptibility to drug and electroshock-induced seizures and a genetic model for epilepsy in rats (the GEPR rat) is characterized by low blood manganese concentrations. It is evident that a deficiency of manganese may contribute to the pathology of epilepsy at multiple points, given that Mn^{2+} is implicated in activation of glutamine synthetase, a Mn^{2+}-specific brain ATPase; production of cyclic AMP; altered synaptosomal uptake of noradrenalin and serotonin; glutamate, GABA, and choline metabolism; and biosynthesis of acetylcholine receptors.

Evidence of widespread manganese deficiency in human populations is lacking. Typically, manganese intakes approximate the 2001 US Institute of Medicine's suggested adequate intakes as follows: 3 μg/day for infants 0–6 months old, 0.6 mg/day for infants 7–12 months old, 1.2–1.9 mg/day for children 1–13 years old, 1.6–2.2 mg/day for older children, and 1.8–2.6 mg/day for adults. The Tolerable Upper Intake Level (UL) is the highest level of a daily nutrient intake that is likely to pose no risk of adverse health effects in almost all individuals. The Institute of Medicine's recommended intakes for manganese set ULs at 2, 3, and 6 mg/day for children 1–3, 4–8, and 9–13 years old, respectively. Values were set at 9 mg/day for adolescents 14–18 years old and at 11 mg/day for adults.

Manganese Toxicity

In domestic animals, the major reported lesion associated with chronic manganese toxicity is iron deficiency, resulting from an inhibitory effect of manganese on iron absorption. Additional signs of manganese toxicity in domestic animals include depressed growth, depressed appetite, and altered brain function.

In humans, manganese toxicity represents a serious health hazard, resulting in severe pathologies of the central nervous system. In its most severe form, the toxicosis is manifested by a permanent crippling neurological disorder of the extrapyramidal system, which is similar to Parkinson's disease. In its milder form, the toxicity is expressed by hyperirritability, violent acts, hallucinations, disturbances of libido, and incoordination. The previous symptoms, once established, can persist even after the manganese body burden returns to normal. Although the majority of reported cases of manganese toxicity occur in individuals exposed to high concentrations of airborne manganese (>5 mg m^{-3}), subtle signs of manganese toxicity, including delayed reaction time, impaired motor coordination, and impaired memory, have been observed in workers exposed to airborne manganese concentrations less than $1\,mg\,m^{-3}$. Therefore, an inhalation reference concentration range for manganese has been established by the US Environmental Protection Agency to be between 0.09 and $0.2\,\mu g\,m^{-3}$. Manganese toxicity has been reported in individuals who have consumed water containing high levels ($\geq 10\,mg\,Mn\,l^{-1}$) of manganese for long periods of time. Recently, there has been concern that the risk for manganese toxicity may be increasing in some areas because of the use of MMT in gasoline as an antiknock agent, although there is little evidence that air, water, or food manganese concentrations have increased where this fuel is used.

In addition to neural damage, reproductive and immune system dysfunction, nephritis, testicular damage, pancreatitis, lung disease, and hepatic damage can occur with manganese toxicity, but the frequency of these disorders is unknown. Although there is a limited body of epidemiological data that suggests that high levels of manganese can result in an increased risk for colorectal and digestive tract cancers, most investigators do not consider manganese to be a carcinogen. In contrast, both divalent ($MnCl_2$) and heptavalent forms ($KMnO_4$) of manganese are recognized to be strong clastogens both *in vitro* and *in vivo*; exposure to high concentrations of either form results in chromosomal breaks, fragments, and exchanges. High concentrations of manganese can also induce forward and point mutations in mammalian cells. High levels of dietary manganese have not been reported to be teratogenic in the absence of overt signs of maternal toxicity. However, there are reports that exposure to high levels of manganese during prenatal development can result in behavioral abnormalities. High levels of brain manganese have been reported in subjects with amyotrophic lateral sclerosis, and it has been suggested that this increase may contribute to the progression of the disease. Similar to the cases in humans, chronic manganese toxicity in rhesus monkeys is characterized by muscular weakness, rigidity of the lower limbs, and neuron damage in the substantia nigra. Findings from a recent study suggest that iron and aluminum, which accumulate in the globus pallidus and the substantia nigra of these animals, induce tissue oxidation that may contribute to the damage associated with manganese toxicity. Neural toxicity is a consistent finding in rats exposed to chronic manganese toxicity. Significant manganese accumulation was accompanied by an increase in cholesterol content in the hippocampal region of manganese-treated rats, which was

associated with impaired learning; this impairment was corrected by an inhibitor of cholesterol synthesis. The development of manganese toxicity in individuals with compromised liver function, or compromised biliary pathways, is well documented. Significantly, these individuals can have abnormal magnetic resonance imaging (MRI) patterns, which improve following the alleviation of the manganese toxicity. For example, in some cases improvements in brain function have been achieved after liver transplant. The mechanisms underlying the toxicity of manganese have not been agreed upon but may involve multiple etiologies, including endocrinological dysfunction, excessive tissue oxidative damage, manganese-mediated disruptions in intracellular calcium and iron metabolism, and mitochondrial dysfunction caused by manganese inhibition of some pathways of the mitochondrial respiratory chain.

Severe cases of manganese toxicity in humans have been reported for adults, as well as isolated cases in other groups of individuals who are vulnerable, including children on long-term parenteral nutrition and parenteral nutrition patients who have cholestasis or other hepatic disease. In many cases, the previously mentioned groups of individuals have been reported to be characterized by high brain manganese concentrations based on MRI. Although no known cases have been reported, infants may be at a high risk for manganese toxicity due to a high absorptive capacity for the element and/or an immature excretory pathway for it. If manganese is taken up by extrahepatic tissues via the manganese–transferrin complex, the developing brain may be particularly sensitive to manganese toxicity due to the high number of transferrin receptors elaborated by neuronal cells during development, coupled with the putative need by neural cells for transferrin for their differentiation and proliferation. Newborn rats given daily doses of dietary manganese at a level equivalent to that of soy formula exhibited significant neurodevelopmental delays as assessed by several behavioral tests. It should be noted that the concentration of manganese in soy formula is relatively modest but approximately 60–100 times higher than that of breast milk. Brain manganese concentration was increased and striatal dopamine concentrations were significantly decreased even 45 days after the supplementation ended, suggesting that the impact of manganese on the brain and behavior was irreversible. Thus, dietary exposure to high levels of manganese during infancy can be neurotoxic to rat pups and result in developmental deficits. Further studies on human infants fed diets with different levels of manganese are needed to assess whether there are any long-term consequences of early manganese exposure of newborns.

Another group of neuropathological conditions that has been associated with elevated levels of brain manganese is transmissible spongiform encephalopathies. These diseases found in animals and humans are also referred to as prion diseases. There is strong evidence that in their native state, prions are normal brain glycoproteins that bind copper and have an antioxidant function. However, it has been suggested that in the disease process an abnormal isoform of the protein is generated in which manganese is substituted for copper. This isoform is proteinase resistant, no longer has antioxidant activity, and may play a role in the etiology of these diseases. Indeed, elevated levels of brain manganese, along with lower than normal levels of brain copper, have been measured in patients with the prion disease, Creutzfeld–Jakob disease. Whether the elevated levels of brain manganese observed in these patients as well as in animal models of these diseases play an important role in their pathogenesis or are secondary to other factors remains to be determined.

Assessment of Manganese Status

Reliable biomarkers for the assessment of manganese status have not been identified. Whole blood manganese concentrations are reflective of soft tissue manganese levels in rats; however, it is not known whether a similar relationship holds for humans. Plasma manganese concentrations decrease in individuals fed manganese-deficient diets and are slightly higher than normal in individuals consuming manganese supplements. Lymphocyte MnSOD activity and blood arginase activity are increased in individuals who consume manganese supplements; however, their value as biomarkers for manganese status may be complicated due to the number of cytokines and disease states that may also increase their expression. Urinary manganese excretion has not been found to be sensitive to dietary manganese intake. With respect to the diagnosis of manganese toxicosis, the use of MRI appears to be promising because the images associated with manganese toxicity are relatively specific. Whole blood manganese concentrations can be correlated with MRI intensity and Ti values in the globus pallidus even in the absence of symptoms of neurological damage. Thus, although it is relatively expensive, MRI

may be particularly useful as a means of identifying susceptible individuals in, or around, manganese-emitting factories. In addition, the method may be useful in the evaluation of patients with liver failure.

Further Reading

Brown DR (2002) Metal toxicity and therapeutic intervention. *Biochemical Society* 30: 742–745.

Crossgrove JS, Allen DD, Bukaveckas BL, Rhineheimer SS, and Yokel RA (2003) Manganese distribution across the blood–brain barrier. I. Evidence for carrier-mediated influx of manganese citrate as well as manganese and manganese transferrin. *Neurotoxicology* 24: 3–13.

Davey CA and Richmond TJ (2002) DNA-dependent divalent cation binding in the nucleosome core particle. *Proceedings of the National Academy of Sciences of the United States of America* 99: 11169–11174.

Garrick MD, Dolan KG, Horbinski C et al. (2003) DMT1: A mammalian transporter for multiple metals. *BioMetals* 16: 41–54.

Gerber GB, Léonard A, and Hantson PH (2002) Carcinogenicity, mutagenicity and teratogenicity of manganese compounds. *Critical Reviews in Oncology/Hematology* 42: 25–34.

Guo H, Seixas-Silva JA, Epperly MW et al. (2003) Prevention of radiation-induced oral cavity mucositis by plasmid/liposome delivery of the human manganese superoxide dismutase (SOD2) transgene. *Radiation Research* 159: 361–370.

Kwik-Uribe CL, Reaney S, Zhu Z, and Smith D (2003) Alterations in cellular IRP-dependent iron regulation by *in vitro* manganese exposure in undifferentiated PC12 cells. *Brain Research* 973: 1–15.

Normandin L and Hazell AS (2002) Manganese neurotoxicity: An update of pathophysiologic mechanisms. *Metabolic Brain Disease* 17: 375–387.

Sabbatini M, Pisani A, Uccello F et al. (2003) Arginase inhibition slows the progression of renal failure in rats with renal ablation. *American Journal of Renal Physiology* 284: F680–F687.

Salvemini D, Muscoli C, Riley DP, and Cuzzocrea S (2002) Superoxide dismutase mimetics. *Pulmonary Pharmacology and Therapeutics* 15: 439–447.

Takagi Y, Okada A, Sando K et al. (2002) Evaluation of indexes of *in vivo* manganese status and the optimal intravenous dose for adult patients undergoing home parenteral nutrition. *American Journal of Clinical Nutrition* 75: 112–118.

Takeda A (2003) Manganese action in brain function. *Brain Research Reviews* 41: 79–87.

Tran T, Chowanadisai W, Crinella FM, Chicz-DeMet A, and Lönnerdal B (2002) Effect of high dietary manganese intake of neonatal rats on tissue mineral accumulation, striatal dopamine levels, and neurodevelopmental status. *Neurotoxicology* 158: 1–9.

Vahedi-Faridi A, Porta J, and Borgstahl GEO (2002) Improved three-dimensional growth of manganese superoxide dismutase crystals on the International Space Station. *Biological Crystallography* 59: 385–388.

Yokel RA, Crossgrove JS, and Bukaveckas BL (2003) Manganese distribution across the blood–brain barrier. II. Manganese efflux from the brain does not appear to be carrier mediated. *Neurotoxicology* 24: 15–22.

MICROBIOTA OF THE INTESTINE

Probiotics

M Gueimonde and S Salminen, University of Turku, Turku, Finland

Introduction

The human gastrointestinal (GI) tract harbors a complex collection of microorganisms. The individual digestive system contains about 1.5 kg of viable (live) bacteria, made up of more than 500 different identified microbial species. Indeed, the total number of bacteria in the gut amounts for more than 10 times that of eukaryotic cells in the human body, and this bacterial biomass can constitute up to 60% of fecal weight. This complex microbiological community is called the intestinal microflora. While most people are familiar with the side-effects of some members of it (e.g., diarrhea), the beneficial effects in stabilizing gut well-being and general health are less well known. These so-called 'friendly' bacteria are naturally present in the GI tract as part of the normal healthy intestinal microflora and ensure the balance that creates a healthy individual. Such beneficial microbes and a healthy intestinal microflora also constitute the main source of probiotics used to improve intestinal and host health.

Fermented products containing living microorganisms have been used for centuries to restore gut health. Such utilization of live microorganisms to improve host health forms the basis of the probiotic concept.

Usually probiotics are taken in the form of dairy products, drinks, or supplements, but in African countries they have traditionally also been ingested in fermented cereal and in fermented vegetables in Asian countries. The claimed benefits of traditional fermented foods range from treatment of diarrheal diseases to alleviation of the side-effects of antibiotics to the prevention of a number of other health problems. In some countries fermented foods have even been associated with benefits to the skin.

Definition of Probiotics

Probiotics have been defined as 'bacterial preparations that impart clinically verified beneficial effects on the health of the host when consumed orally.'

According to this definition the safety and efficacy of probiotics must be scientifically demonstrated. However, as different probiotics may interact with the host in different manners, their properties and characteristics should be well defined. It is understood that probiotic strains, independent of genera and species, are unique and that the properties and human health effects of each strain must be assessed in a case-by-case manner. Most probiotics are currently either lactic acid bacteria or bifidobacteria, but new species and genera are being assessed for future use. The probiotic bacteria in current use have been isolated from the intestinal microflora of healthy human subjects of long-standing good health and thus most of them are also members of the healthy intestinal microflora.

It has been demonstrated that probiotics have specific properties and targets in the human intestinal tract and that they are able to modulate the intestinal microflora.

Intestinal Microflora

Composition of the Intestinal Microflora

The human GI tract hosts a rich and complex microflora that is specific for each person depending on environmental and genetic factors. Different bacterial groups and levels are found throughout the GI tract, as corresponds with the different ecological niches present from mouth to colon. The stomach and the upper bowel are sparsely populated regions (10^3–10^4 CFU per g contents) while the colon is heavily populated (10^{11}–10^{12} CFU g contents). In the small intestine genera such as *Lactobacillus* and *Bacteriodes* are usually found, whereas those considered predominant in the large bowel include *Bacteriodes*, *Bifidobacterium*, *Eubacterium*, *Clostridium*, *Fusobacterium*, and *Ruminococcus* among others. Several health-promoting properties have been attributed to defined members of the intestinal microflora such as lactobacilli and bifidobacteria. A balanced microflora provides a barrier against harmful food components and pathogenic bacteria and has a direct impact on the morphology of the gut. Hence, the intestinal microflora constitutes an important factor for the health and well-being of the human host and a healthy stable microflora affords a potential source of future probiotics.

Development and Succession of Microflora during Life-Time

The human fetus is sterile and the maternal vaginal microflora comprises the first inoculum of microbes. The indigenous intestinal microflora develops over time, determined by an interplay between genetic factors, mode of delivery, contact with the initial surrounding environment, diet, and disease. As a result, every individual has a unique characteristic microflora. The human intestinal microbiota does not exist as a defined entity; this population comprises a dynamic mixture of microbes in each individual.

The establishment of the gut microflora, a process commencing immediately upon birth, provides an early and massive source of microbial stimuli, and may consequently be a good candidate 'infection.' This step-wise succession begins with facultative anaerobes such as the enterobacteria, coliforms, and lactobacilli first colonizing the intestine, rapidly succeeded by bifidobacteria and lactic acid bacteria. The indigenous gut microflora plays an important role in the generation of an immunophysiological regulation of the gut, providing key signals for the development of the immune system in infancy and also interfering with and actively controlling the gut-associated immunological homeostasis later in life. A healthy microflora can thus be defined as the normal individual microflora of a child that both preserves and promotes well-being and absence of disease, especially in the GI tract, but also beyond it. It provides the first step in long-term well-being for later life and the basis for this development lies in early infancy. Failure in the establishment of a healthy microflora has been linked to the risk of infectious, inflammatory, and allergic diseases later in life. Demonstration of this has stimulated researchers to elucidate the composition and function of the intestinal microflora.

Microflora Research

In spite of the recent development of DNA based methods, microbiota development and characterization in the human host still rests largely on the culture-based assessment pioneered by Japanese researchers. The identification of different microbial species and strains has been dependent on microbial characterization, which is usually based on limited phenotypic properties and the metabolic activity of the microbes, for example, sugar fermentation profiles. There are several bacteria, however, that cannot be cultured and isolated or identified by the traditional methods. The culture technique as used in microbial assessments of feces is also hindered by the fact that microbes in the feces will mainly

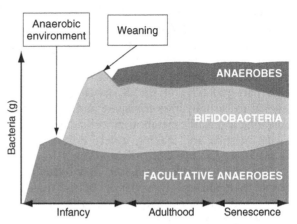

Figure 1 Development of microflora throughout life.

represent the microflora in the lumen of the sigmoid colon, while the composition of the intestinal microflora differs both along the GI tract and between the lumen and the mucosa. For more accurate information on the population elsewhere in the intestine, samples should be taken by endoscopy or during surgery. Most of our current data on microflora are derived from results obtained from fecal samples and culturing. These data indicate that there are several successive phases in microflora development related to age (**Figure 1**). In early infancy the microflora is scant and simple consisting mainly of bifidobacteria. During breast-feeding it remains so, but following weaning its complexity increases, reaching the state observed in adults where the microflora is specific to each person. Aging is related to further changes and the diversity is again decreased. The microflora becomes more unstable and vulnerable to diseases, for example, diarrheal diseases caused by intestinal pathogens.

Current research efforts focus on revealing genomic data on both probiotic microorganisms and certain important intestinal commensals. This has provided information indicating that gut commensals not only derive food and other benefits from the intestinal contents but also have a role in influencing the human host by providing maturational signals for the developing infant and child and providing later signals for alteration to gut barrier mechanisms.

The genomic data on, for instance, *Bifidobacterium longum* and *Bacteroides thetaiotaomicron*, both important members of the human intestinal microflora, give an indication as to how specific bacteria are adapted to the development of the gut by specific genes enabling the use of intestinal mucins and breast milk oligosaccharides as main sources or nutrients.

Genomic information on *B. longum* also gives insight into the adhesive mechanisms that comprise a basis both for populating the infant gut and for communicating developmental signals to specific areas and sites of the gut mucosa. Furthermore, a large part (>8.5%) of the *B. longum* genome is devoted to carbohydrate transport and metabolism, indicating a versatile metabolism well adapted to life in the intestine and making it very different from, for instance, *Lactobacillus johnsonii*.

Bacteroides thetaiotaomicron has also been shown to modulate glycosylation of the intestinal mucus and to induce expression of angiogenins, revealing proposed mechanisms whereby intestinal microbes may influence the gut microecology and shape the immune system. Incorporating such information with host gene expression data from the exposed mucosal sites and beyond them will enable us to understand the role of both microbial transfer and succession and microbe–microbe and host–microbe interactions. Recent information demonstrates that the vast community of indigenous microbes colonizing the human gut also shapes our development and biology.

Role of Microflora in Health and Disease

Major dysfunctions of the GI tract are thought to be related to disturbances or aberrationss of the intestinal microflora. Recent findings confirm that aberrations can be documented and related to disease risk. The microorganisms present in our GI tract thus have a significant influence on our health and well-being.

The development of the intestinal microbiota needs to be characterized to define the composition that helps us to remain healthy. Specific aberrations in the intestinal microflora may predispose to disease. Such aberrations have been identified in allergic disease, including decreased numbers of bifidobacteria and an atypical composition of bifidobacterial microflora. Also, aberrations in *Clostridium* content and composition have been reported to be important. Similar predisposing factors may also exist in the case of microflora and both inflammatory gut diseases and rotavirus diarrhea. Microflora aberrations have also been reported in rheumatoid arthritis, juvenile chronic arthritis, ankylosing spondylitis, and irritable bowel syndrome patients. A thorough knowledge of the intestinal microflora composition will offer a basis for future probiotic development and the search for new strains for human use. Many diseases and their prevention can be linked to the microflora in the gut.

Modulation by Probiotics

In general, probiotic bacteria do not colonize the human intestinal tract permanently, but specific strains are able to transiently colonize or persist for some time in the intestine and may modulate the indigenous microflora. The rationale for modulating the gut microflora by means of probiotics derives from the demonstration that this microflora is important to the health of the host. Specific probiotics have been shown to colonize temporarily the human intestinal tract, thereby modulating the intestinal microflora both locally and at the commensal level. Such modification has not been reported to be permanent; rather it is related to a balancing of aberrant or disturbed microflora to assist it to return to normal metabolic and physiological activities. Such modulation and restoration of the normal state of the microflora activity is a key target for probiotic action. However, the state of the microflora should be well characterized to enable the selection of specific probiotics to counteract the aberration or disturbance in question.

Specific probiotic bacteria can modulate both the intestinal microflora and local and systemic immune responses. Activation of immunological cells and tissues requires close contact of the probiotic with the immune cells and tissue on the intestinal surface. Interestingly, both lactobacilli and bifidobacteria, which colonize mainly the small and large intestine respectively, when given as probiotic supplements were able to modify immunological reactions related to allergic inflammation, whereas lactobacilli were ineffective in protection against cows' milk allergy. In this respect, preferential binding of probiotics on the specific antigen-processing cells (macrophages, dendritic, and epithelial cells) may be even more important than the location of adhesion. It is also known that the cytokine stimulation profiles of different *Bifidobacterium* strains vary and that strains isolated from healthy infants stimulate mainly noninflammatory cytokines.

Results of an increasing number of clinical and experimental studies demonstrate the importance of constituents within the intestinal lumen, in particular the resident microflora, in regulating inflammatory responses. Probiotic bacteria may counteract inflammatory processes by stabilizing the disturbed gut microbial environment, forming a stable healthy microflora and thus improving the intestine's permeability barrier. Another mode of action comprises enhancing the degradation of enteral antigens and altering their immunogenicity. Yet another mechanism for the gut-stabilizing effect could be improvement of the intestine's immunological barrier, particularly intestinal IgA responses. Probiotic effects may also be mediated via control of the balance between pro- and anti-inflammatory cytokines. Such effects may be mediated through changes in the intestinal microflora, especially by modulation of the bifidobacteria microflora.

Importance of Understanding Intestinal Microflora

It is obvious that an understanding of the cross-talk that occurs between the intestinal microflora and its host promises to expand our conceptions of the relationship between the intestinal microflora and health. There is also an increasing amount of information indicating that specific aberrations in the intestinal microflora may render us more vulnerable to intestinal inflammatory diseases and other diseases beyond the intestinal environment. It is likely that some aberrations may even predispose us to specific diseases. Unfortunately, however, we are still far from knowing the qualitative and quantitative composition of the intestinal microflora and the factors governing its composition in an individual.

Probiotic Effects

Living microorganisms have long been used as supplements to restore gut health at times of dysfunction. It is clear that different strains from a given microbial group may possess different properties. It is thus important to establish which specific microbial strain may have a beneficial effect on the host; even closely related strains can have significantly different or even counteracting effects. Their properties and characteristics should thus be well defined; studies using closely related strains cannot be extrapolated to support each other.

Working hypotheses can be supported by studies carried out *in vitro* using cell culture models or *in vivo* using animal models. However, the studies most important for efficacy assessment are carefully planned and monitored clinical studies in humans.

In summary, well-designed human studies are required to demonstrate health benefits. Using the criteria thus obtained it can be concluded that certain specific probiotics have scientifically proven benefits that can be attributed to specific products (see below). Other reported probiotic health-related effects are only partially established (**Figure 2**), and require more data from larger double-blind placebo controlled studies before firm conclusions can be reached.

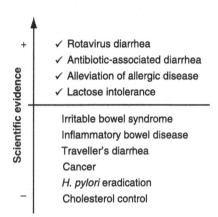

+
✓ Rotavirus diarrhea
✓ Antibiotic-associated diarrhea
✓ Alleviation of allergic disease
✓ Lactose intolerance

Irritable bowel syndrome
Inflammatory bowel disease
Traveller's diarrhea
Cancer
H. pylori eradication
–
Cholesterol control

Scientific evidence

Figure 2 Health benefits of probiotics.

Scientifically Documented Effects

Diarrhea The mechanisms by which probiotics prevent or ameliorate diarrhea may involve stimulation of the immune system, competition for binding sites on intestinal epithelial cells (**Figure 3**), or the elaboration of bacteriocins or binding of virus particles in the gut contents. These and other mechanisms are thought to be dependent on the type of diarrhea being investigated, and may therefore differ between viral diarrhea, antibiotic-associated diarrhea, or traveller's diarrhea.

Viral diarrhea Shortening of the duration of rotavirus diarrhea using *Lactobacillus* GG (LGG) is perhaps the best-documented probiotic effect. A reduction in the duration of diarrhea was first shown in several studies around the world and also

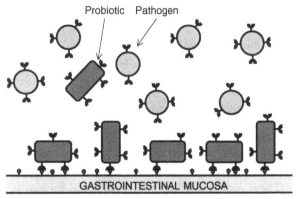

Probiotic   Pathogen

GASTROINTESTINAL MUCOSA

Figure 3 Probiotic adhesion and replacement of pathogenic bacteria.

in a recent multicenter European study on the use of LGG in acute diarrhea. Other investigators demonstrated that supplementation with a combination of *Bifidobacterium bifidum* and *Streptococcus thermophilus* reduces the incidence of diarrhea and shortens the duration of rotavirus shedding in chronically hospitalized children. On average, the duration of diarrhea was shortened by 1 day in both hospitalized children and those treated at home.

Other investigators have studied the immune modulating effects of probiotics as a means of reducing diarrhea, suggesting that the humoral immune system plays a significant role in the probiotics' effect.

From these numerous studies it is clear that probiotics do indeed play a therapeutic role in viral diarrhea. Even meta-analyses have been conducted in this area, showing that probiotic therapy shortens the duration of acute diarrhea in children. However, the exact mechanism of action involved is not clear and is very likely multifactorial.

Antibiotic-associated diarrhea The incidence of antibiotic-associated diarrhea is between 5 and 30%. The success of probiotics in reducing or preventing this form of diarrhea has been convincing, and includes a number of probiotics as well as various antibiotics.

LGG has been shown to prevent antibiotic-associated diarrhea when consumed in both yogurt form or as a freeze-dried product. Also, *Saccharomyces boulardii* has been found to be effective in preventing antibiotic-associated diarrhea. Other microorganisms such as *Enterococcus faecium* or a combination of *L. acidophilus* and *L. bulgaricus* have also been reported to be effective.

Alleviation of symptoms of allergic disease It has been shown that changes in intestinal microflora composition precede the development of some allergic diseases, indicating a potential area for probiotic application. LGG given prenatally to mothers and during the first months to infants with a high risk of atopic disease has reduced the prevalence of atopic eczema to about half in the infants receiving the strain. Furthermore, extensively hydrolyzed whey formula supplemented with LGG or *Bifidobacterium lactis* Bb12 is more effective than unsupplemented formula in eczema alleviation in infants with atopic eczema.

These results indicate a high potential for probiotic application in the treatment and reduction of risk of allergic diseases.

Lactose intolerance Several studies have shown that lactose-intolerant individuals suffer fewer symptoms if milk in the diet is replaced with fermented dairy products. The mechanisms of action of lactic acid bacteria and fermented dairy products include the following: lower lactose concentration in the fermented product due to lactose hydrolysis during fermentation; high lactase activity of bacterial preparations used in production; and increased active lactase enzyme entering the small intestine with the fermented product or within the viable bacteria.

The bacterial enzyme beta-galactosidase, which can be detected in the duodenum and terminal ileum after consumption of viable yogurt, is thought to be the major factor improving digestibility by the hydrolysis of lactose, mainly in the terminal ileum. Another factor suggested to influence lactose digestion is the slower gastric emptying of semisolid milk products such as yogurt.

In conclusion, there is good scientific evidence to demonstrate the alleviation of lactose intolerance symptoms by specific probiotic lactic acid bacteria. However, the strain-specific lactase activities may vary from nil to very high values. Thus, different products may have varying lactose contents and individual strains, when released into the duodenum, vary in their lactase activity.

Potential Effects Requiring Further Clinical Work

Intestinal microecology and cancer A number of studies have focused on the impact of probiotics on intestinal microecology and cancer. *Lactobacillus acidophilus*, *L. casei* Shirota strain, and LGG have been shown to have inhibitory effects on chemically induced tumors in animals. Some specific strains of probiotic bacteria are able to bind carcinogens and to downregulate some microbial carcinogenic enzymatic activities. This phenomenon may then reduce carcinogen production and exert a beneficial effect in the colon, the urinary tract, and the bladder.

The most interesting documentation is that concerning *L. casei* Shirota. There have been several mechanistic studies on the effects of the strain reporting decreased mutagen excretion, and some human clinical studies have been conducted using this strain. In clinical and multicenter studies carried out in Japan, prophylactic effects of oral administration of *L. casei* Shirota on the recurrence of superficial bladder cancer have been reported. Recently, a large Japanese case control study has been conducted on the habitual intake of lactic acid bacteria and risk reduction of bladder cancer. Results suggested that the habitual intake of fermented milk with the strain reduces the risk of bladder cancer in the Japanese population. More studies, and especially human studies in other countries, are needed prior to the establishment of firm conclusions.

Irritable bowel syndrome There is a rationale for investigating the effect of probiotics in the treatment of this common disorder where intestinal motility and dysfunctions in the intestinal microflora are important factors to consider. In a recent study using *L. plantarum* 299v, a reduction of symptoms was reported. *Enterococcus faecium* preparations have also been evaluated for the treatment of patients with irritable bowel syndrome, and although patient-recorded symptoms did not show significant differences, the physician's subjective clinical evaluation revealed an improvement.

Inflammatory bowel disease Inflammatory bowel disease (IBD) comprises a heterogeneous group of diseases of unknown etiology (Crohn's, ulcerative colitis, and pouchitis), but here also factors related to the intestinal microflora seem to be involved, providing a rationale for the application of probiotics. From reviewing studies on the use of probiotics in IBD it can be concluded that, although there are some promising preliminary findings, more well-planned long-term studies are needed before any firm conclusions can be drawn.

Traveller's diarrhea There are a few studies on the prevention of traveller's diarrhea using probiotics and these show a positive outcome for LGG and a combination of *L. acidophilus* LA5 with *B. lactis* Bb-12. The results offer some indication of beneficial effects, even though some studies yielded no reported effects, but information from good and extensive human studies using defined strains for traveller's diarrhea is still largely lacking. The current data on traveller's diarrhea show no scientifically proven effects for any of the strains used. More studies are required for efficacy assessment.

***Helicobacter pylori* eradication** Specific strains of lactic acid bacteria have been reported to inhibit a wide range of intestinal pathogens including *Helicobacter pylori*, which is involved in the process of gastric ulcer development. Lactic acid bacteria are often able to survive acidic gastric conditions and it has therefore been proposed that they may have a beneficial influence during the eradication of *H. pylori*. It has been reported that both the inhibitory substances produced and the specific strains may influence the survival of *Helicobacter*, and studies have been conducted, particularly with a *L.*

johnsonii strain. It has been shown that there is good *in vitro* inhibition and that fermented milk containing the strain has a positive effect when consumed during *Helicobacter* eradication therapy. However, more controlled human studies in different populations need be conducted to verify this effect.

Cholesterol control The cholesterol-lowering effects of probiotics have been the subject of two recent reviews with contradictory results. The first, which focused on short-term intervention studies with one yogurt type, reported a 4% decrease in total cholesterol and a 5% decrease in LDL. Contrary to this, the second review concluded that no proven effects could be found. In this context, it is clear that long-term studies are required before the establishment of any conclusion.

Safety

Safety assessment is an essential phase in the development of any new food. Although few probiotic strains or prebiotic compounds have been specifically tested for safety, the long history of safe consumption of some probiotic strains could be considered the best proof of their safety. Although some lactobacilli and bifidobacteria have been associated with rare cases of bacteremia, usually in patients with severe underlying diseases, the safety of members of these genera is generally recognized due to their long history of safe use and their lack of toxicity. Furthermore, the low incidence of infections attributable to these microorganisms, together with a recent study showing that there is no increase in the incidence of bacteremia due to lactobacilli in Finland despite the increased consumption of probiotic lactobacilli, supports this hypothesis. With regard to other bacteria such as enterococci, *S. boulardii*, *Clostridium butyricum*, or some members of the genus *Bacillus* the situation is more complicated, even though they have been used as probiotics for some time.

In addition to the possibility of infection there are other risks that must be taken into account (**Table 1**). These include those risks associated with the metabolic properties of the strain (capacity for deconjugation/dehydroxylation of bile salts, production of enzymes favoring the invasion/translocation through the epithelium, etc.), with the presence of active substances in the probiotic or product (immunoactive substances, toxic compounds, etc.), or with antibiotic resistance. It is clear that strains harboring transferable antibiotic resistance genes should not be

Table 1 Probiotic action: potential benefits and risks

Action mechanisms	Potential risks
Improvement of gut barrier (immunologic, nonimmunologic)	Proinflammatory effects
Modulation of aberrant gut microbiota	Adverse effects on innate immunity
Modulation of inflammatory response	Infection
Degradation of antigens	Production of harmful substances
Binding/inhibition of carcinogens	Antibiotic resistance (Specific risks related to host, strain characteristics, or interactions)

used. In this context the specific risks related to each probiotic strain must be carefully identified.

Guidelines are needed to test the safety of probiotics. However, taking into account the great diversity of probiotic microorganisms, it is necessary to identify the specific risks associated with the respective strains, as well as the risk factors associated with the host and the possible interactions between probiotic–host–food components in order to assess the safety of these products. Additional epidemiological surveillance and follow-up of novel strains should be conducted. In this context, the specific risks related to each probiotic strain must be carefully identified. With regard to this, knowledge of mechanisms involved is a key factor not only for the assessment of health effects but also for the safety aspects of probiotics.

Future Challenges

Some of the claimed beneficial effects of probiotics are backed by good clinical studies. However, other possible effects call for further investigation in new, well-planned, long-term human clinical studies prior to any firm conclusions being made. Protocols for human studies need to be developed for probiotics. In some cases, even postmarketing surveillance studies on intakes and long-term effects are useful; such studies have in fact already been used for the safety assessment of current probiotics.

The assessment of potential probiotic strains must be based on a valid scientific hypothesis with realistic studies supporting it. In this respect, knowledge of mechanisms of action is a key factor for hypothesis formulation and for the selection of biomarkers appropriate to the specific state of health and well-being or reduction of risk of disease. It is thus important to improve our knowledge of the mechanisms involved and take into account the fact that probiotic mechanisms of action are multifactorial and that each probiotic may have specific functions affecting the host.

It is also of key interest to increase our knowledge of intestinal microflora composition and to understand its role in health and disease, identifying those microorganisms related to the health status of the host, in order to select probiotic strains able to modulate the intestinal microflora in a beneficial manner.

Knowledge accrued regarding the intestinal microflora, nutrition, immunity, mechanisms of action and specific diseases should be carefully combined with genomic data to allow the development of a second generation of probiotics; strains for both site- and disease-specific action.

See also: **Microbiota of the Intestine**: Prebiotics.

Further Reading

Benno Y and Mitsuoka T (1986) Development of intestinal microflora in humans and animals. *Bifidobacteria Microflora* 5: 13–25.

Dai D and Walker WA (1999) Protective nutrients and bacterial colonization in the immature human gut. *Advances in Pediatrics* 46: 353–382.

De Roos N and Katan M (2000) Effects of probiotic bacteria on diarrhea, lipid metabolism, and carcinogenesis: a review of papers published between 1988 and 1998. *American Journal of Clinical Nutrition* 71: 405–411.

Falk PG, Hooper LV, Midvedt T, and Gordon JI (1998) Creating and maintaining the gastrointestinal ecosystem: What we know and need to know from gnotobiology. *Microbiology and Molecular Biology Reviews* 62: 1157–1170.

Guandalini S, Pensabene L, Zikri M, Dias J, Casali L, Hoekstra H, Kolacek S, Massar K, Micetic-Turk D et al. (2000) *Lactobacillus* GG administered in an oral rehydration solution to children with acute diarrhea: a multicenter European trial. *Journal of Pediatric Gastroenterology and Nutrition* 30: 54–60.

Guarner F and Malagelada JR (2003) Gut flora in health and disease. *Lancet* 381: 512–519.

Gueimonde M, Ouwehand AC, and Salminen S (2004) Safety of probiotics. *Scandinavian Journal of Nutrition* 48: 42–48.

He F, Morita H, Hashimoto H, Hosoda M, Kurisaki J, Ouwehand AC, Isolauri E, Benno Y, and Salminen S (2002) Intestinal Bifidobacterium species induce varying cytokine production. *Journal of Allergy and Clinical Immunology* 109: 1035–1036.

Isolauri E, Kirjavainen PV, and Salminen S (2002) Probiotics: a role in the treatment of intestinal infection and inflammation? *Gut* 50(Suppl. 3): iii54–iii59.

Isolauri E, Salminen S, and Ouwehand AC (2004) Probiotics. *Best Practice and Research Clinical Gastroenterology* 18: 299–313.

Jonkers D and Stockbrügger R (2003) Probiotics and inflammatory bowel disease. *Journal of the Royal Society of Medicine* 96: 167–171.

Kalliomäki M, Kirjavainen P, Eerola E, Kero P, Salminen S, and Isolauri E (2001) Distinct patterns of neonatal gut microflora in infants developing or not developing atopy. *Journal of Allergy and Clinical Immunology* 107: 129–134.

Kalliomäki M, Salminen S, Arvilommi H, Kero P, Koskinen P, and Isolauri E (2001) Probiotics in the prevention of atopic diseases: a randomised placebo-controlled trial. *Lancet* 357: 1076–1079.

Ohashi Y, Nakai S, Tsukamoto T, Masumori N, Akaza H, Miyanaga N *et al.* (2002) Habitual intake of lactic acid bacteria and risk reduction of bladder cancer. *Urology International* 68: 273–280.

Pridmore RD, Berger B, Desiere F, Vilanova D, Barretto C, Pittet A-C, Zwahlen M-C, Rouvet M, Altermann E, Barrangou R, Mollet B, Mercenier A, Klaenhammer T, Arigoni F, and Schell MA (2004) The genome sequence of the probiotic intestinal bacterium Lactobacillus johnsonii NCC 533. *Proceedings of the National Academy of Sciences of the United States of America* 101: 2512–2517.

Salminen S, Bouley MC, Boutron-Rualt MC, Cummings J, Franck A, Gibson G, Isolauri E, Moreau M-C, Roberfroid M, and Rowland I (1998) Functional food science and gastrointestinal physiology and function. *British Journal of Nutrition* Suppl 1: 147–171.

Salminen SJ, von Wright AJ, Ouwehand AC, and Holzapfel WH (2001) Safety assessment of probiotics and starters. In: Adams MR and Nout MJR (eds.) *Fermentation and Food Safety*, 1st edn, pp. 239–251. Gaithersburg: Aspen Publishers, Inc.

Schell MA, Karmirantzou M, Snel B, Vilanova D, Berger B, Pessi G, Zwahlen M-C, Desiere F, Bork P *et al.* (2002) The genome sequence of *Bifidobacterium longum* reflects its adaptation to the human gastrointestinal tract. *Proceedings of the National Academy of Sciences of the United States of America* 99: 14422–14427.

Schiffrin EJ, Brassart D, Servin AL, Rochat F, and Donnet-Hughes A (1997) Immune modulation of blood leukocytes in humans by lactic acid bacteria: criteria for strain selection. *American Journal of Clinical Nutrition* 66: 515S–520S.

Shanahan F (2002) Crohn's disease. *Lancet* 359: 62–69.

Sudo N, Sawamura S, Tanaka K, Aiba Y, Kubo C, and Koga Y (1997) The requirement of intestinal bacterial flora for the development of an IgE production system fully susceptible to oral tolerance induction. *Journal of Immunology* 159: 1739–1745.

Tannock GW (2003) Probiotics: time for a dose of realism. *Current Issues in Intestinal Microbiology* 4: 33–42.

Van Niel CW, Fewudtner C, Garrison MM, and Christakis DA (2002) Lactobacillus therapy for acute infectious diarrhea in children: a meta-analysis. *Pediatrics* 109: 678–684.

Vaughan E, de Vries M, Zoentendal E, Ben-Amor K, Akkermans A, and de Vos W (2002) The intestinal LABs. *Antonie Van Leeuwenhoek* 82: 341–352.

Xu J, Chiang HC, Bjursell MK, and Gordon JI (2004) Message from a human gut symbiont: sensitivity is a prerequisite for sharing. *Trends in Microbiology* 12: 21–28.

N

NIACIN

C J Bates, MRC Human Nutrition Research,
Cambridge, UK

This article is reproduced from the previous edition,
pp. 1290–1297, © 1998, Elsevier Ltd.

Absorption, Transport, and Storage

Niacin is a B vitamin that is essential for health in humans and also in most other mammals that have been investigated. Niacin is associated with a characteristic deficiency disease in humans known as pellagra. Pellagra has been described and identified in various communities, notably in Spain and North America, in the last century and the early years of this century. It has persisted in Yugoslavia, Egypt, Mexico, and some African countries. Pellagra is characteristically associated with maize-based diets. The skin lesions found in pellagra are most severe during the summer months because of the effects of the exacerbating sun exposure. However, some countries with a maize diet (e.g., Guatemala) avoid pellagra by means of the niacin present in roasted coffee (**Table 1**). Others avoid it by lime treatment, e.g., in the preparation of tortillas.

Preformed niacin occurs in foods either as nicotinamide (niacinamide) or as the pyridine nucleotide coenzymes derived from it, or as nicotinic acid, without the amide nitrogen, which is the form known as 'niacin' in North America. Both nicotinamide and nicotinic acid are equally effective as the vitamin, but in large doses they exert markedly different pharmacological effects, so it is important, at least in that context, to make and maintain the distinction. In addition to the preformed vitamin, an important *in vivo* precursor is the amino acid L-tryptophan, obtained from dietary protein. Because the human total niacin supply, and hence niacin status, depends on the dietary tryptophan supply as well as on the amount of preformed dietary niacin and its bioavailability, it has become the accepted practice to express niacin intakes as 'niacin equivalents,' which is a combination of mg preformed dietary niacin and mg niacin which can become available by conversion from tryptophan within the body. As discussed later, this calculation involves several assumptions, and is therefore only an approximation to the actual supply to the body for any particular individual; however, it is considered adequate for most practical purposes.

It appears likely that the most important ultimate sources of preformed niacin in most foods, particularly those of animal foods, are the pyridine nucleotides: $NAD(H_2)$ and $NADP(H_2)$. Hydrolases and pyrophosphatases present in biological tissues convert these coenzymes to partly degraded products, which are then available as sources of the vitamin. NAD glycohydrolase and pyrophosphatase enzymes are present in the gut mucosa to assist hydrolysis and absorption of the hydrolyzed products, and these are likely to include both nicotinamide and nicotinamide ribonucleotide, the latter being further degraded to the riboside. Absorption of nicotinamide or nicotinic acid by the mammalian intestine has been shown to consist of a saturable transport component, dominant at low intakes, which is dependent on sodium, energy and pH, and a nonsaturable component, which becomes dominant at high doses or intake levels. Absorption is efficient even at such high discrete doses as 3 g or more: as much as 85% of such a dose is subsequently excreted into the urine. Absorption of test niacin doses introduced directly into the human upper ileum is rapid, with peak levels appearing in blood plasma within 5–10 min.

Transport of niacin between the liver and the intestine can occur *in vivo*, as indicated by radioactive probes in animals, and the liver appears to be a major site of conversion of niacin to its ultimate functional products: the nicotinamide nucleotide coenzymes. Nicotinamide can pass readily between the cerebrospinal fluid and the plasma, thus ensuring a supply also to the brain and spinal cord. Liver contains greater niacin coenzyme concentrations than most other tissues, but all metabolically active tissues contain these essential

Table 1 Niacin equivalents in selected foods[a]

	Niacin equivalents from preformed niacin[b] (mg per 100 g, wet)	Niacin equivalents from tryptophan[c] (mg per 100 g, wet)	Total niacin equivalents (mg per 100 g, wet)
Milk	0.1	0.8	0.9
Raw beef	5.0	4.7	9.7
Raw white fish	2.4	3.4	5.8
Raw eggs	0.1	3.7	3.8
Raw potatoes	0.6	0.5	1.1
Raw peas	2.5	1.1	3.6
Raw peanuts	13.8	5.5	19.3
White bread	0.8	1.7	2.5
Polished rice	0.2	1.5	1.7
Maize	0.1	0.9	1.0
Cornflakes (fortified)	16.0	0.9	16.9
Coffee[d]	24.1	2.9	27.0

[a]Data adapted from: Paul AA (1969) The calculation of nicotinic acid equivalents and retinol equivalents in the British diet. *Nutrition* (*London*) **23**: 131–136,[a] and supplements to *McCance and Widdowson's The Composition of Foods* (Holland B, Welch AA, Unwin ID, Buss DH, Paul AA, and Southgate DAT (1991), The Royal Society of Chemistry and MAFF),[a] and from Bressani R *et al.* (1961) Effect of processing method and variety on niacin and ether extract content of green and roasted coffee. *Food Technology* **15**: 306–308.
[b]Amount available for absorption. In the case of bread, rice, and maize, the total amounts present are 1.7, 1.5, and 1.2 mg per 100 g, but apart from the niacin added in the fortification of white flour, 90% of this is unavailable for utilization by humans.
[c]Assuming that 60 mg tryptophan yields 1 mg niacin equivalent.
[d]Niacin is released from trigonelline in coffee beans by the roasting process.

metabolic components. Both facilitated diffusion (which is sodium- and energy-dependent and saturable), and passive diffusion (which is nonsaturable) contribute to tissue uptake from the bloodstream. With the exception of muscle, brain and testis, within the body nicotinic acid is a better precursor of the coenzyme form than is nicotinamide. The liver appears to be the most important site of conversion of tryptophan to the nicotinamide coenzymes.

Of the two pyridine nucleotide coenzymes, NAD is present mainly as the oxidized form in the tissues, whereas NADP is principally present in the reduced form, $NADPH_2$. There are important homeostatic regulation mechanisms which ensure and maintain an appropriate ratio of these coenzymes in their respective oxidized or reduced forms in healthy tissues. Once converted to coenzymes within the cells, the niacin therein is effectively trapped, and can only diffuse out again after degradation to smaller molecules. This implies, of course, that the synthesis of the essential coenzyme nucleotides must occur within each tissue and cell type, each of which must possess the enzymatic apparatus for their synthesis from the precursor niacin. Loss of nicotinamide and nicotinic acid into the urine is minimized (except when the intake exceeds requirements) by means of an efficient reabsorption from the glomerular filtrate.

Metabolism and Excretion

The conversion of tryptophan to nicotinic acid *in vivo* is depicted in **Figure 1**. The rate of conversion of tryptophan to niacin and the pyridine nucleotides is controlled by the activities of tryptophan dioxygenase (known alternatively as tryptophan pyrrolase), kynurenine hydroxylase, and kynureninase. These enzymes are, in turn, dependent on factors such as other B vitamins, glucagon, glucocorticoid hormones, and estrogen metabolites, and there are various competing pathways which also affect the rate of conversion. For these reasons, a variety of nutrient deficiencies, toxins, genetic and metabolic abnormalities, etc. can influence niacin status and requirements.

For practical purposes, on the basis of studies performed in the 1950s, 60 mg tryptophan is deemed to give rise to 1 mg nicotinic acid; hence 60 mg tryptophan contributes 1 mg niacin equivalent, for dietary intake calculations and food tables (see **Table 1**).

The two pyridine nucleotide coenzymes, formerly known as 'coenzymes I and II,' then for a period as 'DPN and TPN,' and known nowadays as 'NAD' and 'NADP' (nicotinamide adenine dinucleotide and nicotinamide adenine dinucleotide phosphate), are involved in hundreds of enzyme-catalyzed redox reactions *in vivo*. Although a minority of these diverse reactions can use either of the two

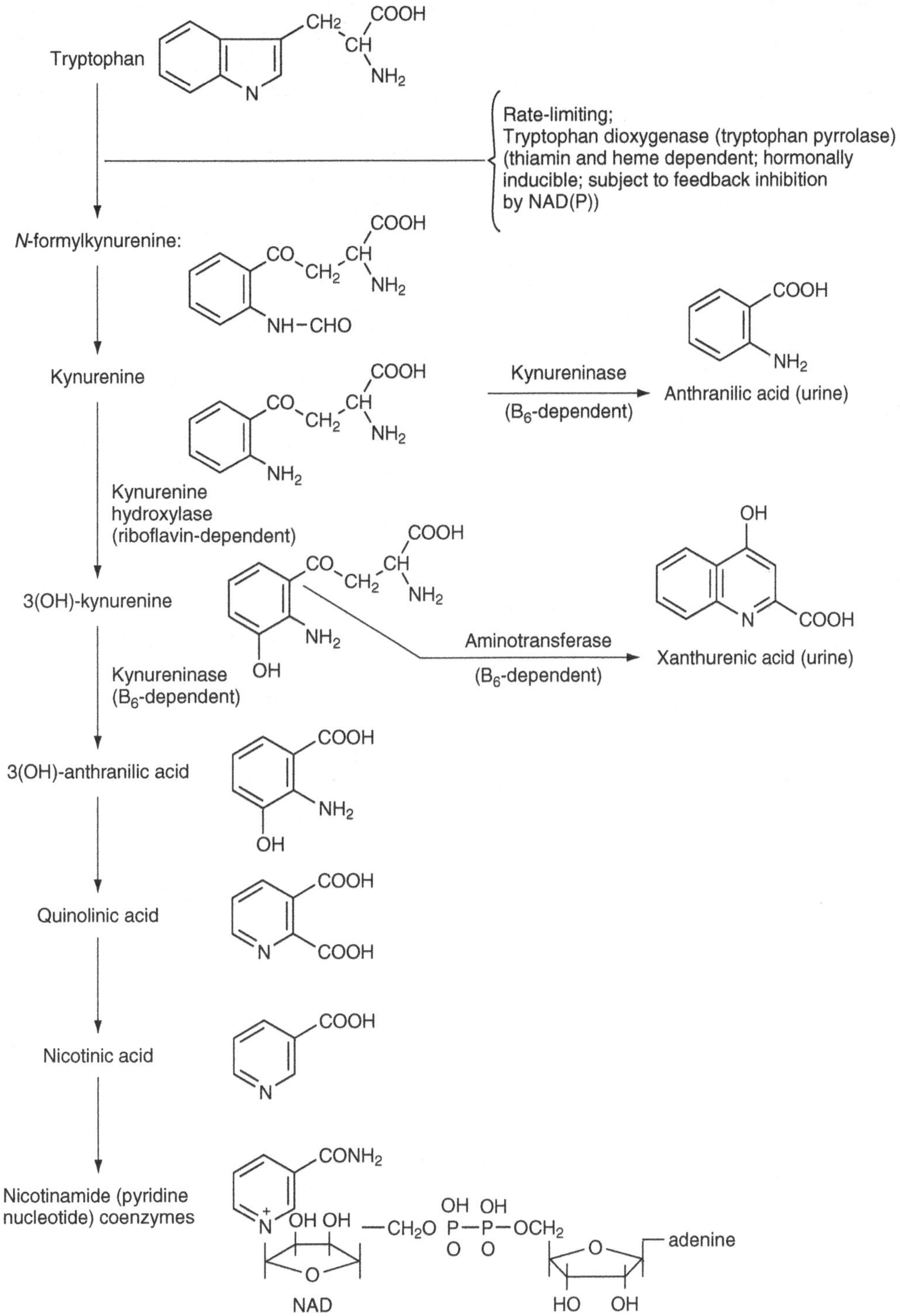

Figure 1 *In vivo* conversion of tryptophan to nicotinic acid and NAD.

niacin-derived cofactors, most are highly specific for one or the other.

Catabolism of the pyridine nucleotide coenzymes *in vivo* is achieved by four classes of enzymes: NAD glycohydrolase, ADP ribosyl transferase, and poly (ADP ribose) synthetase, (all of which liberate nicotinamide), and NAD pyrophosphatase (which liberates nicotinamide mononucleotide which is then further hydrolyzed to nicotinamide). Turnover of nicotinamide then results in the formation of 1-methylnicotinamide (usually described as N^1-methyl nicotinamide or NMN), an excretory product which is excreted in the kidney and appears in the urine, together with some further oxidation products, typically the 1-methyl-2-pyridone-5-carboxamide and 1-methyl-4-pyridone-3-carboxamide (usually referred to as '2-pyridone' and '4-pyridone', respectively). These excretory turnover products can be used as indicators of whole body niacin status (see below). At high intakes of niacin, as much as 85% of the intake may be excreted unchanged; however the excretion of nicotinamide always predominates over that of nicotinic acid.

Hydrolysis of hepatic NAD to yield nicotinamide allows the release of niacin for utilization by other tissues. Relative protection of the pyridine nucleotide within certain key enzymes such as glyceraldehyde 3-phosphate dehydrogenase confers a protection on certain key metabolic pathways, thus ensuring good homeostatic control. By contrast, there is evidence that the enzymes which catalyze pyridine nucleotide turnover may be hyperactivated within cells that have been damaged by carcinogens, including mycotoxins, thus starving these damaged cells of essential cofactors and causing their death, presumably to protect the rest of the organism. This effect may help to explain the otherwise puzzling observation that moldy grain in the diet can increase the risk of pellagra when niacin and tryptophan intakes are marginal. In normal, healthy cells, the compartmentalization of hydrolytic enzymes prevents unwanted coenzyme turnover, and this compartmentalization seems to become breached in damaged or dying cells.

Other urinary excretion products of niacin include nicotinuric acid (nicotinoyl glycine); nicotinamide N-oxide, and trigonelline (N^1-methyl nicotinic acid); the latter may arise from bacterial action in the gut or from the absorption of this substance from foods. The pattern of the different turnover metabolites varies between species, between diets (depending partly on the ratio of nicotinamide to nicotinic acid in the diet), and partly with niacin status; thus there are complex regulatory mechanisms to be considered.

Metabolic Function and Essentiality

The best-known functions of niacin are derived from the functions of its coenzymes: NAD and NADP in the hydrogen/electron transfer redox reactions in living cells. Like most B vitamins, niacin is not extensively stored in forms or in depots that are usually metabolically inactive, but rather those that can become available during dietary deficiency. However, some 'storage' of the coenzymes NAD and NADP in the liver is thought to occur. An inadequate dietary intake leads rapidly to significant tissue depletion within 1–2 months, and then successively to biochemical abnormalities, followed by clinical signs of deficiency, and eventually to death. As with the other B vitamins, rates of turnover and hence the rates of excretion of coenzyme breakdown products decline progressively as dietary deficiency becomes more severe and prolonged, so that the tissue levels are relatively protected and spared. In adult humans a severe deficiency may take many months to develop before it results in the clinical signs of pellagra.

Some of the most important and characteristic functions of NAD manifest in the principal cellular catabolic pathways, responsible for liberation of energy during the oxidation of energy-producing fuels. NADP, however, functions mainly in the reductive reactions of lipid biosynthesis, and the reduced form of this coenzyme is generated via the pentose phosphate cycle. NAD is essential for the synthesis and repair of DNA. NAD has, in addition, a role in supplying ADP ribose moieties to lysine, arginine, and asparagine residues in proteins such as histones, DNA lyase II, and DNA-dependent RNA polymerase, and to polypeptides such as the bacterial diphtheria and cholera toxins. In the nucleus, poly (ADP ribose) synthetase is activated by binding to DNA breakage points and is involved in DNA repair. It is also concerned with condensation and expansion of chromatin during the cell cycle and in DNA replication. Niacin status affects the level of ADP ribolysation of proteins. A high level of poly (ADP ribose) synthetase activity, which is found in some tumors, can result in low levels of NAD. A chromium dinicotinate complex found in yeast extracts may function as a glucose tolerance factor or in detoxification, but this has not yet been proven.

Because the electron transport functions of NAD frequently involve flavin coenzymes, and because both flavin coenzymes and vitamin B_6 coenzymes are involved in the conversion of tryptophan to niacin *in vivo*, there are important metabolic interactions between these B vitamins. A similarity of clinical deficiency signs, making it difficult to distinguish between them, may be encountered in population studies of deficiency.

Because the body's need for niacin can be met completely by dietary tryptophan, it is not, strictly speaking, an essential vitamin. In this respect it resembles carnitine, which can be synthesized entirely from lysine, but for which in some circumstances a dietary requirement exists. Traditionally, however, niacin is classified as an essential vitamin, because some human diets have tended to be lacking in niacin and its precursor, tryptophan. Some animals such as sheep and cattle appear to be able to synthesize sufficient niacin for their needs from tryptophan, and do not therefore need preformed niacin in their diets.

Assessment of Niacin Status

Whereas the measurement of B vitamin status has, in recent years, tended to focus on blood analysis, perhaps mainly because of the convenience of sample collection, the development of blood-based status analysis for niacin has lagged behind that of the other components of the B complex. Some studies have indeed suggested that the erythrocyte concentration of the niacin-derived coenzyme NAD may provide useful information about the niacin status of human subjects; that a reduction in the ratio of NAD to NADP to below 1.0 in red cells may provide evidence of niacin deficiency; and that a decline in plasma tryptophan levels may indicate a more severe deficiency than a decline in red cell NAD levels. These claims now need to be tested in naturally deficient human populations. The niacin coenzymes can be quantitated either by enzyme-linked reactions or by making use of their natural fluorescence in alkaline solution.

At present, niacin status is most commonly assessed by the assay of some of the breakdown products of niacin coenzymes in the urine. Of these, N^1-methyl nicotinamide (NMN) is the easiest to measure, because of a convenient conversion *in vitro* to a fluorescent product, which can then be quantitated without the need for separation. However, more definitive and reliable information can be obtained by the measurement of urinary NMN in conjunction with one or more of the urinary pyridone turnover products (N^1-methyl-2-pyridone-5-carboxamide and N^1-methyl-4-pyridone-3-carboxamide), which can be detected and quantitated by UV absorption following high-pressure liquid chromatography. The Interdepartmental Committee on Nutrition for National Defense (USA) selected the criterion of niacin deficiency in humans as an NMN excretion rate of $<5.8\,\mu mol$ (0.8 mg) NMN per day in 24 h urine samples.

Requirements and Signs of Deficiency

As for most other micronutrients, the requirement of niacin to prevent or reverse the clinical deficiency signs is not known very precisely, and probably depends on ancillary dietary deficiencies or other insults occurring in natural human populations. For the purpose of estimating niacin requirements

for dietary reference values, the criterion of restoration of urinary excretion of NMN during controlled human depletion–repletion studies has been selected, and on this basis, the average adult requirement has been estimated as 5.5 mg (45 μmol) of niacin equivalents per 1000 kcal (4200 kJ). Adding a 20% allowance for individual variation this needs to be increased to 6.6 mg (54 μmol) per 1000 kcal, (4200 kJ), which is the current reference nutrient intake (UK). Niacin requirements were, by convention, expressed as a ratio to energy expenditure. For subjects with very low energy intakes, the daily intake of niacin equivalents should not fall below 13 mg, however. If dietary protein levels and quality are high, it is possible for tryptophan alone to provide the daily requirement for niacin equivalents. Dietary niacin deficiency is now rare in most Western countries.

The appearance of severe niacin deficiency as endemic pellagra, especially in North America in the nineteenth and early twentieth centuries, has been ascribed to the very poor availability of bound forms of niacin (in niacytin, a polysaccharide/glycopeptide/polypeptide-bound form, which is 90% indigestible), together with the relatively low content of tryptophan occurring in grains (see **Table 1**). However, the lack of available niacin and tryptophan may not have been the whole story, since coexisting deficiencies or imbalances of other nutrients, including riboflavin, may also have contributed to this endemic disease. It appears also that the choice of cooking methods may have been critical, since the Mexican custom of cooking maize with lime in the preparation of tortillas helps to release the bound niacin from its carbohydrate complex and to increase the bioavailability of tryptophan-containing proteins, and thus to reduce the prevalence of clinical deficiency disease. In parts of India, pellagra has been encountered in communities whose main staple is a form of millet known as 'jowar', which is rich in leucine. It was proposed, and evidence was obtained from animal and *in vitro* studies, that high intakes of leucine can increase the requirements for niacin. However, other evidence is conflicting (this interaction is not fully understood). In parts of South Africa, iron overload has been reported to complicate the metabolic effects of low niacin intakes.

The average content of niacin in human breast milk is 8 mg (65.6 μmol) per 1000 kcal (4200 kJ), and this is the basis for the recommendations (and dietary reference values) for infants up to 6 months. In the UK, the Reference Nutrient Intake niacin increment during pregnancy is nil, and during lactation it is 2 mg per day.

The most characteristic clinical signs of severe niacin deficiency in humans are dermatosis (hyperpigmentation, hyperkeratosis, desquamation – especially where exposed to the sun), anorexia, achlorhydria, diarrhea, angular stomatitis, cheilosis, magenta tongue, anemia, and neuropathy (headache, dizziness, tremor, neurosis, apathy). In addition to the pellagra caused by dietary deficiency or imbalance, there are also reports of disturbed niacin metabolism associated with phenylketonuria, acute intermittent porphyria, diabetes mellitus, some types of cancer (carcinoid syndrome), thyrotoxicosis, fever, stress, tissue repair, renal disease, iron overload, etc. The picture in other species is not radically different; however, deficient dogs and cats typically exhibit 'black tongue' (pustules in the mouth, excessive salivation) and bloody diarrhea, pigs exhibit neurological lesions affecting the ganglion cells, rats exhibit damage to the peripheral nerves (cells and axons), and fowl exhibit inflammation of the upper gastrointestinal tract, dermatitis, diarrhea, and damage to the feathers. All species exhibit reduction of appetite and loss of weight; however, it is of interest that the skin lesions seen in humans are rare in most other species.

Dietary Sources, High Intakes, and Antimetabolites

As can be seen from **Table 1**, different types of foods differ considerably, not only in their total contribution to nicotinic acid equivalents, but also in the ratio of the contribution from preformed niacin and from tryptophan. In a typical Western diet, it has been calculated that if the 60 mg tryptophan = 1 mg niacin formula is applied, then preformed niacin provides about 50% of the niacin supply in the diet. In practice it seems possible for all of the niacin requirement to be provided by dietary tryptophan in Western diets. As is the case for the other B vitamins, meat, poultry, and fish are excellent sources of niacin equivalents, followed by dairy and grain products, but as noted above, certain grains such as maize, and whole highly polished rice, can be very poor sources and may be associated with clinical deficiency if the diets are otherwise poor and monotonous.

In recent years, both nicotinamide and nicotinic acid have been proposed and tested for possibly useful pharmacological properties at high intake levels. This new phase of interest in the vitamin has, in turn, raised concerns about the possible side effects of high intakes, and the definition of maximum safe intakes.

The greatest interest, in pharmacological terms, has been centered around nicotinic acid, which has been shown to have marked antihyperlipidemic properties at daily doses of 2–6 g. Nicotinamide does not share this particular pharmacological activity. Large doses of nicotinic acid reduce the mobilization of fatty acids from adipose tissue by inhibiting the breakdown of triacylglycerols through lipolysis. They also inhibit hepatic triacylglycerol synthesis, thus limiting the assembly and secretion of very low-density lipoproteins from the liver and reducing serum cholesterol levels. Large doses of nicotinic acid ameliorate certain risk factors for cardiovascular disease: for instance they increase circulating high-density lipoprotein levels. The ratio of HDL_2 to HDL_3 is increased by nicotinic acid; there is a reduced rate of synthesis of apolipoprotein A-II and a transfer of some apolipoprotein A-I from HDL_3 to HDL_2. These changes are all considered potentially beneficial in reducing the risk of cardiovascular disease. If given intravenously, large doses of nicotinic acid can, however, produce side effects such as temporary vasodilatation and hypotension. Other side effects can include nausea, vomiting, diarrhea and general gastrointestinal disturbance, headache, fatigue, difficulty in focusing, skin discoloration, dry hair, sore throat, etc. A large trial for secondary prevention of myocardial infarction, with a 15 year period of follow-up, produced convincing evidence for moderate but significant protection against mortality, which was attributed either to the cholesterol-lowering effect or an early effect on nonfatal reinfarction, or both. Nicotinic acid is still the treatment of choice for some classes of high-risk hyperlipidemic patients, although newer drugs may have fewer side effects and therefore be preferred.

The potential benefits of the lipid-lowering effects of nicotinic acid have to be considered in the light of possibly toxic effects, particularly for the liver. These may manifest as jaundice, changes in liver function tests, changes in carbohydrate tolerance, and changes in uric acid metabolism including hyper-uricemia. There may also be accompanying ultrastructural changes. Hyperuricemia may result from effects on intestinal bacteria and enzymes, and from effects on renal tubular function. Such toxic effects are especially severe if sustained release preparations of nicotinic acid are used.

Nicotinamide does not share with nicotinic acid these effects on lipid metabolism or the associated toxicity. However, it has been shown to be an inhibitor of poly (ADP ribose) synthetase in pancreatic β cells in animal studies. A high-risk group of children aged 5–8 years in New Zealand given large doses of nicotinamide daily for up to 4.2 years had only half the predicted incidence of insulin-dependent diabetes.

Other claims for megadoses of nicotinic acid or nicotinamide, such as the claim that abnormalities associated with schizophrenia, Down's syndrome, hyperactivity in children, etc. can be reduced, have so far failed to win general acceptance. Clearly niacin deficiency or dependency can exacerbate some types of mental illness such as depression or dementia. There have been a number of attempts to treat depression with tryptophan or niacin, or both, on the basis that the correction of depressed brain levels of serotonin would be advantageous. However, these have met with only limited success. Schizophrenics have been treated with nicotinic acid on the basis that their synthesis of NAD is impaired in some parts of the brain, and that the formation of hallucinogenic substances such as methylated indoles may be controlled.

There are various medical conditions and drug interactions that can increase the requirement for niacin. Examples are: Hartnup disease, in which tryptophan transport in the intestine and kidney is impaired; carcinoid syndrome, in which tryptophan turnover is increased; and isoniazid treatment, which causes B_6 depletion and hence interference with niacin formation from tryptophan. Hartnup disease (the name of the first patient being Hartnup) is a rare genetic disease in which the conversion of tryptophan to niacin is reduced, partly as a result of impaired tryptophan absorption. Affected subjects exhibit the classical skin and neurological lesions of pellagra, which can be alleviated by prolonged treatment with niacin. Another genetic disease which may respond to niacin supplements is Fredrikson type I familial hypercholesterolemia; nicotinic acid is effective in reducing the raised blood cholesterol levels associated with this abnormality.

There are several analogs and antimetabolites of niacin that are of potential use or metabolic interest. The closely related isoniazid is commonly used for treatment of tuberculosis; indeed, nicotinamide itself has been used for that purpose. Nicotinic acid diethylamide ('nikethamide') is used as a stimulant in cases of central nervous system depression after poisoning, trauma or collapse. Possible antineoplastic analogs include 6-dimethylaminonicotinamide and 6-aminonicotinamide; however, the latter is also highly teratogenic. These latter compounds inhibit several key enzymes whose substrates are NAD or NADP, by being converted *in vivo* to analogs of these coenzymes. The compound 3-acetyl pyridine, which also forms an analog of NAD, can have either antagonistic or niacin-replacing properties, depending on the dose used. Commonly used drugs such as metronidazole are also niacin antagonists.

See also: **Riboflavin. Vitamin B$_6$**.

Further Reading

Bender DA (1992) Niacin. In: *Nutritional Biochemistry of the Vitamins*, ch. 8, pp. 184–222. Cambridge: Cambridge University Press.

Carpenter KJ (ed.) (1981) *Pellagra: Benchmark Papers in the History of Biochemistry/II.* Stroudsburg, Pennsylvania: Dowden, Hutchinson & Ross Publ. Co.

Di Palma JR and Thayer WS (1991) Use of niacin as a drug. *Annual Review of Nutrition* 2: 169–187.

Fu CS, Swendseid ME, Jacob RA, and McKee RW (1989) Biochemical markers for assessment of niacin status in young men: levels of erythrocyte niacin coenzymes and plasma tryptophan. *Journal of Nutrition* 119: 1949–1955.

Hankes LV (1984) Nicotinic acid and nicotinamide. In: Machlin LJ (ed.) *Handbook of Vitamins*, ch. 8, pp. 329–377. New York: Marcel Dekker Inc.

Henderson LM (1983) Niacin. *Annual Review of Biochemistry* 3: 289–307.

Horwitt MK, Harvey CC, Rothwell WS, Cutler JL, and Haffron D (1956) Tryptophan–niacin relationship in man. *Journal of Nutrition* 60(supplement 1): 1–43.

Jacob RA, Swendseid ME, McKee RW, Fu CS, and Clemens RA (1989) Biochemical markers for assessment of niacin status in young men: urinary and blood levels of niacin metabolites. *Journal of Nutrition* 119: 591–598.

Sauberlich HE, Dowdy RP, and Skala JH (1974) *Laboratory Tests for the Assessment of Nutritional Status*, pp. 70–74. Boca Raton: CRC Press.

Swendseid ME and Jacob RA (1984) Niacin. In: Shils ME and Young VR (eds.) *Modern Nutrition in Health and Disease*, 7th edn., ch. 22, pp. 376–382. Philadelphia: Lea & Febiger.

PANTOTHENIC ACID

C J Bates, MRC Human Nutrition Research, Cambridge, UK

Absorption, Transport and Storage, Status Measurement

A considerable proportion of the pantothenic acid (vitamin B_5, see **Figure 1**) that is present in food eaten by animals or humans exists as derivatives such as coenzyme A (CoA) and acyl carrier protein (ACP). Compared with the crystalline vitamin, only about half of the vitamin in food is thought to be absorbed. The pantothenic acid in its derivatives in food is largely released as free pantothenic acid or pantetheine by pancreatic enzymes, and is then absorbed along the entire length of the small intestine by a combination of active transport and passive diffusion, of which the active transport process seems to predominate at physiological intakes. This active transport process is dependent on sodium, energy and pH and is saturable: the K_m is $c.$ 17 μM and V_{max} is $c.$ 1000 pmol cm^{-2} h^{-1}, with minor variations among species. The transport pathway is shared by biotin in colonic epithelial cells, and it appears to be regulated by an intracellular protein kinase C-mediated pathway. Calmodulin is also implicated in cellular pantothenic acid transport pathways.

In mice, it was found that usual dietary pantothenate levels did not affect the rate of absorption of a standard pantothenate dose, i.e., there was no evidence for feedback adaptation of the absorption pathway to low or high intakes, and it is assumed that the same is true in other species, including humans. However, there is some evidence from rat studies that the extent of secretion of enzymes degrading CoA into the gut lumen may partially limit the availability of pantothenic acid from CoA.

In humans, studies of urinary excretion of pantothenic acid after oral intakes of either free pantothenic acid or of the pantothenic acid present in food have indicated a relative availability of $c.$ 50% from the food-borne vitamin. Urinary excretion of pantothenate was $c.$ 0.8 mg day^{-1} when a pantothenate-deficient diet

was eaten, rising to 40–60 mg day^{-1} at a high daily intake of 100 mg day^{-1}. At intermediate intakes, in the range 2.8–12.8 mg day^{-1}, the urinary excretion rate varied between 4 and 6 mg day^{-1}. Excretion of less than 1 mg day^{-1} is considered low. Urinary excretion rates reflect recent intakes perhaps more closely than most other biochemical indices.

The contribution of the gut flora to the available pantothenate for humans is unknown, but there is some evidence that bacterial synthesis of the vitamin may be important in animals, especially ruminants, since severe deficiency can only be achieved by using antibiotics or antagonists. Clinical conditions such as ulcers or colitis can adversely affect pantothenate status and excretion rates, and dietary fiber may affect its absorption.

After a dose of ^{14}C-labeled pantothenate, about 40% of the dose appears in muscle tissue and about 10% in the liver, with smaller amounts occurring elsewhere. The differential affinities of the various different tissues determines their individual contents of the coenzyme derivatives, CoA and ACP, since there is no other major store of the vitamin anywhere in the body. Most organs, including placenta, exhibit evidence of a unidirectional active transport process for the intracellular accumulation of pantothenate, which is dependent on sodium, energy, and pH. In placenta (and probably elsewhere) this transport process is also shared by biotin and by some of its analogs, which can exhibit competitive inhibition. The only tissues that have been shown to differ with respect to transport mechanisms are red cells and the central nervous system.

The uptake and efflux of pantothenate into and out of red blood cells is unaffected by sodium, energy, or pH. Red cells contain pantothenate, 4-phosphopantothenate, and pantetheine, but they do not contain mitochondria, or carry out CoA-dependent processes. The function of the pantothenate derivatives found in red cells is unknown, but their formation clearly results in higher concentrations of total pantothenate in red cells than in plasma, and red cell (or whole blood) total pantothenate is considered a better status index, and is more predictably related to

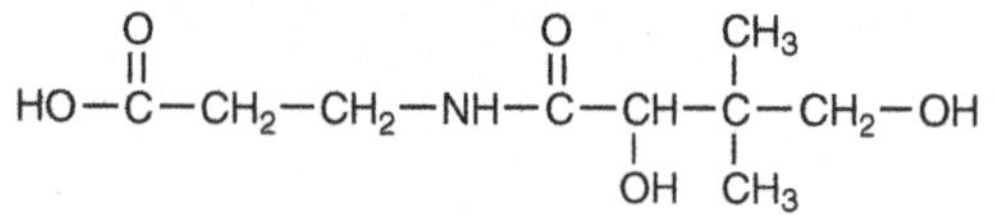

$$HO-\overset{\overset{\displaystyle O}{\|}}{C}-CH_2-CH_2-NH-\overset{\overset{\displaystyle O}{\|}}{C}-\underset{\underset{\displaystyle OH}{|}}{CH}-\underset{\underset{\displaystyle CH_3}{|}}{\overset{\overset{\displaystyle CH_3}{|}}{C}}-CH_2-OH$$

Figure 1 Structure of pantothenic acid.

intake, than is serum or plasma pantothenate. A concentration less than $1\,\mu\text{mol}\,l^{-1}$ of pantothenate in whole blood is considered low; the normal range is $1.6\text{–}2.7\,\mu\text{mol}\,l^{-1}$. Pantothenate in serum appears to be a very short-term marker and it is not well correlated with changes in intake or status.

Concentrations in body fluids are traditionally measured by microbiological assay using *Lactobacillus plantarum*. If CoA is present, enzymatic hydrolysis is needed to liberate free pantothenic acid for the microbiological assay. Other assay methods reported include gas chromatography (after conversion to a volatile derivative), radioimmunoassay (RIA), or enzyme-linked immunoabsorbent assay (ELISA).

Unlike several other B vitamin precursors of cofactors, pantothenate is not entirely converted to coenzyme forms inside the cell, and metabolic 'trapping' is therefore less dominant than it is for some other B vitamins. There is some evidence that the free pantothenate in tissues is more closely related to dietary pantothenate than the coenzyme forms are; the latter are relatively protected during periods of dietary deficiency or of low intakes. Uptake of pantothenate from plasma into most tissues is proportional to the plasma concentration because the active transport process is nowhere near saturated at typical plasma concentrations of $c.\ 10^{-6}\,\text{M}$.

Pantothenate is required for the hepatic acetylation of drugs by its presence in acetyl CoA, and it has been shown that pantothenate deficiency can impair this process; moreover, 20–60% of human populations are slow acetylators, varying with their ethnic grouping. Whether this function can be used to develop a functional test for pantothenate status is an intriguing but unresolved question.

Metabolism and Turnover

The primary role of pantothenic acid is in acyl group activation for lipid metabolism, involving thiol acylation of CoA or of ACP, both of which contain 4-phosphopantotheine, the active group of which is β-mercaptoethylamine. CoA is essential for oxidation of fatty acids, pyruvate and α-oxogutarate, for metabolism of sterols, and for acetylation of other molecules, so as to modulate their transport characteristics or functions. Acyl carrier protein, which is synthesized from apo-ACP and coenzyme A, is involved specifically in fatty acid synthesis. Its role is to activate acetyl, malonyl, and intermediate chain fatty acyl groups during their anabolism by the biotin-dependent fatty acid synthase complex (i.e., acyl-CoA: malonyl-CoA-acyl transferase (decarboxylating, oxoacyl and enoyl-reducing, and thioester-hydrolyzing), EC 2.3.1.85).

The organ with the highest concentration of pantothenate is liver, followed by adrenal cortex, because of the requirement for steroid hormone metabolism in these tissues. Ninety-five per cent of the CoA within each tissue is found in the mitochondria. However, the initial stages of activation of pantothenate and conversion to CoA occur in the cytosol. It was originally believed that the final stages of CoA synthesis must occur within the mitochondria, but later evidence indicated that transport across the mitochondrial membrane is, after all, possible. β-oxidation within the peroxisomes is also CoA-dependent, and is downregulated by pantothenate deficiency.

The pathways of conversion of pantothenic acid to CoA and to ACP are summarized in **Figure 2**. There are three ATP-requiring reactions and one CTP-requiring reaction in the synthesis of CoA. The rate of CoA synthesis is under close metabolic control by energy-yielding substrates, such as glucose and free fatty acids (via CoA and acyl CoA) at the initial activation step, which is catalyzed by pantothenate kinase (ATP: pantothenate 4-phosphotransferase, EC 2.7.1.33). This feedback control is thought to be a mechanism for conservation of cofactor requirements. There are also direct and indirect effects of insulin, corticosteroids, and glucagon, which result in important changes in tissue distribution, uptake, etc. in persons with diabetes. The mechanisms involved here are complex and not yet fully understood; however insulin represses and glucagon induces the enzyme.

A rare genetic disease, Hallervorden-Spatz syndrome, has recently been shown to result from deficiency of pantothenate kinase, and is now alternatively known as pantothenate kinase-associated neurodegeneration (PKAN). Dystonia, involuntary movements, and spasticity occur, and although there is no cure, some palliative treatment is possible.

In genetically normal people, fasting results in a reduction of fatty acid synthase activity with loss of the coenzyme of ACP, which thus achieves the desired objective of a shift away from fatty acid synthesis, towards breakdown. This interconversion of apo-ACP and holo-ACP is thus a very important process for the short-term regulation of fatty acid synthesis.

Deficiency of sulfur amino acids can result in reduced CoA synthesis; likewise copper overload can (by interfering with sulfur amino acid function) also reduce CoA synthesis.

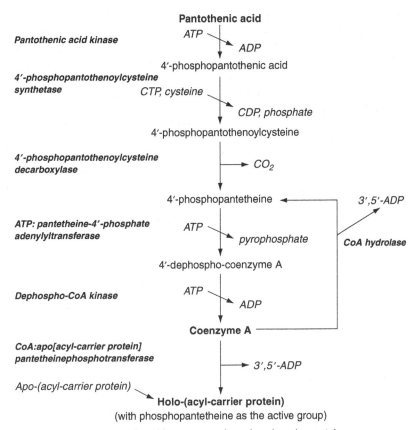

Pantothenic acid

Pantothenic acid kinase   ATP ⟶ ADP

4'-phosphopantothenic acid

4'-phosphopantothenoylcysteine synthetase   CTP, cysteine ⟶ CDP, phosphate

4'-phosphopantothenoylcysteine

4'-phosphopantothenoylcysteine decarboxylase   ⟶ CO_2

4'-phosphopantetheine   ⟵   3',5'-ADP

ATP: pantetheine-4'-phosphate adenylyltransferase   ATP ⟶ pyrophosphate   *CoA hydrolase*

4'-dephospho-coenzyme A

Dephospho-CoA kinase   ATP ⟶ ADP

Coenzyme A

CoA:apo[acyl-carrier protein] pantetheinephosphotransferase   ⟶ 3',5'-ADP

Apo-(acyl-carrier protein)

Holo-(acyl-carrier protein)
(with phosphopantetheine as the active group)

Figure 2   Synthetic pathway between pantothenic acid, coenzyme A, and acyl carrier protein.

Excretion of free pantothenate in the urine is the primary excretion route in humans; in other mammals the glucuronide or glucoside may be excreted. There is little evidence of degradation to simpler products, and pantothenic acid appears to be very efficiently conserved in animals. Some bacteria can cleave it to yield pantoic acid and β-alanine. A potentially useful breakdown product of CoA is taurine, formed via cysteamine. This amino acid is an essential nutrient for some carnivorous animals such as cats.

When dietary intakes are low, the majority of the circulating vitamin, which is filtered in the kidney tubules, is absorbed by the same type of sodium-dependent active transport process that also occurs at most other sites in the body. Retention of a test dose of pantothenate is, as expected, greater in partially depleted subjects, than in saturated ones. Secretion into breast milk is proportional to intake and to blood levels of the vitamin; therefore, dietary supplements taken by the lactating mother generally increase the breast milk content of the vitamin.

Metabolic Function and Essentiality

As noted above, the biochemical functions, and hence the basis for the dietary requirement of pantothenic acid, arise entirely from its occurrence as an essential component of CoA and of ACP, which cannot be synthesized *de novo* in mammals from simpler precursors.

In addition to the now well-established roles of CoA in the degradation and synthesis of fatty acids, sterols, and other compounds synthesized from isoprenoid precursors, there are also a number of acetylation and long-chain fatty acylation processes which seem to require CoA as part of their essential biological catalytic sites, and which are still being explored today. The acetylation of amino sugars, and some other basic reactions of acetyl-CoA and succinyl-CoA in intermediary metabolism, have been known since the 1980s. However, the addition of acetyl or fatty acyl groups to certain proteins in order to modify and control their specific and essential properties is a more recent discovery. The first category of these modifications comprises the acetylation of the N-terminal amino acid in certain proteins, which occurs in at least half of all the known proteins that are found in higher organisms. The specific amino acids that are recipients of these acetyl groups are most commonly methionine, alanine, or serine. The purposes of this terminal acetylation process are not entirely clear and may be multiple, including modifications of function (e.g., of hormone function), of binding and site recognition, of tertiary peptide structure, and of eventual susceptibility to degradation. Another possible site of protein acetylation is the side chain of certain internal lysine residues, whose side chain ε-amino group may become acetylated in some proteins, notably the basic histone proteins of the cell nucleus, and the α-tubulin proteins of the cytoplasmic microtubules, which help to determine cell shape and motility. Its essential role in the synthesis of α-tubulin appears to be a particularly important one.

Proteins can also be modified by acylation with certain long-chain fatty acids, notably the 16-carbon saturated fatty acid, palmitic acid, and the 14-carbon saturated fatty acid, myristic acid. Although structurally very similar to each other, these two fatty acids seek entirely different protein locations for acylation and also have quite different functions. They have recently been explored with particular emphasis on viral and yeast proteins, although proteins in higher animals, in organs such as lung and brain, can also become acylated with palmityl moieties. Palmitoyl CoA is also required for the transport of residues through the Golgi apparatus during protein secretion. It is believed that these protein acylations may enable and control specific protein interactions, especially in relation to cell membranes, and proteins that are palmitoylated are generally also found to be associated with the plasma membrane. Signal transduction (e.g., of the human β_2-adrenergic receptor) is one process that appears to be controlled by palmitoylation, and other palmitoylated proteins possess some structural importance, for example in the case of the protein–lipid complex of brain myelin. Clearly, these subtle protein modifications, all of which depend on CoA and hence on pantothenic acid, have a wide-ranging significance for many biological processes, which is still being actively explored.

Pantothenic acid is essential for all mammalian species so far studied, namely humans, bovines, pigs, dogs, cats, and rodents, as well as for poultry and fish. Pantothenate deficiency signs in animals are relatively nonspecific and vary among species. Deficiency in young animals results in impaired growth, and requirement estimates based on maximum growth rates are between 8 and 15 mg per kg diet. Rats that are maintained on a diet low in pantothenate exhibit reduced growth, scaly dermatitis, alopecia, hair discoloration and loss, porphyrin-caked whiskers, sex organ disruption, congenital malformations, and adrenal necrosis. Deficient chicks are affected by abnormal feather development, locomotor and thymus involution, neurological symptoms including convulsions, and hypoglycemia. Pigs exhibit intestinal problems and abnormalities of dorsal root

ganglion cells, and several species suffer nerve demyelination. Fish exhibit fused gill lamellae, clumping of mitochondria, and kidney lesions. Signs specific for pantothenate depletion are not well characterized for humans. A syndrome that included 'burning feet' has been described in tropical prisoner-of-war camps during World War II, and it was said to respond to pantothenic acid supplements; however this was likely to have been a more complex deficiency. A competitive analog of pantothenate, ω-methyl pantothenate, interferes with the activation of pantothenic acid; it also produces burning feet symptoms, Reye-like syndrome, cardiac instability, gastrointestinal disturbance, dizziness, paraesthesia, depression, fatigue, insomnia, muscular weakness, loss of immune (antibody) function, insensitivity to adrenocorticotrophic hormone, and increased sensitivity to insulin. Large doses of pantothenate can reverse these changes. One of the earliest functional changes observed in mildly deficient rats was an increase in serum triacylglycerols and free fatty acids, presumably resulting from the impairment in β-oxidation. Paradoxically, CoA levels are relatively resistant to dietary pantothenate deficiency; however there are some inter-organ shifts in pantothenate in certain metabolic states.

As noted above, CoA is required for Golgi function, involved in protein transport. Pantothenate deficiency can therefore cause reductions in the amounts of some secreted proteins. Other metabolic responses to deficiency include a reduction in urinary 17-ketosteroids, a reduction in serum cholesterol, a reduction in drug acetylation, a general reduction in immune response, and an increase in upper respiratory tract infection.

Recently, some studies of wound healing and fibroblast growth have indicated that both pantothenic acid and ascorbic acid are involved in trace element distribution in the skin and scars of experimental animals, and that pantothenic acid can improve skin and colon wound healing in rabbits. It is not yet known whether these observations are relevant to wound healing in humans.

Requirements

In the UK, National Food Survey records suggest that during recent decades mean adult daily pantothenate intakes have been consistently in the range of 4–6 mg. Since there is little evidence for the magnitude of minimum requirements in humans, the UK committee responsible for the revision of dietary reference values in 1991 suggested that intakes in the range 3–7 mg day^{-1} can be considered as adequate (although no specific values for the reference nutrient intake, estimated average requirement or lower reference nutrient intake for pantothenate were set). The US adequate intake (AI) for pantothenic acid is currently set at 5 mg day^{-1} for adults; 4 mg day^{-1} for children aged 9–13 years; 3 mg day^{-1} for 4–8 years, and 2 mg day^{-1} for 1–3 years. There was insufficient evidence to set an estimated average requirement (EAR), a recommended daily allowance (RDA), or a tolerable upper intake level (UL).

There are few studies in communities where intakes are likely to be low; indeed, pantothenic acid is so widely distributed in human foods that it is unlikely that any natural diets with a very low content will be encountered. Some variations in status among communities have been described, but these do not define requirements. In a group of adolescents in the USA, daily pantothenate intakes were around 4 mg; total blood pantothenate was in the 'normal' range of c. 350–400 ng ml^{-1}, and intakes were correlated with red cell pantothenate ($r = 0.38$) and with urinary pantothenate ($r = 0.60$), both $P < 0.001$. In adults, these correlations were less strong.

During pregnancy and lactation there is some evidence that requirements may increase. As for most water-soluble vitamins, maternal blood levels do decrease significantly on normal diets during pregnancy, and the mean daily output of the vitamin in breast milk in the US is of the order of 2–6 mg. The adequate intake (AI) in the USA is 6 mg day^{-1} during pregnancy and 7 mg day^{-1} during lactation. It has been suggested that infant formulas should contain at least 2 mg pantothenate per liter and the AI for infants is 1.7 mg day^{-1} from birth to 6 months and 1.8 mg day^{-1} from 7 to 12 months of age.

Dietary Sources and High Intakes

Pantothenate is widely distributed in food; rich sources include animal tissues, especially liver, and yeast, with moderate amounts occurring in whole grain cereals and legumes (see **Table 1**). It is fairly stable during cooking and storage, although some destruction occurs at high temperatures and at pH values below 5 or above 7. Highly processed foods have lower contents than fresh foods. Commercial vitamin supplements containing pantothenate usually contain the calcium salt, which is crystalline and more stable than the acid.

Synthesis by gut flora in humans is suspected but not yet proven; the rarity of diet-induced deficiency has been attributed to contributions from gut flora sources.

There is some evidence that pantothenic acid supplements may be beneficial for treatment of rheumatoid arthritis and for enhancement of athletic performance, specifically in running. Pantethine, the disulfide dimer of pantetheine, may have cholesterol-

Table 1 Pantothenate content of selected foods

Food	mg per 100 g wet wt	mg per MJ
Meat, offal, and fish		
Stewed minced beef	0.36	0.41
Grilled pork chop	1.22	1.58
Calf liver, fried	4.1	5.59
Lamb's kidney, fried	4.6	5.87
Cod, grilled	0.34	0.85
Dairy products		
Cow's milk, full cream	0.58	2.12
Cheese, cheddar	0.50	0.29
Yogurt (whole milk, plain)	0.50	1.50
Boiled chicken's egg	1.3	2.12
Human milk	0.25	0.87
Fruits		
Apples, eating, flesh and skin	trace	trace
Oranges, flesh	0.37	2.34
Pears, flesh and skin	0.07	0.41
Strawberries, raw	0.34	3.01
Dried mixed fruit	0.09	0.08
Vegetables		
Potatoes, boiled, new	0.38	1.18
Carrots, boiled, young	0.18	1.94
Brussel sprouts, boiled	0.28	1.83
Cauliflower, boiled	0.42	3.59
Onions, fried	0.12	0.18
Grains, grain products, nuts		
White bread	0.40	0.43
Wholemeal bread	0.60	0.65
Rice, boiled, white	0.10	0.17
Comflakes	0.30	0.19
Baked beans in tomato sauce	0.18	0.51
Peanuts, plain	2.66	1.14

Compiled from Food Standard Agency (2002) McCance and Widdowson's *The Composition of Foods*, 6th Sixth Summary edn. Cambridge: Royal Society of Chemistry, © Crown copyright material is reproduced with the permission of the Controller of HMSO and Queen's Printer for Scotland.

lowering properties. The mechanisms of these reported effects are unclear and they require further investigation and verification. A homolog of pantothenate, pantoyl γ-aminobutyrate (hopanthenate), which can act as a pantothenate antagonist, has been used to enhance cognitive function, especially in Alzheimer's disease. It acts on GABA receptors to enhance acetylcholine release and cholinergic function at key sites in the brain.

There is little or no evidence for any toxicity at high intakes: at daily intakes around 10 g there may be mild diarrhea and gastrointestinal disturbance, but no other symptoms have been described. Pantothenate has been prescribed for various chronic disorders, but is not known to be useful in high doses.

See also: **Fatty Acids**: Metabolism.

Further Reading

Bender DA (1992) Pantothenic acid. *Nutritional Biochemistry of the Vitamins*, ch. 12, pp. 341–359. Cambridge: Cambridge University Press.

Bender DA (1999) Optimum nutrition: thiamin, biotin and pantothenate. *Proceedings of the Nutrition Society* 58: 427–433.

Institute of Medicine (2000) *Dietary Reference Intakes for Thiamin, Riboflavin, Niacin, Vitamin B6, Folate, Vitamin B12, Pantothenic Acid, Biotin and Choline*, pp. 357–373. Washington, DC: National Academy Press.

Miller JW, Rogers LM, and Rucker RB (2001) Pantothenic acid. In: Bowman BA and Russell RM (eds.) *Present Knowledge in Nutrition*, 8th edn., ch. 24. pp. 253–260. Washington, DC: ILSI Press.

Plesofsky NS (2001) Pantothenic acid. In: Rucker RB, Suttie JW, McCormick DB, and Machlin LJ (eds.) *Handbook of Vitamins*, 3rd edn., ch. 9. pp. 317–337. New York: Marcel Dekker Inc.

Plesofsky-Vig N and Brambl R (1988) Pantothenic acid and coenzyme A in cellular modification of proteins. *Annual Review of Nutrition* 8: 461–482.

Plesovsky-Vig (2000) Pantothenic acid. In: Shils ME, Olson JA, Shike M, and Ross AC (eds.) *Modern Nutrition in Health and Disease*, 9th edn., ch. 25. pp. 423–432. Baltimore: Williams & Wilkins.

Smith CM and Song WO (1996) Comparative nutrition of pantothenic acid. *Journal of Nutritional Biochemistry* 7: 312–321.

Swaiman KF (2001) Hallervorden-Spatz syndrome. *Pediatric Neurology* 25: 102–108.

Tahiliani AG and Beinlich CJ (1991) Pantothenic acid in health and disease. *Vitamins and Hormones* 46: 165–227.

van den Berg H (1997) Bioavailability of pantothenic acid. *European Journal of Clinical Nutrition* 51: S62–63.

PHOSPHORUS

J J B Anderson, University of North Carolina, Chapel Hill, NC, USA

The consumption of a diet sufficient in phosphorus, in the form of phosphate salts or organophosphate molecules, is critical for the support of human metabolic functions. Too much phosphorus, in relation to too little dietary calcium, may contribute to bone loss, and too little phosphorus along with too little dietary calcium may not adequately maintain bone mass, especially in the elderly. Therefore, under normal dietary conditions, dietary phosphorus is used for numerous functions without any concern; it is only when too much or too little phosphorus is ingested that skeletal problems may arise. Certainly, elderly subjects need to consume sufficient amounts of phosphorus, like calcium, to maintain bone mass and density, but too much phosphorus may contribute to inappropriate elevations of parathyroid hormone (PTH) and bone loss. It is not clear where most elderly subjects fall along this continuum of intake patterns. This article discusses the mechanisms by which phosphate ions impact on calcium and also on bone tissue.

Calcium–Phosphate Interrelationships

Although phosphorus in the form of phosphate ions is essential for numerous body functions, its metabolism is intricately linked to that of calcium because of the actions of calcium-regulating hormones, such as PTH and 1,25-dihydroxyvitamin D, on bone, the gut, and the kidneys. Adequate phosphorus and calcium intakes are needed not only for skeletal growth and maintenance but also for many cellular roles, such as energy production (i.e., adenosine triphosphate (ATP)). Phosphate ions are incorporated in many organic molecules, including phospholipids, creatine phosphate, nucleotides, nucleic acids, and ATP.

Dietary Sources of Phosphorus

Animal products, including meats, fish, poultry, eggs, milk, cheese, and yogurt, are especially rich in phosphorus, as phosphates, but good amounts of phosphorus can be obtained from cereal grains and many vegetables, including legumes. Because of the abundance of phosphorus in the food supply, deficiency is highly unlikely except perhaps late in life when some elderly individuals consume little food. An extremely rare deficiency disease, phosphate rickets, in infants has been reported to result from inadequate phosphorus intake.

In the United States, mean phosphorus intakes approximate 1200–1500 mg per day in adult males and 900–1200 in adult females. In addition, phosphate additives used in food processing and cola beverages are also consumed, but the quantities are not required by food labeling laws to be given on the label so that the actual additional amounts consumed can only be estimated. Phosphate additives used by the food industry may be found in baked goods, meats, cheeses, and other dairy products. A conservative estimate is that most adults in the United States consume an extra 200–350 mg of phosphorus each day from these sources and cola beverages. Therefore, the total phosphorus intakes for men and women are increased accordingly. Because the typical daily calcium intake of males is 600–800 mg and that of females is 500–650 mg, the Ca:P ratios decrease from approximately 0.5–0.6 to less than 0.5 when the additive phosphates are included. As shown later, a chronically low Ca:P dietary ratio may contribute to a modest nutritional secondary hyperparathyroidism, which is considered less important in humans than in cats. **Table 1** provides representative values of calcium and phosphorus in selected foods and the calculated Ca:P ratios. Only dairy foods (except eggs), a few fruits, and a few vegetables have Ca:P ratios that exceed 1.0.

Recommended intakes of phosphorus have been set for adults in the United States at 900 mg per day for men and 700 mg per day for women.

Intestinal Absorption of Phosphates

Because phosphate ions are readily absorbed by the small intestine (i.e., at efficiencies of 65–75% in adults and even higher in children), a prompt increase in serum inorganic phosphate (Pi) concentration follows within an hour after ingestion of a meal begins. (Calcium ions or Ca^{2+} are much more slowly absorbed.) The increased serum Pi ($HPO_4^=$) concentration then depresses the serum calcium ion concentration, which in turn stimulates the parathyroid glands to synthesize and secrete PTH. PTH acts on bone and the kidneys to correct the modest decline in Ca^{2+} and homeostatically return it to the set level. Reports suggest that an elevation of serum Pi ionic concentration directly influences PTH secretion independently of hypocalcemia. These meal-associated fluctuations in Pi and Ca^{2+} are part of normal physiological adjustments that occur typically three or more times a day.

Pi ions are thought to be absorbed primarily by transcellular mechanisms that involve cotransport with cations, especially sodium (Na^+). These rapid mechanisms account for the uptake of Pi ions in blood within 1 h after ingestion of a meal. The blood concentration of Pi is less tightly regulated than the serum calcium concentration. Wider fluctuations in serum Pi concentrations reflect both dietary intakes and cellular releases of inorganic phosphates.

Most Pi absorption by the small intestine occurs independently of the hormonal form of vitamin D. The reported role of 1,25-dihydroxyvitamin D in intestinal Pi transcellular absorption is somewhat unclear because of the normally rapid influx of Pi ions after a meal, but this hormone may enhance the late or slower uptake of Pi ions. Paracellular passive absorption of Pi ions may also occur, but the evidence for this is limited.

Phosphate Homeostatic Mechanisms

The blood concentrations of Pi ions are higher early in life and then decline gradually until late life. The normal range for adults is 2.7–4.5 mg/dl (0.87–1.45 mmol/l). The percentage distributions of the blood fractions of phosphorus compared to those

Table 1 Calcium and phosphorus composition of common foods

Food category	Phosphorus mg/serving	Calcium mg/serving	Ca:P ratio (wt:wt)
Milk, eggs, and dairy			
Cheddar cheese, 1 oz.	145	204	1.4
Mozzarella cheese-part skim, 1 oz.	131	183	1.4
Vanilla ice milk, 1 cup	161	218	1.4
Lowfat yogurt, 1 cup	353	448	1.3
Skim milk, 8 oz.	247	301	1.2
Skim milk-Lactose reduced, 8 oz.	247	302	1.2
Vanilla ice cream, 1 cup	139	169	1.2
Vanilla soft-serve ice cream, 1 cup	199	225	1.1
Egg substitute, frozen, 1/4 cup	43	44	1.1
Chocolate pudding, 5 oz.	114	128	1.1
Processed American cheese, 1 oz.	211	175	0.8
Lowfat cottage cheese, 1 cup	300	200	0.7
Processed cheese spread, 1 oz.	257	129	0.5
Instant chocolate pudding, 5 oz.	340	147	0.4
Soy milk, 8 oz.	120	10	0.1

Table 2 Approximate percentage (%) distributions of calcium and phosphate in blood

Serum fraction	Calcium	Phosphate
Ionic	50–55%	55–60%
Protein-Bound	45–50	10–13
Complexed	0.3–0.6	30–35

of calcium are given in **Table 2**. The homeostatic control of this narrow concentration range of Pi is maintained by several hormones, including PTH, 1,25(OH)$_2$ vitamin D, calcitonin, insulin, glucagon, and others, but the control is never as rigorous as that of serum calcium. In contrast to calcium balance, which is primarily regulated in the small intestine by 1,25(OH)$_2$ vitamin D, Pi balance is mainly regulated by the phosphaturic effect of PTH on the kidney, primarily the proximal convoluted tubule. In this sense, Pi regulation is less critical than that of calcium, which may result from the presence of multiple stores of this ion distributed throughout the body (i.e., bone, blood, and intracellular compartments).

A major regulator of Pi is PTH, whose role has been fairly well uncovered. PTH increases bone resorption of Pi (and calcium ions), it blocks renal tubular Pi reabsorption following glomerular filtration (whereas PTH favors calcium reabsorption), and it enhances intestinal Pi absorption (and calcium absorption) via the vitamin D hormone, 1,25(OH)$_2$ vitamin D. Other hormones have more modest effects on serum Pi concentration.

Functional Roles of Phosphates

Several major roles of Pi ions have been briefly noted (i.e., intracellular phosphate groups for cellular energetics and biochemical molecules as well as for the skeleton and teeth (structures)). Other important functions also exist. For example, in bone tissue phosphates are critical components of hydroxyapatite crystals, and they are also considered triggers for mineralization after phosphorylation of type 1 collagen in forming bone. Serum phosphates, $HPO_4^=$ and $H_2PO_4^-$, also provide buffering capacity that helps regulate blood pH and also cellular pH.

Considerable cellular regulation occurs through the phosphorylation or dephosphorylation of Pi ions under the control of phosphatase enzymes, including protein kinases. These cell regulatory roles of Pi ions coexist with regulatory functions involving calcium ions, but Pi ions are much more widely distributed within cells and cell organelles than Ca ions.

Insulin affects Pi ions by increasing their intracellular uptake, although temporarily, for the prompt phosphorylation of glucose. Insulin may also influence the use of Pi ions when insulin-like growth factor-1 acts to increase tissue growth or other functions. Because of the broad uses of Pi ions in structural components, energetics, nucleic acids, cell regulation, and buffering, there is an overall generalization that these versatile yet critical ions support life.

Phosphate in Health and Disease

Phosphate balance in adults is almost always zero, in contrast to calcium balance, which is usually negative, because of the effective action of PTH on renal tubules to block Pi reabsorption. In late life, however, intestinal phosphate absorption decreases and the serum phosphate concentration declines. These physiological decrements may contribute to disease, especially to increased bone loss and osteopenia or more severe osteoporosis. Typically, these changes in Pi balance are also accompanied by similar changes in calcium balance. Too little dietary phosphorus and too little dietary calcium may be determinants of low bone mass and density and, hence, increased bone fragility. The usual scenario invoked to explain osteoporosis in old age, however, is that too little dietary calcium in the presence of adequate dietary phosphorus stimulates PTH release and bone loss (**Figure 1**).

Three human conditions that involve abnormal Pi homeostasis need explanation.

Aging and Renal Function

The serum concentration of Pi increases with a physiological decline in renal function associated with aging (but not renal disease per se). Healthy individuals excrete approximately 67% of their absorbed phosphate via the urine and the remainder via the gut as endogenous secretions. As the glomerular filtration capacity of the kidneys declines, the serum Pi concentration increases and more Pi is retained by the body. PTH secretions increase but the typical serum PTH concentrations, although elevated, remain within the upper limits of the normal range, at least for a decade or so. Thereafter, however, serum Pi and PTH both continue to climb as renal function declines and increased rates of bone turnover lead to measurable bone loss. This situation probably affects millions in the United States each year as they enter the 50s and proceed into the 60s; many of these individuals are overweight or obese and have the metabolic syndrome, which

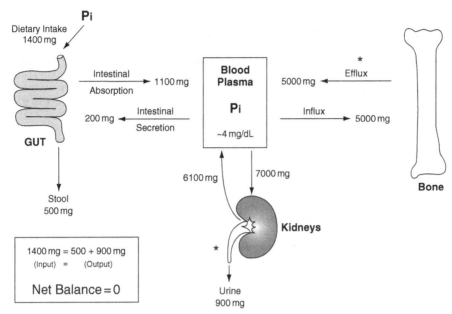

Figure 1 Phosphorus homeostasis and balance. The intestine, kidneys, and bone are organs involved in phosphate homeostasis. Fluxes of phosphate ions between blood and these organs are shown. Note the high fluxes in and out of bone each day. To convert phosphorus values from g to mmol, multiply by 32.29; from mg/dl to mmol/l, multiply by 0.3229. *Steps enhanced by parathyroid hormone. (Adapted with permission from Anderson JJB, Sell ML, Garner SC, and Calvo MS (2001) Phosphorus. In: Bowman BA and Russell R (eds.) *Present Knowledge in Nutrition*, 8th edn, p. 282. Washington, DC: International Life Sciences Institute Press.)

may negatively impact renal function. As the syndrome worsens, many of these individuals will progress to chronic renal failure and renal secondary hyperparathyroidism.

Nutritional Secondary Hyperparathyroidism

This mild condition has not been fully assessed in any longitudinal studies lasting as long as 1 year. The initiating event is a chronic low-calcium and high-phosphorus intake (low Ca:high P ratio) that leads to a chronic elevation of serum PTH. Elevations in PTH stimulate osteoclastic bone resorption and declines in bone mass and density. This condition has only been studied experimentally using human subjects for 28 days, but the chronic increases in PTH and vitamin D hormone suggest that even a lowering of the Ca:Pi ratio below 0.5—in this study to ~0.25—resulted in adverse effects. Longer term studies are needed to determine if bone losses occur under this chronic dietary regimen.

Renal Secondary Hyperparathyroidism

The true secondary hyperparathyroidism of chronic renal failure (CRF) has been extremely difficult to treat by clinicians because of high Pi and PTH concentrations in this condition. Traditional treatment includes the use of binders (chemical) to prevent Pi absorption from the small intestine. In recent years, a calcium-sensing receptor (CaR) in the parathyroid glands has been identified and drugs are being developed that will trick the CaR into thinking that serum calcium is normal rather than depressed, thereby reducing PTH secretion. A reduction in PTH then helps in the conservation of bone tissue since bone loss is such a severe problem in CRF patients.

Conclusions

The general view of dietary phosphorus, supplied in foods as phosphates, is that too much relative to calcium skews the Ca:P ratio to much less than 0.5. Another view, however, has been emerging that suggests that many elderly subjects, especially women, have very low phosphorus intakes in addition to low calcium intakes and that they may benefit from increased consumption of both calcium and phosphate from foods and supplements. In dietary trials designed to reduce fractures of elderly women and men, especially nonvertebral fractures, calcium plus vitamin D has been the treatment, but at least one trial that used calcium phosphate plus vitamin D has shown significant reduction in fractures over 18 and 36 months of follow-up. Further studies are needed to target the role of phosphate ions in reducing fractures among the elderly.

See also: **Calcium**.

Further Reading

Anderson JJB, Sell ML, Garner SC, and Calvo MS (2001) Phosphorus. In: Bowman BA and Russell R (eds.) *Present Knowledge in Nutrition*, 8th edn. Washington, DC: International Life Sciences Institute Press.

Baker SS, Cochran WJ, Flores CA *et al.* (1999) American Pediatrics Committee on Nutrition. Calcium requirements of infants, children, and adolescents. *Pediatrics* **104**: 1152–1157.

Brot C, Jorgensen N, Jensen LB, and Sorensen OH (1999) Relationships between bone mineral density, serum vitamin D metabolites and calcium:phosphorus intake in healthy perimenopausal women. *Journal of Internal Medicine* **245**: 509–516.

Calvo MS, Kumar R, and Heath HH III (1990) Persistently elevated parathyroid hormone secretion and action in young women after four weeks of ingesting high phosphorus, low calcium diets. *Journal of Clinical Endocrinology and Metabolism* **70**: 1340–1344.

Calvo MS and Park YM (1996) Changing phosphorus content of the US diet: Potential for adverse effects on bone. *Journal of Nutrition* **126**: 1168S–1180S.

Chapuy MC, Arlot ME, Duboeuf F *et al.* (1992) Vitamin D$_3$ and calcium to prevent hip fractures in elderly women. *New England Journal of Medicine* **327**: 1637–1642.

Garner SC (1996) Parathyroid hormone. In: Anderson JJB and Garner SC (eds.) *Calcium and Phosphorus in Health and Disease*, pp. 157–175. Boca Raton, FL: CRC Press.

Goulding A, Cannan R, Williams SM *et al.* (1998) Bone mineral density in girls with forearm fractures. *Journal of Bone and Mineral Research* **13**: 1143–1148.

Harnack L, Stang J, and Story M (1999) Soft drink consumption among US children and adolescents: Nutritional consequences. *Journal of the American Dietetic Association* **99**: 436–441.

Institute of Medicine, Food and Nutrition Board (1997) *Dietary Reference Intakes: Calcium, Phosphorus, Magnesium, Vitamin D and Fluoride*. Washington, DC: National Academy Press.

Khosla S, Melton LJ III, Dekutoski MB *et al.* (2003) Incidence of childhood distal forearm fractures over 30 years: A population-based study. *Journal of the American Medical Association* **290**: 1479–1485.

Ritter CS, Martin DR, Lu Y *et al.* (2002) Reversal of secondary hyperparathyroidism by phosphate restriction restores parathyroid calcium-sensing receptor expression and function. *Journal of Bone and Mineral Research* **17**: 2206–2213.

Shea B, Wells G, Cranney A *et al.* (2002) VII. Meta-analysis of calcium supplementation for the prevention of postmenopausal osteoporosis. *Endocrine Reviews* **23**: 552–559.

Slatopolsky E, Dusso A, and Brown A (1999) The role of phosphorus in the development of secondary hyperparathyroidism and parathyroid cell proliferation in chronic renal failure. *American Journal of Medical Sciences* **317**: 370–376.

Uribarri J and Calvo MS (2003) Hidden sources of phosphorus in the typical American diet: Does it matter in nephrology? *Seminars in Dialysis* **16**: 186–188.

Vinther-Paulsen N (1953) Calcium and phosphorus intake in senile osteoporosis. *Geriatrics* **9**: 76–79.

Wyshak G (2000) Teenaged girls, carbonated beverage consumption, and bone fractures. *Archives of Pediatric and Adolescent Medicine* **154**: 610–613.

Wyshak G and Frisch RE (1994) Carbonated beverages, dietary calcium, the dietary calcium/phosphate ratio, and bone fractures in girls and boys. *Journal of Adolescent Health* **15**: 210–215.

PHYTOCHEMICALS

Contents

Classification and Occurrence
Epidemiological Factors

Classification and Occurrence

A Cassidy, School of Medicine, University of East Anglia, Norwich, UK

There is a considerable body of evidence to suggest that populations that consume diets rich in fruits and vegetables, whole-grain cereals, and complex carbohydrates have a reduced risk of a range of chronic diseases. This has led to the suggestion that the diversity of substances found in food, particularly plant-derived or plant-based foods, may underlie the protective effects that are attributed to diets high in fruits and vegetables and other plant foods. Although fruits and vegetables are rich sources of micronutrients and dietary fiber, they also contain a wide variety of secondary metabolites, which provide the plant with color, flavor, and antimicrobial and insecticide properties. Many of these substances have been attributed a wide array of properties but have yet to be recognized as nutrients in the conventional sense. Many of these potentially protective plant compounds, termed phytochemicals, are receiving increasing attention. Phytochemicals, also known as phytonutrients, are plant-based compounds that exert numerous physiological functions in mammalian systems. Many of them are ubiquitous throughout the plant and as a result are present in our daily diet. Among the most important classes are the flavonoids, which are classified based on their chemical and structural characteristics. This article focuses on the different classes of phytochemicals and their relationships to human diseases.

Phytochemicals: General

Plants synthesize a wide array of compounds that play key roles in protecting plants against herbivores and microbial infection and as attractants for pollinators and seed-dispersing animals, allelopathic agents, UV protectants, and signal molecules in the formation of nitrogen-fixing root nodules in legumes. Although they have long been ignored from a nutritional perspective, the function of these compounds and their relative importance to human health are gaining significant interest.

Phytochemicals comprise a wide group of structurally diverse plant compounds, which are predominantly associated with the cell wall and widely dispersed throughout the plant kingdom. They are secondary plant metabolites, characterized by having at least one aromatic ring with one or more hydroxyl groups attached. The nature and distribution of these compounds can vary depending on the plant tissue, but they are mainly synthesized from carbohydrates via the shikimate and phenylpropanoid pathways. They range in chemical complexity from simple phenolic acids, such as caffeic acid, to complex high-molecular-weight compounds, such as the tannins, and they can be classified according to the number and arrangement of their carbon atoms. In plants, they are commonly found conjugated to sugars and organic acids and can be classified into two groups, flavonoids and nonflavonoids. The most researched group of compounds to date is the flavonoids, and this article focuses on this group.

Flavonoids

Flavonoids constitute a large class of phytochemicals that are widely distributed in the plant kingdom, are present in high concentrations in the epidermis of leaves and skin of fruits, and have important and varied roles as secondary metabolites. More than 8000 varieties of flavonoids have been identified, many of which are responsible for the colors of fruits and flower. They are found in fruits, vegetables, tea, wine, grains, roots, stems, and flowers and are thus regularly consumed by humans. Although it has been widely known for centuries that derivatives

of plant origin possess a broad spectrum of biological activities, it was first suggested that flavonoids may be important for human health in the 1930s when it was observed that a fraction from lemon juice could decrease the permeability of arteries and partially prevent symptoms in scorbutic pigs. At the time, it was suggested that these compounds should be defined as a new class of vitamins, vitamin P, and the substance responsible for the effects was identified as the flavonoid rutin. However, the data were not generally accepted and the term vitamin P was abandoned in the 1950s. There was renewed interest in flavonoids when a potentially protective role for flavonoids in relation to heart disease in humans was reported. Since that time, there has been a surge of interest in the potential role of flavonoids in human health, with research suggesting antioxidant effects, hormonal actions, antiinfectious actions, cancer-preventative effects, the ability to induce chemical defense enzymes, and actions on blood clotting and the vascular system. However, concrete evidence that they positively influence human health is lacking, and adverse effects have also been reported for some polyphenols. The main subclasses of flavonoids are flavones, flavonols, flavan-3-ols, isoflavones, flavanones, and anthocyanidins (**Figure 1** and **Table 1**).

Other flavonoid groups that are thought to be less important from a dietary perspective are the dihydroflavones, flavan-3,4-diols, coumarins, chalcones, dihydrochalcones, and aurones. The basic flavonoid skeleton can have numerous constituents; hydroxyl groups are usually present at the 4-, 5-, and 7- positions. Sugars are very common, and the majority of flavonoids exist naturally as glycosides. The presence of both sugars and hydroxyl groups increases water solubility, but other constituents, such as methyl or isopentyl groups, render flavonoids lipophilic.

Although many thousands of different flavonoids exist, they can be classified into different subclasses. The main subclasses that are important from a human health perspective are the flavones, flavonols, flavan-3-ols, isoflavones, flavanones, and anthocyanidins (**Figure 1**).

Flavonols

These are arguably the most widespread of the flavonoids because they are dispersed throughout the plant kingdom. The distribution and structural variations of flavonols are extensive and have been well documented. Extensive information on the different flavonols present in commonly consumed fruits, vegetables, and drinks is available; however, there is wide variability in the levels present in specific foods, in part due to seasonal changes and varietal

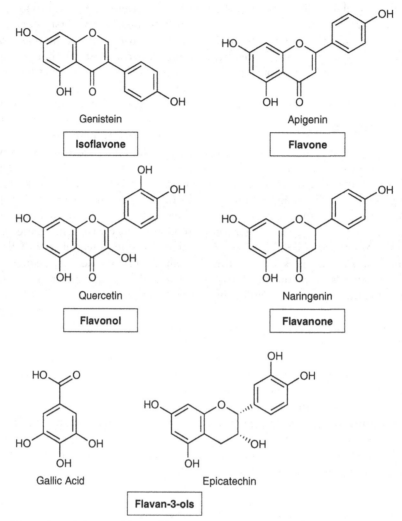

Figure 1 Structures of the major subclasses of flavonoids.

differences. The most common flavonols are kaempferol, quercetin, isorhamnetin, and myricetin.

Flavones

Flavones have a close structural relationship to the flavonols, but unlike flavonols they are not widely distributed in plants. The only significant occurrences in plants are in celery, parsley, and a few other herbs, and they predominantly occur as 7-O-glycosides (e.g., luteolin and apigenin). In addition, polymethoxylated flavones have been found in citrus fruits (e.g., nobiletin and tangeretin).

Flavan-3-ols

Flavan-3-ols, often referred to as flavanols, are the most complex class of the flavonoids because they range from simple monomers (catechin and its isomer epicatechin) to the oligomeric and polymeric proanthocyanidins, which are also known as condensed tannins. Proanthocyanidins can occur as polymers of up to 50 units, and when hydroxylated they can form gallocatechins or undergo esterification to form gallic acid. Red wine contains oligometric proanthocyanidins derived mainly from the seeds of black grapes. Green tea is also a rich source of flavan-3-ols, principally epigallocatechin, epigallocatechin gallate, and epicatechin gallate. However, during fermentation of tea leaves the levels of catechins decline and thus the main components of black tea are high-molecular-weight thearubigins, whose structures are derived from flavonoids but are unknown. The catechins are widespread, but the main sources in the diet come from tea, wine, and chocolate.

Anthocyanins

Anthocyanins are widespread in nature, predominantly in fruits and flower tissues, in which they are responsible for the red, blue, and purple colors.

Table 1 Principal dietary sources of flavonoids

Flavonoid	Compound	Food source
Flavonol	Quercetin, kempferol, myricetin	Onion, apple, broccoli, tea, olives, kale, cranberry, lettuce, beans (green, yellow)
Flavone	Luteolin, apigenin	Olives, celery
Flavan-3-ol	Catechin, epicatechin	Tea, red wine, apple
Flavanone	Naringenin, hesperidin	Citrus fruit
Anthocyanidins	Cyanidin, delphinidin, malvidin, petunidin	Grapes, cherries
Chalcones, dihydrochalcones		Heavily hopped beer, tomatoes (with skins), cider, apple juice
Isoflavone	Genistein, daidzein	Soy

Information from Hollman PC, Katan MB (1997) Absorption, metabolism and health effects of dietary flavonoids in man. Biomed Pharmacother 51(8): 305–10.
Scalbert A, Williamson G (2000) Dietary intake and bioavailability of Polyphenols. J Nutr 130 (8S Suppl): 2073S–85S.

They are also found in leaves, stems, seeds, and root tissue. In plants, they protect against excessive light by shading leaf mesophyll cells. Additionally, they play an important role in attracting pollinating insects. The most common anthocyanins are pelargonidin, cyanidin, delphinidin, peonidin, petunidin, and malvidin, which are predominantly present in plants as sugar conjugates.

Flavanones

The flavanones are the first flavonoid products of the flavonoid biosynthetic pathway. They are characterized by the presence of a chiral center at C2 and the absence of the C2–C3 bond. The flavanone structure is highly reactive, and they have been reported to undergo hydroxylation, glycosylation, and O-methylation reactions. Flavanones are present in high levels in citrus fruits, with the most common glycoside known as hesperidin (hesperetin-7-o-rutinoside), which is present in citrus peel. Interestingly, flavanone rutinosides are tasteless, whereas the flavanone neohesperidoside conjugates (e.g., neohesperidin) from bitter orange and naringenin (naringenin-7-o-neohesperidoside) from grapefruit peel have an intensely bitter taste.

Isoflavones

Isoflavones are flavonoids, but they are also called phytoestrogens because of their oestrogenic activity. Structurally, they exhibit a similarity to mammalian oestrogens and bind to oestrogen receptors α and β. Apart from basic structural similarities, the key to their estrogenic effect is the presence of the hydroxyl groups on the A and B rings. They are classified as oestrogen agonists but also as oestrogen antagonists since they compete with oestrogen for their receptor. They have also been demonstrated to exert effects that are independent of the oestrogen receptor.

Current Estimates of Intake

Diets rich in plant-derived foods can provide more than 1 g of phenolic compounds per day, although there are major international and interindividual differences in exposure. Flavonols, flavones, and flavan-3-ols constitute the three major subclasses of flavonoids, and a significant amount of information on the content of selected flavonoids from these subclasses in fruits and vegetables has been obtained using high-performance liquid chromatography techniques. The other subclasses are flavanones, anthocyanidins, and isoflavones.

Given the differences in dietary intake, particularly for fruits and vegetables, between populations, it is not surprising that the relationships between the predominant flavonoids and their sources will vary between populations, nor is it unexpected that there will be wide inter- and intraindividual variations in intake of the individual subclasses of the flavonoids. Flavonol intake was estimated to be highest in a Japanese population group (64 mg/day) and lowest in Finland (6 mg/day). International comparisons of dietary sources also reflect this variation, but only a few sources of flavonoids are responsible for most of the intake. Red wine was the main source of the flavonol quercetin in Italy, tea was the main source in Japan and The Netherlands, and onions were the most significant contributor to intake in Greece, the United States, and the former Yugoslavia (**Table 1**).

The estimated daily intake of flavonoids, including catechins and anthocyanins, is >50 mg for all the countries presented in **Table 2**, and realistically intake is probably higher than 100 mg/day if data on all flavonoid groups were available. If this intake is compare to daily intakes of other dietary antioxidants, such as vitamin C (80 mg/day), vitamin E (8.5 mg/day), and β-carotene (1.9 mg/day), it is clear that flavonoid intakes exceed or are at least comparable to those of other established

Table 2 Estimated dietary intake of flavonoid subclasses in different countries

Flavonoid subgroup	Estimated intake (mg/day)			
	Denmark	Holland	Finland	Japan
Flavonol	1.5–8.6	1–17	1.1–7	16.4
Flavone	1–2	2	No data	0.3
Flavan-3-ol	45	50	8.3	40
Flavanone	7.1–9.3	No data	8.3–28.3	No data
Isoflavone	<1	No data	No data	50
Anthocyanidins	6–60	No data	No data	No data

antioxidants, indicating that these compounds constitute an important part of dietary intake of antioxidants.

Absorption and Metabolism of Flavonoids

The flavonols and flavones are generally present in plants in the form of glycosides and as such are water-soluble. Thus, some of the flavonol glycosides may be absorbed intact in the small intestine or hydrolyzed by mucosal enzymes and absorbed as aglycones. However, those that pass through the small intestine unabsorbed or reenter the gut from the bile become available for bacterial metabolism in the colon.

The colon contains numerous microorganisms and as a result it has significant capacity for catalytic and hydrolytic reactions. These colonic bacteria produce enzymes that are capable of stripping flavonoid conjugates of their sugar moieties, enabling free aglycones to be absorbed. The enzymes produced by colonic bacteria can also break down the flavonoids into simple compounds, resulting in the production of a range of derivatives, some of which may be more biologically active than the parent compound. This is an important area for future research because the metabolism of flavonoids is influenced by intestinal microflora and these metabolic reactions may result in deactivation of bioactive compounds or activation of previously inactive compounds. It is therefore critical to identify the bacteria involved in these transformation reactions and define their relative importance and occurrence in the human gut to gain a better understanding of the transformation processes.

Other key body compartments that are important in defining the metabolism of flavonoids are the liver and, to a lesser extent, the small intestine and kidney, in which the biotransformation enzymes are located. Flavonols and flavan-3-ols are primarily metabolized in the colon and liver.

The evidence for absorption of intact flavonoid glycosides is weak. Recent data showing β-glucosidase activity in the small intestine, together with the absence of intact glycosides in plasma and urine, strongly suggest that only free flavonoid aglycones are being absorbed. In addition, data also indicate that there is a more rapid and efficient absorption of flavonoids originating from glucosides than from other glycosides or free aglycones. This suggests that dietary sources containing high levels of glucose-bound flavonoids are more likely to have potential health benefits than foods containing other flavonoid glycosides.

Bioavailability of Flavonoids

Critical to a food's 'nutritional' value is whether the 'nutrient' or compound is provided in a bioavailable form from the food. Flavonoids therefore may have to be absorbed from the large intestine if they are to exert a potential health effect. Early data from animal studies suggested that flavonoids were only absorbed to a limited degree because gut microflora preferentially destroyed the heterocyclic rings of the compounds before absorption occurred in the small intestine. However, an increasing number of studies suggest that the bioavailability of flavonoids is greater than was previously recognized, although increases in the concentrations of flavonoids and its associated metabolites in plasma and urine do not necessarily mean that they have significant effects *in vivo*. There are few data on their intracellular location and mechanism of action. Thus, a key area for future research will be to clarify the absorption, bioavailability, and metabolism of a range of flavonoid compounds.

Potential Mechanisms of Action

The effect of flavonoids on enzymatic, biological, and physiological processes has been extensively studied, but few studies have attempted to determine the actual compound or metabolite responsible for the observed effects. Much of the *in vitro* data assume that the biological activity originates from the flavonoid ingested, without taking into consideration the biotransformations that may occur following ingestion and metabolism, as it is well established that following ingestion they are transformed into a range of structurally distinct compounds.

In interpreting the mechanistic data, it is also important to remember that little attention has been paid to the physiological relevance of the concentration used in the *in vitro* model systems. Thus, in some instances biological effects have been shown at concentrations that are unachievable *in vivo*; therefore, the biological relevance of these mechanisms to humans is questionable.

Since flavonoids are complex groups of compounds with variable structures and activities, it is unlikely that they exert their biological effects by common mechanisms. However, since it is also now established that the pathophysiological processes leading to the development of cardiovascular disease and cancer are complex, this means that there are many potential sites and stages at which bioactive plant compounds present in food could act to potentially reduce the formation of cancerous cells or the atherosclerotic plaque in cardiovascular disease. Elucidating the underlying mechanisms of how flavonoids work is a key aim for nutrition research.

In vitro experimental systems suggest that flavonoids can scavenge oxygen-derived free radicals; exert antiinflammatory, antiallergic, and antiviral effects; and have anticarcinogenic properties.

Potential Health Effects

There is substantial epidemiological evidence that populations that consume diets rich in plant foods have a reduced risk of cardiovascular disease and various cancers, and the potential role of bioactive compounds in plants in this association is gaining significant attention within nutrition research. Identification of the role of flavonoids in the primary mechanisms that may protect against cellular damage may yield clues to slowing aspects of the aging process and postpone age-related diseases.

Most research on flavonoids and health has focused on quercetin due to its antioxidant potency and potential role in cardiovascular disease. However, the diverse and broad nature of flavonoids means that subclasses other than the flavonols may be more important to human health since they appear to be more bioavailable and thus have a greater potential to protect against the various mechanisms involved in aging and disease development.

Cardiovascular Health

The stimulus for much of the research on the role of flavonoids in human health was derived from epidemiological studies, particularly a study suggesting that dietary flavonoids may protect against

cardiovascular disease. During the past decade, a significant amount of research has examined the effect of flavonoids in foods and pure flavonoid compounds at various stages in the atherosclerosis process.

A significant proportion of the research on flavonoids has concentrated on their antioxidant actions, and their capacity to act as antioxidants remains their best described biological property to date. Their antioxidant ability is well established *in vitro*, and *in vivo* animal data also suggest that consumption of compounds such as rutin or red wine extracts, tea, or fruit juice lowers oxidative products such as protein carbonyls, DNA damage markers, and malonaldehyde levels in blood and a range of tissues.

The flavones and catechins appear to be the most powerful flavonoids at protecting the body against reactive oxygen species. Although the mechanisms and sequence of events by which free radicals interfere with cellular functions are not fully understood, one of the most important events may be lipid peroxidation, which results in cellular damage. Flavonoids may prevent such cellular damage by several different mechanisms, including direct scavenging of free radicals such as superoxides and peroxynitrite, inhibition of nitric oxide, or antiinflammatory effects.

Cancer

The specific mechanisms by which individual dietary components can alter the cancer process remain poorly understood. However, mechanisms underlying the carcinogenesis process are understood sufficiently so that model systems to evaluate the ability of a specific compound to inhibit or promote processes that may prevent or delay cancer development can be predicted. Phytochemcials can act at a variety of sites relevant to the development of the cancer cells. They may inhibit carcinogen activation, induce hepatic detoxification pathways, exert antioxidant effects/metal chelation properties, enhance immune response, induce apoptosis, and alter hormonal environment.

From a mechanistic perspective, evidence suggests that flavonoids have the potential to alter the cancer development process by several different mechanisms. These include inhibition of the metabolic activation of carcinogens by modifying the expression of specific phase I and II enzymes, acting as antioxidants, inhibiting protein kinase C, interfering with expression of the mutated *ras* oncogene, and influencing other redox-regulated aspects of cell proliferation.

In addition to *in vitro* data, it is also well established that certain flavonoids can protect against chemically induced and spontaneously formed tumors in animal models. However, despite the significant amount of experimental evidence indicating that specific flavonoids have potent anticarcinogenic effects, the available epidemiological data are contradictory. Some ecological, cohort, and case–control studies suggest that tea consumption lowers the risk of developing cancer, whereas other investigations have failed to find such an association. The inconclusive nature may relate to poor information on dietary intake of flavonoids.

Safety

Although flavonoids may have potential health effects, the function of many of these compounds in the plant is to discourage attack by fungal parasites, herbivores, and pathogens. As a result, it is not surprising than many are toxic and mutagenic in cell culture systems, and excessive consumption by animals or humans may cause adverse metabolic reactions. However, the concentrations used in cell culture experiments in general tend to exceed the levels that are achievable *in vivo* following dietary consumption. Results of recent studies using β-carotene supplements should reinforce the need to proceed with caution in using flavonoid supplements, where levels could easily exceed doses obtained from normal dietary intake. For the majority of the identified phytochemicals, there are limited data on the 'safe level' of intake or optimal level of intake for health benefits, and it is critical that these margins be more clearly defined in future research.

Conclusions

There is increasing evidence that flavonoids may be protective against a number of age-related disorders. Data suggest that diets high in flavonoids may not only reduce the risk of cardiovascular disease and cancer but also, by protecting against cellular damage, may slow aspects of the aging process and improve quality of life by postponing age-related diseases. There is still much to be uncovered about their bioavailability, metabolism, mode of action, and optimal doses or, indeed, the actual compounds responsible for the health effect. Research has focused on foods as well as individual components of food to help us further our knowledge. Given the limited information to date, there are no recommended dietary intakes for phytochemicals, but people should consume a wide variety of foods that incorporate the various phytochemicals to maximize disease prevention. Further research is required to define optimal doses for potential health effects and to define safe levels of intakes for many of these phytochemicals. Many of these compounds should be viewed as pharmaceutical compounds because although they occur naturally, they still require the same levels of proof of efficacy and safety in use as synthetic pharmaceutical agents.

See also: **Antioxidants**: Diet and Antioxidant Defense; Observational Studies; Intervention Studies. **Coronary Heart Disease**: Prevention. **Phytochemicals**: Epidemiological Factors. **Whole Grains**.

Further Reading

BNF (2003) Plants: Diet and health. In: Goldberg G (ed.) *The Report of the BNF Task Force*. Oxford: Blackwell. [ISBN 0-632-05962-1].

Bravo L (1998) Polyphenols: Chemistry, dietary sources, metabolism, and nutritional significance. *Nutrition Reviews* 56: 317–333.

Cassidy A, DePascual S, and Rimbach GH (2003) Molecular mechanisms by which isoflavones potentially prevent atherosclerosis. *Expert Reviews in Molecular Medicine* 5: 1–9.

Day AJ and Williamson G (2001) Biomarkers for exposure to dietary flavonoids: A review of the current evidence for identification of quercetin glycosides in plasma. *British Journal of Nutrition* 86(supplement 1): S105–S110.

Dragsted LO (2003) Antioxidant actions of polyphenols in humans. *International Journal for Vitamin and Nutrition Research* 73: 112–119.

Duthie G and Crozier A (2000) Plant-derived phenolic antioxidants. *Current Opinion in Clinical Nutrition and Metabolic Care* 3: 447–451.

Hasler CM and Blumberg JB (1999) Phytochemicals: Biochemistry and physiology. Introduction. *Journal of Nutrition* 129: 756S–757S.

Hertog MG, Kromhout D, Aravanis C *et al.* (1995) Flavonoid intake and long-term risk of coronary heart disease and cancer in the seven countries study. *Archives of Internal Medicine* 155: 381–386.

Hollman PC and Arts ICW (2000) Flavonols, flavones and flavonols—Nature, occurrence and dietary burden. *Journal of the Science of Food and Agriculture* 80: 1081–1093.

Hollman PC and Katan MB (1999) Health effects and bioavailability of dietary flavonols. *Free Radical Research* 31(supplement): S75–S80.

Nielsen SE, Freese R, Kleemola P *et al.* (2002) Flavonoids in human urine as biomarkers for intake of fruits and vegetables. *Cancer Epidemiology Biomarkers and Prevention* 11: 459–466.

Nijveldt RJ, van Nood E, Van Hoorn DE *et al.* (2001) Flavonoids: A review of probable mechanisms of action and potential applications. *American Journal of Clinical Nutrition* 74: 418–425.

Setchell KD and Cassidy A (1999) Dietary isoflavones: Biological effects and relevance to human health. *Journal of Nutrition* 129: 758S–767S.

Epidemiological Factors

H Wiseman, King's College London, London, UK

There is considerable interest in the role that dietary phytochemicals may play in the protection of human health. This article considers the epidemiological evidence for the health protective effects of phytochemicals such as flavonoids, phytoestrogens, glucosinolates, and their derivatives and allium organosulfur compounds, particularly against cancer and heart disease. Possible health benefits of the soya isoflavone phytoestrogens to brain (especially cognitive function) and bone health are also considered together with the importance of their metabolism by the gut microflora (conversion of daidzein to equol) (**Table 1**). The possible mechanisms of action of these phytochemicals and others of related interest are also considered.

Epidemiological Sources of Evidence Indicating Potential Health Benefits of Phytochemicals

Flavonoids

Flavonoids are a group of more than 4000 polyphenolic compounds found in many plant foods. This group includes the flavonols such as quercetin, flavanols (or catechins, including catechin, epicatechin, epigallocatechin, and epigallocatechin gallate), flavones such as apigenin, and flavanones and anthocyanadins.

Until recently, the extent of absorption and bioavailability of flavonoids was somewhat unclear. Studies with ileostomy patients have shown that humans can absorb significant amounts of quercetin and that glycosides can be absorbed from the small intestine. Absorption of quercetin glucosides was

52%, absorption of pure quercetin was 24%, and that of quercetin rutinoside was 17%. This shows that not only can the glycone form of quercetin be absorbed but also absorption of the glucoside was greater than that of both the aglycone and the rutinoside, showing absorption to be enhanced by conjugation with glucose.

Epidemiological evidence suggests that dietary flavonoids, such as the quercetin, kaempferol, myricetin, apigenin, and luteolin found in tea, apples, onions, and red wine (usually as glycoside derivatives of the parent aglycones), may help to protect against coronary heart disease (CHD). The main epidemiological evidence comes from the Zutphen Elderly study and the Seven Countries Study. In the Zutphen Elderly study (805 men aged 65–84 years), the mean baseline flavonoid intake was 25.9 mg daily and the major sources of intake were tea (61%), onions (13%), and apples (10%). Flavonoid intake, which was analyzed in tertiles, was significantly inversely associated with mortality from CHD, and the relative risk of CHD in the highest versus lowest tertile of flavonoid intake ($\geq$28.6 vs <18.3 mg/day) was 0.42 (95% confidence interval, 0.20–0.88).

The Zutphen Elderly study thus suggests that regular flavonoid consumption, as part of the food matrix, may reduce the risk of death from CHD in elderly men. This study also provides evidence for flavonoid-mediated protection against stroke. Dietary flavonoids (particularly quercetin) were inversely associated with stroke incidence. The relative risk of the highest versus the lowest quartile of flavonoid was 0.27 (95% confidence interval, 0.11–0.70). Black tea contributed approximately 70% to flavonoid intake and the relative risk for a daily consumption of 4.7 cups or more of tea versus less than 2.6 cups of tea was 0.31 (95% confidence interval, 0.12–0.84). This study also found that intake of catechins, whether from tea or other sources (e.g., chocolate), may reduce the risk of ischemic

Table 1 Overview of epidemiological data relating to the role of soybean products in breast cancer risk

Study	Soybean product	Findings	Estimate of relative risk
Case–control[a]	Soybean protein	↓ Risk	0.43
	Soybean:total protein	↓ Risk	0.29
Case–control	Soybean	Not significant	[b]
Prospective	Miso soup	↓ Risk	0.46
Prospective	Miso soup	↓ Risk[c]	[b]
	Tofu	↓ Risk[c]	[b]

[a]Premenopausal women only.
[b]Could not be calculated.
[c]Decreased risk was only found to be significant for the baseline period 1971–1975.
Adapted from Messina MJ, Persky V, Setchell KDR and Barnes S (1994) Soy intake and cancer risk: A review of the *in vitro* and *in vivo* data. *Nutrition and Cancer* **21**: 113–131.

Table 2 Data from the Seven Countries Study: Flavonoid (flavonol and flavone) intakes of middle-aged men in various countries in approximately 1960 and contribution of different foods to total flavonoid intake

Country	Flavonol and flavone intake (mg/day)	Quercetin intake (mg/day)	Tea (%)	Fruit and vegetables (%)	Red wine (%)
The Netherlands	33	13	64	36	0
Japan	64	31	90	10	0
United States	13	11	20	80	0
Finland	6	6	0	100	0
Croatia	49	30	0	82	18
Serbia	12	10	0	98	2
Greece	16	15	0	97	3
Italy	27	21	0	54	46

Adapted from Hertog MGL and Hollman PCH (1996) Potential health effects of the dietary flavonol quercetin. *European Journal of Clinical Nutrition* **50**: 63–71.

heart disease but not stroke. In the Rotterdam study (a large population-based study of men and women aged 55 or older), an inverse association was found between tea and flavonoid (quercetin, kaempferol, and myricetin) intakes and the incidence of myocardial infarction.

In 16 cohorts of the Seven Countries Study, the average long-term intake of flavonoids was inversely associated with mortality from CHD (**Table 2**). Surprisingly, flavonoid intake, did not appear to be an important determinant of cancer mortality in this study. This is in contrast to the anticarcinogenic effects observed in animal models and in human cancer cells *in vitro*. An inverse association between tea consumption and the incidence of some cancers has been reported in a prospective cohort study of 35 369 postmenopausal women. Inverse associations with increasing frequency of tea drinking were seen for cancers of the digestive tract and the urinary tract. The relative risk for women who reported drinking ≥2 cups (474 ml) of tea per day compared to those who never or only occasionally drank tea was 0.68 (95% confidence interval, 0.47–0.98) for digestive tract cancers and 0.4 (95% confidence interval, 0.16–0.98) for urinary tract cancers. Another epidemiological study reported a reduced risk of gastric cancer from drinking 10 cups or more daily of green tea. Tea, especially green tea, is particularly rich in catechins, such as epicatechin, epigallocatechin, and epigallocatechin gallate, in addition to flavonols such as quercetin.

The association between flavonoid intake and chronic diseases has been studied in Finland in 10 054 men and women. The incidence of cerebrovascular disease was lower at higher kaempferol, naringinin, and hesperetin intakes. Asthma incidence was lower at higher quercetin, naringinin, and hesperetin intakes. Men with high quercetin intakes had a lower

lung cancer incidence, and men with higher myricetin intakes had a lower prostate cancer risk.

Flavonol and flavone intakes have been studied in the United States in health professionals (37 886 men and 78 886 women) using a semiquantitiative food frequency questionnaire. Of the flavonols and flavones investigated, quercetin contributed 76% in men and 73% in women. The mean flavonol and flavone intake was 20–22 mg/day, and onions, tea, and apples contributed the greatest amounts of flavonols and flavones. This information should prove useful in the investigation of the role of flavonoids in disease prevention.

Phytoestrogens

Phytoestrogens are phytochemicals found in a number of edible plants. The highest levels of dietary intakes of phytoestrogens are found in countries with a low incidence of hormone-dependent cancers. The main phytoestrogens in the human diet are the isoflavonoids and the lignans. Isoflavonoids include the isoflavones genistein, daidzein, and glycitein and occur mainly (as glycosides of the parent aglycone) in soybeans (*Glycine max*), a wide range of soy products, and to a lesser extent in other legumes. The main source of plant lignans are various seeds, such as linseed (secoisolariciresinol), sesame seed (matairesinol), and various grains (matairesinol and secisolariciresinol).

The incidence of breast and prostate cancer is much higher in Western countries than in Far Eastern ones, where there is an abundance of dietary phytoestrogens. Populations in the Far East have been consuming soyabean for centuries. In contrast, Western cultures and diets have only started to adopt soy foods much more recently. Western-style soy foods are produced by modern processing techniques in large soybean-processing plants.

Traditional soy foods, made from soybeans, include both nonfermented and fermented foods. The nonfermented soy foods include soy milk and the soy milk product tofu and also whole-fat soy flour, soy nuts, whole dry beans, and fresh green soybeans. Traditional fermented soy foods include soy sauce, tempeh, natto, miso, and fermented tofu and soy milk products. Soy milk is the name given to the aqueous extract derived from whole soybeans. A cup of soy milk is thought to contain approximately 40 mg of isoflavones. In soybeans, textured vegetable protein, and tofu (soybean curd), there are high levels of the conjugated isoflavones called daidzin and genistin. In contrast, in the fermented soybean products such as miso, nearly all the isoflavones are present in their unconjugated forms called genistein and daidzein.

After ingestion, the glycones daidzin and genistin are hydrolyzed by gut bacterial glucosidases and by mammalian intestinal lactase phlorizin hydrolase to release the aglycones genistein and daidzein. These may be absorbed or further metabolized. Although most studies suggest that the bioavailabilities of genistein and daidzein are similar, some indicate greater bioavailability for genistein. Daidzein can be metabolized by the gut microflora to form the isoflavan equol (oestrogenic and more potent antioxidant than daidzein) or O-desmethylangolensin (O-DMA; nonoestrogenic), whereas genistein is metabolized to the nonoestrogenic p-ethyl phenol. In studies, only approximately 35% of subjects are able to convert daidzein to equol. Interindividual variation in the ability to metabolize daidzein to equol could thus influence the potential health protective effects of soya isoflavones. Equol is produced in greater amounts by subjects who consume diets that are low in fat and high in carbohydrate and fiber. Developmental changes in isoflavone metabolism occur, and although isoflavone absorption and the ability to convert daidzein to O-DMA develop early in infancy, equol production appears much later.

The lignan phytoestrogen precursors matairesinol and secisolariciresinol are present in foods as glycosides and are converted by gut bacteria to the two main mammalian lignans enterolactone and enterodiol, respectively, which are weakly oestrogenic. Matairesinol undergoes dehydroxylation and demethylation directly to enterolactone, whereas secisolariciresinol is converted to enterodiol, which can then be oxidized to enterolactone. After absorption, enterolactone and enterodiol are converted to their β-glucuronides and eventually excreted in urine.

In humans, omniverous subjects usually have quite low levels of isoflavonoid excretion. The Japanese (males and females) have the highest levels of isoflavonoid excretion in subjects following macrobiotic, vegan, and lactovegetarian diets. Urinary lignan excretion is higher in Finland compared to the United States and Japan. In assessing exposure to the protective effects of phytoestrogens, urinary excretion rates should be considered in combination with actual plasma levels. In some Japanese men, the plasma biologically active sulfate + free lignan fraction was similar or even higher than in Finnish men.

Urinary excretion of phytoestrogens can be used as a measure of intake and thus possible exposure and possible protection against cancer. Low urinary excretion of enterolactone in breast cancer patients was found in an epidemiological case–control study in Australia. Prospective studies from Finland and Sweden have shown low plasma concentrations of enterolactone to be associated with a high risk of breast cancer. However, the Swedish study also found a greatly increased risk of breast cancer in the highest quintile of enterolactone concentrations. A plasma enterolactone concentration of 30–80 nmol/l is therefore probably protective against breast cancer. Production of equol is associated with a decreased risk of breast cancer, and production of large amounts of equol is associated with an increased ratio of 2-hydroxyestrone to 16α-hydroxestrone in urine and this has been suggested to decrease breast cancer risk.

Japanese women and women of Japanese origin living in Hawaii but who consume a diet similar to the traditional Japanese diet (rich in soy products) have a low breast cancer incidence and mortality. Women in the Far East who have low rates of breast cancer are thought to consume approximately 30–50 times more soy products than women in the United States. A case–control study in Singapore found that premenopausal women who consumed 55 g of soy per day had a 50% reduced risk of breast cancer compared to women who infrequently consumed soy foods. A high intake of miso soup has been associated with a reduced risk of breast cancer in Japanese women. In prospective trials, a trend toward an inverse association between intake of tofu and subsequent risk of breast cancer and an inverse association between intake of miso soup and development of breast cancer have been found. However, a large prospective study in Japan did not show any effect of soy consumption on breast cancer risk, although this may be because dietary intake was studied in adult women rather than in children or adolescents. A number of studies in rodents have indicated that a protective effect of a soy isoflavone-rich diet may occur only if soya is consumed before puberty or during adolescence. Soy, if consumed throughout life, appears to protect against breast cancer, particularly if consumed before and during adolescence. Soy isoflavones may decrease breast cancer risk by influencing the menstrual cycle and endogenous sex hormone concentrations. In some but not all studies, increased concentrations of sex hormone binding globulin leading to lower free sex hormone concentrations and a longer menstrual cycle were observed.

A trend toward protective effects against prostate cancer of tofu but not miso has been shown in a large group (approximately 8000) of men of Japanese ancestry in Hawaii followed for 20 years. The latency period for prostate cancer appears to be lengthened in these men, who have a low mortality from prostate cancer. However, the incidence of *in situ* prostate cancer in autopsy studies is similar to that of men in Western countries. The consumption of soy isoflavones by these men may be responsible for this long latency period. This probably means that they die of other causes, including old age, before the prostate cancer can develop to a life-threatening stage. The three most recent studies all suggest that soy intake does protect against prostate cancer. Two studies showed that reduced risk is related to consumption of soy foods and one was a prospective study that showed that consumption of soy milk more than once a day was protective against prostate cancer.

Although soy and isoflavonoids appear not to protect against colon cancer, lignans or lignan-rich foods can protect against colon cancer development in animal models. There is also increasing evidence for cardioprotective effects, bone protective effects, and possibly cognitive benefits of phytoestrogens, and these are under investigation. A lower incidence of heart disease has been reported in populations consuming large amounts of soy products, often in combination with oily fish consumption, which also has cardioprotective benefits. Increased bone mineral density has been found in epidemiological studies in women with high dietary intakes of soy isoflavones. The incidence of dementia has been reported to be lower in Asian countries, particularly Japan, where consumption of soy isoflavones is high. Although one epidemiological study found an association between high intakes of tofu and cognitive impairment, other factors, including age and education, may explain this possible increased risk among tofu consumers.

Brassica Glucosinolates and Their Derivatives

Glucosinolates (previously known as thioglucosides) are sulfur-containing phytochemicals found in cruciferous or brassica vegetables, such as broccoli, cabbage, kale, cauliflower, and Brussels sprouts. Although approximately 100 different glucosinolates are found in the plant kingdom, only approximately 10 are found in brassica vegetables. They are also found in other plant foods. Degradation products of glucosinolates include other organosulfur compounds, such as the isothiocyanates and dithiothiols. Glucosinolate degradation products also include indoles.

Epidemiological data suggest that the relatively high content of glucosinolates and related compounds may be responsible for the observed protective effects of brassica vegetables in the majority of the 87 case–control studies and 7 cohort studies that have been carried out on the association between brassica consumption and cancer risk (**Tables 3–5**). In the case–control studies, 67% of studies showed an inverse association between consumption of brassica vegetables and risk of cancer at various sites. If individual brassica vegetables are considered, then the values for the number of studies that showed an inverse association between consumption of brassica vegetables and risk of cancer at various sites are as follows: broccoli, 56%; Brussels sprouts, 29%; cabbage, 70%; and cauliflower, 67%. The cohort studies showed inverse associations between broccoli consumption and the risk of all types of cancer taken together; between the consumption of brassicas and risk of stomach cancer and the occurrence of second primary cancers; and between the consumption of cabbage, cauliflower, and broccoli and the risk of lung cancer. Overall, it appears that a high consumption of brassica vegetables is associated with a decreased risk of cancer. The associations were most consistent for stomach, lung, rectal, and colon cancer. The epidemiological literature also provides some support for the hypothesis that high intakes of brassica vegetables can reduce risk of prostate cancer. Further epidemiological research is required to separate the cancer protective effects of brassica vegetables from those of vegetables in general.

Allium Organosulfur Compounds

There is increasing epidemiological evidence that other organosulfur compounds in addition to those derived from glucosinolates can protect against cancer. Allium species such as garlic (*Allium sativum*) and onions (*Allium cepa*) are a rich source of organosulfur compounds, such as the diallyl sulfides. There is epidemiological evidence from the Netherlands Cohort Study (120 852 men and women 55–69 years of age) for a strong inverse association between onion consumption and incidence of stomach carcinoma. However, the consumption of leeks and the use of garlic supplements were not

Table 3 Case–control studies of stomach, colon, and rectal cancer showing inverse, null, or positive associations for the consumption of different types of phytochemical-rich fruit and vegetables

Fruit or vegetable type	No. of studies								
	Stomach cancer[a]			Colon cancer[b]			Rectal cancer[c]		
	Inverse	Null	Positive	Inverse	Null	Positive	Inverse	Null	Positive
Fruit	14	3	0	5	2	1	3	0	1
Citrus fruit	11	1	0	2	1	3	4	1	0
Tomatoes	9	1	1	4	0	2	3	2	1
Vegetables	11	0	0	8	0	1	2	0	2
Raw vegetables	10	0	0	3	0	1	—	—	—
Allium vegetables	9	1	1	4	1	1	2	0	1
Cruciferous vegetables	—	—	—	8	3	1	5	0	0
Green vegetables	8	0	0	4	1	0	—	—	—
Legumes	7	0	2	1	2	2	—	—	—
Carrots	7	1	1	—	—	—	4	0	1

[a]Data summarize the results from 31 studies (both statistically significant and nonsignificant results included).
[b]Data summarize the results from 21 studies (both statistically significant and nonsignificant results included).
[c]Data summarize the results from 13 studies (both statistically significant and nonsignificant results included).
Adapted from Steinmetz KA and Potter JD (1996) Vegetables, fruit and cancer prevention: A review. *Journal of the American Dietetic Association* **96**:1027–1039.

Table 4 Case–control studies of lung, breast, and pancreatic cancer showing inverse, null, or positive associations for the consumption of different types of phytochemical-rich fruit and vegetables

Fruit or vegetable type	No. of studies								
	Lung cancer[a]			Breast cancer[b]			Pancreatic cancer[c]		
	Inverse	Null	Positive	Inverse	Null	Positive	Inverse	Null	Positive
Fruit	8	0	0	3	0	1	6	1	0
Citrus fruit	—	—	—	1	0	2	1	2	0
Tomatoes	4	0	0	—	—	—	—	—	—
Vegetables	7	0	0	—	—	—	5	1	0
Raw vegetables	—	—	—	—	—	—	2	1	0
Green vegetables	9	0	0	5	1	0	—	—	—

[a]Data summarize the results from 13 studies (both statistically significant and nonsignificant results included).
[b]Data summarize the results from 13 studies (both statistically significant and nonsignificant results included).
[c]Data summarize the results from nine studies (both statistically significant and nonsignificant results included).
Adapted from Steinmetz KA and Potter JD (1996) Vegetables, fruit and cancer prevention: A review. *Journal of the American Dietetic Association* **96**: 1027–1039.

associated with stomach carcinoma risk. The relative risk for stomach carcinoma in the highest onion consumption category (≥ 0.5 onions/day) was 0.50 (95% confidence interval, 0.26–0.95) compared to the lowest consumption category (no onions/day). However, this study did not support an inverse association between the consumption of onions and leeks and the use of garlic supplements and the incidence of male and female colon and rectal carcinoma. There is only limited epidemiological evidence concerning the beneficial influence of garlic organosulfur compounds on cardiovascular disease.

Potential Importance of Flavonoids to Human Health: Molecular Mechanisms of Action

Flavonoids possess a broad spectrum of biological actions ranging from anticarcinogenic to antiinflammatory, cardioprotective, immune-modulatory, and antiviral. The mechanisms by which flavonoids cause these effects may include induction of the activity of some important enzymes while inhibiting the activity of others. Modulation of membrane function, including the activity of membrane-bound

Table 5 Cohort and case–control studies of all types of cancer showing inverse, null, or positive associations for the consumption of different types of phytochemical-rich fruit and vegetables

Fruit or vegetable type	All types of cancer[a]		
	Inverse	Null	Positive
Fruit	29	12	5
Citrus fruit	26	8	6
Tomatoes	35	5	10
Vegetables	55	4	9
Raw vegetables	33	4	2
Allium vegetables	27	3	4
Cruciferous vegetables	38	8	8
Green vegetables	61	5	13
Legumes	14	6	16
Carrots	50	7	7

[a]Data summarize the results from 194 studies (both statistically significant and nonsignificant results included).
Adapted from Steinmetz KA and Potter JD (1996) Vegetables, fruit and cancer prevention: A review. *Journal of the American Dietetic Association* **96**: 1027–1039.

enzymes, through a protective membrane antioxidant action is likely to be of prime importance.

Membrane function is understood to be of vital importance to many cellular processes, including the role of membrane enzymes and receptors in cell growth and signalling. Membrane function may be influenced by dietary components directly by altering membrane fluidity or indirectly by protection against the free radical-mediated process of membrane lipid peroxidation. This can arise from oxidative stress and result in oxidative membrane damage. Flavonoids such as quercetin and myrecetin have been widely found to inhibit membrane lipid peroxidation. Flavonoids inhibit lipid peroxidation *in vitro* by acting as chain-breaking antioxidants: They donate a hydrogen atom to lipid radicals, thus terminating the chain reaction of lipid peroxidation. Additionally, flavonoids can act as metal chelating agents. Furthermore, kaempferol-3-O-galactoside protected mice against bromobenzene-induced hepatic lipid peroxidation. The relative potencies of flavonoids as antioxidants is governed by a set of structure–function relationships: In general, optimum antioxidant activity is associated with multiple phenolic groups, a double bond in C2–C3 of the C ring, a carbonyl group at C4 of the C ring, and free C3 (C ring) and C5 (A ring) hydroxy groups. It is of related interest that consumption of 300 ml of either black or green tea greatly increased plasma antioxidant capacity in 10 volunteers. This suggests that normal levels of tea consumption could provide sufficient flavonoids to achieve a potentially health protective effect.

There is increasing evidence for the role of free radicals in the oxidative DNA damage implicated in carcinogenesis. The ability of flavonoids to act as antioxidants may contribute to the anticancer effects observed in animal models and human cells in culture *in vitro*, which could potentially be important to human health despite the current lack of epidemiological evidence and the finding that consumption of flavonoids in onions and black tea (providing 91 mg/day of quercetin for 2 weeks) by young healthy male and female subjects had no effect on oxidative DNA base damage in leucocytes. Quercetin has been shown to have growth inhibitory effects *in vitro* on breast cancer cells, colon cancer cells, squamous cell carcinoma cell lines, acute lymphoid and myeloid leukemia cell lines, and a lymphoblastoid cell line. These effects appear to be mediated *via* binding to cellular type 2 oestrogen binding sites. Furthermore, when the ability of two citrus flavonoids, hesperetin and naringenin (found in grapefruit mainly as its glycosylated form naringin), and three noncitrus flavonoids to inhibit the proliferation and growth of a human breast cancer cell line was investigated, the concentrations required to achieve 50% inhibition ranged from 5.9 to 56 μg/ml. The effectiveness of the citrus flavonoids was enhanced by using them in combination with quercetin, which is widely distributed in other foods. Quercetin fed to rats in the diet at levels of 2% or 5% inhibited the incidence and multiplicity of chemical carcinogen-induced mammary tumors. Mammary tumorigenesis in rats was delayed in the groups given orange juice (rich in citrus flavonoids together with other phytochemicals and nutrients) or fed the naringin-supplemented diet compared with the other groups. A number of the phenolic compounds of green tea, including the catechins, have been shown to inhibit tumour formation in rats induced by N-methyl-N'-nitro-N-nitrosoguanidine and also mutation induced by aflatoxin and benz(a)pyrene.

Quercetin has been shown to inhibit the activity of two enzymes that play an important role in mammary cell growth and development, tyrosine protein kinase activity and phosphoinositide phosphorylation, and it also inhibits protein kinase C, which is vital in the regulation of cellular proliferation. Blockade of the tyrosine kinase activity of the EGR receptor leading to growth inhibition and apoptosis in pancreatic tumor cells have been reported for quercetin and luteolin. Furthermore, inhibition of tumor growth through cell cycle arrest and induction of apoptosis by quercetin are thought to be functionally related to activation of the tumor supressor protein p53. In addition, quercetin has been shown to regulate the growth of endometrial cancer cells (Ishikawa cell line) via suppression of EGF and the cell cycle protein, cyclin D1. A further mechanism for the antiproliferative action of quercetin may be via perturbation of microtubule functions such as polymerization through the binding of quercetin to tubulin, which induces conformational changes.

A number of mechanisms have been proposed for the protection by flavonoids against CHD, including antioxidant activity. Oxidative damage to low-density lipoprotein (LDL) (particularly to the apoprotein B molecule) is considered to be an important stage in the development of atherosclerosis: It is a prerequisite for macrophage uptake and cellular accumulation of cholesterol leading to the formation of the atheromal fatty streak. Flavonoids such as quercetin are effective inhibitors of in vitro oxidative modification of LDL by macrophages or copper ions. Although consumption of flavonoids in onions and black tea (providing 91 mg/day of quercetin for 2 weeks) by young healthy male and female subjects had no effect on plasma F_2-isoprostane concentrations (a biomarker of in vivo lipid peroxidation) or on resistance of LDL to copper–ion-induced oxidation, flavonoids in red wine have been reported to protect LDL against oxidative damage. The antioxidant properties of flavonoids may contribute to the reduced risk of CHD in wine drinkers, the so-called French paradox. Resveratrol, another phenolic phytochemical found in wine, has been shown to protect LDL against oxidative damage and appears to protect against cancer in animal models. Further studies on this interesting compound are clearly warranted.

Quercetin displays potent antithrombotic effects: It inhibits thrombin and ADP-induced platelet aggregation in vitro, and this may be through inhibition of phospholipase C activity rather than through inhibition of thromboxane synthesis. Flavonoid binding to platelet membranes may inhibit the interaction of activated platelets with vascular endothelium. In addition, quercetin elicits coronary vasorelaxation that is endothelium independent. The antioxidant activity of flavonoids may also prevent the damaging action of lipid peroxides generated by activated platelets on endothelial nitric oxide and prostacyclin, which both inhibit platelet aggregation and have vasodilatory activity.

The activity of flavonoids as inhibitors of the viral enzyme reverse transcriptase also suggests that they may be beneficial in the control of retroviral infections such as AIDS.

Possible adverse effects on human health should also be considered. Quercetin was reported to induce bladder cancer in rats when administered in the diet at a level of 2%. These results were not confirmed in another study, however, which used quercetin at levels reaching 10%. It should be noted that under certain in vitro conditions flavonoids and other phenols can act as prooxidants and cause DNA damage. However, phenols have complex pro- and antioxidant effects in vitro, depending on the assay system used, and it is often difficult to predict their net effect in vivo. For example, many synthetic and dietary polyphenols (including quercetin, catechin, gallic acid ester, and caffeic acid ester) can protect mammalian cells from the cytotoxicity induced by peroxides such as hydrogen peroxide. Although tea is a good source of flavonoids, phenolic compounds including tannins and also polyphenols and phenol monomers are good inhibitors of iron absorption, which could contribute to the nutritional problem of iron deficiency. In general, it is unlikely that sufficiently toxic quantities of any particular flavonoid could be consumed from the diet, which contains many diverse varieties of flavonoids in varying quantities.

Potential Importance of Phytoestrogens to Human Health: Molecular Mechanisms of Action

The probable beneficial effects of phytoestrogens against breast cancer are likely to be mediated via numerous mechanisms. However, it has not been fully established whether the protective effects of soya and cereals result from their phytoestrogen content or from some other effect.

Many studies utilising breast cells in culture such as the oestrogen-sensitive MCF-7 cell line show that phytoestrogens (genistein was used in most of studies) stimulate tumor growth at low concentrations while inhibiting growth at higher concentrations. Genistein is a potent and specific in vitro inhibitor of tyrosine kinase action in the autophosphorylation of the epidermal growth factor (EGF) receptor and is thus frequently used as a pharmacological tool. The EGF receptor is overexpressed in many cancers, particularly those with the greatest ability for metastasis, and it has therefore often been assumed that some of the anticancer effects of genistein are mediated via inhibition of tyrosine kinase activity. However, this is likely to be an oversimplification of the true in vivo situation.

Although genistein is a much better ligand for oestrogen receptor β (ERβ) than for the ERα (20-fold higher binding affinity), it can also act as an oestrogen agonist via both ERα and ERβ in some test systems. Mechanisms other than those involving oestrogen receptors are likely to be involved in the inhibition of cell proliferation by genistein because genistein inhibits both the EGF-stimulated and the 17β-oestradiol-stimulated growth of MCF-7 cells. Although studies have shown that exposure to genistein can reduce the tyrosine phosphorylation of cell proteins in whole cell lysates, studies using cultured human breast and prostate cancer cells have not confirmed that genistein has a direct effect on the autophosphorylation of the EGF receptor. Many other mechanisms of anticancer action for isoflavones and genistein in particular have been suggested, including inhibition of DNA topoisomerases, cell cycle progression, angiogenesis, tumor invasiveness, and enzymes involved in oestrogen biosynthesis. They also include effects on the expression of DNA transcription factors c-*fos* and c-*jun*, on reactive oxygen species, on oxidative membrane damage and oxidative damage *in vivo*, and on the negative growth factor, transforming growth factor-β (TGF-β).

Although cholesterol lowering is probably the best documented cardioprotective effect of soya, vascular protection is also likely to contribute and may be mediated via a number of mechanisms. Soya isoflavones are likely to contribute to the cardioprotective benefits of soya.

ERβ is the predominant ER isoform expressed in the rat, mouse, and human vascular wall. In the rat carotid injury model, following endothelial denudation of rat carotid artery, ERα is expressed at a low level, whereas the expression of ERβ increases by greater that 40-fold and treatment of ovariectomized female rats with genistein provides a similar dose-dependent vasculoprotective effect in this model to that observed with 17β-oestradiol. However, studies in ERβ knockout mice have shown that ERβ is not required for oestrogen-mediated inhibition of the response to vascular injury and suggest that either of the two known oestrogen receptors (or another unidentified one) is sufficient to protect against vascular injury.

Vascular protection could also be conferred by the ability of genistein to inhibit proliferation of vascular endothelial cells and smooth muscle cells and to increase levels of TGF-β. TGF-β helps maintain normal vessel wall structure and promotes smooth muscle cell differentiation while preventing their migration and proliferation. Genistein has been shown to increase TGF-β secretion by cells in culture, and increased TGF-β production may be a mediator of some of the cardioprotective effects of soya isoflavones.

Antioxidant action is one of the mechanisms that may contribute to the vascular protective effects of soya isoflavones. Antioxidant properties have been reported for isoflavones both *in vitro* and *in vivo*. In a randomized crossover study of young healthy male and female subjects consuming diets that were rich in soy that was high (56 mg total isoflavones/day: 35 mg genistein and 21 mg daidzein) or low in isoflavones (2 mg total isoflavones/day), each for 2 weeks, plasma F_2-isoprostane concentrations were significantly lower after the high-isoflavone dietary treatment than after the low-isoflavone dietary treatment. The lag time for copper–ion-induced LDL oxidation was significantly longer.

Increased resistance to LDL oxidation has also been reported in a 12-week single open-group dietary intervention with soy foods (60 mg total isoflavones/day) in normal postmenopausal women. A randomized crossover study in hyperlipidemic male and female subjects consuming soya-based breakfast cereals (168 mg total isoflavones/day) and control breakfast cereals, each for 3 weeks, reported decreased oxidized LDL (total conjugated diene content) following consumption of the soy-based breakfast cereal compared to the control.

Effects of soya isoflavones on arterial function, including flow-mediated endothelium-dependent vasodilation (reflecting endothelial function) and systemic arterial compliance (reflecting arterial elasticity), may contribute to vascular protection and these have been measured in a number of studies. A randomized double-blind study administering either soy protein isolate (118 mg total isoflavones/day) or cesin placebo for 3 months to healthy male and postmenopausal subjects (50–75 years of age) showed a significant improvement in peripheral pulse wave velocity (reflecting peripheral vascular resistance and one component, together with systemic arterial compliance, of vascular function) but worsened flow-mediated vasodilation in men and had no significant effect on the flow-mediated vasodilation in postmenopausal women.

Some beneficial effects following dietary intervention with soy isoflavones have been observed on bone health, and the mechanism is likely to be via an oestrogenic action, particularly because ERβ is highly expressed in bone, although this requires further investigation. Consumption by postmenopausal women (6-month parallel group design) of soy protein (40 g/day providing either 56 mg isoflavones/day or 90 mg isoflavones/day) compared to caesin and nonfat dry milk (40 g/day) produced significant increases in bone mineral content (BMC) and bone mineral density (BMD) in the lumbar spine (but not in any other parts of the body) only in the higher isoflavone (90 mg/day) group compared to the control group. In a long-term study, consumption by postmenopausal women (2-year parallel group design) of isoflavone-rich soy milk (500 ml/day providing 76 mg isoflavones/day) compared to isoflavone-poor soy milk control (providing 1 mg isoflavones/day) resulted in no decline in BMC and BMD in the treatment group compared to significant losses in the control group. The ability to produce equol was associated with a better response to the treatment.

Some beneficial effects following dietary intervention with soy isoflavones have been observed on the cognitive function aspect of brain health, and the mechanism is likely to be via an oestrogenic action, particularly because ERβ, in addition to ERα, is expressed in brain. Although other mechanisms may contribute, they remain to be elucidated. Consumption by young healthy male and female subjects (parallel group design) of a high-soy diet (100 mg isoflavones/day for 10 weeks) compared to a low-soy diet (0.5 mg isoflavones/day) resulted in improved cognitive function, including significantly improved short-term and long-term memory and mental flexibility. These improvements were found in males and females. Consumption by postmenopausal women (parallel group design, placebo controlled) of a dietary supplement (soy extract containing 60 mg isoflavones/day for 12 weeks) resulted in improved cognitive function, particularly improved long-term memory.

Phytoestrogens can cause infertility in some animals and thus concerns have been raised over their consumption by human infants. The isoflavones found in a subterranean clover species (in Western Australia) have been identified as the agents responsible for an infertility syndrome in sheep. No reproductive abnormalities have been found in peripubertal rhesus monkeys or in people living in countries where soy consumption is high. Indeed, the finding that dietary isoflavones are excreted into breast milk by soy-consuming mothers suggests that in cultures in which consumption of soy products is the norm, breast-fed infants are exposed to high levels without any adverse effects. Isoflavone exposure soon after birth at a critical developmental period through breast feeding may protect against cancer and may be more important to the observation of lower cancer rates in populations in the Far East than adult dietary exposure to isoflavones. Although some controversy exists as to whether soy-based infant formulas containing isoflavones pose a health risk, a review of studies on the use of soy milk in infants suggests that there is no real basis for concern. Toxicity from isoflavones may arise from their action as alternative substrates for the enzyme thyroid peroxidase, and people in Southeast

Asia would be protected by the dietary inclusion of iodine-rich seaweed products.

Potential Importance of Glucosinolate Derivatives and Related Compounds to Human Health: Molecular Mechanisms of Action

There may be some important health protective effects of glucosinolate derivatives and related compounds. The hydrolytic products of some glucosinolates have been shown to display anticancer properties. Glucosinolates are hydrolyzed following exposure to the endogenous plant enzyme myrosinase (also found in the gut microflora) to form isothiocyanates. Isothiocyanates are biologically active compounds with anticancer properties and are more bioavailable than glucosinolates.

A metabolite of glucobrassicin (3-indoylmethylglucosinolate), indole-3-carbinol has been shown to inhibit the growth of human tumors of the breast and ovary. Furthermore, indole-3-carbinol may modulate the oestrogen hydroxylation pathway such that a less potent form of oestradiol is produced, thus conferring protection against oestrogen-related cancers.

Consumption of Brussels sprouts (300 g/day of cooked sprouts) for 1 week has been shown to increase rectal glutathione S-transferase -α and -π isoenzyme levels. Enhanced levels of these detoxification enzymes may partly explain the epidemiological association between a high intake of glucosinolates in cruciferous vegetables and a decreased risk of colorectal cancer. It is likely that genetic polymorphisms and associated functional variations in biotransformation enzymes, particularly in glutathione S-transferases, will alter the cancer preventative effects of cruciferous vegetables.

Compounds including the isolated glucosinolate sinigrin and aqueous extracts of cooked and autolyzed Brussels sprouts (rich in glucosinolate degradation products) decreased hydrogen peroxide-induced DNA stand breaks in human lymphocytes and thus exerted a DNA-protective effect. Oral adminiatration of sinigrin has been shown to induce apoptosis and suppress aberant crypt foci in the colonic mucosa of rats treated with 1,2-dimethylhydrazine. Similar effects were observed with oral administration of freshly prepared Brussels sprout juice, rich in glucosinolate breakdown products including isothiocyanates.

Isothiocyanates can prevent the formation of chemical carcinogen-induced tumors of the liver, lung, mammary gland, stomach, and oesophagus in animal models. The anticarcinogenic effects of isothiocyanates may be mediated by a combination of mechanisms, including inhibition of carcinogen activation by cytochromes P450: This could be achieved by both direct inhibition of enzyme catalytic activity and downregulation of enzyme levels and induction of phase 2 enzymes such as glutathione transferases and NAD(P)H:quinone reductase (these detoxify any remaining DNA-attacking electrophilic metabolites generated by phase 1 enzymes). Dietary glucosinolates and their breakdown products have been tested as anticarcinogens in terms of their ability to induce the anticarcinogenic phase 2 enzyme marker quinone reductase in murine Hep a1c1c7 cells, and the relative activities observed were found to be dependent on the nature of the side chain of the parent glucosinolate.

Phenethyl isothiocyanate protects mice against nitrosoamine-induced lung tumorigenesis. It also modulates the activity of phase 1 and phase 2 xenobiotic-metabolizing enzymes, resulting in the inhibition of the oxidative activation of a number of chemical carcinogens.

The isothiocyanate sulforophane is a particularly potent inducer of detoxification enzymes. A novel isothiocyanate-enriched broccoli has been developed that has an enhanced ability to induce phase 2 detoxification enzymes in mammalian cells compared to standard commercial broccoli.

Undesirable goitrogenic effects have been identified for isothiocyanates and other hydrolytic products of glucosinolates. Furthermore, in contrast to the anticancer effects of brassica vegetables discussed previously, a number of genotoxic effects have also been demonstrated in bacterial and mammalian cells. In bacterial assays (induction of point mutations in *Salmonella* TA98 and TA100 and repairable DNA damage in *Escherichia coli* K-12), juices from eight brassica vegetables tested caused genotoxic effects in the absence of metabolic activation. The order of potency was Brussels sprouts > white cabbage > cauliflower > green cabbage > kohlrabi > broccoli > turnip > black raddish. In mammalian cells, structural chromosome aberrations were observed with some of the juices, with the most potent being Brussels sprouts and white cabbage, and genotoxic effects were accompanied by decreased cell viability. The isothiocyanate-containing fraction (and other breakdown products of glucosinolates) of these brassica juices was found to contain 70–80% of the total genotoxic activity of the juices. The flavonoid- and other phenolic-containing fraction had a much weaker effect. In related studies, the isothiocyanates, allyl isothiocyanate and phenethyl isothiocyanate, were found to be more than 1000-fold more cytotoxic in a Chinese hamster ovary cell line than their parent glucosinolates (sinigrin and

gluconasturtiin, respectively). Phenethyl isothiocyanate also induced genotoxic effects (chromosome aberrations and sister chromatid exchanges).

More data are required before an overall recommendation can be made regarding the likely beneficial or otherwise influences of glucosinolates (and their derivatives) on human health.

S-Methyl Cysteine Sulfoxide

S-methyl cysteine sulfoxide is another sulfur-containing phytochemical found in all brassica vegetables, in addition to glucosinolates. Both *S*-methyl cysteine sulfoxide and methyl methane thiosulfinate (its main metabolite) can block genotoxicity, induced by chemicals, in mice. *S*-methyl cysteine sulfoxide is thus likely to contribute to the observed ability of brassica vegetables to protect against cancer in both human and animal studies. It is of interest that a hydrolytic product of *S*-methyl cysteine sulfoxide was linked in the 1960s to the severe hemolytic anemia or kale poisoning observed in cattle in Europe in the 1930s.

Potential Importance of Other Phytochemicals to Human Health: Molecular Mechanisms of Action

Allium Organosulfur Compounds

Allium organosulfur compounds may be phytchemicals of importance to human health by acting as antioxidants, thus protecting against free radical-mediated damage to important cellular targets such as DNA and membranes implicated in cancer and neurodegenerative diseases and aging. Protection against oxidative damage to LDL and cellular membranes could also protect against cardiovascular disease. Aged garlic extract (AGE) inhibits lipid peroxidation and the oxidative modification of LDL, reduces ischemic/reperfusion injury, and enhances the activity of the cellular antioxidant enzymes superoxide dismutase, catalase, and glutathione peroxidase. AGE also inhibits the activation of the oxidant-induced transcription factor NF-κB. Investigation of the major organosulfur compounds in AGE identified highly bioavailable water-soluble organosulfur compounds with antioxidant activity, such as *S*-allylcysteine and *S*-allylmeracptocysteine.

Organosulfur compounds such as diallyl sulfide may also protect against cancer by modulation of carcinogen metabolism, and this may involve altered ratios of phase 1 and phase 2 drug-metabolizing enzymes. Various garlic preparations including aged garlic extract have been shown to inhibit the formation of nitrosamine-type carcinogens in the stomach, enhance the excretion of carcinogen metabolites, and inhibit the activation of polyarene carcinogens. Inhibitory effects of organosulfur compounds on the growth of cancer cells *in vitro*, including human breast cancer cells and melanoma cells, have been observed. Modulation of cancer cell surface antigens, associated with cancer cell invasiveness, has been observed, and in some cases cancer cell differentiation can be induced. AGE can reduce the appearance of mammary tumors in rats treated with the powerful carcinogen dimethyl benz(*a*)anthracene (DMBA), which is activated by oxidation by cytochromes P450 to form the DNA binding form of DMBA diol epoxide, resulting in DNA legions and cancer initiation. The antibacterial activity of these allium compounds may also prevent bacterial conversion of nitrate to nitrite in the stomach. This may reduce the amount of nitrite available for reacting with secondary amines to form the nitrosamines likely to be carcinogenic particularly in the stomach.

Allium organosulfur compounds appear to possess a range of potentially cardioprotective effects. In one study, 432 cardiac patients were divided into a control group (210) and a garlic-supplemented group (222), and garlic feeding was found to reduce mortality by 50% in the second year and by approximately 66% in the third year. Furthermore, the rate of reinfarction was reduced by 30 and 60% in the second and third year, respectively. It should be noted that only a small number of patients in both groups experienced the end event of death or myocardial infarction, and a much larger scale study is needed. AGE lowers cholesterol and triglycerides in laboratory animals and can reduce blood clotting tendencies. It has been suggested that garlic supplementation at a level of 10–15 g of cooked garlic daily could lower serum cholesterol by 5–8% in hypercholestrolemic individuals. However, there may be more important cardioprotective effects of garlic. In animal studies, AGE suppressed the levels of plasma thromboxane B_2 and platelet factor levels, which are important factors in platelet aggregation and thrombosis. In rats, frequent low doses (50 mg/kg) of aqueous extracts of garlic or onions (onion was less potent) produced significant antithromotic activity (lowering of thromboxane B_2) without toxic side effects.

Aqueous extracts of raw garlic also inhibited cyclooxygenase activity in rabbit platelets, again contributing to an antithrombotic effect. In addition, AGE and S-allyl cysteine and S-allyl mercaptocysteine have antiplatelet adhesion effects. Platelet adhesion to the endothelial surface is involved in atherosclerosis initiation. Furthermore, S-allyl mercaptocysteine inhibits the proliferation of rat aortal smooth muscle cells, another important

atherosclerotic process. Indeed, this antiproliferative effect on smooth muscle cells may be indicative of a possible antiangiogenic ability in relation to prevention of tumor growth and metastasis.

Saponins

Saponins are another steroidal phytochemical of interest that may, in addition to isoflavone phytoestrogens, contribute to the health protective effects of soya products. Soyabeans have a high saponin content and soyabean saponins have been shown to have a growth inhibitory effect on human carcinoma cell *in vitro*, probably by interacting with the cell membrane and increasing membrane permeability. The proposed anticarcinogenic mechanisms of saponins include normalization of carcinogen-induced cell proliferation, direct cytotoxicity, bile acid binding, and immune-modulating effects. Of particular interest is the finding that saponins actively interact with cell membrane components: They possess surface active characteristics because of the amphiphillic nature of their chemical structure. Thus, they can act to alter cell membrane permeability and cellular function. Soybean saponins have been reported to inhibit hydrogen peroxide damage to mouse fibroblast cells and thus may protect human health through antioxidant-mediated mechanisms.

Saponins from ginseng root (*Panax ginseng C.A. Mey.*) may also be important. Antioxidant effects have been reported for total ginseng saponins and its individual saponins (ginsenosides Rb1, Rb2, Rc, and Rd; others include Re and Rg1). Furthermore, ginsenosides Rb1 and Rb2 protected cultured rat myocardiocytes against superoxide radicals, and the mechanism for this may involve induction of genes responsible for antioxidant defences rather than radical scavenging. Ginsenosides stimulate endogenous production of nitric oxide in rat kidney, and this may contribute to the observed antinephritic action of these compounds and suggest a protective role in the kidney. Furthermore, it has been suggested that the observed cardioprotective effects of ginsenosides in animal models may be mediated by nitric oxide release. In addition, ginsenoside enhanced release of nitric oxide from endothelial cells, particularly from perivascular nitric oxidergic nerves in the corpus cavernosum of animal models, may partly account for the reported aphrodisiac effects of ginseng. Also, ginsenosides have been shown to have beneficial effects on inferior human sperm motility and progression. It is of interest that regulation of lipid metabolism by ginseng has been reported, and although the mechanism of action remains unclear, it is likely that the peroxisome proliferator-activated receptor-α is involved.

Other Phytochemicals of Interest

A wide range of other phytochemicals may have important beneficial effects on human health if consumed in sufficient amount to be efficacious. In many cases, their full spectrum of molecular actions remains to be elucidated. Nevertheless, the following phytochemicals and their main botanical sources are deemed worthy of mention.

The phytochemicals dihydrophthalic acid, ligustilide, butylidene, phthalide, and n-valerophenone-O-carboxylic acid have been isolated from Angelica root (*Angelica sinensis*). They are likely to contribute to the observed circulatory modulating effects of Angelica root, including increasing coronary flow, modulation of myocardial muscular contraction, and antithrombotic effects.

Phytochemicals extracted from licorice (*Glycyrrhiza glabra L.*) include glycyrrhetic acid, glycyrrhizic acid (the sweet principle of licorice), and an active saponin glycyrrhizin (a 3-O-diglucuronide of glycyrrhetic acid). In rats, dietary supplementation with 3% licorice elevated liver glutathione transferase activity, suggesting a potential detoxification and anticancer effect of these phytochemicals because glutathione transferase catalyses the formation of glutathione conjugates of toxic substances for elimination from the body. Antibacterial, antiviral, antioxidant, and antiinflammatory effects have also been reported for these compounds. Indeed, glycyrrhizin has been reported to inhibit HIV replication in cultures of peripheral blood mononuclear cells taken from HIV-seropositive patients.

Phytochemicals found in ginkgo (*G. biloba*) leaves, including ginkgolic acid, hydroginkgolic acid, ginkgol, bilobol, ginon, ginkgotoxin, ginkgolides (A–C), and a number of flavonoids common to other plants, such as kaempferol, quercetin, and rutin, are currently attracting attention for their possible effects on circulation, particularly cerebral circulation, and this may improve brain function and cognition. Indeed, ginkgo, ginseng, and a combination of the two extracts have been found to improve different aspects of cognition in healthy young volunteers. A number of studies have reported that extracts of ginkgo leaves enhanced brain circulation, increased the tolerance of the brain to hypoxia, and improved cerebral hemodynamics. It has been suggested that these effects are mediated via calcium ion flux over smooth cell membranes and via stimulation of catecholamine release. In addition, protection against free radical-mediated retinal injury has been reported; thus, other antioxidant-mediated protective effects on human health are also possible. Damage to mitochondrial DNA could play a role in neurodegenerative diseases such as Alzheimer's disease and Parkinson's disease. There is limited evidence for significant improvements in CHD patients following treatment with a daily dose equivalent to 12 mg total ginkgetin. Ginkgolide B-activated inhibition of glucocorticoid production has been reported and is likely to result from specific transcriptional suppression of the adrenal peripheral-type benzodiazepine receptor gene in rats. This suggests that ginkgolide B may be useful pharmacologically to control excess glucocorticoid formation.

See also: **Coronary Heart Disease**: Prevention. **Phytochemicals**: Epidemiological Factors.

Further Reading

Adlercreutz CHT (2002) Phyto-oestrogens and cancer. *Lancet Oncology* 3: 32–41.

Arts IC, Hollman PC, Feskens EJ, Bueno de Mesquita HB, and Kromhout D (2001) Catechin intake might explain the inverse relationship between tea consumption and ischemic heart disease: The Zutphen Elderly Study. *American Journal of Clinical Nutrition* 74: 227–232.

Beatty ER, O'Reilly JD, England TG et al. (2000) Effect of dietary quercetin on oxidative DNA damage in healthy human subjects. *British Journal of Nutrition* 84: 919–925.

File SE, Jarrett N, Fluck E et al. (2001) Eating soya improves human memory. *Psychopharmacology* 157: 430–436.

Gupta K and Panda D (2002) Perturbation of microtubule polymerization by quercetin through tubilin binding: A novel mechanism of its antiproliferative activity. *Biochemistry* 41: 13029–13038.

Kim H, Xu J, Su Y et al. (2001) Actions of the soy phytoestrogen genistein in models of human chronic: Potential involvement of transforming growth factor β. *Biochemical Society Transactions* 29: 216–222.

Knekt P, Kumpulainen J, Jarvinen R et al. (2002) Flavonoid intake and risk of chronic diseases. *American Journal of Clinical Nutrition* 76: 560–568.

Mithen R, Faulkner K, Magrath R et al. (2003) Development of isothiocyanate-enriched broccoli and its enhanced ability to induce phase 2 detoxification enzymes in mammalian cells. *Theoretical Applied Genetics* 106: 727–734.

O'Reilly JD, Mallet AI, McAnlis GT et al. (2001) Consumption of flavonoids in onions and black tea: Lack of effect on F_2-isoprostanes and autoantibodies to oxidized LDL in healthy humans. *American Journal of Clinical Nutrition* 73: 1040–1044.

Rowland IR, Wiseman H, Sanders TAB, Adlercreutz H, and Bowey EA (2000) Interindividual variation in metabolism of soy isoflavones and lignans: Influence of habitual diet on equol production by the gut microflora. *Nutrition and Cancer* 36: 27–32.

Shapiro TA, Fahey JW, Wade KL, Stephenson KK, and Talalay P (2001) Chemoprotective glucosinolates and isothiocyanates of broccoli sprouts: Metabolism and excretion in humans. *Cancer Epidemiology Biomarkers and Prevention* 10: 501–508.

Thomson M and Ali M (2003) Garlic [allium sativum]: A review of its potential use as an anticancer agent. *Current Cancer Drug Targets* 3: 67–81.

Wiseman H (2000) The therapeutic potential of phytoestrogens. *Expert Opinion in Investigational Drugs* 9: 1829–1840.

Wiseman H, Goldfarb P, Ridgway T, and Wiseman A (2000) *Biomolecular Free Radical Toxicity: Causes and Prevention.* Chichester, UK: John Wiley.

Wiseman H, O'Reilly JD, Adlercreutz H *et al.* (2000) Isoflavone phytoestrogens consumed in soy decrease F_2-isoprostane concentrations and increase resistance of low-density lipoprotein to oxidation in humans. *American Journal of Clinical Nutrition* 72: 395–400.

POTASSIUM

L J Appel, Johns Hopkins University, Baltimore, MD, USA

The major intracellular cation in the body is potassium, which is maintained at a concentration of approximately 145 mmol/l of intracellular fluid but at much lower concentrations in the plasma and interstitial fluid (3.8–5 mmol/l of extracellular fluid). The high intracellular concentration of potassium is maintained via the activity of the Na^+/K^+-ATPase pump. Because this enzyme is stimulated by insulin, alterations in the plasma concentration of insulin can affect cellular influx of potassium and thus plasma concentration of potassium. Relatively small changes in the concentration of extracellular potassium greatly affect the extracellular/intracellular potassium ratio and thereby affect nerve transmission, muscle contraction, and vascular tone.

In unprocessed foods, potassium occurs mainly in association with bicarbonate-generating precursors such as citrate and, to a lesser extent, with phosphate. In processed foods to which potassium is added and in supplements, the form of potassium is potassium chloride. In healthy people, approximately 85% of dietary potassium is absorbed. Most potassium (approximately 77–90%) is excreted in urine, whereas the remainder is excreted mainly in feces, with much smaller amounts excreted in sweat. Because most potassium that is filtered by the glomerulus of the kidney is reabsorbed (70–80%) in the proximal tubule, only a small amount of filtered potassium reaches the distal tubule. The majority of potassium in urine results from secretion of potassium into the cortical collecting duct, a secretion regulated by a number of factors including the hormone aldosterone. An elevated plasma concentration of potassium stimulates the adrenal cortex to release aldosterone, which in turn increases secretion of potassium in the cortical collecting duct.

Acid–Base Considerations

A diet rich in potassium from fruits and vegetables favorably affects acid–base metabolism because these foods are also rich in precursors of bicarbonate. Acting as a buffer, the bicarbonate-yielding organic anions found in fruits and vegetables neutralize noncarbonic acids generated from meats and other high-protein foods. In the setting of an inadequate intake of bicarbonate precursors, excess acid in the blood titrates bone buffer. As a result, bone becomes demineralized and calcium is released. Urinary calcium excretion increases. This state has been termed a 'low-grade metabolic acidosis.' Increased bone breakdown and calcium-containing kidney stones are adverse clinical consequences of excess diet-derived acids. Diets rich in potassium with its bicarbonate precursors might prevent kidney stones and bone loss. In processed foods to which potassium is added and in potassium supplements, the conjugate anion is typically chloride, which cannot act as a buffer.

Adverse Effects of Insufficient Potassium

Severe potassium deficiency, which most commonly results from diuretic-induced potassium losses, is characterized by a serum potassium concentration of less than 3.5 mmol/l. The adverse consequences of hypokalemia are cardiac arrhythmias, muscle weakness, and glucose intolerance. Moderate potassium deficiency, which commonly results from an inadequate dietary intake of potassium, occurs without hypokalemia and is characterized by increased blood pressure, increased salt sensitivity, an increased risk of kidney stones, and increased bone turnover. An inadequate intake of dietary potassium may also increase the risk of stroke and perhaps other cardiovascular diseases.

Kidney Stones and Bone Demineralization

Because of its effects on acid–base balance, an increased dietary potassium intake might have

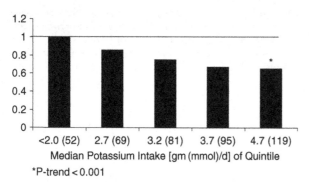

Figure 1 Relative risk of kidney stones during 12 years of follow-up by quintile of potassium intake in 91 731 women. (Data from Curhan GC, Willett WC, Speizer FE, Spiegelman D, and Stampfer MJ (1997) Comparison of dietary calcium with supplemental calcium and other nutrients as factors affecting the risk of kidney stones in women. *Annals of Internal Medicine* **126**: 497–504.)

favorable effects on kidney stone formation. In one large observational study of women (**Figure 1**), there was a progressive inverse relationship between greater intake of potassium and incident kidney stones. At a median potassium intake of 4.7 g/day (119 mmol/day), the risk of developing a kidney stone was 35% less compared to that for women with an intake of <2.0 g/day (52 mmol/day). In the one available trial, an intake of approximately 3.6–4.7 g/day (92–120 mmol/day) of potassium in the form of potassium citrate reduced the risk of recurrent kidney stones.

Epidemiologic studies have consistently documented that increased potassium intake is associated with greater bone mineral density. In trials, supplemental potassium bicarbonate reduced bone turnover as manifest by less urinary calcium excretion and by biochemical evidence of greater bone formation and reduced bone resorption. However, no trial has tested the effect of increased potassium or diets rich in potassium on bone mineral density or clinical outcomes related to osteoporosis.

Elevated Blood Pressure

High levels of potassium intake are associated with reduced blood pressure. Observational data have been reasonably consistent in documenting this inverse relationship, whereas data from individual trials have been less consistent. However, three meta-analyses of these trials have each documented a significant inverse relationship between potassium intake and blood pressure in nonhypertensive and hypertensive individuals. In one meta-analysis, average net systolic/diastolic blood pressure reductions associated with a net increase in urinary potassium excretion of 2 g/day (50 mmol/day) were 4.4/2.4 mmHg. Typically, greater

blood pressure reductions from potassium occur in African Americans compared to non-African Americans. Most of the trials that tested the effects of potassium on blood pressure used pill supplements, typically potassium chloride.

A high potassium intake has been shown to blunt the rise in blood pressure in response to increased salt intake. The term 'salt-sensitive blood pressure' applies to those individuals or subgroups who experience the greatest reduction in blood pressure when salt intake is reduced. One metabolic study of 38 healthy, nonhypertensive men (24 African Americans and 14 non-African Americans) investigated the effect of potassium supplementation on the pressor effect of salt loading (5.7 g/day of sodium (250 mmol)). Before potassium was supplemented, 79% of the African American men and 26% of the non-African American men were termed 'salt sensitive,' as defined by a salt-induced increase in mean arterial pressure of at least 3 mmHg. There was a progressive reduction in the frequency of salt sensitivity as the dose of potassium was increased. In the African Americans with severe salt sensitivity, increasing dietary potassium to 4.7 g/day (120 mmol/day) reduced the frequency of salt sensitivity to 20%, the same percentage as that observed in non-African American subjects when their potassium intake was increased to only 2.7 g/day (70 mmol/day).

Other studies indicate that potassium has greater blood pressure lowering in the context of a higher salt intake and lesser blood pressure reduction in the setting of a lower salt intake. Conversely, the blood pressure reduction from a reduced salt intake is greatest when potassium intake is low. These data are consistent with subadditive effects of reduced salt intake and increased potassium intake on blood pressure.

Cardiovascular Disease

The beneficial effects of potassium on blood pressure should reduce the occurrence of blood pressure-related cardiovascular disease. Potassium may also have protective effects that are independent of blood pressure reduction. This possibility has been tested in experimental studies conducted in rodents. In a series of animal models, the addition of either potassium chloride or potassium citrate markedly reduced mortality from stroke. Interestingly, these reductions occurred when blood pressure was held constant. Such data indicate that potassium has both blood pressure-dependent and blood pressure-independent properties that are cardioprotective.

In many, but not all, epidemiologic studies, an inverse relationship between dietary potassium intake and subsequent stroke-associated morbidity

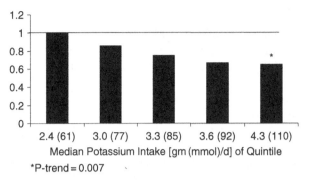

*P-trend = 0.007

Figure 2 Relative risk of ischemic stroke by quintile of potassium intake in 43 738 men. (Data, from Ascherio A, Rimm EB, Hernan MA *et al.* (1998) Intake of potassium, magnesium, calcium, and fiber and risk of stroke among U.S. men. *Circulation* **98**: 1198–1204.)

and mortality has been noted. A few observational studies have also shown an inverse association between potassium intake and coronary heart disease. In a 12-year follow-up of 859 men and women enrolled in the Rancho Bernardo Study, a significant inverse relationship between potassium intake and subsequent risk of stroke-related mortality was documented. Similarly, during the course of 8 years of follow-up in 43 738 US men in the Health Professionals Follow-Up Study, there was a significant inverse relationship between baseline potassium intake and stroke after adjustment for established cardiovascular disease risk factors, including blood pressure and caloric intake (**Figure 2**). In this study, a median potassium intake of 4.3 g/day (110 mmol/day) was associated with a 41% reduced risk of stroke in comparison to those with a median intake of 2.4 g/day (61 mmol/day). Consistent with these studies are other observational studies that have repeatedly documented a reduced risk of stroke from an increased intake of fruits and vegetables.

Adverse Effects of Excess Potassium Intake

In the generally healthy population with normal kidney function, a high potassium intake from foods poses no risk because excess potassium is readily excreted in the urine. In contrast, supplemental potassium can lead to acute toxicity in healthy individuals. Also, in individuals whose urinary potassium excretion is impaire a potassium intake less than 4.7 g/day (120 mmol/day) is appropriate because of adverse cardiac effects (arrhythmias) from hyperkalemia. Drugs that commonly impair potassium excretion are angiotensin converting enzyme inhibitors, angiotensin receptor blockers, and potassium-sparing diuretics. Common medical conditions associated with impaired potassium excretion are diabetes, chronic renal insufficiency, end stage renal disease, severe heart failure, and adrenal insufficiency. Elderly individuals are at increased risk of hyperkalemia because they often have one or more of these conditions or take one or more of the medications that impair potassium excretion.

Recommended Potassium Intake, Current Intake, and Dietary Sources

On the basis of available data, an Institute of Medicine committee set an Adequate Intake for potassium at 4.7 g/day (120 mmol/day) for adults. This level of dietary intake should maintain lower blood pressure levels, reduce the adverse effects of salt on blood pressure, reduce the risk of kidney stones, and possibly decrease bone loss. Current dietary intake of potassium is considerably lower than this level.

Humans evolved on a diet that was rich in potassium and bicarbonate precursors and low in salt. However, contemporary Western-style diets have the opposite pattern—that is, relatively low content of potassium and high content of salt. Based on intake data from the Third National Health and Nutrition Examination Survey (NHANES-III,1988–1994), the percentage of men and women who consumed equal to or more than 4.7 g/day (120 mmol/day) was less than 10 and 1%, respectively. Median intake of potassium in the United States ranged from 2.8 to 3.3 g/day (72 to 84 mmol/day) for adult men and 2.2 to 2.4 g/day (56 to 61 mmol/day) for adult women. The median potassium intake of non-African Americans exceeded that of African Americans. Because African Americans have a relatively low intake of potassium and a high prevalence of elevated blood pressure and salt sensitivity, this subgroup would especially benefit from an increased potassium intake.

Dietary intake surveys typically do not include estimates from salt substitutes and supplements. However, less than 10% of those surveyed in NHANES-III reported using salt substitutes or a reduced-sodium salt. Because a high dietary intake of potassium can be achieved through diet rather than pills and because potassium derived from foods also comes with bicarbonate precursors, as well as a variety of other nutrients, the preferred strategy to achieve the recommended potassium intake is to consume foods rather than supplements.

Dietary sources of potassium, as well as bicarbonate precursors, are fresh fruits, fruit juices, dried fruits,

Table 1 Foods rich in potassium

Food	Portion size	Potassium content, g (meq)
Beans		
Cooked dried beans	1/2 cup	0.4 (10.7)
Lima beans	5/8 cup	0.4 (10.8)
Fruit		
Apple	1 medium	0.1 (2.8)
Apricots	3 medium	0.3 (7.2)
Banana	6 in.	0.4 (9.5)
Cantaloupe	1/4 medium	0.3 (6.4)
Dates	10 pitted	0.6 (16.6)
Orange	1 small	0.3 (7.7)
Peach	1 medium	0.2 (5.2)
Prunes, dried	10 medium	0.7 (17.8)
Raisins	1 tablespoon	0.1 (2.0)
Watermelon	1 slice	0.6 (15.4)
Fruit juices		
Grapefruit	1 cup	0.4 (10.4)
Orange	1 cup	0.5 (12.4)
Pineapple	1 cup	0.4 (9.2)
Tomato	1 cup	0.5 (13.7)
Vegetables		
Corn	1 ear	0.2 (5.0)
Potato		
– White	1 boiled	0.3 (7.3)
– Sweet	1 boiled	0.3 (7.7)
Tomato	1 medium	0.4 (9.4)
Squash, winter	1/2 cup boiled	0.5 (11.9)
Meats		
Hamburger	1 patty	0.4 (9.8)
Rib roast	2 slices	0.4 (11.2)
Fish (e.g., haddock)	1 medium fillet	0.3 (8.0)
Milk		
Skim milk	8 oz.	0.3 (8.5)
Whole milk	8 oz.	0.4 (9.0)

and vegetables. Although meat, milk, and cereal products contain potassium, their content of bicarbonate precursors does not sufficiently balance the amount of acid-forming precursors, such as sulfur amino acids, found in higher protein foods. The typical content of potassium-rich foods is displayed in **Table 1**. Salt substitutes currently available in the marketplace range from 0.4 to 2.8 g/teaspoon (11–72 mmol/teaspoon) of potassium, all as potassium chloride.

Conclusion

Potassium is an essential nutrient that is required for normal cellular function. Although humans evolved on diets rich in potassium, contemporary diets are quite low in potassium. An increased intake of potassium from foods should prevent many of the adverse effects of inadequate potassium intake, which are higher blood pressure levels, greater salt sensitivity, increased risk of kidney stones, and possibly increased bone loss. An inadequate potassium level may also increase the risk of stroke. In view of the high prevalence of elevated blood pressure, stroke, and conditions related to bone demineralization (i.e., osteoporosis and kidney stones) in the general population, individuals should strive to increase their consumption of potassium-rich foods, particularly fruits and vegetables.

Further Reading

Ascherio A, Rimm EB, Hernan MA *et al.* (1998) Intake of potassium, magnesium, calcium, and fiber and risk of stroke among U.S. men. *Circulation* 98: 1198–1204.

Bazzano LA, Serdula MK, and Liu S (2003) Dietary intake of fruits and vegetables and risk of cardiovascular disease. *Current Atherosclerosis Reports* 5: 492–499.

Curhan GC, Willett WC, Speizer FE, Spiegelman D, and Stampfer MJ (1997) Comparison of dietary calcium with supplemental calcium and other nutrients as factors affecting the risk of kidney stones in women. *Annals of Internal Medicine* 126: 497–504.

He FJ and MacGregor GA (2001) Beneficial effects of potassium. *British Medical Journal* 323: 497–501.

Institute of Medicine (2004) *Dietary Reference Intakes for Water, Potassium, Sodium, Chloride and Sulfate.* Washington, DC: National Academy of Sciences.

Lemann J, Bushinsky D, and Hamm LL (2003) Bone buffering of acid and base in humans. *American Journal of Physiology* 285: F811–F832.

Morris RC Jr, Sebastian A, Forman A, Tanaka M, and Schmidlin O (1999) Normotensive salt-sensitivity: Effects of race and dietary potassium. *Hypertension* 33: 18–23.

Whelton PK, He J, Cutler JA *et al.* (1997) Effects of oral potassium on blood pressure. Meta-analysis of randomized controlled clinical trials. *Journal of the American Medical Association* 277: 1624–1632.

RIBOFLAVIN

C J Bates, MRC Human Nutrition Research, Cambridge, UK

Absorption, Transport, and Storage

Riboflavin (vitamin B_2) is not synthesized by higher animals. Therefore, it is an absolute dietary requirement for the synthesis of certain essential coenzymes that are needed for intermediary metabolism in nearly all living cells. Riboflavin must be transported from the food sources within the gastrointestinal tract, across the gut wall into the circulatory system, and thence into the cells of each organ. This transport process occurs against a concentration gradient, in order to ensure the efficient retrieval of the very small amounts that occur in many foods, and from the low concentrations in plasma to higher concentrations inside living cells.

Gut riboflavin transport systems have been studied by partly isolated segments of the small intestine within an anesthetized animal; by an isolated everted gut segment, or by 'vesicles', prepared from the 'brush border.'

Studies with these model systems have shown that the transport of riboflavin at low (e.g., micromolar) concentrations is temperature- and energy-dependent (it is inhibited by inhibitors of ATP production from energy substrates), it becomes saturated as the concentration of riboflavin increases, and it is sodium ion dependent. These characteristics are shared with many other types of small molecules that are actively transported across the gut wall. More specifically for riboflavin, the active transport mechanism involves phosphorylation (to riboflavin phosphate, also known as flavin mononucleotide, or FMN) followed by dephosphorylation, both occurring within the intestinal cells (**Figure 1**). This latter process is not shared by several other B vitamins, but it is one of a number of common strategies which the gut may use to entrap essential nutrients, and then relocate them, in a controlled manner and direction. A similar strategy is employed at other sites in the body, to ensure entrapment of circulating riboflavin by cells whose nascent flavin-dependent enzymes need a supply of the vitamin from beyond their borders.

Although the active transport of riboflavin across the gut wall and across other cell membrane barriers within the animal is a saturable process, if large pharmacological amounts are present then the slower and less efficient but nonsaturable process of passive absorption predominates and contributes significantly to the total mass transfer. The active transport process is increased in riboflavin deficiency and decreased if the riboflavin content of the tissues is high. The transport pathway involves calcium and calmodulin but not sodium. Specific riboflavin receptors have recently been identified, as has a role for microtubules in transport.

Although some of the available riboflavin in natural foods may be present as the free vitamin, ready for intestinal transport, a larger fraction is present in the form of phosphorylated coenzymes: FMN and flavin adenine dinucleotide (FAD), and there may also be very small amounts of a glucoside of the vitamin. These forms are all efficiently converted to free vitamin by enzymes secreted into the gut lumen, and they are therefore highly available for absorption. There are also small amounts of covalently bound forms of riboflavin, present in enzymes such as succinate dehydrogenase (succinate: ubiquinone oxidoreductase EC 1.3.5.1), which cannot be released by the hydrolytic enzymes in the gut and are therefore unavailable for absorption. Also unavailable (or very poorly available) in man is the riboflavin synthesized by the gut flora of the large bowel. Certain animal species such as rodents can utilize this riboflavin source by coprophagy.

A wide variety of artificial analogs of riboflavin have been prepared in order to explore the structural versus functional essentials of the molecule. Some of these analogs have riboflavin-like activity; others are inactive, while a number are antagonists, and can cause functional deficiency. These structural changes

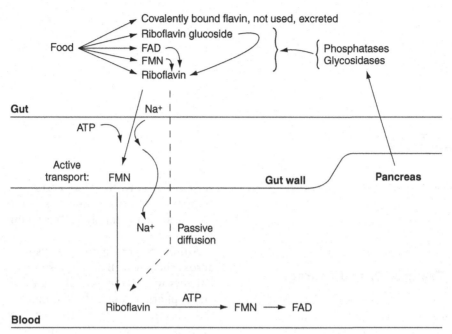

Figure 1 Characteristics of the absorption process for riboflavin and its coenzymes.

can affect absorption or the conversion of riboflavin to its coenzyme forms within the body. Certain drugs that are used for purposes unrelated to riboflavin function, such as the phenothiazines used as antipsychotic drugs, may have sufficient structural similarity to riboflavin to act as antagonists in some situations.

Absorption by Human Subjects

Studies of riboflavin absorption by human subjects require a combination of a test dose, usually taken by mouth, and a sampling procedure to estimate the amount absorbed, and possibly also its subsequent fate. The sampling compartment is generally the urine, since plasma has proved generally unsatisfactory. Fecal sampling is also useless because of the synthesis of riboflavin by bacteria in the large bowel. Although the use of riboflavin labeled with radioactive or stable isotopes is theoretically possible, this has not yet been applied to human studies. The majority of reported studies have relied on relatively large 'bolus' oral doses of riboflavin, comprising at least several milligrams, with urinary monitoring over the subsequent few hours. Riboflavin can be quantitated in urine by its very characteristic fluorescence, or by microbiological assay, or more accurately by high performance liquid chromatography.

For the maximum absorption of a test dose of riboflavin, the duration of exposure within the upper ileum is critical, since this is the region of greatest absorptive efficiency. There is little evidence to suggest that slow-release forms of the vitamin can enhance its absorption, but there does appear to be some absorptive advantage for certain synthetic lipophilic esters, such as the tetrabutyrate ester, which is hydrolyzed to the free vitamin during or after absorption. These have been shown to possess beneficial (e.g., antioxidant) properties in some model systems, but their usefulness in human medicine is still at a very early stage of assessment. The concomitant presence of food can enhance absorption, possibly by increasing the transit time. There is little evidence that the efficiency of absorption varies markedly with age or sex in humans.

Measurements of the plasma pool of riboflavin following test doses is not a viable method of measuring absorption, because redistribution to other tissue sites plus urinary excretion takes place too rapidly for this pool to be representative of the amount absorbed. Although the urinary response to a test dose has been the most commonly used approach to studies of intestinal absorption in humans, it suffers from the potential disadvantage that physiological intakes, and especially low intakes of riboflavin from 'poor' food sources, cannot be measured by this technique. Such studies of small doses are however needed, in order to determine the factors that modulate riboflavin absorption in developing countries, where dietary sources of riboflavin are minimal and clinical signs of riboflavin deficiency are common. A much more sensitive biochemical marker of riboflavin status at low intakes is the index known as 'erythrocyte glutathione reductase activation coefficient' (EGRAC), which will be discussed in greater detail below. It is possible to achieve a graded response to graded intakes of riboflavin, and studies of absorption efficiency using this alternative marker as the outcome measure may become feasible (and useful) in the future.

Riboflavin Transport at other Sites and Storage

As mentioned earlier, nearly all tissues require riboflavin. The free vitamin is trapped as one of its phosphorylated coenzyme forms, which then become specifically associated (and in a few cases covalently linked) to the protein chains of catalytic flavoenzymes. If not already covalently linked, the flavin coenzyme can often be liberated by extremes of pH or by other nonphysiological maneuvers. In a few biological locations, such as the mature red cell, flavoenzymes such as glutathione reductase (NADPH: oxidized glutathione oxidoreductase EC 1.6.4.2) may exist partly in their apoenzyme form, i.e., without the flavin coenzyme and therefore without enzyme activity. An increased supply of riboflavin will permit the depleted coenzyme (in this case FAD) to be synthesized so that enzyme activity can be restored.

Different enzymes and different tissue sites differ in the tenacity with which they can retain flavin coenzymes in times of riboflavin deficiency, so there is a characteristic 'pecking order' for flavoenzyme protection, which appears to reflect the metabolic importance of the different metabolic pathways affected. Apart from this 'pecking order,' however, there is no repository of unused or nonfunctional riboflavin that can act as a 'store' in times of dietary deficiency. Although some organs (such as liver) have relatively high concentrations of flavin enzymes, all of the flavin seems to be present as coenzyme moieties of flavin holoenzymes. Each tissue has a characteristic 'ceiling' level of riboflavin at saturation, and a 'floor' level characteristic of severe depletion, and these are determined, respectively, by the total amount of apoflavoprotein, and the amount of 'resistant' holoenzyme, which cannot be depleted of its cofactor during riboflavin deficiency.

Riboflavin is secreted into milk, the concentration being species specific and to a moderate extent dependent on maternal status and intake. Riboflavin is also required by the developing fetus during pregnancy, which implies a need for active transport from the maternal to the fetal circulation; the flavin concentration being greater on the fetal side. Studies from India have identified a riboflavin carrier protein (RCP) present in bird (e.g., chicken) eggs, which is considered to be specific for riboflavin, and is essential for normal embryological development. If this protein is rendered ineffective (e.g., by immunoneutralization) by treatment of the bird with a specific antibody, then embryonic development ceases and the embryo dies. A genetic mutant lacking RCP is likewise infertile. A homologous protein, which can be rendered ineffective by the antibody to pure chicken riboflavin carrier protein, has been shown to occur in several mammalian species, including two species of monkeys, and also in humans. Very recent studies have suggested that circulating RCP levels and the immunohistochemical staining of RCP in biopsy specimens may provide new markers for breast cancer diagnosis and prognosis. Termination of pregnancy has been demonstrated by immunoneutralization of RCP in monkeys. There remains some controversy over the roles of RCP, however, and other, less specific riboflavin binders in blood, including gamma-globulins, also seem to play an important role. These studies have provided an intriguing example of the role of specific vitamin-transporting mechanisms, designed to ensure that the vitamin needs of the developing embryo will be efficiently met. Further evidence of the special needs of developing embryos has been provided by the demonstration that riboflavin analogs can cause teratogenic changes, even in the absence of any detectable damage to maternal tissues.

Metabolism and Excretion

The interconversions of riboflavin with its coenzyme derivatives are depicted in **Figure 2**. Clearly, the 'high-energy nucleotide' ATP is a cosubstrate and driving force (in energy terms) for both stages of the conversion to FAD. Some flavoenzymes specifically require FAD while others specifically require FMN; it is difficult to account for this dichotomy. **Table 1** lists the broad categories of flavoenzymes found in living tissues: the range of reaction types is considerable, but all of them clearly center around redox processes involving hydrogen transfer. This fact reflects the central biochemical reaction of the flavin coenzymes, which is the interconversion of the reduced, dihydro form of the flavin ring and the more stable oxidized form. One of the most important sites of action of flavoenzymes within higher animals is that of the electron transport chain in the mitochondria. The flavins, which form part of succinic dehydrogenase and NADH dehydrogenase, form an essential redox link between the oxidizable energy-rich substrates of aerobic metabolism, and the cytochrome chain leading to molecular

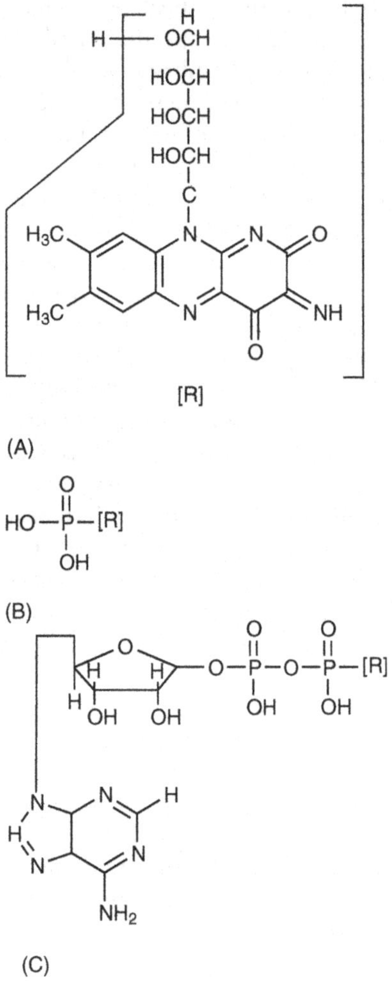

Figure 2 Structure of riboflavin and its coenzyme derivatives. (A) Riboflavin; (B) riboflavin phosphate (flavin mononucleotide, FMN); (C) flavin adenine dinucleotide (FAD).

oxygen, which can generate around 38 moles of energy-rich ATP per mole of glucose oxidized.

Hormone status can affect riboflavin economy in a number of important ways, and there is also some evidence that riboflavin status can affect hormone production. One important control valve for riboflavin economy is thyroid hormone status: hypothyroidism leads to reduced tissue levels of flavin coenzymes, and hence to inactivation of certain flavoenzymes, thus resembling the effects of dietary riboflavin deficiency. Both flavokinase (ATP: riboflavin 5′-phosphotransferase EC 2.7.1.26) and FAD pyrophosphorylase (ATP: FMN adenyltransferase EC 2.7.7.2) are sensitive to thyroid hormone status. In the kidney, synthesis of flavokinase and hence of flavin coenzymes is controlled by aldosterone in a similar manner.

The amount of absorbed riboflavin that can remain within the body and the circulation (in blood plasma) is strictly regulated by glomerular and tubular filtration and tubular reabsorption in the kidneys. The latter is an active, saturable, sodium-dependent transport process, with characteristics similar to those of active transport in the gastrointestinal tract. It is responsible for the very sharp and characteristic transition between minimal urinary excretion of riboflavin at low intakes, and a much higher level of excretion, proportional to intake, at higher intakes. This transition point has been extensively used to define and to measure riboflavin status and requirements (see below), and to permit studies of intestinal absorption *in vivo* (see above). Excretion of riboflavin is affected by some chemicals (such as boric acid, which complexes with it), and by certain diseases and hormone imbalances.

In addition to the excretion of unchanged riboflavin, there are also small amounts of hydroxylated breakdown products of the vitamin, which arise through normal turnover, either within the tissues of the body, or in the gastrointestinal tract from bacterial action, before absorption. The rate of destruction of riboflavin by this turnover pathway is very low in all species examined to date, and

Table 1 Categories of flavoenzymes

Category (subcategory)	Example
1-Electron transferases	Mitochondrial electron-transfer flavoprotein
Dehydrogenases	
Pyridine nucleotide dehydrogenases or reductases	Mitochondrial NADH dehydrogenase
Nonpyridine nucleotide dehydrogenases	Mitochondrial succinate dehydrogenase
Pyridine nucleotide-disulfide oxidoreductases	Glutathione reductase
Dehydrogenase-oxygen reductases	
Flavoprotein oxidases $[O_2 \rightarrow H_2O_2]$	Monoamine oxidase
Flavoprotein monooxygenases (1/2 $O_2 \rightarrow H_2O$)	
Internal (α-hydroxy fatty acid $\rightarrow$ fatty acid (n-1) + CO_2)	Bacterial lactate monooxygenase
External (RH $\rightarrow$ ROH)	Microsomal FAD-containing monooxygenase

Source: Merrill AH, Lambeth JD, Edmondson DE, and McCormick DB (1981) Formation and mode of action of flavoproteins. *Annual Review of Nutrition* **1**: 281–317.

riboflavin within the mammalian body seems to be remarkably efficiently conserved, apparently throughout many cycles of cell turnover.

Metabolic Function and Essentiality

This section will deal in detail with the question: what goes wrong when deficiency of riboflavin is encountered, and how does riboflavin interact with other nutrients, or with biochemical and physiological processes, thus producing characteristic functional effects?

Fatty Acid Oxidation

The first example of serious metabolic disturbance seen in moderate riboflavin deficiency is a disturbance of fatty acid oxidation. The normal first stage in the spiral process of beta-oxidation of fatty acids within the mitochondria is the removal of two hydrogen atoms from the two carbons located alpha- and beta- to the activated carboxyl end of the chain. The fatty acyl coenzyme A substrate is acted upon by one of several fatty acyl CoA dehydrogenase flavoprotein enzymes (e.g., long-chain acyl-CoA:(acceptor) 2,3-oxido-reductase EC 1.3.99.13), each of which is specific for a small range of acyl chains. The second stage in this process involves transfer of the electrons via another flavoenzyme, known as electron transferring flavoprotein dehydrogenase (electron transferring flavoprotein: ubiquinone oxidoreductase EC 1.5.5.1) and thence to the cytochrome chain and to oxygen. These flavoenzymes, unlike the flavoenzymes that are linked to carbohydrate oxidation, are highly sensitive to dietary riboflavin depletion. Characteristic disturbances of lipid metabolism can therefore be detected in riboflavin-deficient tissues and organisms.

Disturbances in fatty acid oxidation by isolated mitochondria, e.g., from livers of deficient animals, have been demonstrated, and one of the most characteristic metabolic changes, observed even in a mild deficiency state in experimental animals, is the appearance of abnormal dicarboxylic acids, and their derivatives, in the urine. These products seem to arise because fatty acyl intermediates become diverted away from the usual pathway of mitochondrial beta-oxidation, towards abnormal partial oxidation in the peroxisomes (which are less severely affected by the riboflavin deficiency state).

Genetically normal human subjects have not yet been shown to accumulate these abnormal urinary products but, in contrast, humans who bear an abnormal gene resulting in dicarboxylic aciduria do quite frequently respond to riboflavin supplements, showing a reduction in their excretion of abnormal fatty acid products. It seems that additional dietary riboflavin can help to overcome the inherent genetic abnormality, presumably by providing more of the coenzyme, and thereby making sure that all of the residual fatty acid oxidation machinery is working at its optimum capacity. Interestingly, the accumulation of dicarboxylic acids in urine is characteristic of riboflavin-deficient mammals but not of birds; chick embryos deprived of riboflavin via the genetic lesion of riboflavin carrier protein seem to die in hypoglycemic shock, but do not exhibit dicarboxylic aciduria.

Iron Economy

An important interaction of riboflavin with iron economy has been suspected for many years, partly because iron-deficient animals failed to respond readily to iron supplements if they were also riboflavin deficient, and also because the redox system involving riboflavin and its coenzymes has been shown to interact very readily with the redox system between ferric and ferrous iron.

Some recent studies in experimental animals have shown that not only is there evidence for some impairment of absorption of iron in riboflavin-deficient animals, and of its distribution between discrete compartments within the body, but also, more surprisingly and strikingly, a major increase in rates of iron loss from the intestinal mucosa, resulting in impaired retention of the body iron stores. This enhanced rate of iron loss is accompanied by hyperproliferation of crypt cells, and increased cellular transit along the villi, leading to an excessive proportion of immature villi, and probably also to a reduction in absorptive area. These studies begin to explain how a combination of iron deficiency and riboflavin deficiency, which is frequently encountered in human populations in many developing countries, may lead to a gradual deterioration of iron status, which is often accompanied by other intestinal lesions and by impaired gut function.

Riboflavin enhances the hematological response to iron, and deficiency may account for at least some of the anemia seen in human populations. Unlike iron-deficiency anemia, the anemia of riboflavin deficiency is reported to be normocytic and normochromic.

Malaria

Low dietary riboflavin intakes are frequently encountered in malarious areas of the world, and in a small number of studies there has arisen the apparently paradoxical observation that biochemical riboflavin deficiency is associated with a lower level of blood cell parasitemia than is encountered in riboflavin-replete subjects. Although neither animal nor human studies have indicated that riboflavin deficiency protects from the life-threatening sequelae of malaria, there does appear to be some interaction between the parasite and flavins within the blood cells, which is not yet fully understood. Interestingly, too, some of the prophylactic drugs used to prevent malaria infection have riboflavin-like structures.

Cataracts and Photoreceptors

Several micronutrients, especially those that can have antioxidant functions in living tissues, have recently been investigated in relation to possible protection against degenerative eye diseases, such as cataract. Studies in animal models have suggested, albeit indirectly, that riboflavin status may be important here, and several recent epidemiological studies, including an intervention study in one region of China, have supported the suggestion that good riboflavin status, or riboflavin supplements, may be protective. Although the evidence must be considered as tentative and incomplete at the present time, this possibility clearly deserves further study.

Another intriguing role of flavoproteins in the eye involves a photoreceptor function that synchronizes circadian rhythms with the solar light–dark cycle, specifically via cryptocromes 1 and 2, which contain FAD and function as blue-light-sensitive photoreceptors.

Interaction with Vitamin B$_6$

There are several metabolic interrelationships between riboflavin and vitamin B$_6$. The conversion of pyridoxine or pyridoxamine phosphates to pyridoxal phosphate is catalyzed by a flavoenzyme (pyridoxaminephosphate oxidase EC 1.4.3.5), so that a deficiency of riboflavin may, at certain key sites, result in a secondary deficiency in B$_6$-dependent pathways. More evidence is needed to clarify the extent and importance of these interactions.

Effect on Folate Metabolism

Riboflavin in the form of FAD is an essential coenzyme for 5,10-methylene tetrahydrofolate reductase, a key enzyme of the folate pathway, which catalyzes the interconversion of 5,10-methylenetetrahydrofolate and 5-methyltetrahydrofolate. Of the known single nucleotide polymorphisms affecting this enzyme, the best known are the C699T and A1298C variants. The former confer thermolability and potentially reduced enzyme activity in the TT homozygote. Marginal riboflavin status may, in some situations, be associated with increased plasma homocysteine levels (possibly predictive of increased

vascular disease risk) that can arise as a result of reduced activity of this key enzyme of folate metabolism in TT subjects. Another example of a common gene polymorphism that affects related pathways is encountered with methionine synthase. These examples of gene–nutrient interactions, which may affect a sizeable proportion of some human populations, illustrate an area of increasing research effort, in which a synergism between a common genetic subtype and a marginal nutrient deficiency or imbalance may confer increased functional risk.

Physical Activity and Neuromuscular Function

Several recent studies have documented an apparent increase in riboflavin requirements accompanying an increase in physical exercise in human subjects. This may reflect the fact that anabolic influences and the accretion of new lean body mass creates a demand for the vitamin, for mitochondrial accretion. Intriguingly, there is also some evidence that indices of neuromuscular function, as illustrated by 'hand-steadiness, may be influenced by riboflavin status in communities where riboflavin deficiency is endemic. If confirmed, this might raise the possibility that peripheral neurological function could be affected by riboflavin status in mammals, including humans, as it is in birds.

Assessment of Riboflavin Status

Assessment of status for specific nutrients such as riboflavin is closely bound up with the estimation of requirements in human individuals and groups of subjects, and with the monitoring of human populations for evidence of the adequacy of their intakes. It is often cheaper, easier, and more accurate to collect a sample of blood or urine from an individual and carry out biochemical analyses that determine status than to carry out reliable measurements of intake over a period of time, since the latter requires considerable cooperation from the subject, and is also affected by uncertainties of food table nutrient values, in relation to specific foods and diets.

Biochemical status estimates are generally based upon urinary excretion or measurements of erythrocyte glutathione reductase (NADPH: oxidized glutathione oxidoreductase EC 1.6.4.2) and its reactivation with flavin adenine dinucleotide (FAD) in red cell lysates. Other biochemical indices, such as plasma or red cell flavin concentrations, have been less widely used, but their potential is increasing with the advent of new assay techniques such as capillary electrophoresis with highly sensitive laser-induced fluorescence detection. Functional indices directed towards the products of flavin-requiring pathways *in vivo* are not in common use except for the investigation of errors of metabolism or rare diseases. The two principal traditional status tests are considered below:

Urinary Excretion

As noted earlier, the amount of riboflavin excreted in the urine is negligible at low intakes of the vitamin. As the dietary level rises there is slow increase to a transition point, above which the slope of the excretion rate increases very sharply, and then remains proportional to intake until absorption is saturated. For population studies it has been found convenient to use the creatinine excretion rate as the denominator, and the suggested interpretation of urinary riboflavin excretion rates is: $<27\,\mu g$ riboflavin per g creatinine for deficient; $27–79\,\mu g\,g^{-1}$ for low; and $>80\,\mu g\,g^{-1}$ for acceptable. Detailed studies of the relation between intake and excretion rate have recently shown that this index is sufficiently sensitive to distinguish riboflavin requirements between people on low-fat, high-carbohydrate diets and the slightly higher requirement associated with high-fat, low-carbohydrate diets. Metabolic states associated with general tissue catabolism can sometimes result in liberation of riboflavin during cell turnover; this increases its urinary excretion, even though dietary intake may be low.

The Glutathione Reductase Test

One rather serious drawback of the urinary excretion index for the assessment of riboflavin status is that it is relatively insensitive at low-to-moderate intakes, because the rate of excretion changes slowly and not very predictably with increasing intake in this region. Another important practical drawback is that 24-h urine samples are not easy to collect and excretion rates may fluctuate over short time periods. A more stable index was therefore sought and was identified in the degree of unsaturation of the red blood cell enzyme, glutathione reductase (NADPH: oxidized-glutathione oxidoreductase EC 1.6.4.2), with respect to its flavin cofactor, flavin adenine dinucleotide (FAD) (**Figure 3**).

As noted earlier, an inadequate supply of dietary riboflavin results in low circulating levels, and hence a gradual progressive loss of cofactor from this red cell flavoenzyme over a period of several weeks. Since the enzyme protein (apoenzyme) remains intact and reactivatable by FAD, it is possible to remove a small sample of blood, collect, wash and hemolyse the red cells, and then measure glutathione reductase activity with and without the FAD cofactor. If the individual is riboflavin replete, then the added FAD has almost no effect and the 'activation coefficient,' or ratio of FAD stimulated to unstimulated activity ('EGRAC') is between 1.0 and 1.3–1.4. If the individual is deficient, then added FAD produces a larger stimulation, and the 'activation coefficient' is higher. For people living in

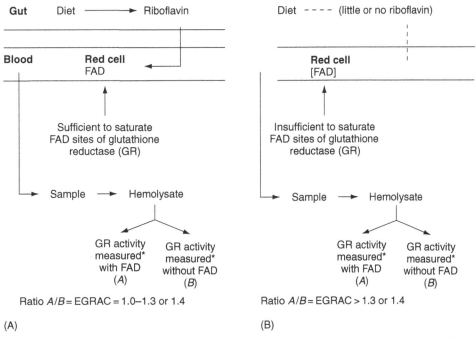

Figure 3 Basis of the glutathione reductase for riboflavin status: (A) riboflavin sufficient; (B) riboflavin deficient. *Reaction of oxidized glutathione with reduced nicotinamide adenine dinucleotide phosphate.

communities with very low intakes of riboflavin and a significant prevalence of clinically recognizable deficiency, activation coefficients as high as 2.0–3.0 are quite common. In Western countries, few values as high as 2.0 are encountered. However, recent population surveys in the UK have indicated that the proportion of values between 1.3 and 1.8 is considerable across all age ranges. Whether this apparent evidence of marginal deficiency has a technical, assay-related explanation, or is a result of decreasing intakes of riboflavin-rich foods, such as cows' milk, is uncertain.

This test has the advantage that it is highly sensitive to, and predictive of, the extent of tissue depletion in the range of severe-to-moderate deficiency; it is robust and requires only a small sample of blood, and it can be automated by modern enzyme rate reaction analyzers. Riboflavin supplements given to deficient subjects result in rapid and reproducible restoration of the saturated condition of the enzyme, and graded supplements can be given to estimate human requirements.

There are minor operational differences among different published versions of the analytical procedure for 'EGRAC,' which result in small between-laboratory differences in the interpretation of the normal range and there are also some instances of specific factors that cause ambiguity of interpretation. The best known of these is the human genetic variant resulting in glucose-6-phosphate dehydrogenase (D-glucose-6-phosphate: NADP+ 1-oxidoreductase EC 1.1.1.49) deficiency. Both homo-and heterozygotes are affected, and in such subjects erythrocyte glutathione reductase becomes almost saturated with FAD, even when they are riboflavin deficient. Other tests of status, such as high-performance liquid chromatography (HPLC) measurement of riboflavin in blood fractions, are then required.

Some groups of people have increased requirements for riboflavin, which is related to special metabolic states. There is, for instance, a progressive increase in requirement during pregnancy, followed by a decrease during lactation. Babies exposed to phototherapy for neonatal jaundice also have increased requirements. In certain circumstances, the use of oral contraceptives may increase requirements, but the evidence is conflicting. The largest and most dramatic increases in requirements have been seen (as noted above) in a subgroup of people with inborn metabolic errors leading to dicarboxylicaciduria and associated clinical abnormalities. Although certain drugs are known to affect riboflavin status indices, there is no clear consensus on the question of the need for supplements by people who are prescribed such drugs – clearly this area needs further study.

Requirements

As with most micronutrients, the evidence on which requirement estimates are based can be subdivided into the following broad classes of criteria:

1. prevention of clinical (pathological) deficiency;
2. attainment of specified blood levels or tissue stores of riboflavin;
3. titration to the urinary excretion threshold;
4. tests based on cofactor saturation of one or more accessible, diet-sensitive, flavin- dependent enzymes, such as erythrocyte glutathione reductase; and
5. physiological function.

Of these five classes of criteria, the first has been useful in defining 'minimum' requirements, but as a practical test of status it has several drawbacks. First, clinical signs of deficiency in human communities tend to be nonspecific and multifactorial. Second, studies resulting in clinical deficiency in controlled trials would be ethically unacceptable. Third, the classical clinical deficiency signs such as angular stomatitis and cheilosis do not always correlate closely with, or respond rapidly to, changes in dietary riboflavin supply or biochemical evidence of deficiency. Additional factors such as local infection are likely to be critical.

Use of physiological functional indices in relation to riboflavin deficiency (analogous to dark adaptation for vitamin A; clotting factors for vitamin K, etc.) has not proved possible, because the analogous riboflavin-sensitive physiological processes are insufficiently specific or easily measurable for use in population studies. Of the biochemical indices, urinary excretion and the flavin-dependent enzyme, erythrocyte glutathione reductase, are generally considered to be the front-runners in the race for acceptance in human studies. These have already been described in the previous section.

For avoidance of clinical deficiency signs in normal healthy adults, the basic requirement for riboflavin is 0.55–0.8 mg day^{-1}. The UK reference nutrient intake for riboflavin is 1.3 mg day^{-1} for men and 1.1 mg day^{-1} for women, rising to 1.6 mg day^{-1} during pregnancy and lactation. For formula-fed infants, the reference intake is 0.4 mg day^{-1}. Requirements may increase to some extent as a result of heavy exercise or dieting, and abnormal status has been observed in the presence of anorexia nervosa.

In the US, the current recommended dietary amounts (RDAs) are 1.3 mg day^{-1} for men and 1.1 mg day^{-1} for women, rising to 1.4 mg day^{-1} in pregnancy and 1.6 mg day^{-1} in lactation, with proportional amounts, based on metabolic body weights and growth requirements, for children and adolescents. RDAs are 20% higher than estimated average requirements (EARs) for each group.

Dietary Sources and High Intakes

Table 2 lists the riboflavin contents of some commonly consumed foods in Western countries. As is the case with most other B vitamins, the richest food sources comprise items such as offal and yeast extract, with meat and dairy products also providing quite generous amounts; fruit and vegetables somewhat less, and the smallest amounts, in relation to their energy content, being present in ungerminated grains and seeds, such as nuts. There is an enormous difference in intakes and in status observed between most Western countries, where the dietary intake tends to be quite generous, and many developing countries, which depend on monotonous and riboflavin-poor staple foods such as polished rice. In developing countries, riboflavin deficiency tends to be widespread. Although even a severe riboflavin deficiency is less obviously life-threatening than some other types of malnutrition that are commonly encountered in the Third World, it can nevertheless cause debility, through skin lesions and metabolic dysfunctions, and riboflavin-nutriture thus deserves an important place in future public health programs.

As with most other B vitamins, riboflavin and its cofactors are remarkably nontoxic even at high intakes. The reasons for this are probably associated with limitations on absorption, once the active transport process has become saturated in the gut; coupled with very effective urinary excretion of any absorbed vitamin that is in excess of cellular requirements.

See also: **Antioxidants**: Diet and Antioxidant Defense. **Fatty Acids**: Metabolism. **Vitamin B$_6$**.

Table 2 Riboflavin content of selected foods

Food	mg per 100 g fresh wt	mg per MJ
Meat, offal, and fish		
Stewed minced beef	0.19	0.22
Grilled pork chop	0.16	0.21
Calf liver, fried	2.89	3.94
Lamb's kidney, fried	3.10	3.95
Cod, grilled	0.06	0.15
Dairy products		
Cows' milk, full cream	0.23	0.84
Cheese, cheddar	0.39	0.23
Yogurt (whole milk, plain)	0.27	0.81
Boiled chicken's egg	0.35	0.57
Human milk	0.03	0.10
Fruits		
Apples, eating, flesh and skin	0.02	0.10
Oranges, flesh	0.04	0.25
Pears, flesh and skin	0.03	0.18
Strawberries, raw	0.03	0.27
Dried mixed fruit	0.05	0.04
Vegetables		
Potatoes, boiled, new	0.06	0.19
Carrots, boiled, young	0.01	0.11
Brussel sprouts, boiled	0.09	0.59
Cauliflower, boiled	0.04	0.34
Onions, fried	0.01	0.01
Grains, grain products, nuts		
White bread	0.08	0.09
Wholemeal bread	0.05	0.05
Rice, boiled, white	Trace	Trace
Cornflakes (Kellogg)	1.3	0.81
Baked beans in tomato sauce	0.06	0.35
Peanuts, plain	0.10	0.04
Other		
Marmite (yeast hydrolysate)	11.9	15.6
Bovril (beef hydrolysate)	8.5	11.2

Compiled and calculated from data in Food Standard Agency (2002) *McCance and Widdowson's The Composition of Foods,* 6th Summary edn. Cambridge: Royal Society of Chemistry.

Further Reading

Bates CJ (1987) Human riboflavin requirements, and metabolic consequences of deficiency in man and animals. *World Review of Nutrition and Dietetics* **50**: 215–265.

Bro-Rasmussen F (1958) The riboflavin requirement of animals and man and associated metabolic relations. 1. Technique of estimating requirement, and modifying circumstances. 2. Relation of requirement to the metabolism of protein and energy. *Nutrition Abstracts and Reviews* **28**: 1–23; 369–386.

Friedrich W (1988) Vitamin B$_2$: riboflavin and its bioactive variants. In: *Vitamins*, ch. 7, pp. 403–471. Berlin: Walter de Gruyter and Co.

Institute of Medicine (2000) *Dietary Reference Intakes for Thiamin, Riboflavin, Niacin, Vitamin B$_6$, Folate, Vitamin B$_{12}$, Pantothenic Acid, Biotin and Choline*, pp. 87–119. Washington DC: National Academy Press.

Massey V. (2000) The chemical and biological versatility of riboflavin. *Biochemical Society Transactions* **28**: 283–296.

McCormick DB (1989) Two inter-connected B vitamins: riboflavin and pyridoxine. *Physiological Reviews* **69**: 1170–1198.

Merrill AH, Lambeth JD, Edmondson DE, and McCormick DB (1981) Formation and mode of action of flavoproteins. *Annual Review of Nutrition* **1**: 281–317.

Powers HJ (1995) Riboflavin-iron interactions with particular emphasis on the gastrointestinal tract. *Proceedings of the Nutrition Society* **54**: 509–517.

Powers HJ (1999) Current knowledge concerning optimum nutritional status of riboflavin, niacin and pyridoxine. *Proceedings of the Nutrition Society* **58**: 435–440.

Rivlin RS (2001) Riboflavin. In: Bowman BA and Russell RM (eds.) *Present Knowledge in Nutrition*, 8th edn, ch. 18, pp. 191–198. Washington, DC: ILSI Press.

Rivlin RS and Pinto JT (2001) Riboflavin (vitamin B$_2$). In: Rucker RB, Suttie JW, McCormick DB, and Machlin LJ (eds.) *Handbook of Vitamins*, 3rd edn, ch. 7, pp. 255–273. New York: Marcel Dekker Inc.

Ross NS and Hansen TPB (1992) Riboflavin deficiency is associated with selective preservation of critical flavoenzyme-dependent metabolic pathways. *Biofactors* **3**: 185–190.

White HB and Merrill AH (1988) Riboflavin-binding proteins. *Annual Review of Nutrition* **8**: 279–299.

S

SELENIUM

C J Bates, MRC Human Nutrition Research, Cambridge, UK

The realization that selenium (Se) may be an essential micronutrient for human diets has arisen only recently, in the second half of the twentieth century. Selenium deficiency, attributable to low soil selenium levels in farm animals, especially sheep that are afflicted by selenium-responsive 'white muscle disease,' has been recognized for at least half a century. However, the more recent identification of Keshan and Kashin–Beck diseases as endemic selenium-responsive conditions, occurring in a central 4000+-km-wide belt of central China and in areas of Russia, demonstrated conclusively that not only is selenium an essential element for man but also deficiencies occur naturally and require public health measures to alleviate them. Selenium incorporation into plants is affected by the acidity of the soil and by the concentrations of iron and aluminum present so that selenium content of human diets is modulated by these components of the environment. The very recent discovery that these diseases probably arise through the interaction of selenium deficiency with enhanced viral virulence has added a further layer of complexity, but it does not alter the fact that selenium is an essential dietary component that cannot be substituted by any other element. Another complicating factor is that moderately increased soil selenium concentrations result in the opposite condition of selenosis, or selenium overload, with equally debilitating consequences. Of all elements, selenium has a very narrow safe intake range, and unlike some other potentially toxic elements, it is absorbed efficiently by the intestine over a wide range of concentrations and across a variety of different molecular forms.

Unlike other elements, selenium can be incorporated in two distinct ways into proteins, either as a functional active center (in specific selenoproteins) via a selective incorporation mechanism that ensures selenocysteine insertion or alternatively by a nonspecific incorporation pathway, in which selenomethionine (or selenocysteine) can replace methionine or cysteine at random, without apparently conferring any special functional characteristics on the recipient proteins. This dichotomy of incorporation complicates the task of measuring status and requirements because the different dietary forms of selenium contribute differently to these two contrasting types of incorporation. Selenomethionine and supplementary selenium in the form of selenium-enriched yeast, in which the incorporated selenium is largely present as selenomethionine, contribute to the random incorporation pathway. This is followed by a gradual turnover of selenium to enrich the specific incorporation pathway. Inorganic selenium, in contrast, feeds directly into the specific incorporation pathway via selenide. Although inorganic selenium may relieve functional selenium deficiency more rapidly than organic selenium, the inorganic forms are potentially more toxic; therefore, selenomethionine supplementation is often preferred because it is safer.

Selenoproteins seem to have a number of functions, comprising various catalytic roles (glutathione peroxidases, thioredoxin reductases, and iodothyronine deiodinases), structural roles, detoxifying functions (e.g., selenoprotein P), and storage and transport activities. Many of these functions are incompletely understood, and advances in this area should help to clarify uncertainties about human requirements and the role of selenoproteins in disease, especially in multifactorial conditions such as cancers. Several controlled intervention trials involving selenium are under way, and these should provide evidence to underpin public health programs in the near future.

Dietary Selenium, Absorption, and Mechanisms of Incorporation of Selenium into Selenoproteins

Rich food sources of selenium in human diets include Brazil nuts, offal, shellfish, and some other types of fish, although there is uncertainty about the extent of selenium bioavailability in some foods, which may in turn be linked to problems of mercury contamination. In the United Kingdom, cereal foods account for approximately 20% of total selenium intake, whereas meat, poultry, and fish account for 30–40%.

Selenium is readily absorbed, especially in the duodenum but also in the caecum and colon. Seleno-amino acids are almost completely absorbed: selenomethionine via the gut methionine transporter and selenocysteine probably via the cysteine transporter. Both selenite and selenate are >50% absorbed, selenite more readily so than selenate, and for these forms there is competition with sulphate transport. Selenite is more efficiently retained then selenate because part of the latter is rapidly excreted into the urine. Vitamins A, E, and C can modulate selenium absorption, and there is a complex relationship between selenium and vitamin E that has not been entirely elucidated for man. A combined deficiency of both nutrients can produce increases in oxidative damage markers (malondialdehyde, F_2 isoprostanes, and breath hydrocarbons) and in pathological changes that are not seen with either deficiency alone. Inorganic Se is reduced to selenide by glutathione plus glutathione reductase and is then carried in the blood plasma, bound mainly to protein in the very low-density lipoprotein fraction. Selenomethionine is partly carried in the albumin fraction.

Figure 1 summarizes the main pathways of interconversion of selenium in mammalian tissues. Selenium appears not to be an essential element for plants, but it is normally taken up readily into their tissues and is substituted in place of sulfur, forming the seleno-amino acids selenomethionine and selenocysteine, which are then incorporated at random in place of the corresponding sulfur amino acids into plant proteins. All branches of the animal kingdom handle selenium in essentially similar ways. When ingested, plant selenium-containing proteins liberate free seleno-methionine and selenocysteine, either for incorporation at random into animal proteins or for metabolic turnover, to liberate inorganic selenide, which is the precursor of active selenium to be inserted at the active site(s) of the selenoproteins. Selenide is also supplied by the reduction of selenite and selenate that enters the diet from nonorganic sources (i.e., from the environment) or from dietary supplements of inorganic selenium. The inorganic forms of the element are absorbed with approximately 50–90% efficiency (i.e., only slightly less than the >90% efficiency of absorption of selenomethionine).

Selenide represents the 'crossroads' of selenium metabolism, from which it may either be committed to specific selenoprotein synthesis or be removed from the body by urinary excretion pathways that involve its detoxification by methylation to methyl selenides, of which the largest fraction is usually trimethyl selenonium. If used for selenoprotein synthesis, selenide combines with a chaperone protein, and the first metabolic step is its conversion to selenophosphate by the ATP-requiring enzyme selenophosphate synthetase, which is a selenoprotein.

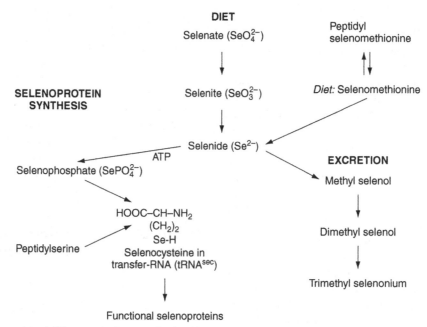

Figure 1 Interconversion of different selenium species in animal and human tissues.

This then becomes the precursor for selenocysteinyl-soluble (or transfer) RNA, which is synthesized from a serine moiety attached to a specific soluble (transfer) RNA identified as tRNA^{sec}. This serine–tRNA complex is first dehydrated to aminoacrylyl–tRNA in a reaction that requires a vitamin B_6 cofactor, pyridoxal phosphate. This product then reacts with selenophosphate in a reaction that requires magnesium and the enzyme selenosynthase. The resulting selenocysteinyl–tRNA then recognizes a UGA codon in the messenger RNA sequence. This codon is also used as a stop sequence; therefore, the adjacent mRNA structure has to provide the correct 'context' (e.g., a stem-loop structure) to direct the incorporation of selenocysteine into the growing polypeptide chain of the selenoprotein. Other gene products are involved, and although the sequence of reactions and the participatory proteins have been studied in detail and largely elucidated for prokaryotes such as *Escherichia coli*, the analogous pathways are only partly understood for eukaryotes such as mammals. Specific selenoprotein synthesis is often tissue specific, with different versions of structurally similar selenoproteins being made at different tissue sites. In liver, for instance, provided that the selenium supply is generous, there is a considerable accumulation of cytosolic glutathione peroxidase type I, which can act as a storage repository of selenium for later liberation and redistribution.

Degradation of selenocysteine is catalyzed by selenocysteine lyase, which releases elemental Se, and this is then reduced to selenide by glutathione or other thiols. The urinary excretion pathway is very important for selenium homeostasis of the tissues. Urinary selenium tends to reflect recent intake rather than tissue status, but it can be a useful source of information about possible selenium overload.

Selenoproteins: Classification and Functions

Table 1 lists the selenoproteins that have been unequivocally identified in mammals, together with a summary of their main locations and known functions. Of the known glutathione peroxidases, three are tetramers and one (the phospholipid hydroperoxide-specific peroxidase) is monomeric in its quaternary structure. It appears to be this class of enzymatic activity that is critical for the action of selenoproteins in maintaining immune function, and indeed, glutathione peroxidase type I knockout mice are susceptible to viral mutation and increased viral virulence, as are selenium-deficient ones. Several other selenoproteins listed in **Table 1** also have antioxidant functions and

activities. Reaction of glutathione peroxidase with peroxides yields selenic or seleninic acid at the active site of the enzyme, which is recycled by glutathione.

The three thioredoxin reductases act in conjunction with the sulfur protein thioredoxin and with NADPH to bind key transcription factors to DNA. The iodothyronine deiodinases modulate the thyroid hormones, helping to ensure an optimal supply of the most active member of the thyroid hormones, triiodothyronine. The different selenoprotein deiodinases are found at different sites in the body. If selenium and iodine are deficient in a human population, the thyroid deficiency is more severe (and goiters are larger) than if only iodine is lacking. This situation is endemic in some areas of central Africa, including Kivu province in the Central African Republic (formerly Zaire).

The sperm mitochondrial capsule selenoprotein has a structural as well as an enzymic role, and it is responsible for both the maintenance of motility and the structural integrity of the tail of the sperm. Both human and other mammals exhibit reduced sperm motility and increased sperm rupture under conditions of low selenium supply. A study in Glasgow, Scotland, recorded enhanced sperm motility and fertility in men who received a selenium supplement.

The precise functional roles of selenoproteins P and W are not well understood. Selenoprotein P contains more selenium (up to 10 atoms per molecule) than any other mammalian selenoprotein, and it can form equimolar selenium–mercury complexes, thereby probably helping to detoxify mercury. It is the major selenoprotein found in plasma and may also act as a selenium transport protein and selenium reserve. Selenoprotein W is found in muscle, and its decline may help explain the molecular basis of white muscle disease in selenium-deficient sheep.

Other selenoproteins have been characterized by their molecular size but not by their functions and health significance (**Table 1**).

Selenium Deficiency, Viral Disease and Mutation, and Immune Function

Initially, Keshan disease was thought to be a deficiency disease alone, involving inadequate intakes of Se and also of Mo, Mg, and thiamin. However, seasonal variations in symptoms suggested that at least one other interacting factor was likely involved. Later, an enterovirus and a Coxsackie virus (strain B4) were isolated from affected individuals. The same Coxsackie virus was able to produce severe heart pathology in mice when they were fed Se-deficient grain from Keshan endemic areas.

Table 1 Selenoprotein description and functions

Selenoprotein	Molecular description	Function
Glutathione peroxidases (GPx)		Removal of potentially harmful peroxides and modulation of eicosanoid synthesis
Type I	Tetramer	>50% of total Se in body; acts as Se buffer/store
Type II	Tetramer	May protect the intestine
Type III	Tetramer	Found in plasma and milk; synthesized in kidney
Type IV	Monomer	Phospholipid hydroperoxide GPx; abundant in testis; resistant to Se deficiency; involved in eicosanoid metabolism
Thioredoxin reductases (types I, II, III)		Transfers protons from NADPH via bound FAD to thioredoxin; regulates gene expression by redox control of binding of transcription factors to DNA; needed for cell viability and proliferation; can reduce dehydroascorbate and ascorbate radical to ascorbate
Iodothyronine deiodinases (types I, II, III)		Type I acts in liver and thyroid gland to convert T_4 to T_3; the other types occur in other tissues and also help to regulate thyroid hormone levels
Selenophosphate synthetase		Synthesizes selenophospate from selenide + ATP as first step in selenocysteine synthesis during Se incorporation into selenoproteins
Sperm mitochondrial capsule selenoprotein		Sperm structural protein required for integrity of sperm tail and its mobility; also an antioxidant, similar to GPx IV
Prostate epithelial selenoprotein	15 kDa	In epithelial cells; possibly redox function, similar to GPx IV
Selenoprotein P		Accounts for 60–80% of plasma selenoproteins; contains up to 10 selenocysteines per molecule; has a transport function; binds mercury; may protect the cardiovascular system and endothelial cells
Selenoprotein W	10 kDa	Small antioxidant protein found in muscle (+ heart); its loss may account for white muscle disease of sheep
18-kDa selenoprotein (SELT)		In kidney and many other tissues; not easily depleted in Se deficiency
SELR, SELN	12.6 and 47.5 kDa, respectively	
Spermatid selenoprotein	34 kDa	In sperm nuclei and in stomach; has GPx activity

There are 30–50 proteins that contain Se, as detected by ^{75}Se-labelling in mammals, only about half of which have been investigated.

Coxsackie virus strain B3, when introduced into Se-deficient mice, produces a myocarditis that is similar to that of human Keshan's disease, and this virus consistently undergoes mutation at six distinct amino acid (= nucleotide) sites in the Se-deficient but not the control animals. These mutated viruses are then able to produce myocarditis even in selenium-replete control mice. Thus, the virulence change has become permanent by mutation, and the increased virulence is no longer dependent on a simultaneous lack of selenium. Comparable selenium limitation-induced mutations in influenza virus have also been shown in Se-deficient mice. It is suggested that in the presence of a low selenium supply, a normally quiescent virus may become activated by increased oxidative stress and host cell apoptosis, the mutation to increased virulence being a survival strategy by the virus.

In HIV-infected individuals, the progression to AIDS and the decline in T helper (CD4) cell counts are accompanied by a parallel decrease in blood selenium levels. Selenium deficiency appears to increase the probability of mortality in HIV-infected subjects.

Human selenium supplementation (e.g., 200 µg/day), even in apparently selenium-replete individuals receiving a diet providing >120 µg Se/day, was able to stimulate the proliferation of activated T cells of the immune system. It elicited an enhanced response to antigen stimulation, an enhanced ability to generate cytotoxic lymphocytes, an enhanced ability to destroy tumor cells, and increased natural killer cell activity. Growth-regulatory interleukin-2 receptors on the surface of activated lymphocytes and natural killer cells became upregulated.

In a study in Liverpool, UK, healthy adult subjects with initial plasma selenium concentrations below

1.2 μmol/l were given placebo or 50 or 100 μg daily supplements of selenium as selenite for 15 weeks. After 6 weeks, they were given oral live attenuated polivirus vaccine, and after 9 weeks, [74]Se stable isotope was given intravenously to measure their body Se pool size. The Se supplements significantly increased the Se pool size, and the supplemented groups cleared the poliovirus more rapidly and their fecal viral RNA products exhibited fewer mutations. Cellular immune response (estimated by interferon-γ and other cytokines) was enhanced and there was an earlier peak of T cell proliferation and numbers in the supplemented groups. This study suggests that selenium supplements can improve a number of indices of immune function, even in individuals whose Se status is not severely deficient.

Selenium Distribution, Status Assays, and Dietary Reference Values

In an adequately supplied adult male human subject, the total body selenium content is on the order of 30–60 mg, of which one-third is found in the skeleton and two-thirds in the soft tissues. A substantial fraction of kidney selenium is retained even when selenium at other sites is severely depleted during deficiency, and renal selenium is more constant between human populations than selenium in other tissues or body fluids. Regulation of selenoprotein synthesis at the transcription level appears to ensure a hierarchy of preservation of individual selenoproteins at critical sites. The cytosolic glutathione peroxidase (GPx I) and selenoprotein P can donate selenium to other sites whenever overall depletion occurs. Selenium crosses the placenta readily, and breast milk selenium concentration is responsive to changes in maternal selenium intake. In the United States, breast milk Se concentrations are generally in the range of 0.19–0.25 μmol/l, but colostrum has levels that are two or three times higher than those of mature breast milk.

Selenium status can be measured in several ways. One recently developed and effective approach toward selenium concentration measurement is the use of inductively coupled plasma mass spectrometry. Older assays are based on the generation of selenium hydrides or fluorescent derivatives of selenium. Selenium status can be measured by its concentration in plasma or serum; in whole blood (a result that can be recalculated to provide red cell selenium concentrations); or in platelets, hair, or nails. The platelet concentration is considered to be a reliable medium-term index, whereas hair and nail concentrations can integrate selenium status, and hence intakes, over a longer term.

Glutathione peroxidase enzymatic assay in plasma or red cells is another frequently used approach to status measurement. In situations of severe to marginal deficiency, this has proven to be a sensitive and responsive index, varying consistently with variations in the selenium supply. However, once an adequate supply is achieved, there is no further capacity for increases in enzyme synthesis, and a plateau of activity is reached that does not respond to further increases in selenium intake. Therefore, if a population exhibits a strong correlation between plasma (or red cell) selenium concentrations and glutathione peroxidase activity in blood fractions, or there is a major increase in GPx activity after selenium supplementation, this can be taken as evidence of suboptimum selenium status in the population. If there is little evidence of such a correlation or of a response to supplementation, then the population is likely to be adequately supplied. The absolute values of GPx activity are more difficult to interpret because there are many different versions of the assay in use in different laboratories, and interlaboratory harmonization has rarely been undertaken for this assay. Recent reappraisal has suggested that the plasma glutathione peroxidase (GPx III) assay may be more reliable than the blood cytosolic (GPx I) enzyme assay because haemoglobin tends to interfere with the reaction in erythrocyte extracts.

A summary of reference values and recommended intakes of selenium from three publications is presented in **Table 2**. Dietary reference values for selenium in the United Kingdom, set in 1991, were based on a number of criteria, including the facts that no evidence of deficiency was detectable in populations with intakes of 40 μg/day and that saturation of GPx in Chinese males occurred at an intake of approximately 41 μg/day (equivalent to 50 μg/day for a UK male based on a body weight comparison). On this basis, the UK Lower Reference Nutrient Intake (LRNI) was set at 40 μg/day for both male and female adults, and the corresponding RNI values were set at 75 μg/day for males and 60 μg/day for females, with lower values, proportional to body weight, for children. No extra increment was considered necessary for pregnancy, but for lactating women an additional 15 μg/day was added to both the LRNI and the RNI.

More recently, selenium recommendations or reference values have been slightly lower. The US committee that set Dietary Reference Intakes in 2000 interpreted the Chinese estimate of 41 μg/day needed to saturate GPx in adult men, and data from New Zealand indicating selenium intake adequacy at 38 μg/day, as supporting an Estimated Average

Table 2 Reference values for intakes of selenium (μg/day)[a]

Population group	UK LRNI	UK RNI	US AI/RDA[b]	WHO/FAO RNI
0–6 months	4–5	10–13	AI:15	6
7–12 months	5–6	10	AI:20	10
1–3 years	7	15	RDA:20	17
4–6 years	10	20	30	22
7–10 years	16	30	30–40	21–26
11–18 years, male	25–40	45–70	40–55	32
11–18 years, female	25–40	45–60	40–55	26
19–65 years, male	40	70	55	34
19–65 years, female	40	60	55	26
65 + years, male	40	70	55	33
65 + years, female	40	60	55	25
Pregnant	40	60	60	26–30
Lactating	55	75	70	35–42

[a]Where a range of values is given, the population group described in this table overlapped across more than one population group in the source table.
[b]The first two age groups are AI; the remainder are RDA.
LRNI, Lower Reference Nutrient Intake; RNI, Reference Nutrient Intake; AI, Adequate Intake; RDA, Recommended Dietary Allowance.
Sources: UK: Department of Health (1991) *Dietary Reference Values for Food Energy and Nutrients for the United Kingdom*, Report on Health and Social Subjects No. 41. London: HMSO. USA: Food and Nutrition Board, Institute of Medicine (2000) *Dietary Reference Intakes for Vitamin C, Vitamin E, Selenium and Carotenoids*. Washington, DC: National Academy Press. WHO/FAO: WHO/FAO (2002) *Human Vitamin and Mineral Requirements. Report of a Joint FAO/WHO Expert Consultation, Bangkok, Thailand*. Rome: WHO/FAO.

Requirement (EAR) of 45 μg/day for adults of both sexes, and hence an Recommended Dietary Allowance (RDA) (with 10% CV of requirements) of 55 μg/day for both sexes, increasing to 60 μg/day for pregnant and lactating women. However, RNI values set by an FAO/WHO committee, published in 2002, were much lower, at only 26 μg/day for women and 34 μg/day for men, based on the premise that full saturation of GPx is unnecessary and two-thirds saturation is probably adequate. Clearly, there has been considerable divergence of opinion between different committees, and this divergence underlies the current uncertainty about the overall adequacy of selenium intakes in many European countries, including the United Kingdom. In the United Kingdom, selenium intakes have declined considerably during the past 25 years because of the substitution of North American wheat imports by European wheat with a much lower selenium content. In contrast, selenium intakes in New Zealand have increased as a result of grain imports from Australia.

There are also recommendations for the upper limit of safe intake of selenium. For the United Kingdom, it was noted that evidence of toxicity was detectable at intakes of approximately 750–900 μg/day, and the UK panel recommended a maximum safe intake of 450 μg for adults (6 μg/kg body weight/day), which was confirmed as an official safe upper

level (SUL) in 2003. In the US Dietary Reference Intakes, the upper level of 400 μg/day was based on a no adverse effect level of 800 μg/day divided by an uncertainty (i.e., safety) factor of 2. The FAO/WHO committee also set an SUL of 400 μg/day for adults. In humans, at intakes of >3 mg/day, overt signs of selenosis include damage to nails and hair, skin and nerve lesions, mottling of teeth, nausea, weakness, and diarrhea. Urinary selenium excretion is high, and a garlic odour may be apparent in the breath.

Selenium Interventions

As noted previously, neither Keshan disease nor Kashin–Beck disease are now thought to be simple dietary deficiency diseases. They probably also involve viral components and may be exacerbated by environmental toxins, including mycotoxins. Thus, they are probably multifactorial, but importantly, public health selenium supplementation interventions have had a dramatically beneficial effect on the prevalence of these diseases. The main clinical features of Keshan disease are cardiac insufficiency and enlargement, electrocardiographic changes, and fibrosis. Those of Kashin–Beck disease are osteoarthropathy and necrosis of the joints and epiphysial plate cartilage. Both diseases occur in school-age children; Keshan disease also occurs in women of child-bearing age, but adult men are less affected.

In hilly and heavily eroded areas of China where these diseases were endemic, the use of selenium-enriched fertilizers was not feasible as an intervention because of the huge geographical areas involved and hence the high cost. Instead, direct human supplementation of at-risk and affected populations was introduced during the 1970s using a 0.5 or 1.0 mg sodium selenite supplement (according to age) per person per week. In Shaanxi province, following supplementation, the prevalence of Keshan disease declined from 12 per 1000 to undetectable levels between 1976 and 1985, and in Heilongjiang province the prevalence of Kashin–Beck disease declined from 44 to 1% of the population between 1970 and 1986.

An alternative approach to intervention, by selenium enrichment of crop and grassland fertilizers, was introduced in the 1970s in Finland. Here, there was no overt evidence of selenium deficiency in the human population, but Se deficiency disease had occurred, and had been successfully eliminated in farm animals, by supplementation of animal feeds during the 1960s. Fertilizer that was Se enriched at 16 mg/kg was then applied to cereal crops for human consumption. Grassland fertilizer was enriched at 6 mg/kg. As a result, adult human Se intake increased from 25–60 to approximately 100 μg/day. Serum Se increased from 65–70 μg/l in 1975 to 120 μg/l in 1989–1991. In 1990, the selenium level was reduced to 6 mg/kg fertilizer for cereal crops as a precaution against possible overload. Selenium intervention by fertilizer enrichment was judged to be a safe, economical, and easily controlled intervention.

New Zealand, which has a similar situation of marginal intakes and status, decided not to intervene on a population or nationwide basis but instead has taken steps to ensure that particular high-risk groups, notably people receiving total parenteral nutrition or children receiving special diets for phenylketonuria prevention, are adequately supplied.

Selenium and Chronic Disease

Several supplementation and epidemiological case–control studies have suggested a possible link between increased selenium intakes or status and protection against certain cancers. First, in intercountry comparisons and studies comparing different regions of the United States having different soil selenium levels, there was a consistent correlation between lower selenium levels and higher risk of cancer. A study of 34,000 male health professionals in the eastern United States

found that toenail selenium levels were inversely proportional to prostate cancer incidence, with diagnoses recorded >2 years later, which helped to reduce confounding by reverse causality (i.e., the presence of cancer causing the low selenium levels). A study in China found that the incidence of hepatocellular carcinoma was lower in a community receiving selenite-fortified salt (15 mg/kg) than in adjacent control communities, and another intervention with selenium + vitamin E + β-carotene supplements seemed to reduce total age-adjusted mortality, especially from cancer. A controlled intervention in the eastern United States recorded an approximately 50% lower cancer mortality in a high-risk group of subjects who were randomized to receive 200 μg selenium/day as Se yeast for several years. Animal model studies have demonstrated reduced susceptibility to cancer induction with increased selenium intakes. Although these studies appear promising, caveats about their design and interpretation imply that none yet conclusively prove the hypothesis that additional dietary selenium is able to reduce human cancer morbidity and mortality. Trials in multiple locations (including Europe)—PRECISE (Prevention of Cancer by Intervention with Selenium) and SELECT (Selenium and Vitamin E Cancer Prevention Trial)—are ongoing and should help to resolve this important question.

Attempts to demonstrate disease-reduction benefit with respect to cardiovascular disease by selenium intervention have proven disappointing, despite the theoretical benefit of lipid peroxide removal by GPx and apparently beneficial changes in intermediate markers such as platelet aggregation, vasoconstriction, and thromboxane:prostacyclin ratios following supplementation. Further studies of high-risk populations are needed, including a focus on the concerted action by combinations of selenium and vitamin E.

Other conditions for which supplementary selenium has been claimed to be beneficial include rheumatoid arthritis, pancreatitis and asthma, and mood alterations. Again, further studies are required.

Conclusion

The essential role of selenium in human nutrition and its discrete biochemical functions are rapidly being characterized. Severe deficiency and selenosis (toxicity) occur in different regions and are manifested by characteristic and life-threatening human diseases. The selenoproteins have a wide variety of roles, both catalytic and noncatalytic. Interactions with redox pathways appear to be common. Selenoprotein P, in particular, appears to play an important detoxification role. Selenium appears to play an important role in cell-mediated immunity. Selenium deficiency can cause viral mutation leading to increased virulence, and such mutation and its consequences appear permanent. Optimum human intakes of selenium are still a matter of debate because some studies have reported benefits (e.g., anticancer and immunological effects) when supplements are given, even to populations that appear to be generously supplied with the nutrient. The distinction between nutritional and pharmacological benefits is unclear, and further trials to determine risk–benefit balance at different intake levels are needed in a range of populations and age and gender groups.

See also: **Antioxidants**: Intervention Studies. **Ascorbic Acid**: Physiology, Dietary Sources and Requirements. **Vitamin A**: Biochemistry and Physiological Role. **Vitamin E**: Metabolism and Requirements.

Further Reading

Allan CB, Lacourciere GM, and Stadtman TC (1999) Responsiveness of selenoproteins to dietary selenium. *Annual Review of Nutrition* 19: 1–16.

Arthur JR, McKenzie RC, and Beckett GJ (2003) Selenium in the immune system. *Journal of Nutrition* 133: 1457S–1459S.

Beck MA, Levander OA, and Handy J (2003) Selenium deficiency and viral infection. *Journal of Nutrition* 133: 1463S–1467S.

Behne D and Kyriakopoulos A (2001) Mammalian selenium-containing proteins. *Annual Review of Nutrition* 21: 453–473.

Broome CS, McArdle F, Kyle JAM *et al.* (2004) An increase in selenium intake improves immune function and poliovirus handling in adults with marginal selenium status. *American Journal of Clinical Nutrition* 80: 154–162.

Brown KM and Arthur JR (2001) Selenium, selenoproteins and human health: A review. *Public Health Nutrition* 4: 593–599.

Driscoll DM and Copeland PR (2003) Mechanism and regulation of selenoprotein synthesis. *Annual Review of Nutrition* 23: 17–40.

Ellis DR and Dalt DE (2003) Plants, selenium and human health. *Current Opinion in Plant Biology* 6: 273–279.

Hatfield DL (ed.) Journal of Trace Elements in Experimental Medicine. *Selenium: Its Molecular Biology and Role in Human Health*. Dordrecht, The Netherlands: Kluwer Academic.

Lyons G, Stangoulis J, and Graham R (2003) High-selenium wheat: Biofortification for better health. *Nutrition Research Reviews* 16: 45–60.

Rayman MP (2000) The importance of selenium to human health. *Lancet* 356: 233–241.

Reilly C (1996) *Selenium in Food and Health*. London: Blackie Academic & Professional.

Schrauzer GN (2000) Selenomethionine: A review of its nutritional significance, metabolism and toxicity. *Journal of Nutrition* 130: 1653–1656.

Tapiero H, Townsend DM, and Tew KD (2003) The antioxidant role of selenium and seleno-compounds. *Biomedicine and Pharmacotherapy* 57: 134–144.

Whanger PD (1998) Metabolism of selenium in humans. *Journal of Trace Elements and Experimental Medicine* 11: 227–240.

WHO Task Group on Selenium (1987) *Selenium*, Environmental Health Criteria 58 Geneva: WHO.

SODIUM

Contents
Physiology
Salt Intake and Health

Physiology

A R Michell, St Bartholomew's Hospital, London, UK

Physiological, Clinical, and Nutritional Importance of Sodium

Despite the fact that the body contains more calcium and potassium, sodium is arguably the most important cation because it dictates the volume of extracellular fluid (ECF) and its concentration affects osmotic concentration of both ECF and intracellular fluid (ICF). Abnormalities of ECF sodium concentration cause movement of water into or out of cells, thus altering the osmotic concentration of ICF in parallel and causing swelling or shrinkage of cells. The main impact of this is on the brain because its cells are rigidly enclosed by the cranium.

Sodium depletion is mainly caused by enteric, renal, or adrenal disease, and sodium retention is caused by renal disease; healthy kidneys are well able to excrete excess dietary salt. However, chronic ingestion of excess salt, whether or not it increases ECF volume, is a predisposing or exacerbating factor in hypertension. Until the 1980s, knowledge of the regulation of body sodium mainly concerned defenses against depletion, while in the 1990s there was a rapid growth in knowledge of the mechanisms that excrete excess sodium. This seems appropriate since most species, especially humans, dogs, and laboratory rats, are exposed to dietary sodium intakes well above their nutritional requirement.

The nutritional requirement is a reflection of obligatory losses (maintenance) and the needs of growth, pregnancy, and lactation. Abnormal losses owing to disease, or in animals such as humans and horses which sweat extensively, raise the requirement. The impact of equine sweating is different from that in humans. Human sweat always contains sodium at concentrations well below plasma levels (and when aldosterone secretion is raised, levels of sweat sodium fall very low); horse sweat is hypertonic but this helps to offset the osmotic effect of the increased respiratory water loss during exertion, i.e., it may be a defense against hypernatremia, rather than a potential cause of sodium depletion. Similarly hypernatremia in many species induces 'dehydration natriuresis' – an appropriate defense.

Consideration of the physiology of sodium thus includes its distribution in the body, regulation of total content and concentration, causes of and responses to depletion or excess, and their nutritional implications.

Distribution

Sodium is a cation, i.e., a positively charged ion; its distribution and physiological effects are fairly independent of the negative ions (anions) that originally accompanied its ingestion though they may affect its absorption and excretion. Most sodium is in ECF (**Table 1**), kept there by the sodium pump, an enzyme system, Na^+/K^+-exchanging ATPase, which uses substantial amounts of energy (adenosine triphosphate; ATP) in maintaining a low intracellular sodium concentration and a high intracellular potassium (K^+) concentration. Sodium transport is

a central issue in the physiology of sodium for a number of reasons:

1. It helps to maintain the ionic environment of ICF and the volume of ECF.
2. It prevents cell swelling (the Na^+ efflux exceeds the K^+ influx).
3. It establishes gradients which, in various tissues, allow transport of other cations in exchange, other anions in parallel or organic solutes – these are often cotransported with sodium down concentration gradients which are secondary to the low sodium environment created by the pump.
4. It establishes the membrane voltages on which excitability and secretory activities frequently depend.
5. The energy expenditure of the pump is a substantial portion of total metabolic activity and contributes to thermogenesis.
6. Sodium transport is not only a key factor in the retention and loss of sodium in the kidney, gut, salivary, and sweat glands but also influences the excretion or retention of many other solutes. Thus, for example, diuretics intended to promote sodium excretion may also cause unintentional losses of potassium and magnesium. Similarly, when renal sodium excretion increases appropriately in response to ingestion of excess salt, there may also be unwanted losses of calcium and in postmenopausal women these may contribute to loss of bone mineral.

Bone also contains substantial quantities of sodium but, as yet, its significance is unknown since it does not appear to be mobilized during sodium depletion. Gut fluids contain considerable amounts of sodium, mostly secretory rather than dietary, and mostly reabsorbed in more distal regions of the intestine.

Extracellular Sodium

Most of the extracellular fluid is interstitial fluid (ISF) in the tissue spaces, providing the transport medium between capillaries and cells. The sodium concentration in plasma is slightly above that in ISF because plasma contains more proteins, notably albumin, which do not readily escape into ISF across the capillary membranes, and the effect of their negative charges is to hold more positively charged ions, notably sodium, in circulation (Gibbs–Donnan equilibrium).

The main effects of excess ECF volume are seen as expanded ISF, visible clinically as edema (or ascites when fluid accumulates in the abdomen rather than

Table 1 Summary of sodium (Na) distribution and requirements

Typical plasma Na concentration (mmol l^{-1})	145 (130–160)
Typical body Na content (mmol kg^{-1})	50–55
Typical proportion (%) of total Na	
ICF	10
ECF	50
Bone	40
Maintenance requirement in mammals (mmol per kg per day)	
Sheep	0.1
Cattle and goats	0.3–0.7
Pigs	0.6
Rats	0.6
Dogs	0.2–0.5
Humans	?<0.6

1 mmol = 23 mg Na^+, 58.5 mg NaCl.

the tissue spaces). Mild edema is merely a cosmetic problem in itself but pulmonary or cerebral edema, or severe ascites, are potentially serious forms. Edema can result from excess ingestion or retention of sodium (overall expansion of ECF) or 'leakage' from plasma to ISF, with plasma volume continuously replenished by renal sodium retention. Such maldistribution of ECF occurs if plasma albumin is very low (renal leakage, hepatic impairment, or severe malnutrition), or with excessive capillary blood pressure (venous blockage, inactivity, heart failure, or arteriolar dilation, e.g., from heat or allergy), capillary damage, or lymphatic blockage. The latter prevents the removal of proteins that have leaked into ISF. Accumulation of protein in ISF undermines the osmotic gradient, normally favors uptake of water at the venous end of the capillary, where the pressure is lower. Since edema involves the expansion of a larger compartment (ISF) from a smaller one (plasma) it is only possible as long as the latter is replenished; hence the kidney, while seldom the primary cause of edema, is always the enabling cause; the use of diuretics is therefore appropriate in the treatment of nonrenal as well as renal causes of edema.

The main effect of inadequate ECF volume is to reduce plasma volume and thus to compromise cardiovascular function, in extreme cases by causing circulatory shock.

Regulation of ECF Sodium

In a mature, nonpregnant, nonlactating, healthy animal, sodium excretion matches sodium intake and is often used to estimate it, although this is not reliable, especially when intake is low. Dietary sodium is readily available, i.e., readily absorbed; thus the traditional view of sodium regulation emphasizes renal regulation of urinary Na^+ loss. This oversimplifies the more subtle interplay seen, for example, in herbivorous animals, where salt appetite may contribute to regulation by intensifying during sodium depletion. Moreover, in many herbivores the feces, rather than urine, may be the major route of sodium excretion and the gut may therefore be an important regulator of sodium balance. Indeed, it is interesting that sodium transport mechanisms in the small intestine show considerable similarities to those of the proximal part of the renal tubules (e.g., linked transport of Na^+, glucose, and amino acids) whereas the colon, like the distal nephron, responds to the salt-retaining (and potassium-shedding) hormone of the adrenal cortex,

aldosterone. Indeed, diarrhea is essentially enteric diuresis; a failure of intestinal sodium and water reabsorbtion, which exceeds the compensatory capacity of the color.

Provided that the adrenal gland is healthy, urinary and fecal sodium loss can be reduced virtually to zero. Sweat loss can also be very low, although with severe exertion in hot climates the volume of sweat may exceed the ability of aldosterone to reduce its sodium concentration and net loss of sodium can occur. Aldosterone also reduces salivary sodium (and raises $[K^+]$).

There are two components to the regulation of ECF sodium: the total amount of sodium retained and its concentration. The former is regulated by mechanisms that directly affect sodium, whereas the latter is essentially regulated via water balance. Thus, whatever sodium is retained in ECF is 'clothed' with the appropriate amount of water to maintain the normal plasma sodium concentration within narrow limits; deviations of less than 1% (hard to measure in the laboratory) trigger corrective responses. Thus, a raised plasma sodium concentration (e.g., after water loss) stimulates both thirst and renal water conservation; antidiuretic hormone (ADH) from the posterior pituitary reduces urine output through its effect on the renal collecting ducts. Even one of these mechanisms can defend body water; thus diabetes insipidus (inadequate production or effect of ADH) does not cause severe dehydration but polydipsia (increased fluid intake; 'thirst' is a sensation).

Excess salt intake does not raise plasma sodium concentration (hypernatremia) if water is available and the patient can drink; the excess sodium is diluted. The resulting increase in ECF volume then stimulates increased sodium excretion. Sodium also enables ECF to hold water against the osmotic 'pull' of the solutes in ICF and sodium thus functions as the 'osmotic skeleton' of ECF; it is the main determinant of its volume.

Plasma sodium concentration is therefore only indirectly related to sodium balance. When ECF volume, notably circulating volume, is severely reduced, this stimulus, rather than Na^+ concentration, becomes the main drive for thirst and ADH secretion. Until ECF volume is restored, water is retained (to protect ECF volume) even though this undermines the protection of ECF Na^+ concentration and, as a result, plasma sodium falls. Thus, during sodium depletion, contraction of ECF volume precedes significant reductions of plasma Na^+, which is therefore a poor index of sodium status.

Sodium-Retaining Hormones

Sodium depletion, by reducing plasma volume and renal perfusion, stimulates the production of renin (from the kidneys), which generates angiotensin in circulation. This hormone is a vasoconstrictor (so protects blood pressure), stimulates thirst (so helps to restore ECF volume), and, above all, stimulates sodium retention both directly (renally) and indirectly (by stimulating adrenal secretion of aldosterone); it thus reduces the sodium concentration of urine, feces, saliva, and sweat, but not milk.

Indices of aldosterone secretion (reduced sodium or potassium concentration in urine, feces, etc.) are often taken as evidence of sodium depletion or inadequate sodium intake, but the following points apply:

1. Aldosterone secretion is also stimulated directly by hyperkalemia (elevated plasma K^+) and promotes potassium excretion.
2. Such interpretations involve a subjective judgement concerning adequate or excessive sodium intake. Because physiologists and clinicians were traditionally more concerned with sodium depletion as well as its consequences and the defenses against it, elevated aldosterone secretion was readily seen as a warning signal. However, if sodium intakes associated with increased aldosterone have no other harmful effects, and especially if excess sodium intakes cause concern, low levels of aldosterone secretion might equally indicate excessive salt intake.

While sodium reabsorption in the distal nephron, influenced by aldosterone, is particularly important because it can produce sodium-free urine and promote potassium loss, the great majority of renal sodium reabsorption occurs elsewhere; about 25% in the loop of Henle and most in the proximal tubule. The loop is also a main site of magnesium reabsorption, hence the tendency for loop diuretics to cause hypomagnesemia.

The factors controlling proximal reabsorption are incompletely understood but their effect is clear: proximal reabsorption of sodium increases or decreases according to the need to enhance or diminish plasma volume. Since the fluid in the proximal tubule is similar to plasma, having been formed from it by glomerular filtration, it has the ideal composition for this purpose.

Natriuretic Hormones

Excretion of excess sodium involves not only suppression of salt-retention mechanisms but also activation of sodium-shedding (natriuretic) mechanisms. Two types of hormones are involved: atrial natriuretic peptide (ANP), produced by the cardiac atria when they are overstretched (reduction of ECF volume being an appropriate response to cardiac overload), and active sodium transport inhibitors (ASTIs), probably produced within the brain. These were probably the original molecules associated with the receptors binding cardiac glycoside drugs and are therefore also called 'endogenous digitalis-like inhibitors' (EDLIs); their exact identity remains uncertain. Atrial natriuretic peptide has various effects that essentially oppose those of the salt retention induced by aldosterone: it increases sodium excretion, lowers arterial pressure, and promotes movement of ECF towards the interstitial compartment.

Other hormones (e.g., sex steroids, parathyroid hormone, calcitonin, thyroid hormone, prolactin) affect renal sodium retention or loss but are not thought to regulate it.

Adequate, Inadequate, and Excess Sodium

It is unlikely that adult daily maintenance requirement exceeds 0.6 mmol per kg body weight and could well be below this in many mammals. Newborn, growing, pregnant, or lactating animals have increased requirements. The appropriate sodium intake for humans remains controversial with some cultures managing on less than 1 mmol per day, while Western intakes may be in the range 200–300 mmol per day, more where processed foods are heavily consumed. There has been insufficient awareness among physicians and human nutritionists of just how high such intakes are, compared with requirements in other animals. Granted that humans are bipeds with a stressful lifestyle quite different from those of animals, there is no real evidence that human obligatory losses or sodium requirements are significantly greater. Rather, there is an ingrained tradition of regarding sodium intake as a benign pleasure, involving a harmless and healthy dietary constituent. The main warnings against this view come from the fact that hypertension is virtually unknown in low-salt cultures and that they do not even have an age-related rise in 'normal' blood pressure. Moreover, there are numerous studies that, when rigorously analyzed, indicate that human arterial pressure and salt intake are positively correlated; sufficiently to anticipate reductions in the prevalence of hypertension in response to manageable reductions in dietary sodium. Unfortunately, such reductions are still handicapped by inadequate food labeling and the fact that most sodium is added by the processor rather than the consumer. Humans, other than vegetarians, also have a very low potassium intake compared with other mammals; potassium may ameliorate the hypertensive effects of sodium.

Because obligatory losses of sodium are so low, dietary sodium depletion is hard to induce and sodium deficiency usually results from losses caused by renal, adrenal, or enteric disease; renal disease may cause either retention or loss of sodium. Globally, both in humans and animals, the most common cause of sodium deficits is acute diarrhea. Fortunately, sufficient gut usually remains unaffected for uptake of sodium and water to be stimulated by suitably formulated oral rehydration solutions. These essentially restore ECF volume (and acid–base balance), allowing natural defenses to overcome the underlying cause of the diarrhea. Despite some species variations, such solutions usually work best if their glucose:sodium ratio (in $mmol\,l^{-1}$) is close to unity and they are virtually isotonic (i.e., they have a similar osmotic concentration to ECF; hypertonic solutions draw water into the gut). The function of glucose in these solutions is to promote sodium uptake; its nutritional contribution is trivial. Anions such as citrate, acetate, propionate, bicarbonate, and amino acids (e.g., glycine and alanine) may further enhance the uptake of sodium and therefore water. These sodium cotransport mechanisms are very similar to those of the proximal renal tubule. More recently, nutritional oral rehydration solutions that provide calories and glutamine (to sustain the form and function of enteric villi) have been successfully used in calves.

Sodium is thus central to the management of two of the most widespread clinical problems; hypertension (in humans) and diarrhea. Indeed, the World Health Organization (WHO) regards the discovery of oral rehydration, which depends on restoration of enteric sodium uptake, as the main life-saving development in twentieth century medicine. This powerful clinical application rests on a simple physiological observation concerning an elementary but vital dietary constituent.

Unresolved Issues

The control of renal sodium excretion is understood in great detail but the regulation of body sodium is not; key questions remaining unresolved e.g., how ECF volume is monitored, granted that most is interstitial rather than intravascular, and how the mechanisms regulating ECF volume and arterial pressure are integrated, granted that both use renal sodium excretion as their effector. The fact is that none of the common forms of general edema, i.e., excess interstitial fluid, is amenable to rigorous explanation, except via abstractions such as 'effective blood volume.'

The key nutritional concern regarding sodium is the human dietary requirement, assuming that excess intake predisposes populations to an age-related rise in arterial pressure. This is regarded as normal but it is not seen in any population whose intake is closer to the likely requirement, compared with other mammals. For many individuals, this rise will ultimately destine them to antihypertensive therapy and predispose them to serious secondary hypertensive damage. While it is encouraging that governments are making serious attempts to reduce salt intake, it remains unlikely that it will be brought below $100\,mmol\,day^{-1}$, whereas if humans are like other mammals, requirement is unlikely to exceed $0.6\,mmol\,kg^{-1}\,day^{-1}$ i.e., $40\,mmol\,day^{-1}$ for a 70-kg human. Those who insist that human requirement is higher must provide evidence that human renal and colonic sodium conservation are uniquely inefficient or that the endocrine responses to lower salt intake, i.e., increased activity of the renin–angiotensin–aldosterone axis, diminished secretion of atrial natriuretic peptide and endogenous active sodium transport inhibitors, have pathological effects that outweigh moderation of the age-related rise of blood pressure.

See also: **Potassium**.

Further Reading

Avery ME and Snyder JD (1990) Oral therapy for acute diarrhea. *New England Journal of Medicine* **323**: 891–894.

Brooks HW, Hall GA, Wagstaff AJ, and Michell AR (1998) Detrimental effects on villus form and function during conventional oral rehydration for diarrhoea in calves: alleviation by a nutrient oral rehydration solution containing glutamine. *Veterinary Journal* **155**: 263–274.

Denton DA (1982) *The Hunger for Salt*. Berlin: Springer-Verlag.

El-Dahr SS and Chevalier RL (1990) Special needs of the newborn infant in fluid therapy. *Pediatric Clinics of North America* **37**: 323–335.

Field M, Rao MC, and Chang EB (1989) Intestinal electrolyte transport and diarrheal disease. *New England Journal of Medicine* **321**: 800–806; 819–824.

Hirschhorn N and Grenough WB (1991) Progress in oral rehydration therapy. *Scientific American* **264**: 16–22.

Law MR, Frost CD, and Wald NJ (1991) By how much does dietary salt lower blood pressure? *British Medical Journal* **302**: 811–815; 815–818; 819–824.

Michell AR (1994) The comparative clinical nutrition of sodium intake: lessons from animals. *Journal of Nutritional Medicine* 4: 363–369.

Michell AR (1995) *The Clinical Biology of Sodium.* Oxford: Elsevier Science.

Michell AR (1996) Effective blood volume: an effective concept or a modern myth? *Perspectives in Biology and Medicine* 39: 471–490.

Michell AR (1997) Pressure natriuresis, diurnal variation and long-term control of blood pressure: what is the baseline? *Perspectives in Biology and Medicine* 40: 516–528.

Michell AR (1998) Oral rehydration for diarrhoea; symptomatic treatment or fundamental therapy? *Journal of Comparative Pathology* 118: 175–193.

Michell AR (2000) Diuresis and diarrhoea: is the gut a misunderstood nephron? *Perspectives in Biology & Medicine* 43: 399–405.

Narins RG (1994) *Maxwell & Kleeman's Clinical Disorders of Fluid and Electrolyte Metabolism,* 5th edn. New York: McGraw-Hill.

Rutlen DL, Christensen G, Helgesen KG, and Ilebekk A (1990) Influence of atrial natriuretic factor on intravascular volume displacement in pigs. *American Journal of Physiology* 259: H1595–1600.

Salt Intake and Health

C P Sánchez-Castillo, National Institute of Medical Sciences and Nutrition, Salvador Zubirán, Tlalpan, Mexico
W P T James, International Association for the Study of Obesity/International Obesity Task Force Offices, London, UK

Introduction

This chapter describes the historical importance of salt use, its production and trade throughout the centuries, and its significance in food preservation, in flavor enhancement and in food processing. Over the years, man has developed complex salt mining and drying systems, which are still in use today as the demand for salt continues to grow. Humans and other animals, exposed throughout evolution to very limited salt sources, have developed an intrinsic biological drive for salt with salt-specific taste receptors and highly effective hormonal and cellular transport systems for minimizing any salt loss from the intestine, kidney, and skin. Unfortunately, the use of highly salted food then induces a series of physiopathological responses including changes in blood volume and hormonal and cellular changes, which lead, in conjunction with other dietary and environmental factors, to a range of disorders including high blood pressure with its increased risks of stroke, coronary heart disease, and heart failure. Excess salt intake also seem to promote the development of osteoporosis, gastric cancer, and bronchial reactivity. The relationship of salt intake to these conditions will be described and the options for limiting intakes will be outlined.

Occurrence in Nature

The terms salt, sea salt, or table salt relate primarily to the compound sodium chloride. Sodium is the sixth most abundant element in the Earth's crust, constituting 2.8%. Sodium is a reactive element and is always found in compound form. There is a huge variety of salts containing sodium and many of these are found in food but in most societies the dominant form of sodium is as sodium chloride. Sodium chloride is very soluble in water and in seawater comprises about 80% of the dissolved matter.

A History of Salt Intake

The fundamental drive to obtain salt can be traced back to the earliest times when humans evolved in a hot African environment with scarce sources of salt. Evidence has been found of salt use during the Neolithic Age, and the Egyptian, Babylonian and Chinese civilizations all had special culinary uses for salt that are well documented. In China, for centuries the production of salt was a major industry. Salt sources were highly valued and were often protected. A tax on salt in the form of a head tax provided the Chinese government with a reliable source of revenue from about 2200 BC onwards. For centuries the only method of extraction practiced by coastal salt-workers was to boil sea water and this technique was employed in every maritime province of China as late as 1830. Solar evaporation was also used; shallow salt fields were filled with seawater which was shifted from field to field daily until salt crystallization began. A third method used in areas either far from the sea or on higher ground involved digging wells to tap sea water or salt-enriched aquifers.

Evidence for the exploitation of saline slicks in the Austrian Tyrol dates from the Bronze Age and to this day the salt mines of Salzburg in Austria and Krakow, Poland are still in use. For the Indians in Central America salt was so precious that to please their gods they abstained from eating salt and Mexican civilizations offered sacrifices to the Goddess of Salt, Vixtocioatl. Arab cultures still offer salt to visitors as a sign that their guest is safe; even a

Bedouin robber will not violate the laws of hospitality once he has tasted his host's salt.

In pre-Roman times, the principal Italian road started at the salt works near the mouth of the Tiber River and cut through the Italian peninsula towards the Adriatic. In North Africa, the caravan route linked the salt oases, while salt roads were a feature of several South American countries. From remote parts of South America, such as the Amazon and Argentina, trails of more than 1500 km were linked to form the famous 'Cerro de Sal.' In the sixteenth century, sea salt crystals were traded from the sea through the Andes, gradually becoming more expensive further from the sea so that at distances of over 300 km only tribal chiefs used it. The common people made do with salt processed from palms and human urine. Salt from springs near Bogota was traded over a distance of 200 km to the north and south. Columbus' voyages were financed by the wealthy proprietors of the Mata Salt region of Spain, and when the first Spaniards arrived in South America in 1537, they found Indians exploiting local salt reserves on a large scale.

The financial structure of Venice was also substantially affected by the salt trade, which contributed to the emergence of Venetian capitalism and the vast fortunes of some Venetian merchants. In France, salt became a political issue in the fourteenth century; the tax on salt was the most hated of all taxes and a major issue prior to the French Revolution. At that time England, Germany, and Italy also taxed salt and in Britain the control of the world salt markets was a substantial contributor to its wealth in the seventeenth and eighteenth centuries. Liverpool, a minor tobacco port in the early eighteenth century, also became a major trading city in part due to its role in the salt trade.

During the earliest period of British rule in India the supply of salt was often tightly controlled and taxed. Gandhi emphasized the essential nature of common salt for human and animal well being, especially in a tropical country like India. Gandhi's 'salt march' to the sea broke the monopoly on salt use and led to his arrest and jailing. The following revolt, with 100 000 arrests, brought a change in the law to allow people to produce salt for their own use.

The production of salt currently depends on the same range of methods that have been used for centuries with substantial amounts being obtained by dry mining and with solution mining still involving water being pumped into rock salt deposits and the resulting brine being pumped back up to the surface for purification and evaporation. Solar evaporations, the oldest of the methods, is still used in hotter climates where salt pools allow the evaporation of sea water in the sun to produce salt. Currently, world salt production is over 210 million tons a year with 60% of the production being used to manufacture chlorine, caustic soda, and synthetic soda ash. About 20% of the world's production is for food use.

Salt in Food Technology

Salt enhances and modifies flavor, controls microbial growth, and alters nutrient availability and the texture/consistency of food. It also aids extraction methods, food formulation, and helps in the malting and fermenting of foods. In the production of some foods, e.g., pickles, cheese and fermented sausages, salt induces the withdrawal of water and various nutrients from the pickled tissue and provides an appropriate environment for growing the specific salt-resistant bacteria required for the fermentation or pickling process.

Sodium is also important in forming the texture of cheese, limiting bacterial growth and dehydrating cheese, thereby helping to form the rind. Most processed meats, e.g., ham and bacon, have added salt to season and cure the meat. Salt also inhibits bacterial growth and helps to emulsify the fat in sausages.

Sodium nitrate is used as a curing agent to prevent botulism as well as to provide the cured taste and red color of such meat products. Sodium polyphosphate is often added to poultry and fish fingers to increase their water-holding capacity and to bind the product. Salt is also effective in binding meat together by altering protein structures and dissolving some proteins. Salting fish has a flavoring and preservative role and fish may be treated in brine before being smoked.

In baking, salt enhances other flavors in the product; it also controls the rate of fermentation of yeast-leavened products and prevents the development of undesirable 'wild' types of yeast, which would lead to uncontrolled fermentation rates and variable products. Salt also strengthens the gluten in bread doughs, thus helping to ensure good dough handling and reducing the rate of water absorption. Sodium acid pyrophosphates are used in many industrial baking powders for specialty products. Salting of canned vegetables is primarily for flavor, but it can be used to separate mature, starchy green beans or peas, which will sink, from the younger, fresher beans, which float.

Processed 'snacks' are often heavily salted as a marketing feature, as are processed cereals and sodium-containing ingredients are added to many processed foods (**Table 1**), with sodium chloride

Table 1 Sodium-containing additives used in food processing

Additive	Use
Sodium citrate	Flavoring, preservative
Sodium chloride	Flavoring, texture preservative
Sodium nitrate	Preservative, color fixative
Sodium nitrite	Preservative, color fixative
Sodium tripoliphosphate	Binder
Sodium benzoate	Preservative
Sodium eritrobate	Antioxidant
Sodium propionate	Preservative
Monosodiumglutamate	Flavor enhancer
Sodium aluminosilicate	Anticaking agent
Sodium aluminum phosphate acidic	Acidity regulatory emulsifier
Sodium cyclamate	Artificial sweetener
Sodium alginate	Thickener and vegetable gum
Sodium caseinate	Emulsifier
Sodium bicarbonate	Yeast substitute

accounting for about 90% of the sodium used by the food industry.

Other Uses of Salt

The universal use of common salt has allowed it to be used as a vehicle for combating widespread iodine deficiency by fortifying the salt with iodine, and fluoride has also been added as a preventive measure against dental caries. Chloroquine or pyrimethamine salt mixtures have been used to suppress the sporozoites responsible for vivax malaria.

The Impact of Refrigeration on Salt Intakes

Salt intake varies widely across the world. Some agricultural communities, e.g., the Yanomano Indians from Brazil and the Chimbus of New Guinea, do not consume salt other than that found in natural food sources. The Kamtschadales and the Tungouses nomadic tribes from the north of Russia and Siberia are also averse to added salt, whereas the Japanese have traditionally consumed large quantities of salt in pickled salted fish and vegetables.

Without some form of food preservation it would be impossible to supply urban populations with food in any systematic way. Refrigerators were introduced on a mass scale from the 1960s onwards and this was accompanied by a fall in salt consumption in most countries (**Table 2**); refrigeration has taken over from salting as a method of preserving food. In Japan, intakes as high as the 60-g intake of a farmer recorded in 1955 and the average of 27–30 g day^{-1} had fallen dramatically to 8–15 g day^{-1} by 1988. In the US, salt intake probably

started to decline in the 1920s as refrigerators became widely available.

Dietary Exposure to Salt in the Young

Table 3 shows the average daily sodium intakes from food consumed by young people in the UK.

Changes in Mineral Composition of Food Induced by Industrialization and Urbanization

The process of industrialization and urbanization has affected the nutritional value of many of the more traditional foods as illustrated for Mexico in **Table 4**. Although home cooked corn (maize) tortillas, together with beans, formed the staple traditional diet, tortillas are now being produced differently: both industrially and by individuals at small market stalls in the cities.

The concentrations of the major nutrients sodium, potassium, calcium, magnesium, and phosphorus in unprocessed foods vary within narrow limits, but in processed or cooked foods, where salt (NaCl) or additions of other sodium-containing ingredients are common, the concentration range of sodium is higher. A large proportion of processed food has salt added; as more processed foods are eaten, the saltier the diet becomes. Table 4 shows that the corn in its original form contains a very small concentration of sodium but is rich in potassium. Once the grain is milled, fractionated, and processed to produce tortillas, then the nutrient composition alters. Potassium is also lost during the initial washing procedure. Limestone is added to release the niacin from its bound form; this also induces a threefold increase in calcium content. Salt is not commonly added during tortilla preparation in the country, but a remarkable 70- to 200-fold increase is found in breakfast cereals and processed corn snacks as well as substantial potassium losses. Almost no calcium is found in modern breakfast cereals whereas traditionally prepared tortillas have almost 60 times more calcium.

Salt and Disease

The Roman word from which the name 'salt' is derived is Salus, Goddess of Health. Gandhi argued that salt was "essential for human well being, specially in a poor country like India where its inhabitants eat vegetables and rice which contain low salt." However, although its name evokes health, over the years a long-term excess intake of salt has come to be recognized as a major cause of hypertension and thus a risk for stroke and coronary heart

Table 2 Salt intake as NaCl (g day^{-1})

Before 1982[a]	Year	Intake	From 1988[b]	Year	Intake
Communities not using added salt					
Brazil (Yanomano Indian)	1975	0.06			
New Guinea (Chimbus)	1967	0.04			
Solomon Island (Kwaio)		1.20			
Botswana (Kung Bushmen)		1.80			
Polynesia (Pukapuka)		3.60			
Alaska (Eskimos)	1961	<4.00			
Marshall Islands in Pacific		7.00			
Salt-using communities					
Kenya (Samburu nomads)		5–8	Mexico (Tarahumara Indians)		3–10
Mexico (Tarahumara Indians)	1978	5–8	Mexico rural, men[d]	1992	6.0
			Mexico rural, women[d]	1992	5.4
			Mexico urban, men[d]	1991	7.7
			Mexico urban, women[d]	1991	6.7
Denmark		9.8	Denmark	1988	8
Canada (New Foundland)		9.9	Canada		8–10
New Zealand		10.1			
Sweden (Gotenburg)		10.2			
USA (Evans County, Georgia)		10.6	USA (Chicago)		7.7
Iran		10.9			
Belgium	1966	11.4	Belgium	1988	8.4
UK (Scotland)		11.5			
UK[c]				1990	9
Australia		12.0			
India (North)		12–15	India		9–11.4
Federal Republic of Germany		13.1			
Finland (East)		14.3	Finland		10.6
Bahamas		15–30			
Kenya (Samburus, Army)	1969	18.6			
Korea		19.9			
Japan					
Japan (farmer)	1955	60.3	Japan	1988	8.15
Japan (Akita)		27–30			
Japan	1964	20.9			

[a]Source: INTERSALT Cooperative Research Group. INTERSALT and international study of electrolyte excretion and blood pressure. Results from 24 hour urinary sodium and potassium excretion. *Br Med J* 1988, **297**: 319.
[b]Source: Pietinen, P (1982) Estimating sodium intake from food consumption data. *Ann Nutr Metab*, **26**:90–99
[c]Gregoy J, Foster K, Tyler H, Wiseman M. The Dietary and Nutritional Survey of British Adults. *HMSO* (London, 1990).
[d]Sánchez-Castillo *et al.* (1996) Salt intake and blood pressure in rural and metropolitan Mexico. *Archives of Medical Research* **27**: 559–566.

Table 3 Sodium consumption in people aged 4–18 years in the UK

Age (years)	Males		Females	
	Sodium intake g day^{-1}(mmol day^{-1})	Estimated salt intake g day^{-1}	Sodium intake g day^{-1}(mmol day^{-1})	Estimated salt intake g day^{-1}
4–6	2.07 (90)	5.3	1.86 (81)	4.7
7–10	2.40 (105)	6.1	2.16 (94)	5.5
11–14	2.70 (118)	6.9	2.27 (99)	5.8
15–18	3.30 (142)	8.3	2.28 (99)	5.8

Source: Gregory J, Foster K, Tyler H, Wiseman M. The Dietary and Nutritional Survey of British Adults. *HMSO* (London, 1990).

Table 4 Effects of industrialization on the composition of Mexican foods

Food	Mineral content (mg per 100 g fresh weight)		
	Na	K	Ca
Corn	4	284	55
Tortilla (traditional)	11	192	177
Processed wheat tortilla	620	73	11
Breakfast cereals	866	101	3
Processed snacks	838	197	102
Beans			
Home cooked	14	470	67
Processed	354	371	26

Source: Sánchez-Castillo CP, Dewey PJS, Reid MD, Solano ML, and James WPT (1997) The mineral and trace element content of Mexican cereals, cereal products, pulses and snacks: preliminary data. *Journal of Food Composition and Analysis.* **10**: 312–333.
Sánchez-Castillo CP, Dewey PJS, Aguirre A, Lara JJ, Vaca R, León de la Barra P, Ortiz M, Escamilla I, and James WPT (1998) The mineral content of Mexican fruits and vegetables. *Journal of Food Composition and Analysis.* **11**: 340–356.

disease. An excess of dietary salt may also affect gastric cancer, osteoporosis, and bronchial hyper-reactivity. Evidence also suggests that high-salt intake causes left ventricular hypertrophy independently of blood pressure effects.

Salt Intake and Blood Pressure

When salt is ingested it is readily absorbed in the small intestine in association with other molecules such as glucose. The intestinal secretions also contain sodium at concentrations similar to those found in the plasma but the colon has a highly effective active transport system for absorbing practically all the sodium in the colonic contents; only about 1 mmol of sodium is normally excreted in the feces except in cases of severe diarrhea Once the sodium is absorbed the body ensures that the tonicity of the body fluids is finely maintained; so water is retained by the kidney and the blood volume tends to expand until the hormonal responses, e.g., from the atrial naturetic hormone (released in response to changes in atrial pressure) and in the renin-angiotensin system, lead to a fall in the kidney and sweat glands' reabsorption of sodium and therefore a greater sodium urinary excretion and loss in sweat. There are also adjustments in vasomotor tone and the neuronal responses as well as changes in the exchange of sodium and potassium across cellular membranes. The blood pressure then rises, as the kidney reflex demands a higher blood pressure in order to limit the body's extracellular volume expansion.

The degree to which the blood pressure rises in response to dietary salt depends on a range of interacting genetic factors and other environmental influences including the intake of potassium, magnesium, and calcium. The suppressive effects of these minerals in part explain the blood pressure-lowering effects of a diet rich in fruit and vegetables. Fat intakes have been shown to amplify resting blood pressures whereas moderately intense exercise is followed by a lower blood pressure. As fat intakes rise and physical activity falls in many modern societies the body weight and body fat of children and adults increase. The greater storage of fat leads to changes in a range of hormonal secretions from the fat cells including angiotensinogen, a precursor of the renin-angiotensin axis affecting the kidney's excretion of sodium. Adiponectin secretion from expanding adipocytes falls thereby making the blood vessels much more sensitive to plaque formation, medial hypertrophy, and fibrosis. Salt-induced increases in blood pressure also involve an array of other hormonal responses including the potent vasoconstrictor endothelin-1 and the vasodilator bradykinin, these being potentially involved in the blood pressure-independent effects of higher salt intake on arterial thickening, cardiac ventricular hypertrophy, and the synthesis of elastin and collagen in the artery. This makes them progressively thicker and less pliable.

Given this complex of interacting factors it is not surprising that the selective effect of salt intake on blood pressure has been hard to define. The role of salt in inducing high blood pressure is based on extensive animal experiments at the cellular and physiological level, on clinical studies and dietary intervention trials, as well as on major population analyses of blood pressure in relation to salt intake. Meta-analyses of longer term intervention trials to investigate the effect of salt reduction on hypertension also demonstrate that a modest reduction in salt intake has a significant effect on blood pressure in normotensive individuals and an even greater effect in those with pre-existing hypertension.

The response of neurohumoral mechanisms to salt loading varies in different individuals and for many years investigators sought to define what they termed 'salt-sensitive' individuals. There are rare genetic mutations associated with extreme salt sensitivity but within the general population there appears to be a more or less continuous variation in responsiveness consistent with multiple gene–environmental interactions. So perhaps it is not surprising that no clear cut-off points have been agreed for defining 'salt-sensitivity.' Patients with advanced renal failure do have an increased response of their blood pressure to salt loading but this is due to a loss of functioning nephrons.

Rural-urban differences in salt intake and blood pressure Migrant studies are useful in assessing the impact of environmental changes on blood pressure in different ethnic groups. Shaper's original study on Samburu men recruited from Kenyan villages to military camps was associated with a 12-mmHg increase in systolic blood pressure within weeks and similar findings were obtained in Ugandan villagers who had migrated to an urban environment. **Table 5** shows some of the differences between individuals living in their original Ugandan environment and those who had migrated to a more complex urban environment. The Ugandan analyses evaluated the rate of rise in blood pressure with age in the two communities and showed marked differences.

Beaglehole also found that the blood pressure of Polynesian children migrating to New Zealand rose simultaneously with dietary changes and this increase was not explained simply by an increase in body weight. More recent studies, e.g., in Mexico (**Table 6**), show the effect of migration on both

Table 5 Migration studies that assessed rural–urban differences in Uganda, Africa

	Villager	Migrant
Systolic blood pressure/age slope[a]	0.15	0.64
Urinary sodium (mmol l^{-1})[a]	82.4	108.6
Urinary potassium (mmol l^{-1})[a]	67.4	38.4

[a]Poulter, NR *et al.* (1990) The Kenyan Luo migration study: Observations on the initiation of a rise in blood pressure. *Br. Med. J.* **300**: 967–972.

Table 6 The urinary 24-h output of electrolytes and the associated blood pressure (BP) differences in rural and urban Mexico

	Men		Women	
	Rural (n = 24)	Urban (n = 19)	Rural (n = 54)	Urban (n = 58)
Sodium (mmol day^{-1})	103.3	133.1	93.3	114.7
Potassium (mmol day^{-1})	41.6	56.7	36.9	50.4
Sodium/potassium ratio	2.64	2.51	2.67	2.44
NaCl (g day^{-1})	5.99	7.72	5.41	6.65
Systolic BP (mmHg)	110.4	114.3	104.4	113.8
Diastolic BP (mmHg)	73.3	75.6	67.0	72.8
BMI	25.5	25.1	24.1	26.6

BP, blood pressure; BMI, body mass index.
From Sánchez-Castillo *et al.* (1996) Salt intake and blood pressure in rural and metropolitan Mexico. *Archives of Medical Research* **27**: 559–566.

sexes. Blood pressure rises in association with increases in urinary sodium but pottasium excretion also rises and the men show a decrease in BMI.

Conversely, Japanese people migrating to the US showed marked reductions in the prevalence of hypertension and stroke mortality consistent with the known markedly lower salt intake in association with other environmental changes in the US.

In all these analyses, several dietary changes as well as altered salt intake have occurred, e.g., in potassium and calcium intakes together with weight gain, altered intensities of physical activity, and doubtless psychosocial stress from entering an unfamiliar environment. Experimental, epidemiological, and clinical evidence suggests that dietary deficiencies of potassium or calcium potentiate the sodium induction of high blood pressure. Potassium loading prevents or ameliorates the development of sodium chloride-induced hypertension in several animal models and epidemiologically the ratio of urinary sodium to potassium (Na:K) is a stronger correlate of blood pressure than either sodium or potassium alone. Results of clinical trials also suggest that an increased potassium intake decreases blood pressure in patients with hypertension and the antihypertensive effect of potassium is more pronounced in persons consuming a high sodium chloride intake. With acculturation, primitive societies tend to increase their sodium intake and reduce the potassium content of their diet; therefore, the combination of a high potassium with a high salt diet is somewhat unusual. High potassium intakes were found, however, in the Aomori prefecture of Japan where there was a lower blood pressure and a reduced mortality from strokes despite high-salt intake.

There is also an inverse association within and among populations between dietary calcium and blood pressure. A low calcium intake may amplify the effect of a high sodium chloride intake on blood pressure, and calcium supplementation blunts this effect. High dietary calcium also preferentially lowers blood pressure or attenuates the development of hypertension in sodium chloride-sensitive experimental models.

Given all these dietary effects discerning the impact of salt intake changes as such is not easy. The migrant studies are crude compared with analyses of controlled dietary changes in the sodium intakes of volunteers. More robust analyses can also be obtained from the relationship between sodium intakes and blood pressure across a whole spectrum of different societies where account is taken of the possible effects of sodium intakes at different ages, of other dietary and environmental effects, as well as of differences in body size. The ability to reduce blood pressure by selectively limiting dietary sodium intake has also been assessed in a series of meticulous meta-analyses.

Genetic influences Primary hypertension has a well-known familial aggregation and has been calculated to be about 40% genetically determined. Children with a family history of hypertension are 30% more likely to remain in the upper quartile of systolic blood pressure than their peers. Young adults from families with hypertension have a greater rate of sodium excretion after a salt load than adults from normotensive families. Studies of twins also provide convincing evidence for a hereditary component to salt responsiveness. However, the effect of family history decreases with age as other environmental factors, e.g., weight gain, modify the risk. Studies have suggested that polymorphisms in certain genes, such as the angiotensinogen gene, might be implicated in the blood pressure response to a high-salt intake and genes whose products function prominently in the renin-angiotensin-aldosterone system are potential candidate genes contributing to essential hypertension. However, two meta-analyses assessed the relation of both insertion/deletion (I/D) polymorphisms of the angiotensin-converting enzyme (ACE) gene and the M235T angiotensinogen gene with primary hypertension and cardiovascular diseases and found no association with hypertension in ACE I/D gene polymorphism. Individuals homozygous for the deletion allele seem to have a higher risk of macrovascular and microvascular complications and the T allele encoding angiotensinogen may be a marker for hypertension, at least in white subjects, but great caution is needed before inferring that a single set of genes has a substantial impact on the development of higher blood pressures in response to increases in salt intake as so many neurohormonal mechanisms are involved.

Age-related changes in blood pressure In most populations, blood pressure increases with age but there are a few small groups who have not been exposed to modern environmental conditions and they do not show a rise in blood pressure with age. The Kuna indigenous population living on islands in the Panamanian Caribbean was among the first communities described showing almost no age-related rise in blood pressure or hypertension. Other populations in Africa, the Americas, Asia, and the Pacific region have the same characteristics. In many of these communities, the primary evidence that the protective factor is environmental rather than genetic was the blood pressure rise following migration to an urban environment. Among the many lines of evidence suggesting a role for salt

intake in the pathogenesis of hypertension, particularly compelling has been the identification of these isolated communities where salt intake is low, hypertension is rare, and blood pressure does not rise with age. Salt intake in such communities generally provided less than 40 mmol of sodium per day, and typically much less. The age-related rise is rare at mean sodium excretion rates of <100 mmol per day but clearly there are many other dietary and environmental differences.

Intersalt studies A major transnational study of over 10 000 men and women described the association between urinary excretion of sodium chloride (as a measure of salt intake) and blood pressure. After adjustments for body weight, alcohol intake, sex, and age, a higher sodium intake of $100 \, \mathrm{mmol \, day^{-1}}$ was linked with a systolic blood pressure rise of 3–6 mmHg in adults aged 40 years but one of 10 mmHg when aged 70 years. Updated results suggest that the association between sodium excretion and blood pressure is stronger when not adjusted for body weight, but the relationship is present whether or not the adjustment is made.

Figure 1 summarizes the relationships between sodium intake and blood pressure in the INTERSALT study. Different populations may show different responses depending on the host of other environmental factors that may be involved. The figure also illustrates the fact that individuals within any population may show very different effects and that appreciable changes in salt intake may be needed before a clear change in blood pressure is evident. Part of the problem in displaying the relationship arises from the difficulty in establishing what the prevailing blood pressure of individuals is given the remarkable variation in blood pressure during the day and night; difficulty also arises because it takes many complete 24-h urinary collections to obtain a reasonable estimate of the customary sodium intakes. The age-related incline also implies longer term amplification of the pathophysiological changes in hormonal controls and in blood vessel reactivity and plasticity; thus, as the blood pressure increases the tendency to further increase is enhanced in an accelerating process. This emphasizes the potential importance of early interventions when the blood pressure is tending to rise. It also implies that interventions to alter the diet of the young may be particularly valuable. This is borne out by the observation in the Netherlands that newborn babies fed a reduced salt content in their formula milk for the first 6 months of life had very much lower blood pressures when reassessed at the age of 15 years.

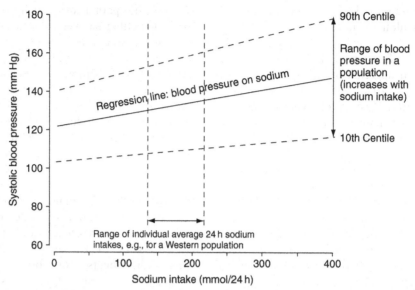

Figure 1 The relationships between sodium intake and blood pressure in the INTERSALT study. Adapted from: Frost CD, Law MR, Wald NJ (1991) Analysis of observational data within populations. *BMJ* **302**: 815–818.

Table 7 shows the estimated changes with age in blood pressures as the salt intake is increased by 100 mmol sodium per day. Epidemiologists concerned with the subtle but substantial population effects are mostly of the opinion that salt is an important causal factor in determining the steady increase in average blood pressure and the prevalence of hypertension in Western societies.

Adults with episodic high blood pressure, e.g., as a response to mental stress, have a greater tendency to develop persisting hypertension. The higher the blood pressure level becomes, the greater the further increase in blood pressure. Thus, the age-dependent increase in blood pressure may be a particularly important factor to measure in both individuals and the community.

On a population basis it has been estimated that in affluent societies, where average population blood pressures are high, a reduction of 2 mmHg in diastolic blood pressure would result in a 15% reduction in the risks of stroke and transient ischemic attacks and a 6% reduction in risk of coronary heart disease. There may also be a reduction independent of the effects on blood pressure on other conditions such as left ventricular hypertrophy.

A higher frequency of salt responsiveness has been observed in adults with hypertension. Estimates of the prevalence of this sensitivity have ranged from 29 to 60% in hypertensive populations and 15–46% in normotensive populations, although the larger studies have indicated that over 50% of a hypertensive population and approximately 25% of a normotensive population are clearly salt responsive. Longer term, e.g., 27-year-long, studies have shown that those with initially normal blood pressure but a marked responsiveness to salt had an increased risk of cardiological events and death as had those with pre-existing hypertension. In the absence of a consensus on defining either the genetic polymorphisms relating to hypertension or the parameters of salt sensitivity the greatest benefits are likely to be achieved by taking a population approach to reducing salt intake.

Table 7 Predicted change in systolic and diastolic blood pressure (mmHg) for each 100 mmol per 24 h change in sodium intake for various centiles of blood pressure distribution

Age (years)	Centile				
	5th	*20th*	*50th*	*80th*	*90th*
Systolic					
15–19	3	4	5	6	7
20–29	2	4	5	6	8
30–39	2	4	6	7	9
40–49	2	4	7	9	11
50–59	4	6	9	12	15
60–69	6	8	10	13	15
Diastolic					
15–19	1	1	2	2	3
20–29	1	2	3	3	4
30–39	1	2	3	4	5
40–49	2	3	4	4	5
50–59	2	3	5	6	7
60–69	2	3	4	6	7

From Law *et al.* (1991) By how much does dietary salt reduction lower blood pressure? III. Analysis of data from trials of salt reduction. *British Medical Journal* **302**: 819–824.

The most recent meta-analysis, which related to studies with modest salt reductions and a duration of at least 4 weeks, showed that there were 17 trials in hypertensives and 11 trials in normotensives for analysis. The combined and pooled estimates found significant reductions in blood pressure of 4.96/2.73 mmHg in hypertensives and 2.03/0.97 mmHg in normotensives, which on a population-wide basis are significant effects.

Recently, new diagnostic thresholds to define hypertension were made available in the Seventh Report of the Joint National Committee on Prevention, Detection, Evaluation, and Treatment of High Blood Pressure. A new category designated 'prehypertension' is defined as systolic blood pressure values between 120 and 139 mmHg and diastolic blood pressure values of 80 to 89 mmHg. Individuals within this group require health-promoting life-style modifications to prevent cardiovascular disease since they are at increased risk for progression to hypertension. The thresholds for stage 1 hypertension are blood pressure values of 140–159 mmHg (systolic) and 90–99 mmHg (diastolic) with stage 2 hypertension being defined when blood pressure values are ≥160 mmHg (systolic) and ≥100 mmHg (diastolic) values, respectively. Both categories require life style modifications as well as drug therapy. Individuals with diabetes, who are recognized as being at greater cardiovascular risk, should keep their blood pressure below 130/80 mmHg.

Salt reduction in pre-existing hypertension Salt deprivation became the major means of treating hypertension in the early part of the twentieth century. The low-salt diets were notoriously unpalatable so patients reduced their food intake and the consequent weight loss helped to reduce the blood pressure further. A large number of trials of salt restriction have been conducted since then on both hypertensive and normotensive subjects and the overall analyses show that the greater the initial blood pressure, the more marked the fall in blood pressure, particularly if the sodium intake reduction persists. These data have been interpreted to suggest that the effect of a universal moderate reduction in dietary salt would substantially reduce a population's mortality from stroke and ischemic heart disease with an impact far greater than that achieved by drug treatment of those with high blood pressure. Thus, the World Health Organization (WHO) and most national dietary guidelines now call for a lowering of salt intake to 5–6 g day⁻¹ on average or less.

More recently, two controlled intervention trials, the Dietary Approaches to Stop Hypertension (DASH) and the follow-up DASH sodium trial, compared three different types of eating patterns: (1) the 'control diet'; (2) extra fruit and vegetables; and (3) the 'DASH or combination diet,' which was lower in saturated fat, total fat, and cholesterol as well as having higher intakes of fruits, vegetables, and low-fat dairy products. All three eating plans used 3 g day⁻¹ sodium. The results of the clinical trials found that the combination diet or 'DASH diet' decreased systolic blood pressure (SBP) by 11.4 mmHg below the control diet and decreased diastolic blood pressure (DBP) by 5.5 mmHg in adults with hypertension. In adults without hypertension the decreases were 3.5 mmHg (SBP) and 2.1 mmHg (DBP).

When the selective effects of salt were examined without weight changes then reducing the salt intake from 9 to 3 g significantly reduced blood pressure by 6.7/3.5 mmHg on the controlled diet and on the higher potassium DASH diet by 3.0/1.6 mmHg. Thus, the combined effects of the DASH diet and low-salt intake on blood pressure were greater than either of the interventions alone. With this combination, mean SBP was 11.5 mmHg lower in participants with pre-existing hypertension, and 7.1 mmHg lower in participants without hypertension. The effects were observed in both sexes and across racial groups. The Seventh Report of the Joint National Committee on Prevention, Detection, Evaluation and Treatment of High Blood Pressure in the USA and the Scientific Advisory Committee on Nutrition from the Food Standards Agency, Department of Health in the UK have acknowledged that the clear and distinct effect of salt on blood pressure shown in the trial indicates that lowering salt intake as part of a healthy whole diet strategy would be most effective as a population-based approach to lowering blood pressures.

Gastric Cancer and Stroke

There is a strong geographical correlation between stomach cancer and stroke mortality, both of which correlate with salt intake. There are four recognized major etiological factors for gastric adenocarcinoma: infection with *Helicobacter* pylori, excessive salt consumption, and low intakes of ascorbic acid, carotenoids or more generically of vegetables and fruits. Sodium chloride induces atrophic gastritis and enhances the mutagenic effect of nitrosated foods. Salt may also play a role in the later steps involving the transformation of mucosal dysplasia to carcinoma. The salted pickles and salted fish of

Japanese cultures appear to be strongly linked to the development of stomach cancers.

Osteoporosis

It has been known for many years that sodium intake is one of the major determinants of urinary calcium excretion. It has been estimated that urinary calcium losses increase by approximately 1 mmol per 100 mmol sodium intake. Experimentally sodium intake increases calcium excretion but also induces markers of bone resorption. It is hypothesized that trabecular demineralization may occur, leading to postmenopausal changes and an increased risk of vertebral fractures and cortical erosions. Further research is required in this area.

Bronchial hyper-reactivity

There have been no large-scale epidemiological studies, but a positive relationship between asthma mortality and regional purchases of table salt per person has been shown. In a randomized double-blind crossover trial in subjects with moderately severe asthma, the airway response to histamine was related to urinary excretion of sodium in a dose-response way, but only in men. A low-salt diet is regarded as having a potentially positive effect in patients with asthma and may help to reduce the need for anti-asthma drugs.

Sources of Salt Intake

Various approaches to measuring the daily salt intake in individuals have been tried. Salt comes from: (1) natural products; (2) salt added during industrial processing; (3) salt from catering; (4) other sodium-containing sources; (5) discretionary use of salt in cooking and table salt; and (6) sodium in drinking water. Traditional methods of estimating salt intake, e.g., with economic data, lead to marked errors and usually substantial overestimates. These have now been replaced by more modern methods.

Estimating Salt Intakes

The principal and most accurate method for estimating sodium intake is to measure sodium excretion rates in individuals who are asked to collect one or more complete 24-h urinary outputs. To measure absolute amounts a marker for completeness of collections is required. Measurement of intake from dietary assessment methods alone is considered unreliable. Until recently, however, there was no way of establishing how much of the 24-h sodium intake was derived from different sources, without the use of traditional weighing and analytical methods. A new technique involving the use of lithium has allowed a new approach; this method involves fusing Li_2Co_4 (used as a tracer) with NaCl. One preliminary 24-h collection and three full 24-h urinary collections are required.

Gains and Losses of Salt during Cooking

Only a small proportion of the salt added to water for cooking foods is eaten. A value of 24% was obtained by the lithium method for the average intake per head of the 'purchased' cooking salt used in cooking in the UK. The only other data using traditional methods come from Hungary where 41% of the salt purchased by households was actually ingested.

Assessment of Total Discretionary Salt Use

Figure 2 compares the traditional and lithium marker techniques for assessing both total salt intake and the distribution of its sources. When table and cooking salt are combined to form a single value, the percentage contribution of these discretionary sources to the total intake measured by the lithium marker technique is significantly lower in the UK compared with that assessed by traditional methods, which do not consider salt losses during cooking and at the table. This intake in the UK seemed unusually low, but when discretionary sources (table and cooking salt) were assessed in various regions of Italy using the lithium marker technique, discretionary salt intake varied between 31 and 41% of total intake. In rural Benin the use of discretionary sources in women was higher (52%) and in rural Guatemala was as much as 77% of total intake. Thus, the more industrialized the food system the greater the proportion of nondiscretionary salt intake, which then makes it more difficult for individuals to reduce their salt intake. In Japan, salt is ingested in large amounts as pickled and salted fish and vegetables but these distinctive items may be considered discretionary sources of salt. Similarly, there are specific discretionary salted meat and vegetable extracts that are used for flavoring in Western societies.

Traditional data on table salt use are given in **Table 8** and new estimates in **Table 9**.

Pore Size in Salt Cellars

The pore size and hole number is important in determining the amount of salt actually shaken onto food. Smaller shaker hole areas lead to a marked fall in salt consumption, for example, to about a quarter of the maximum value.

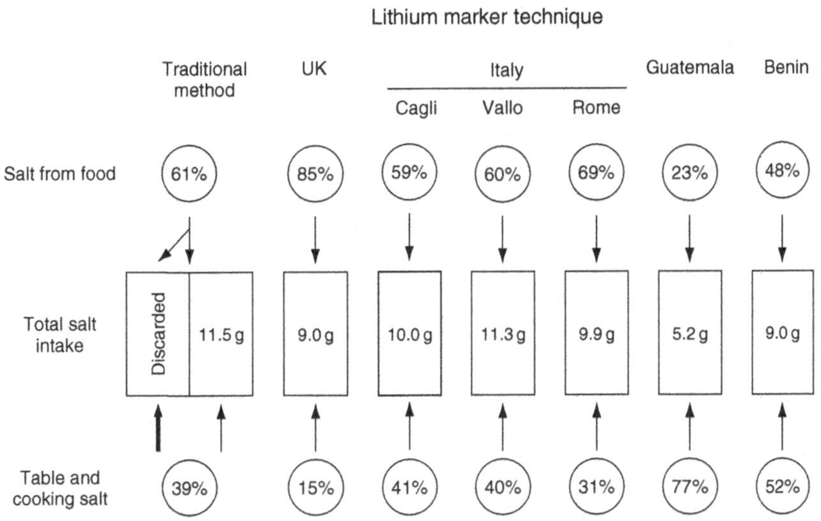

Lithium marker technique

Figure 2 The assessment of total discretionary salt use. (Data from Sánchez-Castillo CP, Branch WJ, and James WPT (1987) A test for the validity of the lithium-marker technique for monitoring dietary sources of salt in man. *Clinical Science* **72**: 87–94; Leclerq C and Ferro-Luzzi A (1991) Total and domestic consumption of salt and their determinants in three regions of Italy. *European Journal of Clinical Nutrition* **45**: 151–159; Melse-Boonstra A, Rozendaal M, Rexwinkel H, Gerichhausen MJ, van den Briel T, Bulux J, Solomons NW, and West CE (1998) Determination of discretionary salt intake in rural Guatemala and Benin to determine the iodine fortification of salt required to control iodine deficiency disorders: studies using lithium-labeled salt. *American Journal of Clinical Nutrition* **68**: 636–641.)

Table 8 Sources of dietary salt in different countries assessed by traditional methods (grams per head per day)

Country	Total	Nondiscretionary sources			Discretionary table/or cooking
		Natural	Processing	Catering	
England	9.5		7.9		1.6
UK	9.7	0.9	5.7	–	3.1
UK	11.7	8.1[a]	–	1.6[a]	2.0
Sweden	11.1	1.0	5.3	–	4.8
USA	14.5	–	8.0	–	6.5
Finland	12.6	1.5	5.3	1.0	4.8
Finland	10.7	1.4	4.7	–	4.6
Finland	11.7	–	7.4	–	4.3
Mexico (State)					7.0

[a]Some cooking salt is included in this value for food consumed at home. For catering and table salt use, a value has been added.

Implications of the Salt-Disease Relationships in Relation to Population and Individual Strategies for Improving Health

A population-based approach to reducing disease by reducing salt intake is a public health strategy directed at the whole population rather than those individuals considered to be at high risk. Such a strategy is based on the observation that a small reduction in risk of a large number of people may result in a large reduction in risk

Table 9 Estimates of the use of table salt

Subjects	Number of subjects	Salt intake (grams per head per day)		
		Total	Table salt	Table salt as % total
Men				
White and black[a]	24	9.8–16.5	1.5 (0.3)	9–15
White[b]	3	11.0	0.44	4
Black[b]	3	8.9	0.27	3
White[d]	33	10.6	1.6 (1.0)[c]	11
Women				
White and black[a]	13	4.4–4.9	0.9 (0.3)	18–20
White[b]	3	6.4	0.64	10
Black[b]	4	6.5	0.13	2
White[d]	50	7.4	0.73 (0.74)[c]	10
White adolescents	8	7.4	0.95	13
Family studies[e]	15	11.7	1.35[c]	11.6

[a]Total intake of the subjects was varied systematically in a metabolic ward.
[b]Salt intake assessed with the use of a dietary history and food model.
[c]Value based on the use of normal, not lithium-tagged salt. Where necessary values are recalculated to give the mean (SD).
[d]Study conducted in England; all other studies conducted in the US.
[e]A complex and less satisfactory approach was used.
Reproduced with permission from James WPT *et al.* (1987) The dominance of salt in manufactured food in the Sodium intake of affluent societies. *Lancet* **1**: 426–429.

for the entire population. This does not mean, however, that individualized strategies cannot be used to help individuals considered at high risk because of pre-existing hypertension. Indeed, the greater reductions in blood pressure in hypertensives on reducing salt intake imply that there should be a special focus on this vulnerable group. So, ideally, both strategies are needed: the whole population strategy because the risk from cardiovascular disease associated with higher blood pressures is not confined to those who are considered clinically hypertensive, but includes large numbers of people in the upper 'normal' blood pressure range. Furthermore, many surveys in different countries show that a large proportion of hypertensives are not in receipt of any treatment. This emphasizes the value of dealing with a population that overall may be at a relatively high risk of premature mortality. Such measures should cause a downward shift in the population distribution of blood pressure, which would also benefit high-risk groups.

Individualized Approaches

Hypertensives can take steps to reduce their salt intake by modifying their diets. If these individuals come from societies where a substantial amount is eaten as discretionary salt then those responsible for adding salt to the cooking either in the home or in catering establishments need to be persuaded to take progressive measures to limit salt use and substitute herbs and other flavors. Individuals can also be asked to eliminate the addition of salt at the table but this can only make a minor contribution in most cases to reducing their salt intake. In theory it is possible for patients to select foods low in salt but this usually means selecting relatively unprocessed foods. Multimineral mixes may also be found to be more acceptable for use in households as these are a mix of different salts with, for example, the addition of potassium and calcium salts to the sodium chloride thereby both diluting the amount of sodium used and adding elements that counter the sodium's effects. Theoretically, food labels can be used to choose lower salted foods but this needs far too much sophisticated understanding for most consumers. The simplest test of an individual's ability to alter their diet and reduce salt intake by avoiding salted and pickled foods, heavily salted breads, prepared meats and snacks is to check their urinary excretion of sodium. The great difficulty in permanently changing diets is shown by longer term analyses of intervention studies, which reveal very modest long-term reductions in urinary sodium.

This emphasizes the need for population approaches such as that developed in Finland where children were taught at school how to select less salted foods and to alter the use of salt in cooking within the home. There was also a multi-pronged drive to persuade catering organizations and restaurants to limit the salt in cooking and the food manufacturing sector was persuaded to alter their product composition and limit salt addition as well as altering their fat and fatty acid content. As a result of these measures the average systolic blood pressure of the adults of North Karelia in Finland fell by 10 mmHg over a 15-year period and this was accompanied by a dramatic fall in stroke and coronary artery disease deaths of over 75%, helped substantially by the simultaneous falls in the average total blood cholesterol levels of the population.

The importance of altering the salt content of foods, especially bread, which is often a major source of salt, was shown in Portugal where a village baker was persuaded to reduce the salt content of his bread. Two years later the average blood pressure of the villagers was significantly lower than that of a neighboring village where no changes had been made.

Thus, governments have a major role in persuading their health services to take a systematic approach to reducing salt in hospital foods and to engage in systematic patient and public health educational initiatives. The problem is that the salt industry and other sectors of the food industry often do their utmost to contest the evidence and find reasons why they should not progressively reduce the salt content of their products. We need to see major improvements in food labels and a traffic light-type warning system so that high-salt products can readily be identified. Several countries are embarking on the exercise of defining high-salt foods and taking steps to counteract the tendency for some soft drink companies to over-salt their snack food products so that they stimulate thirst and increase demand for their drinks! Only when countries follow the Finnish lead can we expect to see an appreciable fall in salt intake and a concomitant reduction in hypertension rates and cardiovascular disease.

Conclusions

Evidence suggests that sodium intake is an important determinant of blood pressure in the population as a whole, and influences the rise in blood pressure with age. The predominant source of salt varies from country to country. In the UK, for example, the greatest potential effect involves reducing the salt content of manufactured food. A different public health approach would apply to Italy, where discretionary intake of salt is two to three times greater than that of the UK and for Guatemala where intakes from these sources are high.

See also: **Calcium**. **Potassium**. **Sodium**: Physiology.

Further Reading

Appel LJ, Moore PJ, Obarzanek E, Vollmer WM, Svetkey LP, Sacks FM, Bray GA, Vogt TM, Cutler JA, Windhauser MM, Lin PH, and Karanja N (1997) A clinical trial of the effect of dietary patterns on blood pressure. DASH Collaborative Research Group. *New England Journal of Medicine* 336: 1117–1124.

Denton D (1982) *The Hunger for Salt.* New York: Springer-Verlag.

Dietary Sodium and Health (1997) *American Journal of Clinical Nutrition* 65(supplement) 2.

Elliot P, Stamler J, Nichols R, Dyer AR, Stamler R, Kesteloot H, and Marmot M (1996) Intersalt revisited: further analyses of 24 hour sodium excretion and blood pressure within and across populations. *British Medical Journal* 312: 1249–1253.

Frost CD, Law MR, and Wald NJ (1991) By how much does dietary salt reduction lower blood pressure? II. Analysis of observational data within populations. *British Medical Journal* 302: 815–818.

Hanneman RL (1996) Intersalt: hypertension rise with age revisited. *British Medical Journal* 312: 1283–1284.

James WPT, Ralph A, and Sanchez-Castillo CP (1987) The dominance of salt in manufactured food in the sodium intake of affluent societies. *Lancet* 1: 426–429.

Joint National Committee on Prevention, Detection, Evaluation and Treatment of High Blood Pressure (2003) The Seventh Report of the Joint National Committee on Prevention, Detection, Evaluation and Treatment of High Blood Pressure. *Journal of the American Medical Association* 289: 2560–2572.

Law MR, Frost CD, and Wald NJ (1991) By how much does dietary salt reduction lower blood pressure? 1. Analysis of observational data among populations. *British Medical Journal* 302: 811–815.

Law MR, Frost CD, and Wald NJ (1991) By how much does dietary salt reduction lower blood pressure? III. Analysis of data from trials of salt reduction. *British Medical Journal* 302: 819–824.

Leclerq C and Ferro-Luzzi A (1991) Total and domestic consumption of salt and their determinants in three regions of Italy. *European Journal of Clinical Nutrition* 45: 151–159.

MacGregor GA and He FJ (2002) Effect of modest salt reduction on blood pressure: a meta-analysis of randomized trials. Implications for public health. *Journal of Human Hypertension* 16: 761–770.

Melse-Boonstra A, Rozendaal M, Rexwinkel H, Gerichhausen MJ, van den Briel T, Bulux J, Solomons NW, and West CE (1998) Determination of discretionary salt intake in rural Guatemala and Benin to determine the iodine fortification of salt required to control iodine deficiency disorders: studies using lithium-labeled salt. *American Journal of Clinical Nutrition* 68: 636–641.

Multhauf RP (1978) *Neptune's Gift.* Baltimore and London: The John Hopkins University Press.

Sacks FM, Svetkey LP, Vollmer WM, Appel LJ, Bray GA, Harsha D, Obarzanek E, Conlin PR, Miller ER 3rd, Simons-Morton DG, Karanja N, and Lin PH (2001) Effects on blood pressure of reduced dietary sodium and the Dietary Approaches to Stop Hypertension (DASH) diet. DASH-Sodium Collaborative Research Group. *New England Journal of Medicine* 344: 3–10.

Scientific Advisory Committee on Nutrition: Food Standards Agency and the Department of Health (2003) *Salt and Health.* Her Majesty's Stationery Office, London.

Sánchez-Castillo CP, Branch WJ, and James WPT (1987) A test for the validity of the lithium-marker technique for monitoring dietary sources of salt in man. *Clinical Science* 72: 87–94.

Sánchez-Castillo CP, Solano ML, Flores J, Franklin MF, Limon N, Martinez del Cerro V, Velazquez C, Villa A, and James WPT (1996)Salt intake and blood pressure in rural and metropolitan Mexico. *Archives of Medical Research* 27: 559–566.

Sánchez-Castillo CP, Warrender S, Whitehead T, and James WPT (1987) An assessment of the sources of dietary salt in a British population. *Clinical Science* 72: 95–102.

SPORTS NUTRITION

R J Maughan, Loughborough University, Loughborough, UK

Introduction

At an international Consensus Conference held at the offices of the International Olympic Committee in 1991, a small group of experts agreed a consensus statement that began with the opening statement: "Diet significantly influences exercise performance." This is a bold and unambiguous statement, leaving little room for doubt. However, the statement went on to add various qualifications to this opening statement. These qualifications reflect the uncertainties in our current knowledge, but are also a consequence of the many different issues that arise in considering the interactions between diet and performance and the diverse needs of athletes in different sports. In the years since that statement was formulated, the world of sport has advanced, with new world records and new champions. The world of science has also moved forward and there have been some important advances in our understanding of the interactions between nutrition and sports performance.

In considering the role of diet in the athlete's life, two main issues must be considered, each of which gives rise to many subordinate questions. The first question is how the demands of training affect the body's requirement for energy and nutrients: this then has implications for body composition (including the body content of fat, muscle, and bone), for the hormonal environment and the regulation of substrate metabolism, and for various disease states that are affected by body fatness, nutrient intake, and other related factors. The second question is how nutritional status influences the responses to and the performance in competition.

Athletes should be encouraged to follow eating plans that maximize the extent of recovery between training sessions, maximize the effectiveness of the adaptations that occur in response to each training session, and minimize the risk of illness and injury that might interrupt training or prevent participation in competition. This involves identification of each athlete's nutritional goals and the formulation of an eating strategy that will allow those goals to be met. There will be special issues in the period before and during competition that will influence nutrition needs, and separate dietary strategies will be necessary for training and for competition.

Nutrition for Training

The training load of athletes varies greatly between individuals, depending on the nature of the sport and the level of competition, and it also varies over time in relation to the competitive season. Training may consist of high-intensity resistance training, brief but intense sprints, prolonged moderate intensity efforts, or technical work. Each places different demands on the muscles, cardiovascular system, and other tissues, and each has different energy requirements. The aim of training is to induce changes in body tissues and organs that will improve exercise performance, but different adaptations are required in different sports. Increasing muscle mass, strength, and power is a key objective in many sports, but in other sports, these changes would hinder, rather than help, performance. The training stimulus, therefore, must be specific to the objectives of the event. Within limits, the greater the training stimulus – consisting of the intensity, duration and frequency of individual training sessions – the greater the adaptation that takes place. As mentioned above, nutrition is important in promoting recovery between training sessions to allow an increase in the training load that can be sustained without succumbing to illness and injury, and also in allowing more effective adaptations to each bout of training. This may be important in complex sports such as soccer, where different training objectives must be achieved and where the training must also accommodate practice of a variety of skills.

Influence of Exercise Training on Energy Balance

Energy must be supplied by the diet to meet immediate energy needs (body functions, energy for activity, and growth) and for the maintenance of body energy stores. Energy stores, consisting primarily of fat, but including the key carbohydrate stores in liver and muscle, play a number of important roles related to exercise performance, since they contribute to size and function (e.g., muscle mass) as well as providing fuel for exercise. Athletes try to manipulate these factors towards the characteristics that offer advantages to their sport: this may mean a change in body mass, a change (usually a reduction) in body fat, a change (usually an increase) in muscle mass, and optimization of muscle and liver carbohydrate stores.

Not all athletes are able to correctly identify goals that are suitable for their sport and for their individual make-up. This can lead to various problems, including excessive restriction of energy intake in an attempt to achieve an unrealistically low body mass. If energy intake is too low, and especially if carbohydrate intake is inadequate, it may not be possible to sustain the training load without the risk of chronic fatigue, injury and illness. If an energy deficit is incurred, it may lead to changes in metabolic and hormonal function, which affect performance, growth and health. One outcome of low energy availability in female athletes is a disturbance of reproductive function and menstrual regularity. Other problems are likely to occur in male athletes. There is a real danger that the focus on achieving a specific body mass and body composition, may become more important than achieving success in competition.

Monitoring of body mass can provide a useful index of energy balance in some situations, but other biomarkers are generally better. Measurement of body fat stores, usually by measurement of skinfold thickness, can be helpful in setting targets and in monitoring progress. Other markers, such as measurement of urinary ketone levels, can identify athletes who are failing to achieve an adequate carbohydrate intake. Problems are most likely to occur when the energy expenditure is either very high or very low. Athletes with very high energy demands are likely to be training at least twice per day, leaving limited opportunities for eating the large amounts of foods that are necessary. Athletes with low energy demands and who must restrict energy intake to achieve a low body mass have two main problems: they must cope with constant hunger and they must also be careful in their selection of foods to ensure that they achieve an adequate intake of essential nutrients.

An athlete's energy requirements are set primarily by the training load and by body mass, although there is also a large interindividual variability even when these factors are constant. Measurements of oxygen uptake, heart rate, and other variables made after exercise show that the metabolic rate may remain elevated for at least 12 h and possibly up to 24 h if the exercise is prolonged and close to the maximum intensity that can be sustained. After more moderate exercise, the metabolic rate quickly returns to baseline level. Therefore, it seems likely that the athlete training at near to the maximum sustainable level and who already has a very high energy demand will find this increased further by the elevation of postexercise metabolic rate: this will increase the difficulties that many of these athletes have in meeting their energy demand. The recreational exerciser, for whom the primary stimulus to exercise is often to control body mass or reduce body fat content, will not exercise hard enough or long enough to experience substantial elevations of metabolic rate after exercise.

Macronutrient Demands

Protein

The idea that protein requirements are increased by physical activity is intuitively attractive, and high-protein diets are a common feature of the diets of sportsmen and women. The available evidence shows an increased rate of oxidation of the carbon skeletons of amino acids during exercise, especially when carbohydrate availability is low. Protein contributes only about 5% of total energy demand in endurance exercise, but the absolute rate of protein breakdown is higher than at rest (where protein contributes about the same fraction as the protein content of the diet, i.e., typically about 12–16%) because of the higher energy turnover. It is often recommended that athletes engaged in endurance activities on a daily basis should aim to achieve a protein intake of about 1.2–1.4 g kg^{-1} day^{-1}, whereas athletes engaged in strength and power training may need as much as 1.6–1.7 g kg^{-1} day^{-1}. Those who take no exercise have an estimated average requirement of about 0.6 g kg^{-1} day and the recommended intake for these individuals is about 0.8–1.0 g kg^{-1} day.

In strength and power sports such as weightlifting, sprinting and bodybuilding, the use of high-protein diets and protein supplements is especially prevalent, and daily intakes in excess of 2–4 g^{-1} kg^{-1} are not unusual. Scientific support for such high intakes is generally lacking, but those involved in these sports are adamant that such high levels of intake are necessary, not only to increase muscle mass but also to maintain muscle mass. This apparent inconsistency may be explained by Millward's adaptive metabolic demand model, which proposes that the body adapts to either high or low levels of intake, and that this adjustment to changes in intake occurs only very slowly. This means that individuals such as strength and power athletes who consume a high-protein diet over many years will find that any reduction in protein intake will result in a loss of muscle mass. This is because of an upregulation of the activity of the enzymes involved in protein oxidation to cope with the high intake: activity of these enzymes remains high when there is a sudden decrease in intake, leading to a net catabolic effect.

Protein synthesis and degradation are both enhanced for some hours after exercise, and the net effect on muscle mass will depend on the relative magnitude and duration of these effects. Several recent studies have shown that ingestion of small amounts of protein (typically about 35–40 g) or essential amino acids (about 6 g) either before or immediately after exercise will result in net protein synthesis in the hours after exercise, whereas net negative protein balance is observed if no source of amino acids is consumed. These observations have led to recommendations that protein should be consumed immediately after exercise, but the control condition in most of these studies has involved a relatively prolonged (6–12 h) period of fasting, and this does not reflect normal behavior. Individuals who consume foods containing carbohydrate and proteins in the hour or two before exercise may not further increase protein synthesis if additional amino acids or proteins are ingested immediately before, during, or after exercise.

Various high (30%) protein, high (30%) fat, low (40%) carbohydrate diets have been promoted for weight loss, and some diets even suggest almost complete elimination of carbohydrate from the diet. Some of these diets have been specifically targeted at athletes, accompanied by impressive claims and celebrity endorsements. Proposed mechanisms of action of these diets include reduced circulating insulin levels, increased fat catabolism, and altered prostaglandin metabolism, but it seems more likely that these diets achieve weight loss simply by restricting dietary choice. These diets can be effective in promoting short-term weight loss, primarily by restricting energy intake (typically to 1000–2000 kcal day^{-1}). There is no evidence to support improvements in exercise performance, and what evidence there is does not support the concept.

Carbohydrate

Carbohydrate is an essential fuel for the brain, red blood cells, and a few other tissues. Fat and carbohydrate are the main fuels used for energy supply in muscle during exercise. In low-intensity exercise, most of the energy demand can be met by fat oxidation, but the contribution of carbohydrate, and especially of the muscle glycogen, increases as the rate of energy demand increases. Carbohydrate oxidation rates of $3-4\,\mathrm{g\,min^{-1}}$ may be sustained for several hours by athletes in training or competition. When the glycogen content of the exercising muscles reaches very low levels, the work rate must be reduced to a level that can be accommodated by fat oxidation. In high-intensity exercise, essentially all of the energy demand is met by carbohydrate metabolism. Therefore, repeated short sprints place high demands on the muscle carbohydrate store, most of which can be converted to lactate within a few minutes.

Carbohydrate is stored in the body in the form of glycogen, primarily in the liver (about $70-100\,\mathrm{g}$ in the fed state) and in the skeletal muscles (about $300-500\,\mathrm{g}$, depending on muscle mass and preceding diet). These stores are small relative to the body's requirements for carbohydrate. Carbohydrate supplies about 45% of the energy in the typical Western diet. This amounts to about $200-300\,\mathrm{g\,day^{-1}}$ for the average sedentary individual, and is adequate for normal daily activities. In an hour of hard exercise, however, up to $200\,\mathrm{g}$ of carbohydrate can be used, and sufficient carbohydrate must be supplied by the diet to replace the amount used. Replacement of the glycogen stores is an essential part of the recovery process after exercise: if the muscle glycogen content is not replaced, the quality of training must be reduced, and the risks of illness and injury are increased. Low muscle glycogen levels are associated with an increased secretion of cortisol during exercise, with consequent negative implications for immune function.

When rapid recovery is a priority, replacement of carbohydrate should begin as soon as possible after exercise with carbohydrate foods that are convenient and appealing. Thereafter, the diet should supply sufficient carbohydrate to replace the amount used in training and to meet ongoing demands of other tissues. Some recommendations for carbohydrate intake after training or competition are shown in **Table 1**. For athletes preparing for competition, a reduction in the training load and the consumption of a high-carbohydrate diet in the last few days are recommended. This maximizes the body's carbohydrate stores and should ensure

Table 1 Suggested carbohydrate intakes for athletes in training

Immediate postexercise recovery (0–4 h): 1 g per kg body mass per h, consisting of several small snacks
Daily recovery (moderate duration/low intensity training): $5-7\,\mathrm{g\,kg^{-1}\,day^{-1}}$
Daily recovery (moderate–heavy endurance training): $7-12\,\mathrm{g\,kg^{-1}\,day^{-1}}$
Daily recovery (extreme training: 4–6 h or more per day): $10-12\,\mathrm{g\,kg^{-1}\,day^{-1}}$

optimum performance, not only in endurance activities, but also in events involving short-duration high-intensity exercise and in field games involving multiple sprints.

The high-carbohydrate diet recommended for the physically active individual coincides with the recommendations of various expert committees that a healthy diet is one that is high in carbohydrate (at least 55% of energy) and low in fat (less than 30% of energy). However, where energy intake is either very high or very low, it may be inappropriate to express the carbohydrate requirement as a fraction of energy intake. With low total energy intakes, the fraction of carbohydrate in the diet must be high, but the endurance athlete with a very high-energy intake may be able to tolerate a higher fat intake. Recommendations, as in **Table 1**, should be framed in absolute amounts relative to body mass, i.e., grams of carbohydrate per kilogram body mass.

The type of carbohydrate eaten is less important than the amount. It is valuable to choose nutrient-rich carbohydrates and to add other foods to recovery meals and snacks to provide a good source of protein and other nutrients. The presence of small amounts of protein in recovery meals may promote additional glycogen recovery when carbohydrate intake is less than optimal or when frequent snacking is not possible. Protein taken at this time may also stimulate protein synthesis in muscles, as described above. Carbohydrate-rich foods with a moderate to high glycemic index (GI) provide a readily available source of carbohydrate for glycogen synthesis, and should be the major fuel choices in recovery meals.

Fat

Fat is an important metabolic fuel in prolonged exercise, especially when the availability of carbohydrate is low. One of the primary adaptations to endurance training is an enhanced capacity to oxidize fat, thus sparing the body's limited carbohydrate stores. Studies where subjects have trained on high-fat diets, however, have shown that a high-carbohydrate diet during a period of training brings about greater improvements in performance. Even when a high-carbohydrate diet is fed for a few days to allow normalization of the muscle glycogen stores before exercise performance is measured, the exercise capacity remains less after training on a high fat diet. It must be recognized, though, that these short-term training studies usually involve relatively untrained individuals and may not reflect the situation of the highly trained elite endurance athlete where the capacity of the muscle for oxidation of fatty acids will be much higher. For the athlete with very high levels of energy expenditure in training, the exercise intensity will inevitably be reduced to a level where fatty acid oxidation will make a significant contribution to energy supply and fat will provide an important energy source in the diet. Once the requirements for protein and carbohydrate are met, the balance of energy intake can be in the form of fat.

Fat also serves other important functions in the diet. As well as providing essential fatty acids, it acts as a vehicle for the transport of fat-soluble nutrients. Some athletes try to minimize their fat intake, but this is not wise.

Micronutrients and Physical Activity

Many micronutrients play key roles in energy metabolism, and high rates of energy turnover (up to 20–100 times the resting rate) may be required in the active muscles during hard exercise. Although an adequate vitamin and mineral status is essential for normal health, marginal deficiency states may only be apparent when the metabolic rate is high. Prolonged strenuous exercise performed on a regular basis may also result in increased losses from the body or in an increased rate of turnover, resulting in the need for an increased dietary intake. An increased food intake to meet energy requirements will increase dietary micronutrient intake, but not all athletes have high-energy intakes. Athletes who restrict food intake to control or reduce body fat levels may have low-energy intakes over prolonged periods. Athletes may also eat monotonous diets, with a limited range of foods, thus increasing the risk of an inadequate micronutrient intake. Supplementation with micronutrients may be warranted in some instances, but normally only where specific deficiencies have been demonstrated by biochemical investigations and where dietary modification is not an option. Individuals who are very active may need to pay particular attention to their intake of iron and calcium.

Iron deficiency anemia affects some athletes engaged in intensive training and competition, but it seems that the prevalence is the same in athletic and sedentary populations, suggesting that exercise *per se* does not increase the risk. The implications of even mild anemia for exercise performance are, however, significant. A fall in the circulating hemoglobin concentration is associated with a reduction in oxygen-carrying capacity and a decreased exercise performance. Low serum ferritin levels are not associated with impaired performance, however, and iron supplementation in the absence of frank anemia does not influence indices of fitness. Routine iron supplementation is not wise, as too much may be harmful.

Osteoporosis is now widely recognized as a problem for both men and women, particularly so in women, and an increased bone mineral content is one of the benefits of participation in an exercise program. Regular exercise results in increased mineralization of those bones subjected to stress and an increased peak bone mass may delay the onset of osteoporotic fractures; exercise may also delay the rate of bone loss. Estrogen plays an important role in the maintenance of bone mass in women, and prolonged strenuous activity may result in low estrogen levels, causing bone loss. Many very active women also have a low body fat content and may also have low energy (and calcium) intakes in spite of their high activity levels. All of these factors are a threat to bone health. The loss of bone in these women may result in an increased predisposition to stress fractures and other skeletal injury and must also raise concerns about bone health in later life. It should be emphasized, however, that this condition appears to affect only relatively few athletes, and that activity is generally beneficial for the skeleton.

Water and Electrolyte Balance

Few situations represent such a challenge to the body's homeostatic mechanisms as that posed by prolonged strenuous exercise in a warm environment. Only about 20–25% of the energy available from substrate catabolism is used to perform external work, with the remainder appearing as heat. At rest, the metabolic rate is low: oxygen consumption is about $250\,\text{ml}\,\text{min}^{-1}$, corresponding to a rate of heat production of about 60 W. Heat production increases in proportion to metabolic demand, and reaches about 1 kW in strenuous activities such as marathon running (for a 70-kg runner at a speed that takes about 2.5 h to complete the race). To prevent a catastrophic rise in core temperature, heat loss must be increased correspondingly and this is achieved primarily by an increased rate of evaporation of sweat from the skin surface. In hard exercise under hot conditions, sweat rates can reach $3 \, l \, h^{-1}$, and trained athletes can sustain sweat rates in excess of $2 \, l \, h^{-1}$ for many hours. This represents a much higher fractional turnover rate of water than that of most other body components. In the sedentary individual living in a temperate climate, about 5–10% of total body water may be lost and replaced on a daily basis. When prolonged exercise is performed in a hot environment, 20–40% of total body water can be turned over in a single day. In spite of this, the body water content is tightly regulated, and regulation by the kidneys is closely related to osmotic balance.

Along with water, a variety of minerals and organic components are lost in variable amounts in sweat. Sweat is often described as an ultrafiltrate of plasma, but it is invariably hypotonic. The main electrolytes lost are sodium and chloride, at concentrations of about $15–80 \, mmol \, l^{-1}$, but a range of other minerals, including potassium and magnesium, are also lost, as well as trace elements in small amounts. Some athletes may lose up to 10 g of salt (sodium chloride) in a single training session, and may train in these conditions twice per day. These substantial salt losses must be replaced from foods and drinks, though the use of salt supplements is seldom necessary.

Failure to maintain hydration status has serious consequences for the active individual. A body water deficit of as little as 1–2% of total body mass can result in a significant reduction in exercise capacity. Endurance exercise is affected to a greater extent than high-intensity exercise, and muscle strength is not adversely affected until water losses reach 5% or more of body mass. Hypohydration greatly increases the risk of heat illness, and also abolishes the protection conferred by prior heat acclimation.

Many studies have shown that the ingestion of fluid during exercise can significantly improve performance. Adding carbohydrate to the fluid confers an additional benefit by providing an energy source for the working muscles. Addition of small amounts (perhaps about 2–8%) of carbohydrate in the form of glucose, sucrose, or maltodextrin will promote water absorption in the small intestine as well as providing exogenous substrate that can spare stored carbohydrate. The addition of too much carbohydrate will slow gastric emptying and, if the solution is strongly hypertonic, may promote secretion of water into the intestinal lumen, thus delaying fluid availability. Voluntary fluid intake is seldom sufficient to match sweat losses, and palatability of fluids is therefore an important consideration. It is not necessary to consume enough fluid during exercise to match sweat losses, as a body mass deficit of 1–2% is unlikely to have adverse consequences. If exercise is prolonged and sweat losses high, the addition of sodium to drinks may be necessary to prevent the development of hyponatremia. Ingestion of large volumes of plain water is also likely to limit intake because of a fall in plasma osmolality leading to suppression of thirst.

Replacement of water and electrolyte losses incurred during exercise is an important part of the recovery process in the postexercise period. This requires ingestion of fluid in excess of the volume of sweat lost to allow for ongoing water losses from the body. Re-establishment of water balance requires replacement of solute, especially sodium, losses as well as volume replacement. If food containing electrolytes is not consumed at this time, electrolytes, especially sodium, must be added to drinks to prevent diuresis and loss of the ingested fluid.

Dietary Supplements

The use of nutritional supplements in athletes and in the health-conscious recreationally active population is widespread, as it is in the general population. A very large number of surveys have been published. A meta-analysis of 51 published surveys involving 10 274 male and female athletes of varying levels of ability showed an overall prevalence of supplement use of 46%, but the prevalence varied widely in different sports, at different levels of age, performance etc., and in different cultural backgrounds.

Many different supplements are used by athletes with the aim of improving or maintaining general health and exercise performance. In particular, supplement use is often aimed at promoting tissue growth and repair, promoting fat loss, enhancing resistance to fatigue, and stimulating immune function. Most of the supplements that are sold to athletes have not been well researched, and both safety and efficacy remain open to question for many of these products. Anyone seeking to improve health or performance would be better advised to ensure that they consume a sound diet that meets energy needs and contains a variety of foods. A recent development of concern to athletes is the finding of various prohibited doping agents in what should be legitimate sports nutrition products. Supplements for which there is good evidence of beneficial effects on performance include caffeine, creatine, and bicarbonate, but the risk of an inadvertent positive doping result must always be considered.

See also: **Anemia**: Iron-Deficiency Anemia.
Carbohydrates: Requirements and Dietary Importance;
Resistant Starch and Oligosaccharides. **Fatty Acids**:
Metabolism; Monounsaturated; Omega-3
Polyunsaturated; Omega-6 Polyunsaturated; Saturated;
Trans Fatty Acids. **Supplementation**: Role of
Micronutrient Supplementation; Developing Countries.

Further Reading

American College of Sports Medicine, American Dietetic Association, and Dietitians of Canada (2000) Joint Position Statement: Nutrition and athletic performance. *Medical Science in Sports and Exercise* 32: 2130–2145.

Ivy J (2000) Optimization of glycogen stores. In: Maughan RJ (ed.) *Nutrition in Sport*, pp. 97–111. Oxford: Blackwell.

Kiens B and Helge JW (1998) Effect of high-fat diets on exercise performance. *Proceedings of the Nutrition Society 57*: 73–75.

Maughan RJ (1999) Nutritional ergogenic aids and exercise performance. *Nutrition Research Reviews* 12: 255–280.

Maughan RJ, Burke LM, and Coyle EF (eds.) (2004) *Foods, Nutrition and Sports Performance*, vol. 2. London: Routledge.

Maughan RJ and Murray R (eds.) (2000) *Sports Drinks: Basic Science and Practical Aspects*. Boca Raton: CRC Press.

Millward DJ (2001) Protein and amino acid requirements of adults: current controversies. *Canadian Journal of Applied Physiology* 26: S130–S140.

Nieman DC and Pedersen BK (1999) Exercise and immune function. *Sports Medicine* 27: 73–80.

Noakes TD and Martin D (2002) IMMDA-AIMS advisory statement on guidelines for fluid replacement during marathon running. *New Studies in Athletics* 17: 15–24.

Shirreffs SM and Maughan RJ (2000) Rehydration and recovery after exercise. *Exercise and Sports Science Reviews* 28: 27–32.

Wolfe RR (2001) Effects of amino acid intake on anabolic processes. *Canadian Journal of Applied Physiology* 26: S220–S227.

SUPPLEMENTATION

Contents

Developed Countries

M F Picciano, National Institutes of Health, Bethesda, MD, USA
S S McDonald, Raleigh, NC, USA

A dietary supplement is a product that is intended to supplement the diet and contains at least one or more of certain dietary ingredients, such as a vitamin, mineral, herb or other botanical, or an amino acid. These products may not be represented as conventional foods; rather, they are marketed in forms that include capsules, tablets, gelcaps, softgels, and powders. Although manufacturers must have evidence to support their claims of a dietary supplement's safety and efficacy, US Food and Drug Administration (FDA) approval is not required before a product is marketed. Micronutrient dietary supplements (vitamins and minerals for purposes of this discussion) are commonly purchased and consumed in developed countries, even though taking greater quantities of micronutrients than recommended may not have proven benefits for the general population and, for some micronutrients (e.g., vitamin A), may have harmful effects. It may seem logical to assume that the majority of people who live in developed countries can use food sources to obtain the amounts of micronutrients required to maintain overall good health. However, the possibility of helping to prevent chronic diseases through micronutrient supplementation is attracting the interest of many people. A rigorous research approach must be used to determine in what circumstances micronutrient dietary supplements can have beneficial, including preventive, health effects. Special attention must be given to possible differences in micronutrient requirements at different life cycle stages. These stages include infancy (birth to 12 months), childhood (1–18 years), adulthood, and older adulthood (70 years and older). Evidence supporting dietary supplementation at different lifestyle stages is summarized here for several micronutrients.

Prevalence of Micronutrient Supplement Use

In the United States, vitamins and minerals are the most widely used dietary supplements. Between 1993 and 2003, total retail sales of vitamins and minerals more than doubled, increasing from approximately $3 billion to $6.7 billion for vitamins and from approximately $0.6 billion to $1.8 billion for minerals. These figures include sales of multivitamin and multimineral combinations as well as individual vitamins and minerals. Multivitamin/mineral preparations, accounting for almost half of micronutrient purchases, consistently have been the best-selling micronutrient supplements, with sales increasing from $2.64 billion in 1997 to $3.68 billion in 2003.

Findings by several research groups show that micronutrient supplement use generally is more common among people with higher education levels, higher incomes, and better diets. Survey results in The Netherlands indicate that micronutrient supplements are used by approximately 20% of adults in that country, fewer than in the United States. Data collected in the 1988–1994 National Health and Nutrition Examination Survey (NHANES III) showed that approximately 40% of the US population 2 months of age and older (44% females versus 35% males) were taking a vitamin, mineral, or other type of dietary supplement during the month before the NHANES III interview. Data from NHANES 1999–2000 (post-DSHEA) indicate that 52% of U.S. adults were taking at least one dietary supplement. Supplement users were more likely to be toddlers and preschool-aged children and middle-aged and older adults. Across all age groups, vitamin/mineral combinations and multivitamins were the most common types of supplements used by individuals who took only one supplement. Collection of these type of data is important to monitor use, identify usage trends, and help understand the popularity of micronutrient supplement use.

Motivation for Micronutrient Supplement Use

People choose to use micronutrient supplements for various reasons. Survey data indicate that many individuals decide to take micronutrient supplements based on advice from health professionals, family, and friends. A majority of supplement users regard micronutrient supplements as 'insurance' against general poor health or becoming ill, even though they recognize that scientific evidence for this belief may be lacking. Generally, people report that they use supplements either because they think that it is difficult to consume a balanced diet or because they believe that even consuming a balanced diet cannot supply the quantity of micronutrients they need for optimal good health.

Major health reasons given for taking supplements include a sense of well-being and 'feeling better' (especially multivitamins/minerals), preventing colds and flu (especially vitamin C), preventing chronic disease (especially vitamin E and calcium), increasing 'energy,' coping with stress, and improving the immune system. Many vitamin E users believe that the vitamin helps prevent heart disease, and most calcium users know that calcium use helps prevent osteoporosis. Using micronutrient supplements is one way by which people who may be at high risk for certain diseases try to gain some degree of personal control over their health outcomes. Ironically, many individuals who take supplements regularly report that they do not discuss the supplement use with their physicians because they believe that physicians are biased against supplements and are not knowledgeable about the products.

Research Approach for Determining the Health Impact of Micronutrient Supplements

A micronutrient supplement will be beneficial to a person's health only when the person's normal dietary micronutrient intake is lower than the amount required for maximum biological benefit. Every person does not have the same micronutrient requirements. The amount of micronutrients required by any person is determined by metabolic, genetic, and environmental factors unique to that person. It may not be readily apparent when micronutrient supplements are needed by certain groups of people. Therefore, as new information becomes available, recommendations for supplementation must be revised. For example, it was observed that pregnant women with periconceptual folate intake at the low end of the range of recommended intake, which was still considered adequate, had an increased risk of giving birth to an infant with neural tube defects (NTDs) such as spina bifida. NTDs originate during the first 4 weeks of pregnancy, before a woman may even realize that she is pregnant. United States survey data (1988–1994) indicated that typical dietary folate intake by women of reproductive age was less than the 400 μg/day believed to be required to reduce the risk of NTDs. Therefore, in 1992, the Centers for Disease Control and Prevention recommended that all women who could become pregnant should take a daily 400 μg folic acid supplement as a preventive measure. In addition, the FDA mandated that, as of January 1998, enriched grain products must be fortified with folic acid, adding an estimated 100 μg folic acid/day to the average diet of US women. Fortification refers to adding nutrients to commonly consumed foods at levels greater than the levels that are part of the standards of identity for the foods; other examples of fortification are vitamin D in milk and calcium in orange juice.

Any recommendations for supplementation must be based on scientific evidence that the supplements are both effective and safe. Ideally, a rigorous systematic research approach (**Table 1**) is carried out and the results are evaluated to assess whether a micronutrient supplement is beneficial to health and whether its recommendation is warranted. All available evidence, including epidemiologic and survey data, as well as preclinical evidence from in vitro laboratory research and in vivo animal studies, is reviewed thoroughly and objectively to determine whether the evidence regarding effectiveness and safety justifies proceeding to clinical trials. If so, the trials are normally conducted in three phases: (1) human safety trials; (2) small efficacy trials, usually in defined target groups; and (3) large-scale trials that are essential in moving from the basic science to evidence-based recommendations that have human health benefits. In fact, the large-scale, double-blind, randomized, placebo-controlled clinical trial, which is designed to eliminate all possible bias, is considered to be the gold standard of scientific intervention research. In such trials, some people receive the substance being tested (e.g., drug, micronutrient, or other dietary constituent) and

Table 1 Components of a research approach to evaluate dietary micronutrient supplements

Basic biomedical laboratory research
  In vitro experiments (e.g., in cell culture and tissue culture)
  In vivo animal experiments (e.g., in mice and rats)
Human observational epidemiologic studies to identify possible links between micronutrients and nutrition/health status (includes surveys of micronutrient intake)
Hypothesis development: Evaluation of existing laboratory and epidemiologic evidence on micronutrient safety and effectiveness as related to human health benefits (decision point: proceed or do not proceed)
If proceeding
  Human safety trials to identify adverse side effects and determine safe doses
  Small trials in defined populations to measure micronutrient effectiveness at various safe doses (e.g., vitamin D supplementation in elderly Scandanavians with low serum 25-hydroxy-vitamin D)
  Large-scale, double-blind, placebo-controlled, randomized clinical intervention trials to test whether micronutrient supplementation has the hypothesized human health benefit
After health benefits are confirmed, develop recommendation for supplementation

some receive an inactive placebo. These trials may not be possible in all circumstances, however, because of ethical issues that make it inappropriate to withhold the substance being tested from any trial participants. For example, now that it is established that low periconceptual folate intake by women is linked to NTDs, a placebo-controlled intervention trial to test the minimum effective supplemental amount would be unethical. In such cases, all available evidence from in vitro laboratory research and in vivo animal studies, as well as epidemiologic studies and surveys, must be reviewed systematically and objectively to draw conclusions about the possible effectiveness and safety of the substance of interest and to make recommendations for supplementation. However, convincing evidence is currently unavailable to indicate that lowering homocysteine through folate and other vitamin (vitamin B-6 and B-12) supplementation will reduce risk of CVD. A number of randomized, placebo-controlled clinical trials are on-going to test the effects of vitamin supplementation on primary and secondary prevention of CVD and stroke.

Research to determine a possible impact of micronutrient supplements on the nutritional status and health status of people has been under way for many years. Considerable preclinical evidence related to human health effects from in vitro laboratory research and in vivo animal studies exists for many micronutrients. In addition, many epidemiologic studies throughout the world have focused on the possible relationship between specific micronutrients and chronic disease. Small clinical studies related to chronic disease also have been carried out for many micronutrients, and human safety data are available for most micronutrients. A comprehensive review of epidemiologic studies and randomized controlled trials of vitamin supplementation to prevent either cancer or cardiovascular disease (CVD) was conducted by the US Preventive Services Task Force. The Task Force concluded that findings did not demonstrate a consistent or significant effect of any single vitamin or combination of vitamins on either incidence of CVD or death from this disease. Also, the Task Force concluded that β-carotene supplements and combinations including β-carotene appeared to be harmful to those at risk for lung cancer but not to the general population.

Important issues to be addressed in research aimed at determining the effects of micronutrient supplements on health include developing better methods to measure the contribution of micronutrient supplements to total micronutrient intake for various population groups and to monitor these contributions over time to identify usage trends. Having accurate data for micronutrient supplement intake and intake trends is essential to help identify possible associations between supplements and health outcomes; such associations can then be tested for validity in future randomized, controlled trials. Collecting data to measure and ultimately monitor consumer use of micronutrient supplements can be expensive and time-consuming, however, particularly if detailed data are required. Currently, in the United States, NHANES interviewers collect the most detailed information about micronutrient supplement intake, including data on supplement brand, labeled ingredients, dose, and frequency of dose. Available dietary supplement databases are based on values declared on product labels rather than direct analysis. Evidence suggests, however, that supplement labels may not always give the true supplement content; this can decrease the accuracy of survey results.

A major concern associated with clinical trials designed to evaluate the health effects of micronutrients (as well as other dietary supplements and drugs) is that participants might take additional micronutrient supplements, which could influence trial outcomes. In the Prostate Cancer Prevention Trial (PCPT) of the drug finasteride, for example, almost half of the participants reported using a multivitamin/mineral supplement, about one-third used single supplements of either vitamin C or E, and one in five used calcium supplements. Very little evidence is available on how individual micronutrient substances may interact with one another to influence health outcomes. For minerals, particularly, supplementation with one mineral may compromise the bioavailability of another. Also, much remains to be learned about how individual genetic susceptibilities may influence the health-related effects of micronutrient supplements. This issue also must be addressed when designing clinical trials.

Evidence Supporting Recommendations for Micronutrient Supplement Use

Importance of Life Cycle

Evaluation of existing evidence related to effects of micronutrient supplements on nutrition and health, aimed at formulating recommendations for supplementation, must take into account the influence of a person's stage of life and general health status on the absorption, usefulness, and need for any particular micronutrient. Physiological needs for specific micronutrients and, consequently, for micronutrient supplements differ at various stages in the life cycle. For example, infants require additional iron after 6 months of age, women who may become pregnant benefit from additional folate, and elderly people who lose their ability to absorb naturally occurring vitamin B_{12} in food require an alternative source of the vitamin. When studies are designed to investigate the relationship between micronutrient supplements and specific health outcomes, the outcomes that are chosen to be measured usually depend on the specific life cycle stage of the study participants. For any life cycle stage, a person's genetic makeup and lifestyle behaviors will also influence his or her individual micronutrient requirements (**Figure 1**).

Infants

Iron Iron is a component of a number of proteins including hemoglobin, which is essential for transporting oxygen to tissues throughout the body for use in metabolic processes. The most well-known consequence of iron deficiency is anemia. A full-term infant normally has a high hemoglobin

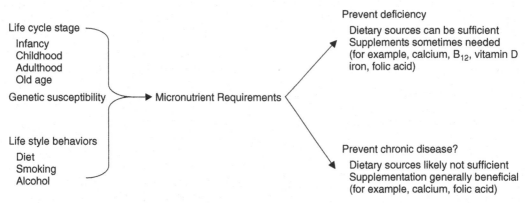

Figure 1 Factors that influence micronutrient requirements.

concentration and a large amount of stored iron. Based on research evidence, this stored iron plus the iron provided in human milk is assumed to be adequate for solely breast-fed infants during the first 6 months after birth. Even though the amount of iron in human milk is low, its bioavailability is greater (>50%) than that of the iron in infant formula (<12%). The body stores of iron in infants decrease during the fourth through sixth months after birth. After 6 months of age, most of the infant's iron needs must be met from food intake. In Western countries, the primary food introduced after 6 months is infant cereal, usually fortified with iron that has low bioavailability. Evidence suggests that infants benefit from iron supplementation after 6 months, and that administration of iron drops between 6 and 9 months has a significant influence on iron status. The American Academy of Pediatrics (AAP) discourages using low-iron infant formulas. AAP recommends that infants who are not breast-fed or who are only partially breast-fed should receive an iron-fortified formula from birth to 12 months of age.

Vitamin D Vitamin D enhances the efficiency of the small intestine to absorb calcium and phosphorus from the diet and thus helps to maintain normal serum levels of these minerals. Vitamin D deficiency in infants and children results in inadequate mineralization of the skeleton, causing rickets, which is characterized by various bone deformations. The major source of vitamin D is its formation in the skin as a result of exposure to sunlight. Dietary sources include fortified foods, such as milk and cereals, and certain fish. Infant formula is fortified with vitamin D in many countries. Because human milk contains only low amounts of vitamin D, breast-fed infants who do not receive either supplemental vitamin D or adequate exposure to sunlight are at risk for developing vitamin D deficiency. Subclinical vitamin D deficiency can be assessed by measuring serum 25-hydroxyl-vitamin D; deficiency occurs months

before rickets is obvious on physical examination. Rickets in infants continues to be reported in the United States as well as in other countries. Epidemiologic evidence indicates that African American infants and children are more likely to develop nutritional rickets than Caucasian infants and children. In the US, the AAP recommends that all breastfed infants receive a daily supplement of 200 IU vitamin D/day, beginning within the first two months of life, unless they are weaned to at least 500 mL per day of vitamin D-fortified formula (<1 year old) or milk (>1 year old).

Children

Calcium Bone is a dynamic tissue that is constantly being formed and resorbed; in children, bone formation is greater than resorption. Adequate calcium intake during childhood is essential for bone mass development. Data for calcium intake, presented in **Table 2**, indicate that for children in the United States, only those younger than 8 years of age are meeting their recommended intake. Factors that may contribute to low calcium intake are restriction of dairy products, low vegetable consumption, and high intake of low-calcium beverages such as juices and sodas. The highest calcium intake levels are required during the preteen and adolescent years to support the rapid growth and bone mineralization associated with pubertal development. In girls, peak calcium absorption and deposition takes place at or near menarche; at this life cycle stage, the bone calcium deposition rate is five times greater than that in adults. During peak bone mass development, calcium intakes of less than 1000 mg/day are associated with lower bone mineral density. Epidemiologic studies have found a direct correlation between calcium intake and bone density in children. Evidence suggests that low intake of dairy products during childhood and adolescence may result in less bone mass and greater risk of fracture as an adult. In addition, evidence from randomized trials suggests that increasing the calcium intake of girls is

Table 2 Average calcium intake and recommended adequate intake levels for US children

	Age/gender					
	1–3 years/ M and F	4–8 years/ M and F	9–13 years/ F	9–13 years/ M	14–18 years/ F	14–18 years/ M
Average intake (mg)	793	838	918	1025	753	1169
Adequate intake (mg)	500	800	1300	1300	1300	1300

F, female; M, male.
From Institute of Medicine (1997) *Dietary Reference Intakes for Calcium, Phosphorus, Magnesium, Vitamin D, and Fluoride.* Washington, DC: National Academy Press.

associated with increased bone mineral deposition, especially during prepuberty. Although it is best to obtain as much calcium as possible from foods, because calcium-rich foods also provide nutrients involved in calcium utilization, calcium supplements may be necessary for children who do not eat calcium-rich foods.

Adults

Vitamin E Vitamin E (α-tocopherol) functions as an antioxidant that promotes normal formation of red blood cells and normal function of the nervous and immune systems. The main dietary sources of vitamin E are vegetable oils; normally, it is possible, unless people consume a very low-fat diet, to obtain amounts of vitamin E intake from foods that are sufficient to prevent signs of deficiency. However, vitamin E is a commonly consumed supplement, likely because of its hypothesized role in decreasing risk of CVD, prostate cancer, and various other chronic diseases.

Evidence from epidemiologic studies suggests that vitamin E supplementation is beneficial for reducing CVD risk. Nevertheless, data from randomized clinical trials, in populations both with and without a history of CVD, generally do not support the epidemiologic findings. The review of evidence by the US Preventive Services Task Force included five well-designed, large cohort studies that investigated the association between vitamin supplementation and CVD mortality, three clinical trials of primary prevention of CVD, and seven clinical trials of secondary prevention of cardiac events. As stated earlier, the Task Force concluded that findings did not demonstrate a consistent or significant effect of vitamin E on either incidence of CVD or death from this disease. Four large clinical trials are currently in progress in the United States to study the effect on CVD of vitamin E supplements alone or combined with other antioxidants: the Women's Health Study, the Women's Antioxidant and Cardiovascular Study, the Physicians' Health Study II, and the Heart Protection study.

Laboratory studies suggest that vitamin E can inhibit the growth of human prostate cancer cell lines. Results of epidemiologic studies, however, do not consistently support a beneficial effect of vitamin E on risk for prostate cancer. Findings from the Alpha-Tocopherol, Beta-Carotene Cancer Prevention (ATBC) study, a large, randomized clinical trial conducted in Finland, suggest a substantial benefit of vitamin E in decreasing prostate cancer risk. This study reported a decrease of 32% in prostate cancer incidence and a decrease of 41% in deaths from prostate cancer among current and former

male smokers who received supplemental vitamin E (50 mg/day). Additional information on the relationship between vitamin E supplementation and prostate cancer likely will be available from the Prostate Cancer Prevention Trial (PCPT), which was stopped in June 2003 when analysis showed that the test drug, finasteride, reduced the risk of developing prostate cancer by 25%. In PCPT, 35% of the study population took vitamin E supplements, and study analyses will include interactions between vitamin E and other supplements and between vitamin E and finasteride. The Selenium and Vitamin E Prevention Trial (SELECT), described later, is also expected to help clarify the association between vitamin E and prostate cancer.

Selenium Selenium, a strong antioxidant, also shows other biological activity, such as enhancing the immune response and inhibiting cell growth. Laboratory and epidemiologic studies support a beneficial effect of selenium on cancer risk. In a large clinical trial, selenium supplementation did not prevent the recurrence of nonmelanoma skin cancer, but it did significantly decrease the total number of deaths and deaths from cancer. In addition, the incidences of prostate, colorectal, and lung cancers all were significantly decreased in the group that received selenium supplements. These findings and the results of the ATBC study linking vitamin E supplementation with decreased prostate cancer risk led to the development of SELECT. Started in 2001, SELECT is a randomized, double-blind trial designed to test whether selenium (200 µg/day) alone, vitamin E (400 mg/day) alone, or selenium and vitamin E combined reduce the risk of prostate cancer among healthy men. Men who join SELECT are required to stop taking any purchased vitamin supplements that contain either selenium or vitamin E. An ongoing intervention trial in France, the Supplementation en Vitamines et Mineralaux AntioXydants (SU.VI.MAX) study, is testing nutritional levels of both selenium and vitamin E, as well as vitamin C, β-carotene, and zinc, for reducing incidence of cancer and CVD. In addition to cancer and CVD, French researchers are investigating a possible beneficial role for selenium in arthritis and HIV/AIDS.

Folate Folate, a B-complex vitamin, includes the naturally occurring form found in foods as well as the synthetic form (folic acid) found in fortified foods and supplements. The rationale for the recommendation that all women who may become pregnant should take a daily 400 µg folic acid supplement, a preventive measure to reduce the risk of NTDs, has already been discussed. Folate intake is important throughout pregnancy because of its key role in nucleic acid synthesis, which is essential for cell growth and replication.

A deficiency of folate, vitamin B_{12}, or vitamin B_6 may increase the level of homocysteine, an amino acid normally found in the blood. Evidence indicates that a high homocysteine level increases the risk for CVD and stroke, possibly by either damaging coronary arteries or making it easier for blood platelets to clump together and form a clot. However, no evidence is available to suggest that lowering homocysteine through vitamin supplementation will reduce the risk of CVD. Clinical intervention trials to test the effects of vitamin supplementation on CVD and stroke are needed.

Because folate is involved in the synthesis, repair, and functioning of DNA, some have hypothesized that a deficiency of folate may result in DNA damage that can lead to cancer. A comprehensive review of epidemiologic, preclinical, and clinical evidence linking folate deficiency with increased cancer risk concluded that the evidence is strongest for colorectal cancer. Also, it has been suggested that folate deficiency may increase the effects of other cancer risk factors. Researchers are continuing to investigate whether increasing folate intake from foods or folic acid supplements may reduce cancer risk.

Folate is important for cells and tissues that divide rapidly; therefore, high-dose methothrexate is often used to treat cancer because this compound interferes with folate metabolism. Methothrexate, however, has undesirable side effects, including inflammation in the digestive tract. It is not known whether folic acid supplementation can help control these side effects without decreasing the effectiveness of methrothrexate. Low-dose methothrexate is used to treat a variety of diseases, such as rheumatoid arthritis, lupus, psoriasis, asthma, and inflammatory bowel disease. Low-dose treatment can deplete folate stores and cause side effects similar to folate deficiency. In this case, supplemental folic acid may help reduce the undesirable effects of low-dose methothrexate without decreasing treatment effectiveness.

Calcium Bone formation and resorption are balanced in healthy adults, but formation becomes slower than resorption after menopause and also with aging in both men and women. In menopausal women, decreased estrogen production is associated with accelerated bone loss in the first 5 years after menopause, particularly from the lumbar spine. Evidence indicates that although increasing calcium intake at menopause does not prevent this bone loss, it is beneficial for reducing bone loss in compact bones (e.g., hips, legs, and arms). Furthermore, data suggest that calcium supplementation also

reduces lumbar spine bone loss in women who are more than 5 years beyond menopause. In the United States, the recommended calcium intake is 1000 mg/day for men and women ages 19–50 years and 1200 mg/day for men and women ages 51–70 years. People who are not able to obtain this amount of calcium from foods should consider taking calcium supplements to help decrease the risk of reduced bone mass and osteoporosis.

Elderly

Physiological changes that may occur during the natural course of aging can affect micronutrient requirements. Given the same amount of sun exposure, the skin of young adults synthesizes much more vitamin D than the skin of the elderly; thus, choosing good dietary sources of vitamin D becomes essential. Vitamin D deficiency can be a factor in reduced calcium absorption in the elderly. Furthermore, it is estimated that atrophic gastritis, a change in gastrointestinal physiology that results in low-acid conditions in the stomach, is present in approximately 20% of elderly people. Atrophic gastritis has been related to infection with the bacterium *Helicobacter pylori* and is not necessarily a result of normal aging. The low-acid conditions, however, can decrease the absorption of vitamin B_{12} from food and of folate and calcium in general.

Vitamin D Vitamin D is important in the elderly for enhancing calcium absorption, inhibiting cellular growth, and activating lymphocyte function. Vitamin D deficiency may lead to osteoporosis and osteomalacia and possibly increase the risk for some cancers; it has been associated with increased incidence of hip fractures. More than 50% of elderly people have been reported to be vitamin D deficient in some studies. In addition to the skin's decreased ability to synthesize vitamin D as people age, the kidneys, which help to convert vitamin D to its active form, sometimes do not function as well when people age. All elderly people, particularly people with limited sun exposure, such as those who are either homebound or live in northern latitudes, should include vitamin D-fortified foods and fish in their diets. If elderly people are unable to meet their vitamin D needs using dietary sources, they may require a supplement. Evidence suggests that vitamin D supplementation may reduce the risk of osteoporotic fractures in elderly people with low serum levels of vitamin D.

Vitamin B_{12} Vitamin B_{12} is essential for proper brain and nerve development and for DNA synthesis; also, it improves learning and supports methylation metabolism. Dietary vitamin B_{12} must be separated from food proteins before the vitamin can be bound to intrinsic factor and then be absorbed by the body. Under low-acid conditions in the stomach, neither the separation from protein nor the binding to intrinsic factor can take place, significantly decreasing the bioavailability of vitamin B_{12}. Elderly adults with atrophic gastritis and low stomach acid should consume a source of unbound vitamin B_{12} such as that found in supplements or food that has been fortified with the vitamin to ensure adequate intake. In addition, evidence suggests that the use of antibiotics can improve vitamin B_{12} absorption in these elderly adults.

Folate Atrophic gastritis greatly reduces the ability of elderly people to absorb folate. This problem can be corrected by administering folic acid with dilute hydrochloric acid to increase stomach acidity and thus increase absorption. There is concern, however, about the possibility that supplemental folic acid could mask the signs of vitamin B_{12} deficiency. Folic acid can remedy the anemia that results from vitamin B_{12} deficiency, its key diagnostic sign. It cannot, however, correct the permanent nerve damage that is possible if vitamin B_{12} deficiency is not treated. Intake of supplemental folic acid should not be greater than 1000 µg per day to prevent the masking of signs of vitamin B_{12} deficiency.

Calcium Adequate calcium intake is required to maintain bone mineral density and reduce the risk of osteoporosis in the elderly. In addition to the reduced absorption of calcium by elderly people that results from age-related changes in vitamin D metabolism, the elderly also show a reduced ability to increase the efficiency of calcium absorption as an adaptive response to low-calcium diets. Also, as noted earlier, the low-acid conditions resulting from atrophic gastritis can reduce calcium absorption. Dietary calcium reacts with hydrochloric acid in the stomach to form soluble calcium chloride, which is absorbed in the small intestine. In the United States, the recommended calcium intake is 1200 mg/day for men and women older than age 70. Many elderly people may benefit from calcium supplements.

See also: **Folic Acids. Supplementation:** Dietary Supplements; Role of Micronutrient Supplementation; Developing Countries.

Further Reading

Blendon RJ, DesRoches CM, Benson JM, Brodie M, and Altman DE (2001) Americans' views on the use and regulation of dietary supplements. *Archives of Internal Medicine* **161**: 805–810.

DeJong N, Ocké MC, Branderhorst HAC, and Friele R (2003) Demographic and lifestyle characteristics of functional food consumers and dietary supplement users. *British Journal of Nutrition* **89**: 273–281.

Ervin RB, Wright JD, and Kennedy-Stephenson J (1999) Use of dietary supplements in the United States, 1988–94. National Center for Health Statistics. *Vital Health Statistics* Series 11, No. 244.

Institute of Medicine (1997) *Dietary Reference Intakes for Calcium, Phosphorus, Magnesium, Vitamin D, and Fluoride.* Washington, D.C.: National Academy Press.

Institute of Medicine (1998) *Dietary Reference Intakes for Thiamin, Riboflavin, Niacin, Vitamin B_6, Folate, Vitamin B_{12}, Pantothenic Acid, Biotin, and Choline.* Washington, D.C.: National Academy Press.

Institute of Medicine (2000) *Dietary Reference Intakes for Vitamin C, Vitamin E, Selenium, and Carotenoids.* Washington, D.C.: National Academy Press.

Institute of Medicine (2001) *Dietary Reference Intakes for Vitamin A, Vitamin K, Arsenic, Boron, Chromium, Copper, Iodine, Iron, Manganese, Molybdenum, Nickel, Silicon, Vanadium, and Zinc.* Washington, D.C.: National Academy Press.

Kim Y-I (1999) Folate and carcinogenesis: Evidence, mechanisms, and implications. *Journal of Nutritional Biochemistry* **10**: 66–88.

Morris CD and Carson S (2003) Routine vitamin supplementation to prevent cardiovascular disease: A summary of the evidence for the U.S. Preventive Services Task Force. *Annals of Internal Medicine* **139**: 56–70.

Ritenbaugh C, Streit K, and Helfand M (2003) *Routine vitamin supplementation to prevent cancer: A summary of the evidence from randomized controlled trials for the U.S. Preventive Services Task Force.* Rockville, MD: Agency for Healthcare Research and Quality. Available at www.ahrq.gov/clinic/3rduspstf/vitamins/vitasum.htm.

Russell RM (2001) Factors in aging that affect the bioavailability of nutrients. *Journal of Nutrition* **131**: 1359S–1361S.

Special Supplement (2003) Dietary supplement use in women: Current status and future directions. *Journal of Nutrition* **133**(6): 1957S–2013S.

U.S. Preventive Services Task Force (2003) Routine vitamin supplementation to prevent cancer and cardiovascular disease: Recommendations and rationale. *Annals of Internal Medicine* **139**: 51–55.

Zeisel SH (2000) Is there a metabolic basis for dietary supplementation? *American Journal of Clinical Nutrition* **72**: 507S–522S.

Developing Countries

R Shrimpton, Institute of Child Health, London, UK

Micronutrient supplementation is the distribution of specially formulated preparations of one or more nutrients, usually in the form of a pill, a capsule, or syrup. It seems to be the Cinderella of nutrition interventions, more than capable of dancing but not quite good enough to be invited to the Ball. It is often described as a 'short-term' option and a 'medical' approach and considered more appropriate for the treatment of severe micronutrient deficiencies in those most affected than to prevent deficiencies in whole populations. However, for the half of humanity affected by micronutrient deficiencies, the overwhelming majority of whom are the poor concentrated in the developing world, solving these problems through food-based approaches is only likely to happen in the very long term. The immune system is compromised by vitamin A deficiency in 40% of children younger than 5 years old in the developing world, leading to approximately 1 million deaths each year. In the 6- to 24-month-old age group, mental development is impaired due to iron deficiency in 40–60% of the developing world's children. Severe iron deficiency also causes more than 60 000 deaths of women during pregnancy and childbirth every year. Approximately 18 million infants per year are born mentally impaired as a result of iodine deficiency during pregnancy. Providing vulnerable groups, such as children and women of childbearing age, with low-cost vitamin and mineral supplements is the least that governments can do to protect the growth and development of the next generation as a first step toward realizing the right of every individual to be adequately nourished.

Experience in achieving high coverage of those most at risk with micronutrient supplements is quite varied, with both successes and failures. A good communication strategy is an essential part of achieving high levels of adherence in micronutrient supplementation programs, but these aspects are not particular to nutrition programs and are not considered here. Deficiencies of iodine, iron, vitamin A, and folate are the most commonly recognized deficiencies for which there are programs, but in practice most of those affected have multiple vitamin and mineral deficiencies that overlap and interact at great cost. This article reviews the policy dimensions of the efforts to establish programs aimed at eliminating iodine deficiency, iron deficiency anemia, and vitamin A deficiency through supplementation, and it provides a perspective on zinc supplementation and multiple micronutrient supplementation as future components of nutrition programs in developing countries.

Iodine Supplementation

Today, approximately 70% of the world's salt is iodised, compared to just 10% in 1990, and therefore iodine supplementation programs are greatly reduced. Until universal salt iodization is guaranteed in the third of the world in which iodized salt is not yet available, especially in remote populations in which goiter is endemic, supplements should be used during pregnancy and early childhood. In the past, it was common to provide annual intramuscular injections of iodized oil to women of reproductive age in order to ensure iodine status during the first months of pregnancy when the risk of cretinism is greatest. In more recent years, oral iodized oil capsules have proven to be as efficacious and more effective in controlling iodine deficiency in both women of reproductive age and schoolchildren. Oral iodine supplements initially based on expensive poppy seed oil have since been replaced by cheaper rapeseed and peanut oil preparations, which are equally effective.

Vitamin A Supplementation

The use of supplements to eliminate vitamin A deficiency is a notable success, with remarkable advances achieved within the past decade. Although the elimination of vitamin A deficiency by year 2000 was one of the goals set at the World Summit for Children in 1990, little progress was evident at mid-decade. Clinical vitamin A deficiency was estimated to affect approximately 3.3 million children younger than the age of 5 years in 1995, with an additional 100 million subject to subclinical deficiency. The periodic distribution of high-dose vitamin A supplements, originally employed in Indonesia during the 1970s for the prevention of blindness in children, was shown in the 1980s to also impact young child mortality. The supplements have the advantage of ensuring requirements for 4–6 months after administration, such that two or three capsules per year can meet vitamin A requirement of preschool children.

The lack of perception of vitamin A deficiency as a problem was a substantial barrier to establishing large-scale preventive supplementation programs. The prevalence of clinical signs of frank vitamin A deficiency, such a Bitot's spot and corneal lesions, that make it a 'public health problem' is very small at just 0.5%. Since clinical signs are often more common in rural populations, a significant vitamin A deficiency problem can easily go undetected. National representative surveys were thus a prerequisite for taking action. Another barrier is the voice of those who advocate for food-based approaches and view supplements as technical fixes or golden bullets that are of questionable sustainability promoted by the pharmaceutical sector. In reality, of course, these are not either/or options.

Convincing proof of the efficacy of vitamin A capsules for child mortality reduction in the early 1990s helped to create increased momentum for populationwide preventive supplementation programs. The turning point for increasing the coverage of vitamin A supplements was undoubtedly the publication of a meta-analysis of the efficacy trials of massive-dose vitamin A capsules. The analysis of eight mortality trials indicated that improving the vitamin A status of children aged 6 months to 5 years by massive-dose capsule distribution reduced child mortality rates by approximately 23%. The important conclusion of the meta-analysis was that increased risk of mortality from vitamin A deficiency was not just limited to those portions of the population with severe vitamin A deficiency problems but was present across the whole population distribution.

What consisted of 'the justification' for carrying out vitamin A supplementation programs evolved rapidly during the latter half of the 1990s. Many of these discussions were held at the meetings of the International Vitamin A Consultative Group and the working group on vitamin A of the Standing Committee on Nutrition of the United Nations. A broad technical consensus was finally accepted that even in the absence of survey data, it was highly likely that the benefits of vitamin A supplements would be evident in populations in which the mortality rates for those younger than 5 years old were higher than 70 per 1000. Prior to this, vitamin A supplements were targeted to those children with illnesses such as measles and diarrhea. The most recent programmatic recommendations are that if mortality for those younger than 5 years old is higher than 50 per 1000, then supplements should be employed routinely as a preventive measure for all young children. Subsequent to this consensus, a global policy to integrate vitamin A capsule distribution into regular immunization schedules, and also to incorporate vitamin A capsules into the national immunization campaign days being promoted to achieve the eradication of polio, was rapidly adopted.

Programmatic vitamin A interventions received considerable impetus from the Vitamin A Global Initiative, an informal interagency advocacy group that worked to promote the adoption of vitamin A supplementation programs. The initiative included WHO and UNICEF, together with CIDA from Canada, DIFID from the United Kingdom, USAID from the United States, and the Micronutrient Initiative (MI). Through their networks, these various organizations worked together to convince governments with high mortality rates for children younger than age 5 years to introduce periodic vitamin A capsule distribution programs. Vitamin A capsules were made available by CIDA through UNICEF to any developing country that wanted them, and UNICEF and MI with USAID and DIFID funds developed a global communication campaign.

By the end of the 1990s, vitamin A supplementation programs had seen a remarkable expansion. Most countries with high mortality rates for children younger than 5 years old adopted vitamin A supplementation programs, with the most notable exception being India. The number of countries with vitamin A programs increased from 10 in 1995 to 72 in 2000. The ways in which the vitamin A capsule programs were developed and implemented varied by country, but the most common strategy was to use national immunization days for polio eradication to piggyback vitamin A supplements. The use of this approach doubled from 30 countries in 1997 to 60 in 1999. Because the polio eradication strategy requires two nationwide campaigns not more than 2 months apart, some countries also promoted separate micronutrient days, or child health days, so that children would get at least two capsules during the course of a year, 6 months apart. UNICEF procured through its central warehouse in Copenhagen and supplied through its country programs an average of 289 million capsules per year from 1993 to 1998, which was estimated to be only 38% of the worldwide need.

Estimates of the coverage of vitamin A capsules indicate a remarkably high coverage of supplements by the turn of the century, with remarkable saving of life. Based on multiple sources, UNICEF estimates that in 1999 half of all children aged 6–59 months in developing countries outside of China, and 80% of such children in the least developed countries, received a vitamin A capsule within the past 6 months. Coverage was highest in sub-Saharan Africa, where 70% of children aged 6–59 months received a capsule in the past 6 months. Extrapolation of the protective effect of a 23% reduction in child mortality shown by the meta-analysis to the increased coverage of capsules achieved between 1998 and 2000 suggests that 1 million lives were saved in this short period.

The challenge that remains for vitamin A supplementation is one of sustainability. Although supplements are traditionally viewed as a short-term solution, in reality they need to be maintained during at least the medium term if continued gains in mortality reduction are to be realised. Increases in other sources of vitamin A, be it through diet and/or fortification, are unlikely to be achieved in the short term. The eventual phasing out of national immunization days, as polio eradication becomes a reality, will cause problems for maintaining the high coverage of vitamin A capsules. Alternate strategies are needed and are being put in place in many countries. Bangladesh and Nepal are two examples of countries that successfully promote biannual micronutrient days with large-scale social mobilisation efforts. Sustaining the provision of the vitamin A capsules is also likely to become a problem. Until now, supplements have predominantly been provided by the Canadian government and supplied through UNICEF, and how long this will be sustained is not known. The costs for individual governments to take on are small, however, and the benefits in terms of lives saved will likely remain enormous for many decades.

Iron/Folate Supplementation

Although iron deficiency is the most widespread of nutritional problems, supplementation with iron has not proven to be a very successful intervention. Global policy recommendations to routinely provide iron/folate supplements for women during pregnancy and lactation have changed little in almost three decades, and all anemic pregnant women should receive such supplements in almost all contexts. Approximately half of the developing countries in the world are reported to have national iron supplementation policies. The World Summit for Children's goal to reduce anemia in women by one-third was given little or no priority by the principal actors involved such that no progress was made during the past decade. Anemia still affected 44% of nonpregnant women and 56% of pregnant women in developing countries at the end of the twenty first century.

Although there is ample evidence that iron deficiency and the anemia associated with it are a great burden on society, especially the poor, the advocacy base for pushing for program implementation is still weak. The link of iron deficiency to maternal and child survival has not been concretely proven. The effect of iron deficiency on cognitive deficits in children and on adults later in the life course has been established. The absolute losses in Southeast Asia are estimated to be approximately $5 billion annually, and for India the median value of productivity losses due to iron deficiency alone is approximately $4 per capita or 0.9% of gross domestic product. The efficacy of iron/folate supplements for controlling anemia is well documented, and there is a considerable amount of descriptive evidence linking maternal anemia to both low birth weight and maternal mortality.

Despite high cost-effectiveness, little or no priority has been given to iron deficiency anemia reduction programs. At $0.002 per tablet, the iron supplement is relatively cheap, and the cost per disability adjusted life year of $13 makes the supplementation of pregnant women with iron a very cost-effective intervention. At the national level, despite the existence of national policies, rarely is there a budget for the provision of supplements and/or supervision of iron deficiency anemia programs. Although UNICEF is a major supplier of iron/folate supplements to the developing world, the level of supply is far lower than that believed to be needed. In the period 1993–1996, 2.7 billion tablets were shipped to 122 countries at a cost of $7.5 million as part of UNICEF assistance to programs aimed at eliminating maternal anemia. This was less than 5% of that needed to cover all pregnancies in developing countries. There have been few, if any, attempts to gauge the coverage of iron/folate supplements at any level, be it district, national, or international. Neither has there been any effort put into creating political accountability to ensure high coverage.

Many meetings and publications during the past few decades that have examined the causes and solutions of iron deficiency anemia conclude that lack of effectiveness of iron supplementation programs for anemia control is largely related to problems with supply of the supplement. Although the side effects of iron pills are often cited as the reason why iron supplementation programs do not work, this rarely seems to be the case. One of the major causes of nonadherence seems to be lack of understanding of the benefits the supplements can bring among health staff that deliver the tablets. Most of the program reviews have concluded that where supportive community-level delivery mechanisms are put in place that encourage adherence, and the supply of supplements is ensured, high levels of coverage can be achieved and sustained. It is often the case, however, that in health systems in developing countries, nutrition is everybody's business and nobody's responsibility, and iron supplements have ended up low on the list of things to do.

Despite an international consensus that supplementation has a key role to play in the control of iron deficiency anemia, there are still those that question such programs. In 1998, a technical consensus meeting on what was needed to solve the problem of iron deficiency made the recommendation that although the interventions already existed for reducing both iron deficiency and iron deficiency anemia, more work was needed to develop large-scale programs with packages of interventions delivered through multiple sectors. Despite the consensus, there are still those who question the advisability of iron supplementation programs, suggesting that hemoglobin cutoffs may be set too high and/or that receiving excessive amounts of iron is dangerous for those who are iron replete. Another complicating factor is undoubtedly related to the fact that adequate coverage of iron supplements alone will not ensure anemia control in many settings. A global review of anemia causality revealed that perhaps only half of anemia is solely due to iron deficiency, with other micronutrient deficiencies such as vitamin A contributing as well. Infections such as malaria and helminth are also important causes. Programs to eliminate anemia thus require packages of interventions, of which iron supplements are but a part.

Zinc Supplementation

There is strong evidence for the efficacy of therapeutic zinc in improving the prognosis of children being treated for diarrheal disease, and a new WHO/UNICEF recommendation is to give supplemental zinc for 10 days as part of the treatment of diarrhea. A pooled analysis of randomized controlled therapeutic zinc trials in children with diarrhea showed that zinc-supplemented children with acute diarrhea had a 15% lower probability of continuing diarrhea on a given day, and in those with persistent diarrhea there was a 24% lower probability. In addition, children with persistent diarrhea had a 42% lower rate of treatment failure or death if zinc supplemented. The WHO/UNICEF recommendation is to give zinc in the form of a tablet for 10 days to all children that are treated for diarrhea. Given that even the current interventions included in child health programs for diarrheal disease treatment, such as oral rehydration therapy, face enormous barriers to achieving and maintaining high levels of coverage, the challenge for achieving high levels of coverage of zinc supplements in the treatment of diarrhea is likely to be considerable. If these efforts are successful, however, then the impact is likely to be great.

The most effective way to give preventive zinc supplements is an ongoing research question.

Multiple Micronutrient Supplementation

In recent years, the case has increasingly been made for providing multiple micronutrient supplements instead of iron supplements for young children and women of reproductive age in developing countries. A woman's or an infant's diet that is deficient in iron is likely to be deficient in many other micronutrients. Outside of emergency situations, such as natural catastrophes, famine, and civil strife, poor dietary quality rather than quantity is the determinant of inadequate micronutrient status among infants and women. The nutrient-to-energy ratios of iron, zinc, folate, vitamins B_6 and B_{12}, vitamin A, riboflavin, and calcium are commonly below the recommended levels needed, assuming energy needs are met.

Although the incremental cost of distributing a multiple micronutrient supplement is likely to be small, the increased benefits may be large. The main cost of the delivery of a nutrient supplement for women of reproductive age is not the cost of the supplement but the cost of the delivery system. Although it may not be working very well, a delivery system already exists for the iron/folate supplements that could be used to provide these other micronutrients. There has been much speculation about the costs of a multiple micronutrient supplement compared to the iron/folate tablet currently procured and provided by UNICEF. Adding the extra nutrients to the iron/folate tablets will not add more than 20% to the cost of the tablet, as long as they are procured in bulk on the international market, as is the case for the current iron/folate tablets supplied by UNICEF.

The potential benefits for pregnant women from improving not only iron and folate but also zinc, vitamin A, and other antioxidant nutrient status are likely to be great. Providing women with vitamin A supplements together with iron supplements has been shown to improve the hematinic effects of the iron supplements. The findings that vitamin A supplements to women of reproductive age reduced maternal mortality by approximately 40% in Nepal and that zinc supplementation improved birth weight among poor women in the United States point to the possible multiple benefits, beyond anemia reduction, of introducing a multiple micronutrient supplement for use by women in developing countries.

The composition of a multiple micronutrient supplement for use in trials among pregnant and lactating women in developing countries has recently been agreed on. The proposed formulation contains physiological doses of the micronutrients based on the recommended daily allowance (RDA). The US/Canadian recommendations were used since they are the most recent and best documented. The selection of nutrients included in the supplement was based on evidence of deficiencies, possible consequences of deficiencies for mother and child, weighing of risks and advantages, and interaction between nutrients. Furthermore, information about toxicity levels, cost of nutrients, the size of the resulting supplement, and possible side effects related to supplement intake were considered. The formulation agreed upon includes 15 micronutrients (vitamins A, D, E, B_1, B_2, B_6, B_{12}, and C, niacin, and folic acid and minerals Fe, Zn, Cu, I, and Se), all at the RDA level, except for folic acid, which was included at the 400-μg level—considered sufficient to prevent neural tube defects if taken periconceptually.

The multiple micronutrient tablet formulation for supplementation during pregnancy was developed with various users in mind. For pregnant women, the tablet should be taken on a daily basis for as long as possible during pregnancy. For lactating women, the supplement should be taken daily until at least 3 months postpartum. The tablet can also be taken by adolescent girls on a once-a-week basis as a way of improving micronutrient status before getting pregnant. Another possible target group is refugees, who can take the supplement according to their biological state (pregnant or not) and, in case of severe deficiency, can take two tablets per day.

Although the supplement is not considered a dangerous product, it was still recommended for use in trials, with special attention to monitoring and evaluation. Tablets of similar composition are regularly prescribed by physicians and/or purchased by mothers in developed countries, and they can be found in the pharmacies of the capitals of most developing countries and are widely consumed by the richer segments of the population. Despite the relative safety of the supplement, it was recognized that many issues related to multiple micronutrient supplements remain to be investigated. Research topics identified included the assessment of risks as opposed to benefits of regular supplement intake in environments in which many disease agents are present. Factors that influence adherence to tablet intake were also considered a crucial area for investigation.

The need to carry out both efficacy and effectiveness studies of the multiple micronutrient supplements in various different populations is well recognized. The need for micronutrient supplementation in pregnancy is likely to be great because of widespread maternal malnutrition. However, it has to be recognized that public health resources are always limited and priority is given to interventions that are both efficacious and effective. Proving the efficacy of multiple micronutrient supplements is thus essential for being able to advocate for their widescale use. However, multiple micronutrient supplements are almost always going to be part of a package of interventions, especially in developing countries. Indeed, the micronutrient supplements will likely be most effective as part of a package that also seeks to control the major diseases afflicting the mothers, be that malaria, sexually transmitted diseases, or intestinal parasites. Being part of a package obviously makes it difficult in field conditions to test the relative merits of the individual pieces, including the micronutrient supplement. For these reasons, both 'plausibility'- and 'probability'-based approaches are recommended for measuring performance of the multiple micronutrient supplements so that experience can be gained on how to develop programs that promote fetal and infant growth and it can be determined whether micronutrient supplements are truly efficacious in developing countries.

UNICEF has incorporated the multiple micronutrient supplements into ongoing programs as part of an initiative to prevent low birth weight. A total of 18 million infants are born low birth weight (<2.5 kg) every year, accounting for approximately 14% of all live births. These infants are at increased risk of infections; to have weakened immunity, learning disabilities, and impaired physical development; and of dying soon after birth. UNICEF has started promoting programs to reduce the prevalence of low birth weight in Indonesia, the Philippines, Vietnam, China, Bangladesh, India, Pakistan, Nepal, Tanzania, Mozambique, and Madagascar. Low birth weight prevention programs are being fashioned to fit local circumstances, in accordance with the nutrition strategy approved by the UNICEF executive board. The approach being developed in each country elaborates on the 'care for women' element of the care initiative that has been developed to facilitate improvements in caring practices among families and communities. In addition to the multiple micronutrient supplements, other interventions that form part of low birth weight prevention efforts include promoting increased child spacing, increased rest and food for the mother during pregnancy, improved reproductive health, deworming, and malaria control during pregnancy as appropriate. Reducing teenage pregnancy rates is also part of the package, but it is a major challenge since, although the mortality risks for both the teenage mother and her child are known to be considerably increased, teenage pregnancy rates are very high in most developing countries. Prepregnancy weight, weight gain during pregnancy, and birth weight all receive special attention as the principal evaluative indicators of program success.

WHO and UNICEF recommend the use of syrup and/or tablets containing iron for the treatment of anemia in young children, and such products are available through UNICEF supply division in Copenhagen. These products have very little penetration considering the size of the infant anemia problem in most developing countries, where half of all children are commonly affected. Despite the recognition that iron deficiency often coexists with zinc deficiency, together with inadequate intakes of other B vitamins (B_6, riboflavin, and niacin) in infant dietaries, there is no multiple micronutrient supplement available for infants. UNICEF has also been testing the efficacy of a foodlet (a large crumbly pastille that is a cross between a tablet and a food) containing multiple micronutrients during infancy through the Infant Research on Infant Supplementation trials. Trials of multiple micronutrients as preventive supplements are also being carried out by many different groups using supplements provided in the form of sprinkles, tablets, and even as a beverage. Preliminary results of these trials point to a greater impact on anemia and enhancement of multiple micronutrient status by the multiple micronutrient supplements than that of iron supplements, as well as small improvements in growth.

There is a need to bring all of this broad spectrum of experimental and programmatic work together to reach conclusions and achieve consensus before policy and program recommendations can be made on how best to include multiple micronutrient supplements in programs to improve maternal and child health in developing countries. Whether this happens will depend on the continued efforts of the agencies interested in and responsible for promoting maternal and health, to champion the importance of micronutrient supplementation in their programs.

See also: **Anemia**: Iron-Deficiency Anemia. **Folic Acid**. **Iodine**: Physiology, Dietary Sources and Requirements; Deficiency Disorders. **Supplementation**: Role of Micronutrient Supplementation; Developed Countries. **Vitamin A**: Biochemistry and Physiological Role. **Zinc**: Physiology; Deficiency in Developing Countries, Intervention Studies.

Further Reading

Gillespie S, Kevanny J, and Mason J (1991) *Controlling Iron Deficiency*, ACC/SCN State of the Art Series, Nutrition Policy Discussion Paper No. 9. Geneva: SCN.

Gross R, Dwivedi A, and Solomons NW (2003) Supplement: Proceedings of the International Workshop on Multimicronutrient Deficiency Control in the Life Cycle, Lima Peru May 30–June 1, 2001. *Food and Nutrition Bulletin* 24(3):S3–S61.

Huffman SL, Baker J, Shumann J, and Zehnaer ER (1998) *The Case for Promoting Multiple Vitamin/Mineral Supplements for Women of Reproductive Age in Developing Countries*. Washington, DC: The Linkages Project, Academy for Educational Development.

Institute of Medicine (1998) *Prevention of Micronutrient Deficiencies: Tools for Policy Makers and Public Health Workers*. Washington, DC: National Academy Press.

Mason JB, Lotfi M, Dalmiya N, Sethurman K, and Deitchler M (2001) *The Micronutrient Report: Current Progress and Trends in the Control of Vitamin A, Iron, and Iodine Deficiencies*. Ottawa, Ontario, Canada: Micronutrient Initiative, International Development Research Centre.

Ramakrishnan U and Huffman SL (2001) Multiple micronutrient malnutrition: What can be done? In: Semba RD and Bloem MW (eds.) *Nutrition and Health in Developing Countries*, pp. 365–391. Totowa, NJ: Humana Press.

Shrimpton R and Schultink W (2002) Can supplements help meet the micronutrient needs of the developing world? *Proceedings of the Nutrition Society* 61: 223–229.

UNICEF/UNU/WHO (2001) *Iron Deficiency Anaemia: Assessment, Prevention and Control. A Guide for Programme Managers*. Geneva: World Health Organization.

UNICEF/UNU/WHO/MI (1999) *Preventing Iron Deficiency in Women and Children: Background and Consensus on Key Issues. Report of a Technical Workshop, UNICEF, New York 7–9 October 1998*. Ottawa, Ontario, Canada: Micronutrient Initiative and International Nutrition Foundation.

WHO/UNICEF/IVACG (1997) *Vitamin A Supplements: A Guide to Their Use in the Treatment and Prevention of Vitamin A Deficiency and Xerophthalmia*, 2nd edn. Geneva: World Health Organization.

Dietary Supplements

S S Percival, University of Florida, Gainesville, FL, USA

In 2004, global sales of dietary supplements represented a significant business. Worldwide sales have been estimated at $70–250 billion. The demand for herbal products worldwide increased at an annual rate of 8% from 1994 to 2001, although this growth has slowed in recent years.

Issues and controversies in the dietary supplement market are related to defining exactly what is a dietary supplement, understanding how sales and marketing data are derived, defining the regulatory environment, safety issues, product quality issues, labeling and health claim issues, and scientific evidence for benefit. This article describes some of these controversies and provides examples to illustrate these issues.

How Is the Sales Data Derived?

Global sales have been estimated to be between $70 billion and $250 billion. This approximately 3-fold difference in estimates is due to the variation in what products are actually included in product sales results. As will be discussed, the definition of dietary supplements varies greatly from country to country; therefore, deriving sales data is complex.

Another difficulty in assessing sales of dietary supplements is the source from which sales data are gathered. Many business surveys rely on only one or two of the following sales outlets to derive their results:

- Supermarkets and mass merchandisers
- Natural food and health food stores
- Direct sales from Internet, mail order, practitioners, and multilevel marketing
- Pharmacies and drugstore chains

What Is a Dietary Supplement? How Are They Regulated in Different Countries?

Each country has developed regulatory definitions and systems that place dietary supplements, particularly botanicals, into categories of drugs, traditional medicines, or foods. However, in the late 1980s, many countries launched major changes in regulations that may or may not have been approved at the time of this writing. Many regulations are still in draft form.

The US Congress defined the term 'dietary supplement' in the Dietary Supplement Health and Education Act (DSHEA) of 1994. A dietary supplement is a product, taken orally, that contains a 'dietary ingredient' that is intended to supplement the diet. The dietary ingredient includes vitamins, minerals, herbs or other botanicals, amino acids, a dietary substance for use by man to supplement the diet by increasing the total dietary intake (e.g., enzymes or tissues from organs or glands), or a concentrate, metabolite, constituent, or extract. Dietary supplements may be found in many forms, such as tablets, capsules, softgels, gelcaps, liquids, or powders. They may also be produced in other forms, such as a beverage, spread, or bar, in which case information on the label must clearly state that the product is a dietary supplement and it is not represented as a conventional food or a sole item of a meal or diet.

Whatever their form, DSHEA places dietary supplements in a special category under the general umbrella of 'foods,' not drugs, and requires that every supplement be labeled a dietary supplement and carry a Supplement Facts Label.

In the United Kingdom, there is a distinct separation of food supplements and herbal medicines. The Food Standards Agency developed the Food Standard Act of 1999 and is responsible for protection of public health. The Food Supplement Directive 2002/46/EC, which harmonizes European Community legislation on food supplements, was published in 2002. This directive is stricter than existing UK standards and regulations but is relatively more liberal than what exists in other European countries. The directive defines the term 'food supplements,' contains a list of vitamin and mineral sources that may be used in the manufacture of food supplements, states labeling requirements, and, in the future, will provide a framework for maximum and minimum levels for vitamins and minerals in food supplements. Herbals and botanicals are not discussed in this directive.

The Foods Supplement Directive defines a food supplement as any food the purpose of which is to supplement the normal diet and which is a concentrated source of a vitamin or mineral or other substance with a nutritional or physiological effect, alone or in combination, and is sold in dose form. Dose form means capsules, pastilles, tablets, pills, and other similar forms, and also powders, ampoules, drops, or other similar forms of liquids or powders, designed to be taken in small measured quantities. Because the directive defines a food supplement as something to supplement the diet, products that are not meant to supplement the diet (e.g., a weight loss product) are outside the scope of the regulations. There remains a complex legal area between food supplements and medicinal products, although the directive indicates that if a product is used for treating or preventing disease, or restoring, correcting, or modifying a physiological function, then it falls under the Medicines Directive 2001/83/EEC, Medicines Act 1968, or Medicines for Human Use Regulations 1994.

The *Trans*-Atlantic Business Dialogue (TABD) approved a position statement regarding dietary supplements in 2002. The TABD is a group of corporations that promote closer commercial ties between the European Union and the United States. This position statement established industrywide consensus on standards and definition of permissible claims, as well as defining what is necessary for substantiation of those claims. In keeping with the Foods Supplement Directive, the TABD dealt only with vitamins and minerals, with the understanding that some of the conclusions may be revisited when warranted for herbals, botanicals, or other dietary supplements.

Herbal medicines, on the other hand, are regulated by the Medicine and HealthCare Products Regulatory Agency based in London. A herbal remedy is defined as

a medicinal product consisting of a substance produced by subjecting a plant or plants to drying, crushing or any other process, or of a mixture whose sole ingredients are two or more substances so produced, or of a mixture whose sole ingredients are one or more substances so produced and water or some other inert substance.

There are two alternative regulatory routes in the United Kingdom for herbal medicines: licensing and exemption from licensing requirements:

- Licensed herbal medicines: To receive a product license prior to marketing, herbal medicines are required to meet safety, quality, and efficacy criteria in a similar manner to any other licensed medicine.
- Herbal remedies exempt from licensing requirements: The exemption applies to herbal remedies meeting certain conditions set out in Section 12 of the Medicines Act 1968. Section 12 allows a person to make, sell, and supply a herbal remedy during the course of his or her business provided the remedy is manufactured or assembled on the premises and that it is supplied as a consequence of a consultation between the person and his or her patient. Section 12 also allows the manufacture, sale, or supply of herbal remedies where the processing of the plant consists only of drying, crushing, or comminuting; the remedy is sold without any written specification as to its use; and the remedy is sold under a designation that only specifies the plant and the process and does not apply any other name to the remedy.

Canada has been estimated to have approximately 3% of the market share of the global nutritional market. Health Canada established the Office of Natural Health Products. Premarket assessment, labeling, licensing, and monitoring of herbal supplements are items in its mandate. The definition of a natural health product includes products for the use in "diagnosis, treatment, mitigation, or prevention of a disease, disorder, or abnormal physical state or its symptoms in humans; restoring or correcting organic function in humans; or modifying organic functions in humans, such as modifying those functions in a manner that maintains or promotes health." These products include homeopathic preparations, substances used in traditional medicine, a mineral or trace element, a vitamin, an amino acid, an essential fatty acid or other botanical-, animal-, or microorganism-derived substance. Foods are not included in this product category called natural health products. Canada's Food and Drugs Act of 1953 regulates foods and drugs but does not specifically deal with natural health products. Therefore, these types of products are regulated as either a food or a drug depending on the type and concentration of active ingredient and whether claims are made on the products.

Germany regulates vitamins and minerals as food if they are sold to complement the nutritive value of the diet and do not exceed safe levels. However, if the vitamin or mineral is used for disease treatment or prevention and is used at pharmacological levels, then it is considered a drug. Safety and efficacy of drugs must be established by clinical research. Medicinal plants are regulated differently depending on what plant and in what form it is sold. In general, extracts of plants are considered drugs and must be prescribed. Teas, on the other hand, are sold over-the-counter in pharmacies. Other teas, such as those that contain alkaloids, must be sold by prescription only. Beginning in 1980, an extensive analysis of the literature on more than 300 herbal remedies was undertaken by the German Kommission E. Approximately two-thirds of the herbals were listed as safe and at least minimally effective. The results were published as a series of monographs by the German Kommission E, and this body of work was summarized and translated into English by the American Botanical Council. These substances are generally purchased at the pharmacy and are reimbursable through health insurance. One caveat regarding the German herbal preparations is that they are not likely to be the same preparations that are produced by other countries; thus, the safety and efficacy statements in the Kommission E are only for the preparations that are prepared in German pharmacies.

Australia regulates therapeutic goods under the Therapeutic Goods Act of 1989. Therapeutic goods include vitamins, minerals, plants and herbals, nutritional food supplements, naturopathic and homeopathic preparations, and some aromatherapy. The Therapeutic Goods Administration (TGA) developed the Office of Complementary Medicine to evaluate new substances and products. Basically, the TGA regulates these therapeutic goods as they do pharmaceutical products, and thus their criteria are more rigorous than the criteria of other countries. Most of the therapeutic goods are 'generally listed' rather than regulated. Listed medicines are considered to be relatively harmless, so the regulations allow for manufacturers to 'self-assess' their products in some situations. The majority of listed medicines are self-selected by consumers and used for self-treatment, and they are all manufactured with well-known established ingredients, such as vitamin and mineral products or sunscreens. These are assessed by the TGA for quality and safety but not efficacy. This does not mean that they do not work; rather, it means that the TGA has not evaluated them individually to determine if they work. It is a requirement under the act that sponsors have information to substantiate all of their product's claims.

The Japanese Ministry of Health and Welfare does not define or recognize a distinct category known as dietary supplements. Instead, there are only two classifications, food and drugs. In 1993, Japan defined a group of foods known as Foods for Specific Health Use (FOSHU). As of 2004, approximately 342 foods had been approved as FOSHU. The dietary ingredients are sold in the form of foods, not in the form of capsules, tablets, or powders.

The herbal supplements market in Japan has been strongly influenced by the practice of Kampo. Kampo (or Kanpo) is the adaptation of Chinese herb formulas to Japanese medicine. Approximately 25 years ago, the Japanese Ministry of Health formally recognized that certain traditional Chinese herb formulas (and a few formulas of similar nature developed in Japan) were suitable for coverage by national health insurance. These formulas are prepared in factories under strict conditions.

In summary, developing global data on dietary supplement sales depends on how they are defined. Table 1 summarizes the differences in regulatory categories of different countries.

Product Quality and Safety Issues

Product quality is an issue derived from the explosive growth of the industry in the post-DSHEA world. Quality issues revolve around products that contain wrong ingredients, incorrect claims, contamination, or incorrect amounts—either too much or not enough.

An example plant misidentification was published in 1998 by Slifman et al. Two patients were admitted to hospital emergency rooms with palpitations, vomiting, nausea, and chest pressure, among other symptoms. Both individuals, having been admitted 1 month apart, had each consumed a program of dietary supplements, one containing 14 herbs, a tablet containing 11 herbs, liquid clay, a bulking powder, and capsules containing microorganisms. Of the five supplements, the one made up of 14 herbs tested positive for cardiac glycosides. The investigators determined that *Digitalis lanata* was present in the supplement. *Digitalis lanata* contains cardiac glycosides, which resulted in the cardiac symptoms. Further investigation revealed that raw material labeled as plantain (genus *Plantago*)

Table 1 Regulatory categories of different countries

Country, act	Definition
United States, DSHEA	Vitamins, minerals, herbal, other botanical, amino acid, enzymes, organs, glands
Europe, Food Supplement Act	Vitamin and minerals
United Kingdom, Medicine and Health Care	Medicinal plants
Canada, Office of Natural Products	Mineral; trace element; vitamin; amino acid; essential fatty acid; botanical-, animal-, or microorganism-derived substances; homeopathic preparation; traditional preparations
Germany, Kommission E	Vitamin and mineral as both foods and drugs, botanicals (approved and not approved), teas as prescription and as over-the-counter
Australia, Therapeutic Goods Administration	Vitamin and mineral, plants, herbs, nutritional food supplements, naturopaths and homeopathic preparations, aromatherapies
Japan, Ministry of Health and Welfare	No definition of dietary supplements, regulations for foods, drugs, and Kampo

had been contaminated with *D. lanata* due to mis-identification in the field.

Another quality issue that has safety manifestations was an incorrect claim on a product. PC-SPES, a combination of eight herbs, is claimed to be a nonestrogenic treatment for prostate cancer. However, several of the herbs used in this preparation do in fact have estrogenic activity. In 1998, DiPaola *et al.* showed a significant amount of estrogenic activity in both *in vitro* (yeast) and *in vivo* studies (mice and humans) with PC-SPES. Use of the supplement by men with prostate cancer resulted in similar side effects as would develop with estrogen therapy and theoretically could confound the results of standard therapy.

By law (DSHEA), the manufacturer is responsible for ensuring that its dietary supplement products are safe before they are marketed. Unlike drug products that must be proven safe and effective for their intended use before marketing, there are no provisions in the law for the US Food and Drug Administration (FDA) to 'approve' dietary supplements for safety or effectiveness before they reach the consumer. Also unlike drug products, manufacturers and distributors of dietary supplements are not required by law to record, investigate, or forward to the FDA any reports they receive of injuries or illnesses that may be related to the use of their products. Under DSHEA, once the product is marketed, the FDA has the responsibility to show that a dietary supplement is 'unsafe' before it can take action to restrict the product's use or remove it from the marketplace.

In 2003, the FDA banned all products containing ephedra alkaloids. Ephedra-containing products were, until the ban, marketed in conjunction with enhancing athletic performance and/or promoting weight loss. Recent studies provided enough additional evidence that ephedra presents a significant and unreasonable risk of illness and injury that the FDA banned all ephedra-containing products from the market and advised consumers to stop taking such supplements. Strong statements were issued cautioning about the use of ephedra-containing products, especially when strenuously exercising or in combination with other stimulants, such as caffeine.

Interactions

An issue that has become of concern is the interaction of dietary supplements with herbs and other dietary supplements, drugs, foods, lab tests, and diseases or other conditions. There are literally hundreds of potential interactions that have not yet been recognized. Both practitioners and consumers must be aware of the possibilities. In some cases, knowledge about interactions comes from documented reports. However, in other cases, the knowledge is theoretical, based on the pharmacological profile or mechanism of action of the supplement and the drug, food, test, or condition. For example, ginkgo biloba contains ginkgolides in the leaf that competitively inhibit platelet-activating factor (PAF). PAF inhibition decreases platelet aggregation among other many other physiological effects. Inhibition of PAF may increase cardiac contractility and coronary blood flow. Concomitant use of herbs and supplements that affect platelet aggregation could theoretically increase the risk of bleeding in some people due to ginkgo's effects on platelet aggregation. Spontaneous hematomas (broken blood vessels) and hemorrhaging in the anterior chamber of the eye have been reported in ginkgo users, although it is not known what other drugs or supplements these individuals were taking.

Herbs and supplements that promote platelet inhibition include angelica, anise, capsicum, celery, chamomile, clove, fenugreek, feverfew, fish oil, garlic, ginger, horse chestnut, horseradish, licorice, meadowsweet, onion, Panax ginseng, red clover, vitamin E, and willow. Similarly, concomitant administration of drugs, including aspirin, clopidogrel (Plavix), dalteparin (Fragmin), enoxaparin (Lovenox), heparin, indomethacin (Indocin), ticlopidine (Ticlid), and warfarin (Coumadin), may increase the risk of bleeding in some people. This is just one example of the interactions between drugs with herbals and herbals with other herbals. There may be an infinite number of interactions.

Currently, there are no mandated US federal guidelines to report adverse events or consumer health complaints associated with the use of dietary supplements. MedWatch reporting is voluntary. In 2004, the Life Sciences Research Office published a report, *Recommendations for Adverse Event Monitoring Programs for Dietary Supplements*.

Label Claims

Label claims regarding dietary supplements are a complex issue that varies from country to country. Yet no matter what specific claims are allowed or disallowed by a country, it is reasonable to assume that any global regulation requires that the claim be true, not misleading, and be clear to the consumer. A summary of US label claims follows.

The Nutrition Labeling and Education Act (NLEA) was passed in 1990 as a result of a pre-1984 FDA position that prohibited making any therapeutic or disease-related claims on a food or dietary supplement label. The NLEA permits certain claims describing a positive relationship between a supplement and a health-related condition (or disease). These claims are considered 'health claims' in order to distinguish them from nutrient content claims. A health claim must be authorized by the FDA, and the FDA can only authorize a claim if there is "significant scientific agreement among qualified experts" or by the 1997 amendment that permits a manufacturer to rely on a statement from an "authoritative scientific body" of the US government or the National Academy of Sciences. This is a rigorous assessment and only 14 claims have been authorized to date.

In addition to health claims, dietary supplement labels are permitted to have qualified health claims or structure-function claims. The rationale behind the development of a qualified health claim was the idea that the First Amendment should allow disclaimers to be considered as solutions to making claims nonmisleading (Pearson v. Shalala). In other words, the First Amendment does not allow the FDA to reject health claims unless it shows that disclaimers would fail to remedy harm from misleading statements. The criteria for a qualified health claim were released in 2003 and in this context the FDA will not take enforcement action against a manufacturer using the following specified qualifiers provided the FDA is satisfied that the qualifiers are not misleading:

- "Although there is scientific evidence supporting the claim, the evidence is not conclusive."
- "Some scientific evidence suggests .... However, FDA has determined that this evidence is limited and not conclusive."
- "Very limited and preliminary scientific research suggests .... FDA concludes that there is little scientific evidence supporting this claim."

Qualified health claims for dietary supplements recognized by the FDA as part of its enforcement discretion include such examples as the relationships between phosphatidylserine and cognitive function, B vitamins and cardiovascular disease, omega-3 fatty acids and cardiovascular disease, selenium and cancer, and antioxidant vitamins and cancer.

Dietary supplements are not permitted to carry labeling statements that imply such issues as 'cure,' 'mitigate,' 'treat,' or 'prevent disease' because these statements are considered within the definition of a drug and drugs are subjected to a rigorous premarket approval process. However, under DSHEA, structure-function claims are permitted on dietary supplements because dietary supplements may have effects on the structure or function of the body without the implication that they act as a drug and/or are

related to disease. Structure-function claims include those that describe the role of the dietary supplement in affecting the structure or function in humans or the documented mechanism in which a dietary supplement acts to maintain such structure or function. In addition, dietary supplement label claims allow statements of benefits related to classical nutritional deficiency or statements regarding the general feeling of well-being derived from consumption.

Potential Benefits of Dietary Supplements

The 2000 *Dietary Guidelines for Americans* (new release due 2005) emphasizes choosing foods sensibly, maintaining a healthy weight, and exercising regularly. It acknowledges that some people may need a vitamin–mineral supplement to meet specific needs. Similarly, the Food and Nutrition Board and the American Dietetic Association also recognize that dietary supplements may be desirable for some nutrients and for some individuals. The following is a compilation of recommendations by these groups:

- Folic acid supplements for women of childbearing age due to the risk of neural tube defects
- Vitamin B_{12} supplements for people older than age 50 years due to inefficient absorption
- Vitamin B_{12} supplements for vegans who eat no animal products
- Calcium for people who seldom eat dairy products
- Vitamin D for elderly people who do not consume fortified dairy products and for others with little exposure to sunlight
- Iron supplementation for pregnant women
- Multivitamin–mineral supplement for people who are following a severely restricted weight-loss diet

Specifically for athletes, the position of the American Dietetic Association, Dietitians of Canada, and the American College of Sports Medicine is that physical activity, athletic performance, and recovery from exercise are enhanced by optimal nutrition. These organizations recommend appropriate selection of food and fluids, timing of intake, and supplement choices for optimal health and exercise performance. In sports, athletes who are at greatest risk of micronutrient deficiencies are those who restrict energy intake or use severe weight-loss practices, eliminate one or more food groups from their diet, are sick or recovering from injury, or consume high-carbohydrate diets with low micronutrient density. In practice, athletes should consume diets that provide at least the RDAs/DRIs for all micronutrients from food. It follows that, in general, no vitamin and mineral supplements are required if an athlete is consuming adequate energy from a variety of foods to maintain body weight. Supplementation may be necessary under conditions of inadequate food intake. Athletes, as for the general population, should follow supplementation recommendations unrelated to exercise, such as folic acid in women who may become pregnant.

Conclusions

One of the difficulties in assessing the nature of the worldwide dietary supplement industry and its regulations is largely in understanding what products are considered dietary supplements. In the United States, only pills, capsules, tablets, and the like are considered dietary supplements. Globally, it is sometimes difficult to discuss dietary supplements without discussing functional foods or nutraceuticals. Functional foods are similar in appearance to conventional foods but have demonstrated physiological benefits beyond the traditional nutritional value. Nutraceuticals may to go so far as to declare not only health benefits but also medical benefits that reduce the risk of chronic disease beyond basic nutritional functions. Canada regulates functional foods, nutraceuticals, and dietary supplements under one regulatory agency. The United States clearly distinguishes between foods and dietary supplements, although both fall under the category of food, which is distinct from drugs. The United Kingdom distinguishes between herbal medicines and dietary supplements containing vitamins and minerals. Japan regulates functional foods as FOSHU and has no regulatory definition for dietary supplements as defined in the United States. Moreover, these regulations are in a constant state of flux as the industry changes and develops over time. Issues that must be monitored regarding dietary supplements consumption are product quality and potential harmful interactions among supplements, foods, and drugs. Health claims that have been approved by regulatory agencies worldwide stress that the claims be truthful, clear, and not misleading to the ultimate consumer. Current scientific expertise acknowledges that dietary supplements, specifically some of the vitamins and minerals, have potential benefits in certain populations.

See also: **Folic Acid**. **Supplementation**: Role of Micronutrient Supplementation; Developing Countries; Developed Countries.

Further Reading

Anonymous (2000) Nutrition and athletic performance. Position of the American Dietetic Association, Dietitians of Canada, and the American College of Sports Medicine. *Journal of the American Dietetic Association* **100**: 1543–1556.

Huang SM and Lesko LJ (2004) Drug–drug, drug–dietary supplement, and drug–citrus fruit and other food interactions: What have we learned?. *Journal of Clinical Pharmacology* **44**(6): 559–569.

Percival SS and Turner RE (2000) Applications of herbs to functional foods. In: Wildman R (ed.) *Handbook of Functional Foods*. Boca Raton, FL: CRC Press.

Turner RE, Degnan FH, and Archer DL (2005) *Nutrition in Clinical Practice* **20**: 21–32.

U.S. Department of Agriculture (2000) *Dietary Guidelines for Americans*. Washington, DC: U.S. Department of Agriculture. Available at www.health.gov/dietaryguidelines/dgac.

Role of Micronutrient Supplementation

R D W Klemm, Johns Hopkins University, Baltimore, MD, USA

Introduction

Globally, almost two billion people (one-third of the human race) are affected by vitamin A, iron, iodine, and/or zinc deficiencies that put them at an increased risk of poor growth, morbidity, intellectual impairment, and/or mortality. Since the mid-1980s micronutrient supplementation has been a major public-health strategy in developing countries to prevent and control deficiencies in vitamin A, iron, and, to a lesser extent, iodine. More recently, zinc supplementation has come to be considered as an efficacious adjunctive therapy for diarrhea in populations with an elevated risk of zinc deficiency. This article will define micronutrient supplementation, examine the role of supplementation as a strategy for the prevention and control of micronutrient deficiencies, and examine evidence for vitamin A, iron, iodine, and zinc supplementation interventions with respect to efficacy, recommended dose, frequency of administration, safety, and program effectiveness.

Definition of Micronutrient Supplementation

Supplementation refers to the provision of added nutrients in pharmaceutical form (such as capsules, tablets, or syrups) rather than in food. Micronutrients are substances required by the body in small amounts for vital physiological functions. They cannot be synthesized by the body and therefore must be consumed in foods and/or in supplements.

Choice of Interventions

Micronutrient supplementation is one of three major categories of nutrition intervention strategies – the other two being fortification and dietary change. The choice of strategy or mix of strategies will depend on multiple factors including the magnitude, severity, and distribution of the micronutrient deficiency in the population, the relative intervention efficacy, the in-country resources available to deliver the intervention to the target group effectively, the target groups' acceptance of the intervention, and the ability to sustain the intervention.

The theoretical relative advantages of micronutrient supplementation over fortification and dietary-improvement interventions include rapid coverage of a high-risk population, the ability to provide directly a controlled and concentrated dose of the micronutrient(s) to the target group, an immediate impact on micronutrient status and associated functional outcome(s), the relatively low cost of training workers compared with nutrition counselling for diet improvement, and high coverage if supplements are delivered using existing services that already reach a high proportion of the target group. Most supplementation programs have been shown to be cost-effective in achieving their nutritional goals and health impacts, although sustaining large-scale programs over the long-term may be more costly than either fortification or dietary improvement.

Generally, prophylactic micronutrient supplementation is intended as a short-term means of rapidly preventing nutrient deficiency in high-risk individuals and populations until adequate and sustainable food-based programs become effective. However, in many cases, supplementation programs may be the only effective means of reaching specific vulnerable groups, particularly those who have limited or no access to processed fortified foods or those, such as young children and pregnant women, who have high micronutrient requirements that may not be met even with fortification and dietary-improvement interventions. In these situations and populations, supplementation should be sustained over a longer period until nutrient intake from fortified and non-fortified food is adequate.

Based on experiences from vitamin A, iron, and iodine supplementation programs, the key limitations of supplementation are inadequate targeting or coverage (where deficient individuals are missed or reached irregularly), an inability to sustain high

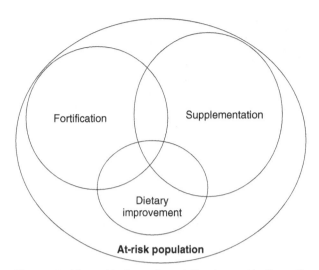

Figure 1 Micronutrient supplementation in combination with other nutrition-focused interventions to prevent micronutrient deficiencies in a target population.

coverage over long periods of time as financial, political, or other health priorities change, and poor compliance by target individuals who are expected to take a daily supplement for extended periods of time (e.g., iron supplementation during pregnancy). As illustrated in **Figure 1**, in many countries – particularly those with high regional variability in socio-economic status, food availability, and market-access – a mix of strategies, rather than any single strategy, is more likely to reach a greater proportion of the at-risk population.

Cost of Micronutrient Interventions

The World Bank's World Development Report 1993 found micronutrient programs to be among the most cost-effective of all health interventions. The cost of micronutrient supplementation needs to be balanced against the cost of other food-based and public-health interventions as well as against the cost of not addressing the insidious effects of micronutrient deficiencies. Costs are likely to vary depending on the scope of the program, existing delivery mechanisms, the nutrient involved, and other factors. Based on World Bank estimates, the costs of vitamin A, iron, and iodine supplementation programs are relatively modest, ranging from US$0.20 to US$1.70 per beneficiary per year. These costs are slightly higher than the estimated relative costs of fortification (US$0.05–0.15 per beneficiary per year) but are considerably lower than the unit costs of education programs (US$5–10) and feeding programs (US$70–100 per beneficiary per year).

Prophylactic Micronutrient Supplementation

Micronutrient supplementation has been the method of choice for the treatment of severe clinical nutrient deficiencies for several decades. Prophylactic supplementation, however, gained wider acceptance only in the late 1980s with the publication of results from a randomized trial in Aceh, Indonesia, showing a 34% reduction in young-child mortality among preschoolers given vitamin A supplements. The introduction of routine vitamin A supplementation to preschool children in developing countries has encouraged this approach and the development of other micronutrient supplementation programs. Each single-nutrient or multiple-micronutrient supplementation strategy should be evaluated separately for efficacy, feasibility, safety, cost, and appropriateness for the cultural and political context in which it will be implemented.

Vitamin A Supplementation

Periodic distribution of high-dose vitamin A supplements, either universally to all preschool children or to targeted high-risk groups, has been the most widely practiced intervention for the prevention and treatment of vitamin A deficiency throughout the world. Giving a high dose of vitamin A every 4–6 months is based on the assumption that vitamin A is stored in the liver and mobilized, as needed, to meet the demands of target tissues. This is in contrast to iron supplements, which need to be given on a daily or weekly basis.

Efficacy of Prophylactic Supplementation

Preschool children Giving children living in areas where vitamin A deficiency is prevalent a large dose (i.e., 200 000 IU or 60 mg Retinol Equivalent (RE)) of vitamin A every 4–6 months has been shown to reduce the risk of both noncorneal and corneal xeropthalmia by 90%, increase serum retinol levels for 1–2 months following supplementation, and reduce young-child mortality by an average of 23% when coverage levels of at least 80% are achieved in deficient populations. In populations deficient in vitamin A, prophylactic supplementation of preschool children is one of the most cost-effective public-health interventions to improve the survival of children aged between 6 months and 6 years.

Post-partum women High-dose vitamin A supplementation is also recommended for post-partum mothers within 6 weeks of delivery, when the chance of pregnancy is remote, because the physiological demands of pregnancy and lactation deplete the mother's vitamin A stores. The provisional recommendation of the International Vitamin A Consultative Group is to give two doses of 200 000 IU at least 24 h apart to all women living in areas where vitamin A deficiency is prevalent and to give the supplement as soon as possible after delivery in order to maximize the beneficial effects on maternal vitamin A status, breast-milk vitamin A concentrations, and subsequent infant vitamin A status. Spacing the two doses by at least a day minimizes the risk of raising breast-milk retinoic acid (a short-lived metabolite of vitamin A) to potentially toxic levels.

Newborns and young infants Two randomized controlled trials in Asia that provided 50 000 IU of vitamin A to infants in the first 2 days of life found significant reductions in infant mortality among the vitamin A supplemented newborns. A third, confirmatory, trial is currently underway in Bangladesh, which, depending on the findings, may lead to newborn dosing recommendations. The current World Health Organization (WHO) recommendation is to provide 50 000 IU of vitamin A to infants with each of the three doses of diphtheria, pertussis, and tetanus at 6, 10, and 14 weeks of age to improve vitamin A status. Further trials, however, are needed to confirm the benefit of implementing this recommendation for early infant vitamin A status, morbidity, and survival.

Pregnant women Where maternal night blindness or biochemical vitamin A deficiency is highly prevalent, prophylactic supplementation with up to 10 000 IU daily or 25 000 IU weekly has been given safely. The efficacy of low-dose maternal supplementation is still under investigation, but a recent community-based randomized placebo-controlled study in Nepal reported a 40% reduction in pregnancy-related maternal mortality among women given low doses of vitamin A or β-carotene, provided as a weekly supplement, during pregnancy and for 3 months post-partum. This is the first trial to link vitamin A supplementation and maternal survival. Confirmatory efficacy trials are underway in Bangladesh and Ghana and should provide guidance on future maternal vitamin A supplementation recommendations.

Form of Supplement

Vitamin A in the form of a gelatinous capsule is the overwhelming choice of delivery mode used in large public-health programs, although there are reports of the successful use of liquid vitamin A in a bottle using a calibrated dispenser. Vitamin A has also been dispensed from an inhalation device in children with parasitic infections as an alternative delivery mode in the very small number of children who exhibit extreme intestinal malabsorption of vitamin A.

Safety

High doses of vitamin A are safe and well accepted by preschool children, although evidence from program evaluations and a randomized trial in the Philippines suggests that up to around 9% of preschool children may experience acute transient side-effects including nausea, vomiting, headache, and/or fever after dosing. Most episodes begin within 24 h of capsule receipt and resolve spontaneously within 12–24 h of onset.

Earlier animal experiments linked high doses of vitamin A to birth defects; however, experimental data proving the teratogenic effect of vitamin A in pregnant women are limited and, for ethical reasons, very difficult or even impossible to obtain rigorously. Nonetheless, high doses of vitamin A should be avoided during pregnancy because of the theoretical risk of teratogenesis.

Delivery Mechanisms

There are a variety of ways to deliver high-dose vitamin A supplements to at-risk populations including restricting delivery to clinic settings for treatment purposes, integrating delivery with existing services such as immunization contacts or routine growth monitoring, or universal delivery, to attain the widest coverage of preschool children, through semi-annual campaigns that specifically promote vitamin A capsule distribution or that are combined with other national programs such as national immunization days or child-health weeks. Each delivery mode has advantages and disadvantages. Restricted delivery targets those most likely to be deficient in vitamin A and requires few additional resources (apart from the supplements); however it may result in poor coverage if those who are most at risk do not regularly access health clinics. 'Piggy-backing' vitamin A distribution onto existing community services can be cost-effective but may also miss the children at greatest risk of vitamin A deficiency if their access to and use of these services is limited. Finally, universal distribution requires strong community mobilization and social marketing to attain coverage levels of at least 80%. Sustaining this coverage level every 4–6 months can be challenging, but there are numerous examples of countries where such levels have been sustained for at least 5–8 years.

Iron Supplementation

Globally, supplementation with iron tablets is the most widely used strategy for the prevention and control of iron-deficiency or anemia in pregnancy. Pregnant women require nearly three times as much iron as non-pregnant women owing to the physiological demands of pregnancy (expanded red-blood-cell volume, the needs of the fetus and placenta, and blood loss at delivery). This high requirement is unattainable by most pregnant women in developing countries, especially those who struggle to meet the $1.5 \, \text{mg day}^{-1}$ requirement when not pregnant, and therefore iron supplementation is recommended during pregnancy.

Efficacy

Pregnancy The rationale for iron supplementation during pregnancy in developing countries is based on a combination of considerations including the high prevalence of anemia in pregnancy (the majority of which is probably associated with iron deficiency), carefully conducted trials that show that consuming iron tablets during pregnancy improves maternal iron status, the higher maternal mortality risks associated with severe anemia, and the postulated risks of iron deficiency in pregnancy (i.e., increased risk of fatigue, cardiovascular stress, impaired resistance to infection, and poor tolerance to heavy blood loss and surgical interventions at delivery) and for fetal development. Although evidence supports the efficacy of iron supplementation in improving the iron status of pregnant women, no trials have examined the impact of iron supplementation on maternal mortality in severely anemic women. Also, there is a lack of causal evidence from controlled studies linking mild-to-moderate iron-deficiency anemia – which is much more prevalent than severe anemia – with an increased risk of low birth weight, preterm delivery, or obstetrical or perinatal complications.

Infancy Iron supplementation in infants is sometimes advised to prevent iron deficiency, even in populations with a relatively low prevalence of iron-deficiency anemia. The US Institute of Medicine, for example, recommends iron drops for exclusively breast-fed infants between 4 and 6 months of age. There is ample evidence from well-designed and controlled studies to show that iron supplementation in infancy significantly improves hemoglobin and ferritin levels, and studies are currently investigating the impact of iron supplementation on dimensions of cognitive development. The benefits and risks of infant iron supplementation, however, remain controversial, particularly in iron-replete children. This is because, although iron is an essential nutrient for adequate infant growth, immune function, and development, it may also contribute to a greater risk of infection if the excess iron increases a pathogen's access to free iron for its own growth and reproduction. Some studies have reported a higher prevalence of diarrhea in iron-supplemented infants, which calls into question the appropriateness of existing hemoglobin and ferritin cut-offs for defining true deficiency in infants and points to the need to clarify the cut-off issue in order to determine an appropriate age for starting iron supplementation.

Low-birth-weight infants   Low-birth-weight infants are born with low iron stores and have higher iron requirements for growth. Their iron needs cannot be met from breast milk alone, and, therefore, they are a priority target for iron supplementation.

Preschooler and school-age children   Several, but not all, placebo-controlled supplementation trials have demonstrated that iron supplements improve hemoglobin concentrations in preschoolers in developing countries, and there is substantial evidence that iron supplementation of anemic children improves their school performance and verbal and other skills.

Dose

The WHO has published global guidelines for iron supplementation and recommends daily prophylactic iron supplementation with 60 mg of iron for all women in developing countries in the second and third trimesters of pregnancy (**Table 1**). In other countries, iron supplementation is recommended only for women with proven iron-deficiency anemia (in Great Britain) or for women with low pre-pregnancy iron stores (in Canada). The efficacy of maternal iron supplementation increases with daily iron doses of up to 60 mg. The WHO also recommends providing low-birth-weight infants with supplemental iron drops from 2 months of age.

Multiple Micronutrient Supplements with Iron

Currently, folic acid is added to most iron supplements for women of fertile age because it reduces the risk of neural-tube defects and because lack of folic acid may limit the hemoglobin response to iron supplements. In the absence of these nutrients such as vitamin A, vitamin B_{12}, and riboflavin may also limit the efficacy of iron supplements, and studies are underway to assess the effect of multiple micronutrient supplements on anemia.

Safety

Iron supplements can cause unpleasant gastrointestinal symptoms (e.g., nausea, constipation, vomiting, and diarrhoea), which may contribute to poor compliance, but these usually occur at higher doses. When iron tablets are taken with meals or if slow-release tablets are used, any side-effects may be mitigated. Complications of excessive iron storage, including hemochromatosis and hemosiderosis, are possible but uncommon in women consuming iron tablets. Another potential danger of iron supplements is accidental overdosing by children in the home, and therefore supplements should be kept out of the reach of children.

Frequency

A perceived concern about the side-effects, compliance, and potential toxicity of a daily regimen of iron supplementation generated research to assess the relative efficacy of weekly versus daily supplementation in pregnant women, adolescents, and children. A review of these studies concluded that both daily and weekly iron supplementation reduces the prevalence of iron deficiency and anemia, daily supplementation is more effective than weekly supplementation in increasing hemoglobin and ferritin, and while daily supplementation produces only a slightly higher average hemoglobin response (approximately $2 \, g \, l^{-1}$) than weekly supplementation, its relative impact on reducing anemia risk is 34%, largely because daily supplementation is more effective at increasing low hemoglobin concentrations.

From the results of two other studies, in Bangladesh and Indonesia, that carefully monitored the number of iron tablets consumed, it appears that the size of the hemoglobin response to iron appears to depend on the total amount of iron consumed. In these studies, most of the hemoglobin response was produced by the first 20–50 tablets consumed. But more research is needed before recommendations can be made about consuming a fixed number of tablets over a defined period of time while permitting flexibility about the consumption interval (i.e., daily, two or three times per week, weekly, etc.).

Taken together, the available evidence suggests that iron supplements should be taken daily to treat iron-deficiency anemia, especially in pregnant women. Weekly supplementation may offer a more feasible preventive strategy, particularly if it reduces costs, improves compliance, and reduces side-effects; however, more information is needed to assess the relative effectiveness of daily versus weekly supplementation under program conditions.

Table 1 Micronutrient supplementation: target groups and prevention schedules

Micronutrient	Target group	Dosage	Frequency and duration
Vitamin A[a]	Children at risk of vitamin A deficiency		
	<6 months	50 000 IU	One dose at 4, 10, and 14 weeks[e]
	6–11 months	100 000 IU	One dose every 4–6 months[f]
	1–5 years	200 000 IU	One dose every 4–6 months
	Post-partum women	400 000 IU[g]	One dose before 8 weeks post-partum
Iron (plus folate)[b]	Pregnant women (living in areas where anemia prevalence is less than 40%)	60 mg iron and 400 μg folic acid[i]	Daily for 6 months[h] in pregnancy
	Pregnant women (living in areas where anemia prevalence is at least 40%)	60 mg iron and 400 μg folic acid[i]	Daily for 6 months[h] in pregnancy, and continuing to 3 months post-partum
	6–24-month-old children of normal birth weight (living in areas where the prevalence of anemia in children is less than 40%)	12.5 mg iron and 50 μg folic acid	Daily to 6–12 months of age
	6–24-month-old children of normal birth weight (living in areas where the prevalence of anemia in children is greater than or equal to 40%)	12.5 mg iron and 50 μg folic acid	Daily to 6–24 months of age
	2–24-month-old children of low birth weight (less than 2500 g)	12.5 mg iron and 50 μg folic acid	Daily to 2–24 months of age
Iodine[c]	Pregnant women in areas where iodine deficiency is endemic[j]	300–480 mg	One dose annually
	Non-pregnant fertile women[j]	400–960 mg	One dose annually
	Children in areas where iodine deficiency is endemic[j]	240 mg iodine	One dose annually
Zinc[d]	Children with persistent diarrhea[k]	10–20 mg	Daily for 14 days
	Children with an elevated risk of zinc deficiency; children who are severely stunted, or have low plasma zinc, or both	Further research needed on relative efficacy of different frequencies and doses	

[a]Adapted from World Health Organization (1997) *Vitamin A Supplements: A Guide to Their Use in the Treatment and Prevention of Vitamin A Deficiency and Xerophthalmia*, 2nd edn. Geneva: World Health Organization.

[b]Adapted from Stoltzfus RJ and Dreyfus JL (1998) *Guidelines for the Use of Iron Supplements to Prevent and Treat Iron Deficiency Anemia*. INACG ILSI Press, Washington DC.

[c]Adapted from World Health Organization (1996) Safe Use of iodized oil to prevent iodine deficiency in pregnant women – a Statement by the WHO. *Bulletin of the World Health Organization* **74**: 1–3.

[d]Adapted from the recommendations of an expert group: Fontaine O (2001) Effect of zinc supplementation on clinical course of acute diarrhoea. *Journal of Health Population and Nutrition* **19**: 339–346.

[e]Give at the time of each of the three diphtheria–pertussis–tetanus vaccinations.

[f]Immunization against measles provides a good opportunity to give one of these doses.

[g]Provisional recommendation of the International Vitamin A Consultative Group, Annecy, France, 30 October–2 November, 2000.

[h]If 6 months' duration cannot be achieved in pregnancy, continue to supplement during the post-partum period for 6 months or increase the dose to 120 mg iron in preganancy.

[i]Where iron supplements containing 400 μg of folic acid are not available, an iron supplement with less folic acid may be used. Supplementation with less folic acid should be used only if supplements containing 400 μg are not available.

[j]Where access to iodine-fortified salt is limited and immediate attention is needed.

[k]In areas where there is an elevated risk of zinc deficiency in the population.

Form of Iron

In tablets, the most common form of iron is ferrous sulphate (which contains 20% iron), but ferrous fumarate (33% iron) and ferrous gluconate (12% iron) are also used. Infant supplements are usually in liquid form and more costly, but when crushed or mixed with food, tablets can also be used.

Effective Iron-Supplementation Programs

Reviews of large-scale iron-supplementation programs in developing countries have reported limited effectiveness in reducing maternal anemia. The limited effectiveness is often attributed to implementation constraints including low compliance, short intervention duration, inadequate supplement supply, or poor coverage of pregnant women. For iron-supplementation programs to achieve improved effectiveness, careful attention must be given to ensuring an adequate supply of iron tablets at the distribution points, access of pregnant women to the distribution points, promotion of the benefits of iron supplementation, counselling about managing possible side-effects, and communication strategies to encourage pregnant women to consume the supplement.

Iodine Supplementation

Salt iodization is the recommended means of population-based intervention to prevent and control iodine deficiency disorders, but, in isolated communities with an urgent need for iodine prophylaxis, direct supplementation of priority groups can be rapidly implemented as an interim measure while salt iodization is being established.

Efficacy

Intramuscular iodine injections Numerous studies have confirmed that iodine supplementation by injection before a woman becomes pregnant can prevent endemic cretinism and that a single injection can prevent goitre for up to 3–4 years. Other documented benefits of maternal supplementation observed in several controlled studies include reduced infant and young-child mortality, improved birth weight, and better manual function in children born to iodine-supplemented mothers.

Oral iodized oil Although efficacious, injections of iodized oil have largely been replaced by oral iodized oil owing to the concern over the AIDS pandemic and use of needles as well as the higher cost of supplies (syringes) and personnel (skilled injectors). Oral delivery of iodized oil appears to be as effective as intramuscular injection but is less costly, carries no infection risk (through a contaminated needle), is painless, and can be administered by untrained personnel. Oral iodized oil is considered to be safe for pregnant women and can be given at any time during pregnancy; however, it appears to protect against moderate and severe neurological abnormalities in the infant only when given during the first two trimesters. The best outcomes are likely to occur when supplementation is given during the first trimester, but even if it is given in late pregnancy or to the infant after birth slight improvements in brain growth and developmental quotients, but not neurological status, are evident.

Dose

Owing to the fact that damage to the developing brain is the most severe consequence of iodine deficiency, women of child-bearing age and children are the first priorities for receiving iodized oil. Recommendations are to give a single dose of 460 mg of iodine to all females below the age of 40 years. A single annual dose of 240 mg of iodine appears to be adequate for children. Larger doses do not necessarily provide longer protection because of increased urinary loss after administration. It is possible that smaller more frequent doses may be more effective, although this issue requires further study. Evidence from studies using 200–500 mg of iodized oil suggests that the protective effect lasts for between 6 months and 2 years.

Safety

Oral iodine supplementation is safe, although side-effects can include transient submandibular swelling and subclinical hypothyroidism.

Zinc Supplementation

During the past decade, zinc supplementation has received increasing attention as results from research trials reveal the extent of zinc deficiency in developing countries and the role of zinc supplementation in reducing intrauterine growth retardation and disease incidence and severity and improving children's cognitive development, growth, and survival. However, most of what is known about zinc supplementation is based on the results of research trials and not of large-scale programs that deliver zinc supplements.

Efficacy

Diarrhoea and pneumonia Short-term treatment of diarrhoea and possibly pneumonia with zinc supplementation has proven efficacious in numerous randomized controlled trials. A pooled analysis of nine randomized controlled trials reported an 18% lower incidence and a 25% reduction in prevalence of diarrhoea in zinc-supplemented children regardless of age, baseline zinc status, wasting prevalence, or sex, suggesting that zinc supplementation may benefit many subgroups of children living in areas at high risk of zinc deficiency. Studies have also investigated the efficacy of a combination of micronutrients given together with zinc and have shown that zinc alone is just as efficacious as a multiple micronutrient that includes zinc in reducing the severity of acute diarrhoea.

There is growing evidence that zinc supplementation reduces the risk of pneumonia. A pooled analysis of five randomized controlled trials reported a 34% reduction in the incidence of pneumonia in zinc-supplemented children, but evidence from three short-course zinc-supplementation trials suggests a non-significant reduction in the incidence of pneumonia and in hospitalization rates for acute lower respiratory infection.

Other outcomes Evidence from a limited number of trials suggests a potential benefit of zinc supplementation on morbidity related to *Plasmodium falciparum* infections, child survival, weight gain in low-birth-weight infants and severely malnourished children, length gain in stunted children, and a host of maternal health and pregnancy outcomes; however, more research is required to determine the benefits of a large-scale zinc-supplementation program targeted at groups of infants, children, and pregnant women.

Dose

There is a need for systematic studies to determine the appropriate dose of supplemental zinc for preventing zinc deficiency in different age groups and under different clinical conditions. However, based on therapeutic studies, giving zinc supplements in doses ranging between one and four times the recommended dietary allowance per day ($15\,mg.day^{-1}$ for children aged less than 1 year, and $20–30\,mg.day^{-1}$ for children aged more than 1 year) for 14 days is efficacious in reducing the severity of diarrhoea and the duration of the episode significantly. In hospitalized children, zinc can be given as two or three divided doses each day, although in community interventions a single dose of $20\,mg.day^{-1}$ appears both safe and efficacious. Studies are underway to determine the feasibility and efficacy of adding zinc to oral rehydration solution.

Form of Zinc

There are many zinc compounds that can be used to produce zinc supplements. They differ in color (from colorless, to white, grey, or yellowish white), taste (bitter, astringent, slightly sour, or bitter), odour (odourless, vanilla odour, or faint odour of acetic acid), solubility in water (insoluble, slightly soluble, or soluble), cost, side-effects, and safety. Water-soluble compounds (e.g., zinc acetate, zinc sulfate, and zinc gluconate) are more easily absorbed and therefore preferred. Zinc supplements have been prepared in flavored syrups, chewable tablets, single-dose 'sachets' to be added to food, as a high-fat spread to be consumed alone or with other food for infants and young children, and as dry supplements (tablets, capsules, or powders) alone or with other nutrients. The choice of supplement form will depend on the age of the target group, preference, and whether other nutrients will be included.

Effectiveness of Zinc-Supplementation Programs

There is little information about the effectiveness of zinc-supplementation programs implemented on a large scale. There is a need to conduct such studies to assess the best ways to deliver zinc supplements to children with diarrhoea, paying particular attention to the feasibility, sustainability, and cost-effectiveness of different zinc-delivery mechanisms.

Summary

The feasibility of micronutrient supplementation and the degree to which it should be pursued in combination with other strategies to prevent and control micronutrient deficiencies depend on the local needs, resources, capabilities, commitment, and evidence of benefit. The successful prevention and control of vitamin A, iron, and zinc deficiencies will probably result from a combination of repetitive distribution of high-dose nutrient supplements, fortification of staple foods, and behavioral change, whereas fortification of salt alone with iodine has already achieved much success in combating iodine deficiency disorders. The adoption of supplementation approaches should be guided by evidence of a need for targeting, impact potential, costs, and potential sustainability.

See also: **Folic Acid. Iodine**: Physiology, Dietary Sources and Requirements; Deficiency Disorders. **Supplementation**: Developing Countries; Developed Countries. **Vitamin A**: Deficiency and Interventions. **Zinc**: Deficiency in Developing Countries, Intervention Studies.

Further Reading

Allen LH (2002) Iron supplements: scientific issues concerning efficacy and implications for research and programs. *Journal of Nutrition* 132(suppl 4): 813S–819S.

Angermayr L and Clar C (2004) Iodine supplementation for preventing iodine deficiency disorders in children (Cochrane Review). In: *The Cochrane Library*, Issue 2, 2004. Chichester: John Wiley & Sons, Ltd.

International Zinc Nutrition Consultative Group (IZiNCG) (2004) Assessment of the risk of zinc deficiency in populations and options for its control. Hotz C and Brown KH (eds.) *Food and Nutrition Bulletin* 25(suppl 1): S91–S204.

Mahomed K (2004) Iron and folate supplementation in pregnancy (Cochrane Review). In: *The Cochrane Library*, Issue 2, 2004. Chichester: John Wiley & Sons, Ltd.

Mahomed K and Gülmezoglu AM (2004) Maternal iodine supplements in areas of deficiency (Cochrane Review). In: *The Cochrane Library*, Issue 2, 2004. Chichester: John Wiley & Sons, Ltd.

Sommer A and West KP Jr (1996) *Vitamin A Deficiency: Health, Survival and Vision*. New York: Oxford University Press.

Stoltzfus RJ and Dreyfuss ML (1998) *Guidelines for the Use of Iron Supplements to Prevent and Treat Iron Deficiency Anemia.* International Nutritional Anemia Consultative Group (INACG)/WHO/UNICEF. Geneva: World Health Organization.

World Health Organization (1996) Safe use of iodized oil to prevent iodine deficiency in pregnant women: a statement by the World Health Organization. *Bulletin of the World Health Organization* 74: 1–3.

World Health Organization (1997) *Vitamin A Supplements: A Guide to Their Use in the Treatment and Prevention of Vitamin A Deficiency and Xerophthalmia*, 2nd edn. Geneva: World Health Organization.

T

THIAMIN

Contents
Beriberi
Physiology

Beriberi

D I Thurnham, University of Ulster, Coleraine, UK

Beriberi is caused by a deficiency of thiamin (also called thiamine, aneurin(e), and vitamin B_1). Classic overt thiamin deficiency causes cardiovascular, cerebral, and peripheral neurological impairment and lactic acidosis. The disease emerged in epidemic proportions at the end of the nineteenth century in Asian and Southeast Asian countries. Its appearance coincided with the introduction of the roller mills that enabled white rice to be produced at a price that poor people could afford. Unfortunately, milled rice is particularly poor in thiamin; thus, for people for whom food was almost entirely rice, there was a high risk of deficiency and mortality from beriberi. Outbreaks of acute cardiac beriberi still occur, but usually among people who live under restricted conditions. The major concern today is subclinical deficiencies in patients with trauma or among the elderly. There is also a particular form of clinical beriberi that occurs in patients who abuse alcohol, known as the Wernicke–Korsakoff syndrome. Subclinical deficiency may be revealed by reduced blood and urinary thiamin levels, elevated blood pyruvate/lactate concentrations and α-ketoglutarate activity, and decreased erythrocyte transketolase (ETKL) activity. Currently, the *in vitro* stimulation of ETKL activity by thiamin diphosphate (TDP) is the most useful functional test of thiamin status where an acute deficiency state may have occurred. The stimulation is measured as the TDP effect.

Epidemiology

Beriberi presents in several different clinical forms (**Table 1**). Beriberi became endemic following the introduction of steam-powered rice mills, which enabled milled rice to be produced cheap enough so that almost everybody could afford it and consume it. It was particularly serious at the end of nineteenth and the beginning of the twentieth centuries when seasonal epidemics of wet beriberi occurred with many deaths. The disease affected mainly the Chinese and Japanese populations, although outbreaks were reported in India and among settlers in the New World during the long cold winters, and the disease was not necessarily confined to rice-eating populations. Where acute cardiac beriberi occurred, dry beriberi was also present but usually in the older members of the community.

Milled rice has a thiamin concentration that is particularly poor ($80\,\mu g/100\,g$), but social conditions at the time of the large epidemics contributed to the problems. Bonded labor was common, with workers living on the work premises most of the time and paid mainly in the form of rice. In addition, reports at the time suggest that the rice was of uncertain freshness and quality, and that it could be so mouldy, matted, and lumpy that it had to be remilled and washed, with a further loss of thiamin. The social conditions prevented natural eating practices because workers had little money to purchase additional food and they were dependent on what they were given. Likewise, badly stored cereals can lose up to 90% of the thiamin content, and toxins associated with mould growth have been implicated in causing sickness that may well precipitate clinical beriberi.

Reports suggest that the acuteness of the outbreak of beriberi and the interrelationship of thiamin

Table 1 Forms of beriberi in man

Subclinical beriberi	Identified by transketolase activity or other biochemical tests of thiamin status. May be associated with early subjective symptoms such as anorexia, weakness, dysthesie, and depression. Responds rapidly to treatment with thiamin.
Wet beriberi	Subacute or cardiac beriberi frequently having muscular pains, oedema of feet and legs, enlarged heart, and tachycardia.
	Responds rapidly to treatment with thiamin. Major form and was typically seasonal in endemic areas.
	Acute fulminant type of beriberi in which the main feature is dominated by insufficiency of the heart and blood vessels. Responds rapidly to treatment with thiamin.
Dry beriberi	Chronic, atrophic type of polyneuropathy in which the main features are of a weak wasted person, with painful musculature making walking difficult, impaired sensory nerves and tendon reflexes, and flaccid paralysis of the motor nerves. Poor or no response to treatment with thiamin.
Infantile beriberi	Usually acute wet beriberi. Responds rapidly to treatment with thiamin.
Wernicke–Korsakoff syndrome	Predominantly neurological, affecting walking and vision in most and memory and cardiac function in over 50% of patients. Wernicke or ocular component responds rapidly to treatment but the Korsakoff psychosis responds slowly or not at all.

Modified from Thurnham DI (1978) Thiamin. In: Rechcigl M Jr (ed.) *Nutrition Disorders*, pp. 3–14. West Palm Beach, FL: CRC Press.

deficiency with deficiencies of other nutrients probably had a major role in determining the nature of the pathological changes and lesions produced. For example, it is reported that protein energy malnutrition almost always accompanied subacute beriberi, reflecting the link between impoverishment and the disease. In contrast, it is also suggested that severe beriberi more often affected the more active, stronger, or supposedly better nourished members of the community. The younger, stronger rickshaw puller was most likely to suffer severe beriberi. Likewise, infantile beriberi appeared to affect the male infant who 'tended to be overfed.' This enigma may be due to thiamin intakes from a diet containing a high proportion of rice being insufficient to meet the thiamin requirement posed by the higher calorie intakes of the more active community members. In the case of infantile beriberi, slightly deficient mothers probably produced milk that was only marginally adequate in thiamin and/or infants were given supplements of thiamin-poor rice. It is a common habit even today for rural mothers to give very young infants, even beginning at 1 week of age, a bolus of masticated rice to supplement the milk intake. The inability to match thiamin intake to energy needs may also explain why nonspecific pyrexia was a precipitating factor for beriberi. A 1 °C rise in body temperature is associated with a 10% increase in basal metabolic rate. It has been suggested that more than half the mild cases of beriberi were associated with a nonspecific bout of fever, and such cases responded less readily to treatment with thiamin.

Parboiled rice is partially cooked before milling, and this prevents beriberi because the thiamin is dispersed through the grain (190 μg/100 g). The advantages of this were clearly seen in Malaya, where at the end of nineteenth century there were large-scale immigrations of young, able-bodied Chinese to work in the tin mines and Indians to work on the rubber estates. In both cases, immigrants often lived in remote regions where there was little opportunity to purchase local food and they were dependent on imported rice. It was the Chinese who, because of their dietary preference for milled rice, died in enormous numbers.

Although ways of avoiding the disease were known to the Japanese navy at the end of the nineteenth century, since the director general of the medical department had demonstrated that the disease was almost eradicated if the traditional rice diet was supplemented with fish, vegetables, meat, and barley, this information was not widely available, and supplementation was not feasible by the vast majority of people. It was widely believed that the cause of beriberi was an infection or toxin resulting from bad food. In particular, Pasteur's work on the microbiological cause of infections led many to search for an infectious agent, but none could be consistently identified. The scale of the problem for the colonial powers in Southeast Asia in the latter part of the nineteenth and early twentieth centuries should not be underestimated. Labour was cheap but the death toll posed enormous problems. Extracts from reports at the time are illuminating: In 1887, there were 690 deaths out of 1931 native government officers in Sumatra, infant mortality was 445 per 1000 live births in the Philippines in 1910, and one report stated that there were so many deaths that "there was insufficient earth to bury the corpses."

The Dutch government sought to resolve the situation by appointing a medical bacteriologist, Christiaan

Eijkman, to travel to Indonesia to investigate the problem. Working in Java, he showed within 6 years that beriberi was a nutritional problem and that a paralytic condition closely resembling the polyneuritic symptoms of beriberi could be produced in chickens by feeding them both stale and freshly cooked polished rice. However, it was Funk in 1911 who first reported the isolation of a 'vital amine' from rice polishings that had anti-beriberi properties. Funk was the first person to coin the word 'vitamine' as a substance essential for life. The structure and synthesis of thiamin were reported in 1936.

Currently, clinical beriberi no longer occurs with the devastating effects of former years. Considerable improvements have occurred in nutrition worldwide, the diversity of foods available, the quality of food due to improved storage methods, and social and economic structures in many countries, especially in Southeast Asia. However, sporadic outbreaks do occur, which are usually of the acute, fulminating type of beriberi, and deaths still occur often in young men aged 20–40 years. Usually, a combination of factors is responsible, but once the cause is identified, treatment is cheap and readily available and, if given rapidly, tragic circumstances can be averted.

Two iatrogenic causes of subclinical beriberi are known, namely that associated with diuretic treatment and one resulting from alcohol abuse. Both are of concern because the use of diuretics is introduced to manage cardiovascular disease, a condition that will deteriorate if thiamin status is impaired, and alcohol abuse can lead to Wernicke–Korsakoff syndrome, which can have many of the features of both wet and dry beriberi.

Severe multisystem trauma, endotoxemia, or situations in which there is a raised metabolic demand for thiamin, such as pregnancy, thyrotoxicosis, and intercurrent illness or impaired absorption (e.g., alcohol abuse or gastrointestinal disease or resection), can produce subclinical evidence of thiamin deficiency or more severe life-threatening aspects of beriberi, such as renal and/or cardiovascular failure. The elderly may be particularly at risk of subclinical thiamin deficiency. One Belgian study on patients with a mean age of 83 years reported that 40% had a raised TDP effect (>15%), in whom there was a high proportion of Alzheimer's disease, depression, cardiac failure, and falls. The diuretic furosemide was also more frequently taken by the thiamin-deficient patients.

Etiology

The factors associated with the various forms of beriberi are listed in **Table 2**. Beriberi is caused by a lack of thiamin in the diet, but the onset of the

Table 2 Aetiological factors contributing to thiamin deficiency

Dietary thiamin deficiency	Commonly milled rice
High dietary carbohydrate to fat ratio	Metabolism of carbohydrate requires thiamin, whereas metabolism of fat spares thiamin requirements
Heavy physical activity	Predisposes to beriberi when accompanied by low intake of thiamin
Protein energy malnutrition	Older literature reports sometimes accompanies subacute beriberi indicating importance of impoverished diet
Poor storage conditions for food	Fall 6- to 10-fold in thiamin content of cereals. Moulds may accelerate decay as well as increase risk of toxins
Thiaminases	Two known, but only of importance when uncooked foods are consumed
Anti-thiamin factors	Factors in food that chelate with thiamin and potentially reduce bioavailability
Alcohol abuse	Alcohol impairs the active absorption mechanism for thiamin
Infection and trauma	Increase requirements for thiamin to support increased carbohydrate metabolism and energy production
Diuretics, long-term use	Accelerate thiamin excretion and appear to block thiamin control mechanism
Seasonal factors	Combination of heavy work load, impoverished diet, and last season's (badly stored) cereals
Male sex	Some evidence that men have higher thiamin requirements than women but more likely to be a combination of the first three factors listed here

disease and the symptoms associated with the disease are influenced by one or more of the other etiological factors. Wet beriberi (i.e., cardiac beriberi) and Wernicke's encephalopathy are conventionally described as acute manifestations of the disease and respond most rapidly to treatment. In contrast, dry beriberi is described as due to a chronic deficiency of thiamin and does not respond well to treatment. However, experimental acute deficiency studies, which very rapidly produced subjective feelings of malaise and weakness at the slightest exertion, very rarely produced evidence of oedema and peripheral pain. These observations suggest that all forms of beriberi are probably preceded by an indeterminate period of chronic thiamin deficiency during which pathophysiological adaptations to the marginal nutritional state occur. Thus, physiological adaptations to the vascular system may well have occurred particularly in those who did heavy physical work and needed to overcome the weakness and malaise imposed by a low thiamin diet. The factor(s) that precipitated the clinical disease may not be thiamin at all. Platt, in his descriptions of beriberi in China, recounts how humid weather and infections such as malaria increased the number of cases of wet beriberi. The extra energy needed to cool the body in hot conditions or fuel the rise in temperature during infection may have imposed a critical burden on energy production that the system could not meet, and beriberi ensued.

However, the increased number of cases associated with heat, humidity, and malaria may also be due to a seasonal decline in the quality of food. A 6- to 12-fold decline in thiamin content is reported for millet when stored under traditional thatched storage houses in the Gambia, and reports suggest that much of the rice consumed late in the season was not in the best condition. Some of the products introduced by mould growth may possess anti-thiamin properties that impair thiamin bioavailability. Thus, the ratio of thiamin to calories is likely to fall during the agricultural year and to be at its worst when calorie requirements are at their highest for land preparation and weeding. Land preparation also takes place just prior to or at the beginning of the rainy season, when the prevalence of malaria and diarrhoeal diseases increases.

Thiaminases are inactivated by cooking; thus, the enzymes are only a problem where certain foods are eaten raw. It has been suggested that in northern Thailand, where consumption of fermented raw fish products is widely practised and raw molluscs are eaten, thiamin status may be impaired by these food habits. Even as recently as 2001, marginal thiamin status was reported in more than 50% of women 3 months postpartum despite thiamin supplements of 100 mg/day during pregnancy. The deficiencies were found in Karen refugee women living on the Thai–Burmese border and whose diet contained fermented fish, tea leaves, and betel nuts—substances suspected of containing thiaminases. Polyphenol compounds in tea and many vegetables may also posses anti-thiamin properties and impair bioavailability, but their etiological importance in causing thiamin deficiency is difficult to assess.

Alcohol is an important factor in causing thiamin deficiency because it inhibits the active transport of thiamin across the gut and when abused it impairs the quality of the diet consumed. Diuretics accelerate the excretion of thiamin and appear to override the renal conservation mechanism. Their use is of potential concern in elderly people whose diet may be poor for other medical reasons and their physicians may be unaware of their need for supplemental nutrient.

Both sexes are vulnerable to the effects of thiamin deficiency, but in many of the sporadic outbreaks that have been reported, there appears to have been a male excess. This may be due to higher thiamin requirements in men than women because of their higher lean body mass or to hormonally driven sex differences. However, it is also possible that the cause is due to a higher risk of a thiamin:calorie imbalance in men compared to women. In many rural communities, men traditionally eat first and may satisfy their calorie requirements, whereas their womenfolk make do with the leftovers. Because of their greater physical strength, men frequently do heavier work than women, requiring more energy (i.e., more food to meet their requirements). Thus, men may consume more of the thiamin-depleted cereals in the diet to satisfy calorie needs and in so doing achieve a poorer thiamin:calorie ratio than women.

Experimental Thiamin Deficiency in Man and Measurement of Thiamin Status

In young and healthy nonalcoholic subjects, subjective symptoms appear after 2 or 3 weeks of deficient diet but urinary thiamin will already be falling (Table 3). Characteristic early symptoms include anorexia, weakness, dysthesiae, and depression. At this stage, urinary thiamin will be almost zero, ETKL activity depressed, and the TDP effect approximately 15–30%. After 6–8 weeks the only objective signs at rest may be a slight fall in blood pressure and moderate weight loss, although urinary thiamin will now be negligible and the TDP effect $\geq 35\%$. After 2 or 3 months, apathy and weakness become extreme, calf muscle tenderness develops, and there is loss of recent memory, confusion, ataxia, and sometimes persistent vomiting. Urinary thiamin will be negligible and the TDP effect may be normal (because apo-ETKL is unstable even *in vivo*), but ETKL activity should be considerably depressed.

The clinical symptoms resulting from experimental thiamin deficiency in man have usually responded rapidly to treatment with thiamin. In one feeding study, however, two mental patients were kept for 110 days on a diet providing 200 μg thiamin daily and 1 mg of thiamin by injection 1 day each week; thus, their overall weekly average was 350 μg/day. They developed a polyneuropathy characterised by defects in the sensory nervous pathways, loss of tendon reflexes, and paralysis of the legs, which took many weeks to respond to large doses of thiamin, and in one case response was still incomplete after 4 months of treatment. The slow cure suggested that degeneration of peripheral nerves had occurred, as is

Table 3 Effects of thiamin deficiency on urinary thiamin, the erythrocyte transketolase TDP effect, and early clinical symptoms of thiamin deficiency in human volunteers

Days of deficiency	Urinary thiamin (μg/day)[a]	TDP effect (%)[a]	Clinical signs of deficiency following diets containing 150–350 μg thiamin/day[b]
5	50	0–10	Mostly studies report no signs but one study (360 μg/day) found within 1 week chest
10	25	~15	pains, extreme lassitude, anorexia, palpitation, and burning feet
21–28	<25	~30	Loss of body weight, anorexia, general malaise, insomnia, increased irritability, fatigue on slightest exertion
30–40	Negligible	≥40	Increased malaise, loss of body weight, intermittent claudication and polyneuritis, bradycardia, peripheral oedema,[a] cardiac enlargement,[a] ophthalmoplegia
>45	10–20	>40	Additional signs of nausea and dizziness appeared
~75	10–20	>40	Additional signs of vomiting, low blood pressure, and tenderness of calves

[a]Biochemical data and report of oedema and cardiac enlargement from Brin (1964), in which healthy male medical students were fed 200 μg thiamin per day for 6 weeks. TDP effect is a measure of thiamin status obtained by measuring the activity of erythrocyte transketolase in the presence and absence of added thiamin diphosphate.
[b]Clinical signs adapted from several studies. Investigators were impressed by the rapid degree of debility induced by the specific withdrawal of thiamin from the diet. In one group (150 μg/day for 75 days, four female mental patients), the authors reported that the condition more closely resembled 'neurasthenia' than beriberi and noted that oedema, cardiac dilation, and peripheral pain characteristic of classic beriberi were all absent (reported by Carpenter, 2002).

indicated in the dry form of beriberi, in which the neurological lesions are irreversible.

Clinical Features of Beriberi

Depletion and repletion studies suggest that intakes >300 μg/4.2 MJ are compatible with normal biochemistry and good health, and clinical signs of thiamin deficiency occur at intakes of thiamin below 200 μg/4.2 MJ (1000 kcal). The disease as studied from the 1880s onward in Asians subsisting on white rice began typically with weakness, 'wandering pains' in the legs, and lack of feeling in the feet. Some patients then developed oedema (the presence of excessive amounts of fluid in the intercellular tissue spaces of the body) of the legs, trunk, and face. In severe cases, sufferers found it increasingly difficult to catch their breath and would die of heart failure. The clinical features of subacute and acute wet beriberi are summarized in **Table 4**. The main form was subacute beriberi, which was typically seasonal in endemic areas. There are reports that the peripheral muscles most severely affected were those most frequently used; thus, in male laborers it was the legs. Aching pain, tightness, and cramps in the calf and associated muscles were usually a first cause of complaint, and pain on squeezing the calves was one of the most useful diagnostic tests for beriberi. In women who performed repetitive tasks involving hands and arms, a loss of sensation in the fingers was frequently a first cause of complaint.

Dry beriberi is essentially a chronic condition showing muscular atrophy and polyneuritis and frequently occurring in older adults. Walking is usually difficult because of the weak wasted and painful musculature, and in the later stages feeding and dressing may also become impossible. When bed-ridden and cachetic (extreme state of malnutrition and wasting), patients become very susceptible to infections. Sensory nervous function is impaired (hypoesthesia) almost to the point of anesthesia. Hypoesthesia is particularly evident in the extremities and progressively extends over the outer aspects of the legs, thighs, and forearms. Motor nerve disturbances also begin in the extremities and ascend progressively. Flaccid paralysis of the extensor muscles precedes that affecting the flexors and results in 'wrist drop' and 'foot drop'. Loss of the Achilles tendon reflex usually precedes an impaired patellar reflex.

Mortality from infantile beriberi mainly affected breast-fed infants between the second and fifth months of life, when solid foods were often first introduced. The introduction of white rice porridges, poor in thiamin, to a rapidly growing child and/or the increased exposure to infections when solids are introduced may both have contributed to infantile beriberi. The onset of the disease was rare in the first month and early signs could be mild and somewhat subjective (e.g., vomiting, restlessness, anorexia, and insomnia). Early signs could progress to subacute infantile beriberi, the acute and usually fatal condition, or a chronic form. Features of acute infantile beriberi are presented in **Table 5**. The subacute form was characterized by slight oedema in the form of puffiness, vomiting, abdominal pain, oliguria, dysphagia, and convulsions. In addition, aphonia (soundless cry) was often a feature of subacute infantile beriberi and may have been due to nerve paralysis or

Table 4 Common features of wet beriberi

	Subacute beriberi	Acute fulminating beriberi[a]
Digestive system	Anorexia is common; constipation more frequent than diarrhea	Vomiting is common, often with intense thirst Liver enlarged and tender and the epigastric region spontaneously painful
Neurological	Aching pain, stiffness, tightness, or cramps in calf or associated muscles Increasing muscular tenderness and weakness with fatigue pains resembling muscular ischemia, especially at night Pain on squeezing calves Inability to rise from squatting position without use of hands Diminished reflexes of ankle and knees usually bilaterally Hypoesthesia or paraesthesia presenting as 'pins and needles,' numbness particularly over the tibia, formication (like ants running on the skin) or itching	Pupils dilated with anxious expression on face Aphonia frequently present and patient moans with cries of a special kind as a result of hoarseness produced by paralysis of laryngeal muscles Reflexes of ankle or knee lost or diminished
Cardiac	Oedema of feet and legs often appearing first on dorsa of feet and extending up legs but may also appear on back of hands and as puffiness in face Heart enlarged with tachycardia and bounding pulse Raised venous pressure (see **Figure 1**) with percussion sometimes revealing dilation of right auricle and ventricle Heart murmurs if present are usually systolic Apex beat is downward and outwardly displaced Neck vein possibly distended showing visible pulsations Dyspnea upon exertion Palpations, dizziness, and giddiness Extremities possibly cold and pale with peripheral cyanosis but where circulation is maintained, skin warm due to vasodilatation Electrocardiograms often undisturbed but QRS complex may show low voltage and inversion of T waves indicating disturbed conduction	Patients severely dyspneic, have violent palpitations of the heart, are extremely restless, experience intense precordial agony but accessory muscles of respiration on slightly brought into action Widespread and powerful undulating pulsations visible in the region of the heart, epigastrium, and neck due to a tumultuous heart action Facial cyanosis more marked during inspiration Pulse is moderately full, regular, even with frequency of 120-150/min A wavelike motion may be felt over the heart On percussion, the heart is enlarged both to the left and right but mainly the latter, and the apex beat may reach the axilla Raised systolic pressure and low diastolic pressure give the 'pistol shot' sound on auscultation over the large arteries Rapidly increasing oedema may extend from legs to trunk and face with associated pericardial, pleural, and other serous effusions
Urine	Nocturia; no albuminuria	Oliguria or anuria; no albuminuria or glycosuria

[a]The whole picture of acute fulminating beriberi is dominated by insufficiency of heart and blood vessels and this tends to mask all other features of the subacute form, although these are often present and accentuated. Death is accompanied by a systolic pressure falling to 70–80 mm, the pulse becomes thinner, and the veins dilate. The rough whistling respiration deteriorates and rales appear. The patient dies intensely dyspneic but usually fully conscious.

oedema of vocal cords. Vomiting was also a feature of chronic infantile beriberi and could be accompanied by inanition, anemia, aphonia, neck retraction, opisthotonus, oedema, oliguria constipation, and meteorismus (swelling of the abdominal cavity from gas in the intestine). Opisthotonus is a characteristic of acute thiamin deficiency in birds and is described as due to a tetanic spasm in which the spine and extremities are bent backwards.

In alcoholic and other malnourished subjects, one of the early signs of thiamin deficiency is anorexia.

In alcohol abuse, the overwhelming desire for alcohol may outweigh all other interest in food, leading to generalized malnutrition. Alcohol specifically blocks the active absorption of thiamin and alcohol abuse can progress to the potentially fatal condition known as Wernicke–Korsakoff syndrome. The typical clinical features of Wernicke's encephalopathy comprise ophthalmoplegia, nystagmus (usually horizontal), ataxic gait, and an abnormal mental state that can range from mild delirium to global confusion. Liver disease and tachycardia occur in more than 50% of cases. Korsakoff's psychosis is

Table 5 Features of acute infantile beriberi and frequency of occurrence

	Features	Frequency (%)
Appearance	Pale and cyanotic appearance, oedematous, ill-tempered with abdominal distension	40
Voice	Hoarseness	80
	Sometimes groaning	50
Digestive system	Vomiting	80
	Dyspepsia	46
Cardiac	Tachycardia, <200 beats/min	83
	Heart dilated	31
	Femoral sound on ascultation	5
Lungs	Rapid breathing	83
	Accentuation of the 2nd pulmonary sound	
Neurological	Tendon reflex usually increased	74
	Less frequently decreased	26
	Convulsions	17
Urinary	Oliguria	65
Other	Slight fever	50
	Uneasiness	50

Modified from Thurnham DI (1978) Thiamin. In: Rechcigl M Jr (ed.) *Nutrition Disorders*, pp. 3–14. West Palm Beach, FL: CRC Press.

characterized by a profound amnesia, disorientation, and often confabulation. The clinical features of Wernicke–Korsakoff syndrome are listed in Table 6.

Management/Treatment

Patients in whom cardiac and renal signs of thiamin deficiency are identified usually respond well to treatment. The dose given and route used will vary with the seriousness of the deficiency. Intravenous doses as high as 250 mg/day for 14 days and intramuscular doses of 25 mg followed by thrice daily oral doses of 10 mg have been reported for wet beriberi and are followed by a marked increase in urinary output and improvement in cardiac function. Peripheral neuropathy (dry beriberi) is more resistant to treatment. Patients with the ocular signs of Wernicke's disease usually respond to two or three daily injections of 50 mg thiamin. Long-term oral treatment of other manifestations of Wernicke–Korsakoff syndrome with doses up to 50 mg/day is reported, although benefit is variable and considerably influenced by patients' ability to avoid further alcohol consumption. It is unlikely that patients receiving oral thiamin will absorb more than 5–7 mg/day, but in patients likely to abuse alcohol, absorption by passive diffusion of high thiamin doses is the only way to ensured that the patient will receive any thiamin. In addition, as in all patients who show evidence of nutritional deficiency, the likelihood of other coexisting deficiencies should not be overlooked and multinutrient treatment is probably desirable. Finally, it is important to realise that untreated thiamin deficiency can result in sudden death.

Table 6 Clinical features of Wernicke–Korsakoff syndrome and frequency of occurrence

	Features	Frequency (%)[a]
Ocular disorders	Nystagmus (ocular ataxia — rhythmical oscillation of the eyeballs), almost always horizontal and in 50% of cases associated with vertical nystagmus on upward gaze	85
	Paralysis of one or more of the ocular muscles	50
	Sluggish reaction by pupils to light	19
Ataxia (inability to coordinate muscles)	Gait	87
	Legs	20
	Arms	12
	Speech	87
Polyneuropathy	Limbs only affected, mainly the legs only	82
	Of arms and legs	18
	Common symptoms include weakness, paresthesia, pain, loss of tendon reflexes and of sensation and motor power	
	Some cases of foot drop or wrist drop or both	
Cerebral function	Global confusional state, profound disorientation, apathy, deranged perception and of memory, drowsiness, inattentiveness, indifference	56
	Disorder of memory: both retrograde and ante-retrograde amnesia, confabulation	57
	Alcohol abstinence syndrome	16
Cardiac	Tachycardia	51
General medical abnormalities	Disorders of skin and mucous membranes	36
	Redness and/or papilliary atrophy of the tongue	29
	Liver disease	60

[a]Percentages based on 188–245 cases.
Modified from Thurnham DI (1978) Thiamin. In: Rechcigl M Jr (ed.) *Nutrition Disorders*, pp. 3–14. West Palm Beach, FL: CRC Press.

Lipid-Soluble Thiamin Derivatives

In recent years, several lipid-soluble derivatives of thiamin have been introduced, of which the best known is benfotiamine. Advantages of these compounds appear to be increased absorption, but by the diffusion mechanism only, and greatly increased transketolase activity. Transketolase is the rate-limiting enzyme of the nonoxidative branch of the pentose phosphate pathway. Benfotiamine has been shown to be useful for the management of rare genetic disorders in thiamin transport and may also prove useful to prevent damage from diabetic hyperglycemia. One study demonstrated that benfotiamine prevented experimental retinopathy. Diabetic hyperglycemia is accompanied by an increase in the potentially pathogenic glycolytic metabolites glyceraldehyde-3-phosphate and fructose-6-phosphate. Benfotiamine, by increasing transketolase activity, stimulates the pentose phosphate pathway to metabolise these glycolytic intermediates into pentose-5-phosphates and prevent the intracellular increase of potentially toxic products.

Case Study

A good example of the specific effect of thiamin in the treatment of beriberi is illustrated by the response of a 29-year-old male who was admitted with an unexplained acute renal failure and had been anuric for 24 h. The physicians' report on his symptoms should be compared with the common clinical features of wet beriberi shown in **Table 4**. The patient's physical state and voice were extremely weak but speech was copious and confused. He complained intermittently of severe central chest and epigastric pain. A central cyanosis was present and he had a respiratory rate of 36 beats per minute. His temperature was normal and peripheries were lukewarm. He had gross generalised oedema. The jugular venous pressure became grossly elevated (**Figure 1**). Pulse rate was 100 beats per minute, regular, and weak at the wrist, although the carotid pulses were visibly bounding. Blood pressure was 80/60. There was a marked parasternal heave present, with a loud pulmonary second heart sound. The chest was clear; the abdomen was obese.

The father reported that the patient's usual beer intake was 6–12 pints daily and his one regular meal was usually no more than a sausage roll or a pie. Prior to admission, for 6 weeks he had felt too tired to go out in the evening, and for 2 weeks he had suffered epigastric discomfort and had eaten nothing. Eight days before admission, he developed painful calf stiffness and he became too weak to go to work. He had a painful dry cough and dyspnoe on

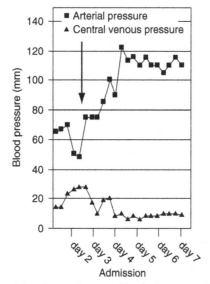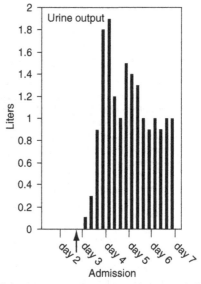

Figure 1 (Left) Arterial and central venous blood pressure and (right) urine output of a patient who was admitted with unexplained acute renal failure in a very weak physical state and whose speech (although very weak) was copious and confused. The patient was discovered to be a regular beer drinker consuming 6–12 pints daily, and his usual food intake amounted to no more than a sausage roll or pie. He had become progressively weaker over the past 8 weeks and had eaten nothing at all in the past 2 weeks. After excluding other diagnoses, it was suspected that the patient had fulminant beriberi and he was treated with thiamin after 36 h. The figures display the rapidly increasing arterial pressure, fall in venous pressure, and a rapid resumption in renal function following thiamin treatment. The patient lost ~20 l of urine during the first 7 days in the hospital. (Modified from Anderson SH, Charles TJ and Nicol AD (1985) Thiamine deficiency at a district general hospital: Report of five cases. *Quarterly Journal of Medicine* **55**: 15–32.)

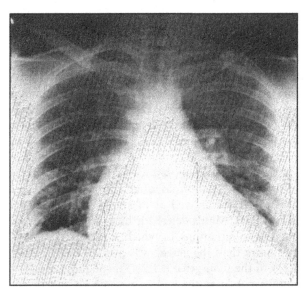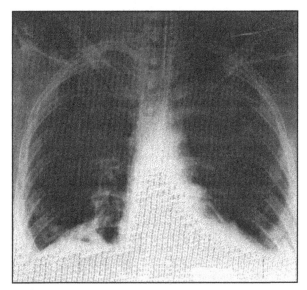

Figure 2 Chest radiographs of the patient described in **Figure 1** obtained on admission (left) and 14 days after high-dose, parenteral thiamin treatment (right). On admission, the heart was grossly enlarged, extending downward and to the right, with a cardiothoracic ratio of 0.63. After treatment for 14 days, the cardiothoracic ratio was 0.44. (Modified from Anderson SH, Charles TJ and Nicol AD (1985) Thiamine deficiency at a district general hospital: Report of five cases. *Quarterly Journal of Medicine* **55**: 15–32.)

the slightest exertion. Finally, confusion, cyanosis, and intermittent vomiting led to admission.

The first diagnoses considered were myocardial infarction, pulmonary embolism, and overwhelming septicaemia, and he was placed on dialysis and received appropriate treatments. His lack of response at 36 h, continuing low systolic pressure (70 beats per minute), increasingly gross hyperdynamic precordial signs, and moribund appearance led to a diagnosis of beriberi. Treatment with intravenous thiamin (250 mg for 14 days) brought about a dramatic response (**Figure 1**). Within 6 h peripheral pulses were strong, blood pressure had risen to 105 systolic, and central venous pressure had fallen by half. By 12 h the parasternal heave was less marked and diuresis of up to 6 l per day ensued. After 24 h, plasma urea concentration peaked at 50.4 mmol/l and creatinine at 832 μmol/l, and thereafter there was a steady fall over the next 2 weeks during which thiamin treatment continued and dialysis stopped. He lost a net 20 l of fluid over the first 7 days in the hospital and creatinine clearance 3 weeks after admission was 178 ml/min, indicating a return to normal kidney function. Other biochemical abnormalities resolved over the 2 weeks on high-dose thiamin, including the chest radiograph (**Figure 2**). It is interesting to note, however, that when he was discharged 3 months after admission, he was walking with a calliper because of a right-sided foot drop. The persistence of the foot drop is a further indication of

the greater difficulty in reversing neurological consequences, in contrast to the cardiac effects, of thiamin deficiency.

Toxicity

Chronic intakes in excess of 50 mg/kg, or more than 3 g/day, are toxic to adults with a wide variety of clinical signs, including headache, irritability, insomnia, rapid pulse, weakness, contact dermatitis, pruritis, and, in one case, death. Early researchers also indicated that regular administration or contact with thiamin occasionally led to allergic response, contact dermatitis, or hypersensitivity.

See also: **Fish**. **Thiamin**: Physiology.

Further Reading

Anderson SH, Charles TJ, and Nicol AD (1985) Thiamine deficiency at a district general hospital: Report of five cases. *Quarterly Journal of Medicine* **55**: 15–32.

Brin M (1964) Erythrocyte as a biopsy tissue for functional evaluation of thiamine adequacy. *Journal of the American Medical Association* **187**: 762–766.

Burgess RC (1958) VI Special problems concerning beriberi. B. Infantile beriberi. Proceedings of a conference on beriberi, endemic goitre and hypervitaminosis A entitled 'Nutritional Disease.' *Proceedings of the Federation of Association of Societies of Experimental Biology* **17**(supplement 2): 39–46.

Carpenter KJ (2002) Acute versus marginal deficiencies of nutrients. *Nutrition Reviews* **60**: 277–280.

Fehily L (1940) Infantile beriberi in Hong Kong. *Caduceus* 19: 78–93.

Friedemann TE, Kmieciak TC, Keegan PK, and Blum Sheft B (1948) The absorption, excretion and destruction of orally-administered thiamin by human subjects. *Gastroenterology* 11: 101–114.

Hammes H-P et al. (2003) Benfotiamine blocks three major pathways of hyperglycemic damage and prevents experimental diabetic retinopathy. *Nature Medicine* 9: 294–299.

Ibner FL, Blass JP, and Brin M (1982) Thiamin in the elderly, relation to alcoholism and to neurological degenerative disease. *American Journal of Clinical Nutrition* 36: 1067–1082.

Luyken R (ed.) (1990) *Polyneuritis in Chickens, or the Origin of Vitamin Research* [First English edition of papers by Christian Eijkman published 1890–1896]. Basle: Roche.

McConachie I and Haskew A (1988) Thiamine status after major trauma. *Intensive Care Medicine* 14: 628–631.

Pepersack T, Garbusinski J, Robberecht J et al. (1999) Clinical relevance of thiamine status amongst hospitalised elderly patients. *Gerontology* 45: 96–101.

Tang CM, Rolfe M, Wells JC, and Cham K (1989) Outbreak of beri-beri in the Gambia. *Lancet* 2: 206–207.

Thurnham DI (1978) Thiamin. In: Rechcigl M Jr (ed.) *Nutrition Disorders*, pp. 3–14. West Palm Beach, FL: CRC Press.

Thurnham DI (2004) An overview of interactions between micronutrients and of micronutrients with drugs, genes and immune mechanisms. *Nutrition Research Reviews* 17: 211–240.

Victor M, Adams RD, and Collins GH (1971) The clinical findings. In: F Plum and FH McDowell (eds.) *The Wernicke–Korsakoff Syndrome*, pp. 16–34. Oxford: Blackwell.

Williams RR (1961) *Towards the Conquest of Beriberi* Cambridge, MA: Harvard University Press.

Physiology

D I Thurnham, University of Ulster, Coleraine, UK

Thiamin is a water-soluble vitamin and the structure comprises a pyrimidine and a thiazole ring linked by a methylene bridge (**Figure 1**). In its metabolically active forms, the hydroxyl group on the thiazole moiety is replaced by one, two, or three phosphate groups to form three phosphorylated coenzymes. A well-nourished human adult body contains approximately 30 mg of thiamin—approximately 80–90% as thiamin diphosphate (TDP), 10% as thiamin triphosphate (TTP), and a small amount of thiamin monophosphate (TMP) and thiamin. Like most water-soluble vitamins, there is no definable store in the body; the only reserves are thiamin coenzymes that are present in most cells in combination with appropriate thiamin-requiring enzymes. The predominant need for thiamin is linked to energy production but there is increasing evidence that thiamin is also needed for additional neurological functions. Thiamin is found in the aleuron layer of cereal grains as well as in animal food products such as liver. Man's desire for high-extraction cereal products in situations in which the diets contained little more than the cereal was a main contributory factor to the scourge of beriberi throughout much of Southeast Asia at the end of nineteenth and beginning of the twentieth century. Thiamin is relatively unstable and destroyed by poor cooking habits, and it is susceptible to degradation in foods that are not stored properly. Thiamin turnover is also quite rapid, and the absence of stores means that a continuous supply of thiamin is required. So thiamin status can be fairly rapidly impaired by factors affecting intake (e.g., vomiting and alcohol abuse) or excessive excretion (e.g., induced by diuretics). Thus, thiamin deficiency is sometimes a problem in pregnancy, in alcohol abuse, and in the elderly. Seasonal outbreaks can also occur in poor developing countries when energy output is high and cereals may have been stored for many months and food supplies are restricted.

Dietary Sources of Thiamin

Thiamin is present in most foods but cereal products provide most thiamin for most people in the world, although the source is fundamentally different in developing and more industrialized countries. In the developing world, unrefined cereal grains and/or starchy roots and tubers provide 60–85% of dietary thiamin, whereas most dietary thiamin in industrialized countries is obtained from fortified cereal products. In the United Kingdom, for example, wheat

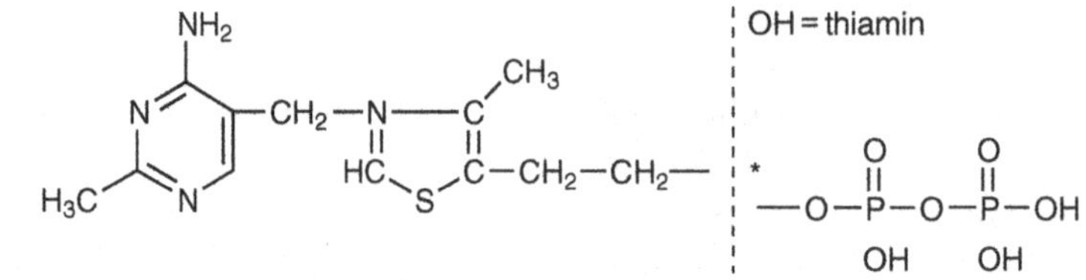

Figure 1 Thiamin and thiamin diphosphate (asterisk). Thiamin monophosphate and triphosphate are formed by the similar addition of one or three phosphate groups at the asterisk.

flour is fortified with 2.4 mg thiamin per kilogram and many breakfast cereals contain 30% or more of the daily thiamin requirement per portion. Thiamin is present in greatest amounts in brewers yeast, the germ and aleuron layers of fresh wheat, egg yolk, and mammalian liver. It is also present in meat flesh, particularly pork, and vegetables, nuts, and legumes (**Table 1**). Milk from both humans (0.49–0.79 μmol/l; 0.23 μg/4.2 MJ (1000 kcal)) and cows (1.18–1.48 μmol/l) is a poor source of thiamin. Thiamin is actively secreted into milk by the lactating mother, and it is of interest that the amount of thiamin in human milk is not increased by supplements, but the concentration and of course the volume consumed increase during the first 6 weeks of lactation.

Refined foods in general, such as fat, sugar, and alcohol, are poor sources of thiamin. Polished rice is particularly low in thiamin (80 μg/100 g) and is especially important because of its widespread consumption and importance as a source of calories. Cereal grains lose thiamin during refining, but the process of parboiling rice before milling enables most of the thiamin to be retained (190 μg/100 g) since it migrates into the starchy endosperm during the

procedure. Proper storage of cereal grains is also important to maintain thiamin activity. Studies in The Gambia, West Africa, found that old season millet, which had been stored under thatch and in high humidity, when consumed in the middle of the rainy season had thiamin concentrations (11 μg/100 g) that were 6–12 times lower than cooked samples obtained immediately postharvest. Imported rice used in the village likewise only contained 10 μg/100 g at the time of consumption.

Because of the water-soluble properties of thiamin, it can be leached from food during cooking. Thiamin is stable in slightly acid water up to boiling point but is unstable in alkaline solution that oxidizes it quantitatively to thiochrome (**Figure 2**). In addition, anti-thiamin factors in food can accelerate thiamin losses. Paralysis in foxes fed raw carp led to the discovery of the thiaminase enzymes. Two thiaminases are found in food. Thiaminase I is found in fish, shellfish, ferns, and some bacteria and catalyzes a base exchange reaction between thiazole and another base. Thiaminase II is a hydrolytic enzyme that cleaves the vitamin at the methylene bridge and is found mainly in bacteria. The thiaminases are heat labile, so only food that is eaten raw or fermented may loose thiamin during its preparation or in the gastrointestinal tract. There are also heat-stable anti-thiamin factors that are found in ferns, tea, betel nuts, large numbers of plants and vegetables, and some animal tissues. Anti-thiamin factors bind with varying degrees of attachment to thiamin and may or may not interfere with the bioavailability of thiamin. Diphenols, especially those with the hydroxyl groups in the *ortho* position, tend to react to give products that are both thiochrome negative and microbiologically inactive (i.e., thiamin is deactivated). Thus, in areas of northern and northeastern Thailand where tea

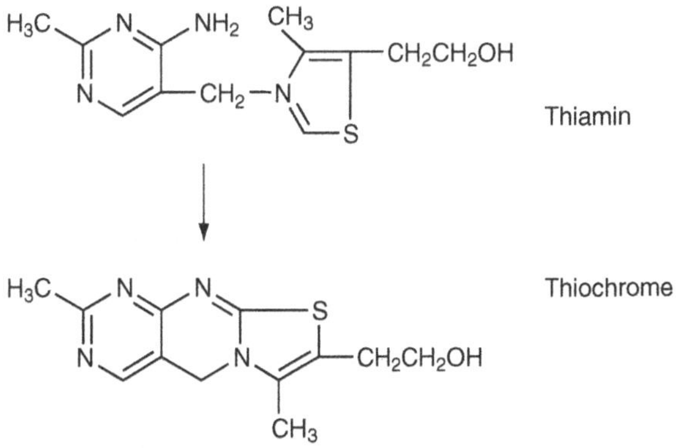

Table 1 Thiamin content of common foods

Food group	Food item	Thiamin content (mg/100 g)
Bread	Wholemeal	0.26
	White	0.18
	Hovis	0.52
Breakfast cereals	Cornflakes (fortified)	1.8
	Rice Krispies	2.3
	Weetabix	1.0
Flour	Wholemeal (100%[a])	0.46
	Brown (85%)	0.42
	White (fortified) (70%)	0.28–0.33
Milk, cheeses		0.03–0.06
Eggs	Cooked (various)	0.07–0.09
	Yolk raw	0.30
Vegetables (cooked)	Various leaf and root types	0.02–0.07
	Dahl, chick peas, green, beans, etc.	0.05–0.14
Pork products	Gammon rashers (lean)	1.0
	Bacon (various)	0.36–0.55
	Pork meat	0.5–0.88
	Liver (stewed)	0.21
Other meats	Beef (various)	0.03–0.09
	Lamb (various)	0.04–0.14
	Lamb liver	0.56
	Chicken (various)	0.04–0.10
	Game	~0.30
Yeast (dried)		2.33

[a]Percentages indicate the level of extraction in flour preparation.
Source: Paul AA, Southgate DAT (1978) *McCance & Widdowson's The composition of food*, 4th edn. London: HMO.

Figure 2 Structures of thiamin and thiochrome.

drinking, chewing fermented tea leaves, chewing betel nuts, and consuming raw/fermented fish are common practices, thiamin deficiency still occurs despite thiamin intakes of 0.44–0.50 mg/4.2 MJ.

Absorption and Ethyl Alcohol

In food, thiamin occurs mainly as phosphate coenzymes and the predominant form is TDP (also called thiamin pyrophosphate and cocarboxylase). The phosphate coenzymes are broken down in the gut by phosphatases to give free thiamin for absorption. Thiamin is absorbed mainly from the upper intestine, and less thiamin is absorbed on an empty stomach than when taken with a meal. The latter could be due to the alkaline conditions in the duodenum, which are prevented by the presence of food. Absorption of up to 2 mg per meal occurs by an active saturable process involving a sodium-dependent adenosine triphosphatase and against a concentration gradient. During absorption, thiamin is phosphorylated to the monophosphate ester (TMP). Thiamin is absorbed via the portal venous system. Further phosphorylation to TDP occurs on entry into all tissues. TDP can cross the blood–brain barrier, where a portion is converted to TTP, although even in the brain, TDP is the predominant form of thiamin. A second passive absorption process operates when intakes of thiamin are >5 mg but the maximum that can be absorbed from an oral dose is 2–5 mg.

The active process of absorption is impaired by ethyl alcohol. For example, 55% of a 5 mg dose of orally administered, labeled thiamin was recovered over 72 h in healthy adults, but this was reduced by 25–40% if they were previously given 1.5–2 g alcohol/kg. In people with fatty livers who had previously been abusing alcohol, mean thiamin absorption was reduced by 60%. However, the passive absorption of thiamin is not inhibited by alcohol, nor does it block entry of thiamin into the liver or interfere with thiamin metabolism in the tissues. Absorption of thiamin may also be reduced by gastrointestinal disturbances, such as vomiting and diarrhea, ulcerative colitis, and neoplasia, and in patients with hepatic disease and achlorhydria.

Transport, Storage, and Excretion

Thiamin with some TMP (19–75 nmol/l) circulates in the blood bound to albumin. When the binding capacity of plasma albumin is exceeded, or thiamin is in excess of tissue needs, it is rapidly excreted in the urine. Most thiamin in erythrocytes is present as TDP principally bound to the enzyme transketolase.

Likewise, in most other tissues, there is very little free thiamin and it is mostly present as TDP (90%) in coenzymes bound to respective enzymes and a smaller amount of TTP (10%) in nervous tissues. The concentration of thiamin in specific tissues is on the order of 2–3 μg/g for heart muscle; 1 μg/g for brain, liver, and kidney; and 0.5 μg/g in skeletal muscle. Thiamin supplements can increase these concentrations slightly and prolonged febrile illnesses are likely to reduce them. Thiamin is mainly excreted intact in the urine but there are small amounts of thiochrome (**Figure 2**) and other thiazole and pyrimidine metabolites. A linear relationship exists between intake and excretion of thiamin until intake falls to an amount approaching minimum requirements when excretion decreases rapidly indicating a renal conservation mechanism.

There is concern that the long-term use of diuretics in the management of chronic congestive heart failure (CHF) may impair thiamin status and, as a consequence, impair myocardial function. The diuretic drug furosemide has been the subject of much attention. In healthy volunteers, a dose-dependent increase in urine flow accompanied by an increase in the urinary thiamin excretion rate have been demonstrated. In furosemide-treated patients, the concomitant presence of thiamin in the urine and biochemical deficiency of thiamin from measurements in blood has been shown. These results suggest that furosemide treatment can override the renal conservation mechanism. In one study, 23 patients with chronic CHF receiving 80–240 mg furosemide daily for 3–14 months were studied along with 16 age-matched controls without heart failure and not taking diuretics. No subjects in either group were identified as consuming inadequate thiamin intake or having increased thiamin requirements. However, biochemically, 21 of the 23 CHF patients and 2 of the controls were thiamin deficient. Furthermore, 5 of the CHF patients were treated with intravenous thiamin (100 mg thiamin HCl twice daily for 7 days). Biochemical thiamin status normalized and echocardiographic assessment of left ventricular ejection fraction increased in 4 of the 5 patients. Because no other changes were made in the patients' therapeutic regimen, the results suggest that the improvement in cardiac contractility was due to the correction of the thiamin deficiency.

Biological Functions

Thiamin functions as the coenzyme TDP in the metabolism of carbohydrates and branched-chain amino acids (α-keto-isocaproic, α-keto-β-methyl valeric, and α-keto-isovaleric acids). In association with Mg^{2+} ions, TDP is important (1) in various dehydrogenase complexes for the oxidation of α-keto acids (pyruvate, α-ketoglutarate, and the branched-chain α-keto acids) and (2) in the formation of α-ketols among the hexose and pentose phosphates catalyzed by transketolase (EC 2.2.1.1). Thus, a deficiency of thiamin has severe consequences for energy generation and amino acid interconnections, and these have important links with lipid metabolism, cell replication, and neural activity.

Two principal dehydrogenase complexes that require the participation of TDP are pyruvate dehydrogenase, which generates acetyl-CoA, and the oxidative decarboxylation of α-ketoglutarate to succinyl-CoA (**Figure 3**). Pyruvate dehydrogenase is situated at the junction of the glycolysis pathway, where it enters the tricarboxylic acid cycle. Acetyl-CoA is a key source of energy for mitochondrial oxidation and the production of adenosine triphosphate (ATP) as well as an important precursor in lipid metabolism. The impaired functioning of pyruvate dehydrogenase leads to a lactic acidosis, with increased concentrations of serum pyruvate and/or lactate especially as a result of exercise. The lactate acidosis can be explained by the fact that ATP

depletion stimulates glycolysis, thus generating more pyruvate. As pyruvate concentrations increase, lactate dehydrogenase converts some of the pyruvate to lactate, producing the lactic acidosis. The increases in these compounds formed the basis of the earliest biochemical test for thiamin deficiency, which was later made more reproducible by taking the blood soon after moderate exercise (e.g., climbing a few steps).

Many features of beriberi indicate that thiamin plays an important role in neural tissues. TTP is specifically found in nervous tissues, but although this triphosphorylated metabolite of thiamin has been known for approximately 30 years, its precise role is still in doubt. TDP in the dehydrogenase complexes is undoubtedly also required for normal function. Some of the earliest biochemical studies on the brain documented abnormalities in the oxidative metabolism of glucose and a disruption in energy supply may underlie many of the neurochemical changes and structural lesions associated with thiamin deficiency. For example, acetyl-CoA produced by pyruvate dehydrogenase is a precursor of the parasympathetic transmitter molecule acetylcholine, but the obligatory requirement of glucose as an energy source for nervous tissue indicates the essentiality of TDP. Likewise, the cytosolic enzyme

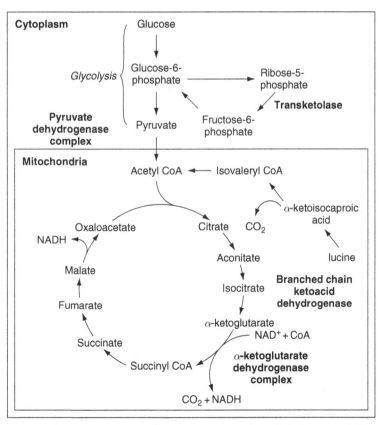

Figure 3 The four principal sites of action of thiamin diphosphate coenzyme in carbohydrate metabolism.

transketolase is also present in nervous tissue, and as a key enzyme in the HMS it may be important in minimizing oxidant stress. The HMS generates NADPH, which is required to maintain glutathione in the reduced state.

The cellular and subcellular localization of the enzymes responsible for metabolism of thiamin phosphates in nervous tissues may indicate possible sites of action of the specific metabolites. Thiamin that enters the brain is phosphorylated by thiamin pyrophosphokinase to form TDP. The concentration of thiamin phosphates is 3 or 4 times higher in neurons than in neuroglia, and the activity of thiamin diphosphatase (TDPase), which converts TDP to TMP, is 20 times higher in neurons than neuroglia. Thiamin monophosphatase is only detected in neuroglia. Within the neuron, TDPase is mostly localised in the microsomal fraction. Thiamin triphosphatase (TTPase), which converts TTP to TDP, is particularly enriched in presynaptic terminals. Stimulation of nerves or treatment with certain neuroactive drugs result in decreases in TDP and particularly TTP in the nerve, with an increase in free TMP in the surrounding fluid. It is postulated that TTP plays an essential role in nerve transmission involving a gating mechanism for sodium and potassium ion transport via the specific ATPase. Some evidence for this comes from patients with Leigh's disease (pathologically similar to Wernicke–Korsakoff syndrome), in whom severe neurological disease is accompanied by a deficiency in TTP but normal TDP concentrations.

The well-documented role of mitochondria in programmed cell death and the importance of thiamin for oxidative metabolism have stimulated investigators to examine brain thiamin homeostasis in neurodegenerative diseases. Diminished thiamin-dependent processes, abnormal metabolism, and oxidative stress accompany the neurodegeneration of Alzheimer's disease (AD), Huntington's disease, Wernicke–Korsakoff syndrome, progressive supranuclear palsy, and the adult-onset neurodegenerative diseases that are caused by genes containing variable numbers of CAG repeats within their coding regions. Abnormalities in the thiamin-dependent processes have also been linked with thiamin-responsive maple syrup urine disease, Leigh's disease (a subacute necrotizing encephalomyelopathy), sudden infant death syndrome, cerebellar degeneration, thiamin-responsive anemia, ataxia, and disorders of energy metabolism including pyruvate dehydrogenase deficiency. The extent to which disturbances in thiamin metabolism are a cause or a consequence of the disease process is still under examination.

Assessment of Thiamin Status

Thiamin status can be assessed using methods that measure thiamin or its metabolites in plasma, erythrocytes and urine (**Table 2**). Samples are acidified to stabilize the thiamin and precipitate any protein. Usually, thiamin is oxidized to thiochrome (**Figure 2**) using cyanogen bromide in alkaline solution and measured by fluorescence with or without chromatography. Concentrations of thiamin in urine and plasma tend to reflect dietary intake, being high when intake is adequate and low when dietary sources are poor. Erythrocyte thiamin is mainly in the form of the coenzyme TDP, which can be extracted from washed erythrocytes, derivatized as described previously, and quantified by high-performance liquid chromatography. The most popular test, however, is the erythrocyte transketolase (ETKL) stimulation test, which measures enzyme activity with and without added TDP. The reference range for ETKL activity in well-nourished, thiamin-adequate people is reported to be 570–830 mU/g hemoglobin. The stimulation test measures the proportion of the apoenzyme in red cell homogenate (i.e., the proportion that is not bound to TDP and represents the degree of thiamin deficiency). Studies have shown that results from the urinary assay for thiamin agree reasonably well with those obtained by the ETKL stimulation test.

One of the reasons for the popularity of the ETKL stimulation test is that sensitivity is still good even in the presence of thiamin deficiency. In all other measurements of thiamin status, as deficiency approaches, the quantity of thiamin or its metabolites diminishes in the biological fluid. Low

Table 2 Biochemical assessment of thiamin status

Test	Acceptable	Marginal risk	High risk
Urinary thiamin (μmol/mol creatinine)[a]			
1–3 years	>66	45–66	<45
4–6 years	>45	32–45	<32
Adults	>25	10–25	<10
Erythrocyte transketolase activity			
Activity coefficient	<1.11	1.11–1.25	>1.25
TDP effect (%)	<11	11–25	>25
Red cell thiamin concentrations (nmol/l)	749 ± 196		~560[b]
Whole blood thiamin concentrations (nmol/l)	166–266		<133

[a]Converted from μg/g creatinine using the factor (×0.376).
[b]Based on a decrease of 25% in red cell thiamine diphosphate (TDP).

concentrations of a product are usually more difficult to measure and precision deteriorates, or the amount of sample has to be increased to provide sufficient material to detect. In contrast with the ETKL stimulation test, in an acute thiamin deficiency, ETKL activity is maintained and only the amount of TDP decreases, so the test becomes more sensitive. However, in chronic thiamin-deficient states, the apoenzyme of ETKL is reported to be unstable *in vivo*, and in the absence of the coenzyme, concentrations of the apoenzyme decrease, with the result that *in vitro* stimulation may show normal thiamin status. Thus, in situations in which chronic thiamin deficiency is suspected as a result of a long-term marginal thiamin intake, alcohol abuse, or use of diuretics for many months, one or more of the concentration tests may be useful as an adjunct to the stimulation test.

Certain precautions should be taken in handling samples for thiamin analysis. Urine should be acidified to avoid degradation and stored below −20 °C. Heparinized whole blood should be collected and immediately put on ice. For total erythrocyte TDP measurements, cells are separated from plasma within 2 h when possible, washed in saline, and diluted 1:1 with saline prior to acidification. Centrifugation of the acidified mixture provides a clear extract that can be stored for no more than 5 days at 4 °C or longer at ≤−20 °C. Washed red cells are also used for the ETKL assay. Duplicate tubes of the red cells in saline suspension with and without added TDP are mixed and can be stored at −70 °C prior to enzymatic analysis of ETKL activity. Even at −70 °C, however, storage should be for no more than a few weeks. The ETKL apoenzyme is unstable, and even in the tubes to which TDP has been added, if mixing did not thoroughly expose all apoenzyme to the added coenzyme, deterioration will occur and results will be unreliable.

Recommended Dietary Allowances

Quantifying thiamin requirements is based on a variety of biochemical data. Early results indicated that a thiamin intake of 0.4 mg/day on a low-energy intake was close to the absolute minimum requirement. Epidemiological evidence suggested that beriberi occurred when the intake of thiamin was <0.2 mg thiamin per 4.2 MJ (1000 kcal); however, when 0.188 mg/4.2 MJ was fed to sedentary elderly men for 2 years, no indisputable alteration in clinical state occurred. Thiamin requirements are strongly influenced by physical activity and at higher energy intakes with liquid formula diets containing 11.76 and 15.12 MJ (2800 and 3600 kcal),

there was good agreement between thiamin excretion and ETKL stimulation to interpret thiamin status at different levels of thiamin intake. Increasing intake from 0.2 to 0.23 mg/4.2 MJ moved first the urinary excretion and then ETKL activation out of the deficient range. Both measurements were normalized at intakes of 0.3 mg/4.2 MJ, and to allow for variance the recommended nutrient intake adopted by the Department of Health in the United Kingdom was 0.4 mg/4.2 MJ. This amount is recommended for all groups of the population since additional needs in pregnancy and lactation are met by increased energy intakes. It was recommended that formula feed should contain not less than 0.3 mg/4.2 MJ.

Women are less affected by beriberi than are men even when they are consuming the same diet, but there is no consistent indication that men have greater needs than women. Differences between the sexes that may affect susceptibility to beriberi need further investigation (e.g., the amount of food eaten by the sexes when supplies are short or of poor quality, metabolic responses to infection during illness, and differences in energy requirements). The close association between thiamin metabolism and carbohydrate metabolism means that thiamin requirements are determined by basal metabolic rate (BMR) and physical activity. BMR of men is slightly higher than that of women of the same weight, but total energy expenditure can vary 1.4 to 2.5 times BMR depending on physical activity.

Drug–Nutrient Interactions

Mention has already been made of the influence of alcohol and diuretics on thiamin status. Oral contraceptives are reported to have no effects on thiamin status.

Toxicity

High intakes of thiamin administered orally are nontoxic. The rapidly saturable thiamin absorption mechanism limits the amount taken up from a single dose to ~2.5 mg, and thiamin present in excess of protein binding capacity is excreted. However, there are reports of toxicity from chronic intakes in excess of 50 mg/kg or >3 g/day with a wide variety of clinical signs, including headache, irritability, insomnia, rapid pulse, weakness, rapid pulse contact dermatitis, pruritus, and, in one case, death.

See also: **Thiamin**: Beriberi.

Further Reading

Bender DA (1984) B vitamins in the nervous system. *Neurochemistry International* 6: 297–321.

Department of Health (1991) *Dietary Reference Values for Food Energy and Nutrients for the United Kingdom*, Report on Health and Social Subjects No. 41. London: HMSO.

Gibson GE and Zhang H (2002) Interactions of oxidative stress with thiamine homeostasis promote neurodegeneration. *Neurochemistry International* 40: 493–504.

Hoyumpa AMJ, Nichols SG, Wilson FA, and Schenker S (1977) Effect of ethanol on intestinal (Na,K) ATPase and intestinal thiamin transport in rats. *Journal of Laboratory & Clinical Medicine* 90: 1086–1095.

Sauberlich HE, Herman YF, Stevens CO, and Herman RH (1979) Thiamin requirements of the adult human. *American Journal of Clinical Nutrition* 32: 2337–2248.

Seligmann H, Halkin H, Rauchfleisch S *et al.* (1991) Thiamine deficiency in patients with congestive heart failure receiving long-term furosemide therapy: A pilot study. *American Journal of Medicine* 91: 151–155.

Sinclair HM (1982) Thiamin. In: Barker BM and Bender DA (eds.) *Vitamins in Medicine*, 4th edn., pp. 114–167. London: Heinemann Medical Books.

Suter PM and Vetter W (2000) Diuretics and vitamin B_1: Are diuretics a risk factor for thiamin malnutrition? *Nutrition Reviews* 58: 319–323.

Thurnham DI (2004) An overview of interactions between micronutrients and between micronutrients with drugs, genes and immune mechanisms. *Nutrition Research Reviews* 17: 211–240.

WHO/FAO (2002) *Human Vitamin and Mineral Requirements; Report of a Joint FAO/WHO Expert Consultation*. Rome: WHO/FAO.

ULTRATRACE ELEMENTS

F Nielsen, Grand Forks Human Nutrition Research Center, Grand Forks, ND, USA

This article is reproduced from the first edition, pp. 1884–1897, © 1998, Elsevier Ltd., with revisions made by the Editor.

Definition

In the earlier part of this century, scientists could qualitatively detect small amounts of several mineral elements in living organisms. In reports, these elements were described as being present in 'traces' or 'trace amounts.' It is not surprising that these elements soon became known as trace elements. Today, sophisticated analytical techniques have permitted the accurate measurement of the amount of many mineral elements, some at very low concentrations, in biological material. The trace elements found in living organisms may be essential, that is, indispensable for growth and health, or they may be nonessential, fortuitous reminders of our geochemical origins or indicators of environmental exposure. Some of the nonessential trace elements can be beneficial to health through pharmacological action. All of the trace elements are toxic when intake is excessive.

Trace elements are those elements of the periodic table that occur in animals or humans in amounts measured in mg per kg of body weight or less. The trace elements essential for health are usually required by humans in amounts measured in mg per day; these elements include copper, iron, manganese, and zinc. The individual trace elements are discussed elsewhere in the encyclopedia. Since 1980, the term 'ultratrace element' has appeared in the nutritional literature. Ultratrace elements have been defined as those elements with estimated dietary requirements usually less than $1\,mg\,kg^{-1}$, and often less than $50\,\mu g\,kg^{-1}$ of diet for laboratory animals. For humans, the term often is used to indicate an element with an established, estimated, or suspected requirement of less than $1\,mg$ per day or generally indicated by μg per day. At least 18 elements could

be considered ultratrace elements: aluminum, arsenic, boron, bromine, cadmium, chromium, fluorine, germanium, iodine, lead, lithium, molybdenum, nickel, rubidium, selenium, silicon, tin, and vanadium. Emerging evidence indicates that silicon should be categorized as a trace element instead of an ultratrace element. However, knowledge about the practical importance or beneficial actions of silicon is in a state similar to that for most of the ultratrace elements; thus, it is considered as one of them here. Cobalt perhaps also belongs in the ultratrace category; however, it is required only in the form of vitamin B_{12} and thus is usually discussed as a vitamin.

The quality of the experimental evidence for nutritional essentiality varies widely for the ultratrace elements. The evidence for the essentiality of three elements, iodine, molybdenum and selenium, is substantial and noncontroversial; specific biochemical functions have been defined for these elements. The nutritional importance of iodine and selenium are such that they have separate entries in this encyclopedia. Molybdenum, however, is given very little nutritional attention, apparently because a deficiency of this element has not been unequivocally identified in humans other than individuals nourished by total parenteral nutrition or with genetic defects causing disturbances in metabolic pathways involving this element. Specific biochemical functions have not been defined for the other 15 ultratrace elements listed above. Thus, their essentiality is based on circumstantial evidence, which most often is that a dietary deprivation in an animal model results in a suboptimal biological function that is preventable or reversible by an intake of physiological amounts of the element in question. Often the circumstantial evidence includes an identified essential function in a lower form of life, and biochemical actions consistent with a biological role or beneficial action in humans. The circumstantial evidence for essentiality is substantial for arsenic, boron, chromium, nickel, silicon, and vanadium. The evidence for essentiality for the other elements is generally limited to a few gross observations in one or two species by one or two research groups. However, it should be noted that two of these ultratrace elements have beneficial actions when ingested in high (pharmacological) amounts: they are fluorine, which prevents tooth caries, and lithium, which is used to treat manic-depressive disorders.

Although aluminum has a separate article, and the elements cadmium, lead, and nickel are discussed in the entry the focus in those entries is toxicity; thus, these elements will be included in the following discussion. Chromium, however, which also has a separate entry, will not be included.

Absorption, Transport, and Storage

Homeostasis (maintenance of a steady optimal concentration of an element in the body) regulation involves the processes of absorption, storage, and excretion. The relative importance of these three processes varies among the ultratrace elements. The amount absorbed from the gastrointestinal tract is often the controlling mechanism for positively charged ultratrace elements such as aluminum, nickel, and tin. With these trace elements, if the body content is low, or if intake is low, the percentage of the element absorbed from the gastrointestinal tract is increased, and vice versa. Elements that exist mainly as negatively charged ions or oxyanions, such as arsenic, boron, and fluoride, are usually absorbed quite freely and completely from the gastrointestinal tract. Excretion through the urine, bile, swear, and breath is, therefore, the major mechanism for controlling the amount of these ultratrace elements in an organism. By being stored at inactive sites or in an inactive form, some ultratrace elements are prevented from causing adverse reactions when present in high quantities. An example of this homeostatic process is the binding of cadmium by the cysteine-rich protein called metallothionein. Release of an ultratrace element from storage forms also can be important in preventing deficiency.

Absorption of ultratrace elements from the intestinal lumen can occur in three ways. These are described below.

1. Passive diffusion – passive transport driven by a difference in concentration of the element between the two sides of the luminal membrane and the mucosa. Transmembrane movement of ions occurs through pores or channels within the membrane and is an energy-independent process. A significant amount of passive transport across the intestinal mucosa may occur through a paracellular pathway, or the transport between cells across intercellular right junctions.

2. Facilitated diffusion – the transfer of an element across the membrane by carrier proteins embedded in the membrane. Facilitated transport resembles simple diffusion because it is not energy dependent and is driven by a difference in the ion concentration between two sides of a membrane. Facilitated transport occurs much more rapidly than simple diffusion and is saturable because of a finite number of carrier proteins.

3. Active transport – the accumulation within, or the extrusion from, a cell of an element in opposition to a concentration gradient. Active transport is saturable, is energy dependent and involves a carrier protein that usually is quite specific for an element. The mechanisms of absorption for the various ultratrace elements are given in **Table 1**; this table also lists the known transport and storage vehicles for these elements.

Metabolism and Excretion

Knowledge about chemical changes that must occur before excretion for most of the ultratrace elements is quite limited. Perhaps the best characterized is inorganic arsenic, which is methylated into monomethylarsonic acid and dimethylarsinic acid, and organic arsenic, which is converted into, or remains mostly as, arsenobetaine before being excreted in the urine. Other ultratrace elements that are known to be incorporated into biochemical metabolites for transport and/or excretion include aluminum bound to transferrin, cadmium incorporated into metallo-thionein, nickel as the α-2-macroglobulin nickeloplasmin or bound to albumin and L-histidine, and vanadium converted into vanadyl-transferrin and vanadyl-ferritin (see **Table 1**). A known important metabolite of molybdenum is a small nonprotein cofactor containing a pterin nucleus that is present at the active site of molybdoenzymes. More than 40% of molybdenum not attached to an enzyme in liver also exists as this cofactor bound to the mitochondrial outer membrane. This form can be transferred to an apoenzyme of xanthine oxidase or sulfite oxidase, which transforms it into an active enzyme molecule. Molecules of biological importance for the ultratrace elements are shown in **Table 2**. The ultratrace elements are excreted from the body mainly via the feces and urine. Fecal excretion of absorbed ultratrace elements

Table 1 Absorption, transport, and storage characteristics of the ultratrace elements

Element	Major machanism(s) for homeostasis	Means of absorption	Percentage of ingested absorbed	Transport and storage vehicles
Aluminum	Absorption	Uncertain; some evidence far passive diffusion through the paracellular pathway; also, evidence for active absorption through processes shared with active processes of calcium; probably occurs in proximal duodenum; citrate combined with aluminum enhances absorption	Less than 1%	Transferrin carries aluminum in plasma; bone a possible storage site
Arsenic	Urinary excretion: Inorganic arsenic as mostly dimethylarsinic acid and organic arsenic as mostly arsenobetaine	Inorganic arsenate becomes sequestered in or on mucosal tissue, then absorption involves a simple movement down a concentration gradient; organic arsenic absorbed mainly by simple diffusion through lipid regions of the intestinal boundary	Soluble inorganic forms, >90%; slightly soluble inorganic forms, 20–30%; inorganic forms with foods, 60–75%; methylated forms, 45–90%	Before excretion inorganic arsenic is converted into monomethyl arsonic acid and dimethylarsinic acid; arsenobetaine not biotransformed; arsenocholine transformed to arsenobetaine
Boron	Urinary excretion	Ingested boron is converted into $B(OH)_3$ and absorbed in this form, probably by passive diffusion	Greater than 90%	Boron transported through the body as undissociated $B(OH)_3$; bone a possible storage site
Bromine	Urinary excretion	Probably passive diffusion because no apparent saturable component	75–90%	None identified
Cadmium	Absorption	May share a common absorption mechanism with other metals (e.g., zinc) but mechanism is less efficient for cadmium	5%	Incorporated into metallothionein, which probably is both a storage and transport vehicle
Fluorine	50% daily intake excreted in urine; about 50% daily intake stored in bone and developing teeth	Absorption by passive diffusion and inversely related to pH. Significant portion absorbed as hydrogen fluoride from stomach; absorption of fluoride also occurs throughout the small intestine	76–90%	Exists as fluoride ion in plasma; hydrogen fluoride is the form in diffusion equilibrium across cell membranes. Stored in bone
Germanium	Urinary excretion	Has not been conclusively determined but most likely is by passive diffusion	Greater than 90%	None identified

Continued

Table 1 Continued

Element	Major mechanism(s) for homeostasis	Means of absorption	Percentage of ingested absorbed	Transport and storage vehicles
Lead	Absorption	Uncertain; thought to be by passive diffusion in small intestine, but evidence has been presented for an active transport, perhaps involving the system for calcium	Adults 5–15% Children 40–50%	Bone is a repository for lead
Lithium	Urinary excretion	Passive diffusion by paracellular transport via the tight junctions and pericellular spaces	Lithium chloride highly absorbed – greater than 90%	Bone can serve as a store for lithium
Molybdenum	Urinary and biliary excretion	Uncertain, possible that molybdate is moved both by diffusion and by active transport, but at high concentrations active transport is a small portion of flux; absorption occurs rapidly in stomach and continues throughout the small intestine	50–93%	Molybdate in blood loosely attached to erythrocytes and tends to bind α_2-macroglobulin. Liver and kidney retain highest amount of molybdate
Nickel	Both absorption and urinary excretion	Uncertain, evidence both for passive diffusion (perhaps as an amino acid or other low molecular weight complex) and for energy driven transport; occurs in the small intestine	<10% with food	Transported in blood principally bound to serum albumin with small amounts bound to L-histidine and α_2-macroglobulin; no organ accumulates physiological amounts of nickel
Rubidium	Excretion through kidney and intestine	Resembles potassium in its pattern of absorption; rubidium and potassium thought to share a transport system	Highly absorbed	None identified
Silicon	Both absorption and urinary excretion	Mechanisms involved in intestinal absorption have not been described	Food silicon near 50%; insoluble or poorly soluble silicates = 1%	Silicon in plasma believed to exist as undisassociated monomeric silicic acid
Tin	Absorption	Mechanisms involved in intestinal absorption have not been described	About 3%. Percentage increases when very low amounts are ingested	None identified. Bone might be a repository
Vanadium	Absorption	Vanadate has been suggested to be absorbed through phosphate or other anion transport systems; vanadyl has been suggested to use iron transport systems. Absorption occurs in the duodenum	<10%	Converted into vanadyl-transferrin and vanadyl-ferritin; whether transferrin is the transport vehicle and ferritin is the storage vehicle for vanadium remains to be determined. Bone is a respository for excess vanadium

Table 2 Excretion, retention, and possible biological roles of the ultratrace elements

Element	Organs of high content (typical concentration)	Major excretory route after Ingestion	Molecules of biological importance	Possible biological role
Aluminum	Bone ($1-12\,\mu g\,g^{-1}$) Lung ($35\,\mu g\,g^{-1}$)	Urine; also significant amounts in bile	Aluminum binds to proteins, nucleotides, and phospholipids; aluminum-bound transferrin apparently is a transport molecule	Enzyme activator
Arsenic	Hair ($0.65\,\mu g\,g^{-1}$) Nails ($0.35\,\mu g\,g^{-1}$) Skin ($0.10\,\mu g\,g^{-1}$)	Urine	Methylation of Inorganic oxyarsenic anions occurs in organisms ranging from microbial to mammalian; methylated and products include arsenocholine, arsenobetaine, dimethylarsinic acid, and methylarsonic acid; arsenite methyltransferase and monomethylarsonic acid methyltransferase use S-adenosylmethionine for the methyl donor	Metabolism of methionine, or involved in labile methyl metabolism; regulation of gene expression
Boron	Bone ($1.6\,\mu g\,g^{-1}$) Fingernails ($15\,\mu g\,g^{-1}$) Hair ($1\,\mu g\,g^{-1}$) Teeth ($5\,\mu g\,g^{-1}$)	Urine	Boron biochemistry essentially that of boric acid, which forms ester complexes with hydroxyl groups, preferably those adjacent and *cis*, in organic compounds. Five naturally occurring boron esters (all antibiotics) synthesized by various bacteria have been characterized	Cell membrane function or stability such that it influences the response to hormone action, transmembrane signaling or transmembrane movement of regulatory cations or anlons
Bromine	Hair ($3.0\,\mu g\,g^{-1}$) Liver ($4.0\,\mu g\,g^{-1}$) Lung ($6.0\,\mu g\,g^{-1}$) Testis ($5.0\,\mu g\,g^{-1}$)	Urine	Exists as Br Ion *in vivo*, binds to proteins and amino acids	Electrolyte balance
Cadmium	Kidney ($14\,\mu g\,g^{-1}$) Liver ($4\,\mu g\,g^{-1}$)	Urine and gastrointestinal tract	Metallothionein, a high sulfhydryl-containing protein involved in regulating cadmium distribution	Involved in metallathionein metabolism and utilization
Fluorine	Bones ($1-5\,mg\,g^{-1}$) Teeth ($500\,\mu g\,g^{-1}$)	Urine	Exists as fluoride ion or hydrogen fluoride in body fluids; about 99% of body fluorine found in mineralized tissues as fluoroapatite	Role in biological mineralization
Germanium	Bone ($9\,\mu g\,g^{-1}$) Liver ($0.3\,\mu g\,g^{-1}$) Pancreas ($0.2\,\mu g\,g^{-1}$) Testis ($0.5\,\mu g\,g^{-1}$)	Urine	None identified	Role in immune function
Lead	Aorta ($1-2\,\mu g\,g^{-1}$) Bone ($25\,\mu g\,g^{-1}$) Kidney ($1-2\,\mu g\,g^{-1}$) Liver ($1-2\,\mu g\,g^{-1}$)	Urine; also significant amounts in bile	Plasma lead mostly bound to albumin; blood lead binds mostly to hemoglobin but some binds a low molecular weight protein in arythrocytes	Facilitates iron absorption and/or utilization

Continued

Table 2 Continued

Element	Organs of high content (typical concentration)	Major excretory route after Ingestion	Molecules of biological importance	Possible biological role
Lithium	Adrenal gland (60 ng g^{-1}) Bone (100 ng g^{-1}) Lymph nodes (200 ng g^{-1}) Pituitary gland (135 ng g^{-1})	Urine	None Identified	Regulation of some endocrine function
Molybdenum	Kidney (0.4 μg g^{-1}) Liver (0.6 μg g^{-1})	Urine; also significant amounts in bile	Molybdoenzymes of aldehyde oxidase, xanthine oxidase/ dehydrogenase and sulfite oxidase in which molyldenum exists as a small nonprotein factor containing a pterin nucleus; molybdate ion (MoO$_4^{2+}$), the form that exists in blood and urine	Molybdoenzymes oxidize and detoxify various pyrimidines, purines, and pteridines; catalyze the transformation of hypoxanthine to xanthine and xanthine to uric acid; and catalyze the conversion of sulfite to sulfate
Nickel	Adrenal glands (25 ng g^{-1}) Bone (33 ng g^{-1}) Kidney (10 ng g^{-1}) Thyroid (30 ng g^{-1})	Urine as low molecular weight complexes	Binding of Ni^{2-} by various ligands including amino acids (especially histidine and cysteine), proteins (especially albumin), and a macroglobulin called nickeloplasmin important in transport and excretion. Ni^{2+} component of urease; Ni^{3-} essential for enzymatic hydrogenation, desulfurization, and carboxylation reactions in mostly anaerobic microorganisms	Cofactor or structural component in specific metalloenzymes; role in a metabolic pathway involving vitamin B$_{12}$ and folic acid. Role similar to potassium; neurophysiological function
Rubidium	Brain (4 μg g^{-1}) Kidney (5 μg g^{-1}) Liver (6.5 μg g^{-1}) Testis (20 μg g^{-1})	Urine: also significant amounts excreted through intestinal tract	None identified	Role similar to potassium; neurophysiological function
Silicon	Aorta (16 μg g^{-1}) Bone (18 μg g^{-1}) Skin (4 μg g^{-1}) Tendon (12 μg g^{-1})	Urine	Silicic acid (SiOH$_4$) is the form believed to exist in plasma; magnesium orthosilicate is probably the form in urine. The bound form of silicon has never been rigorously identified	Structural role in some mucopolysaccharide or collagen; role in the initiation of calcification and in collagen formation
Tin	Bone (0.8 μg g^{-1}) Kidney (0.2 μg g^{-1}) Liver (0.4 μg g^{-1})	Urine; also significant amounts in bile	Sn^{2+} is absorbed and excreted more readily than Sn^{4+}	Role in some redox reaction
Vanadium	Bone (120 ng g^{-1}) Kidney (120 ng g^{-1}) Liver (120 ng g^{-1}) Spleen (120 ng g^{-1}) Testis (200 ng g^{-1})	Urine; also significant amount in bile	Vanadyl (VO^{2+}), vanadate (H$_2$VO$_4^-$ or VO$_3^-$) and peroxovanadyl [V–OO]; VO^{2+} complexes with proteins, especially those associated with iron (e.g., transferrin, hemoglobin)	Lower forms of life have haloperoxidases that require vanadium for activity; a similar role might exist in higher forms of life

None of the suggested biological functions or roles of any of the ultratrace elements have been conclusively or unequivocally identified in higher forms of life except for those of molybdenum.

usually results from biliary excretion, but may be of nonbiliary origin (e.g., through the pancreas or intestine). Ultratrace elements may also be excreted through sweat and breath. Ultratrace elements also are removed from the body through the loss of blood (e.g., menses), skin, hair, semen, saliva, and nails. **Table 2** gives the major routes of excretion for the ultratrace elements.

Requirements and High Intakes

As already mentioned, the ultratrace elements other than selenium and iodine are a disparate group in terms of their possible requirement or nutritional importance for human health and well-being. Although molybdenum has known essential functions, it has no unequivocally identified practical nutritional importance. The other 14 ultratrace elements discussed here have been suggested to be essential based on circumstantial evidence. This evidence is presented below along with some indication of possible requirement (extrapolated from the deficient animal intakes shown in **Table 3**), and some indication as to what constitutes a high intake.

Aluminum

A dietary deficiency of aluminum in goats reportedly results in increased abortions, depressed growth, incoordination and weakness in hind legs, and decreased life expectancy. Aluminum deficiency has also been reported to depress growth in chicks. Other biochemical actions that suggest aluminum could possibly act in an essential role include the *in vitro* findings that it activates the enzyme adenylate cyclase, enhances calmodulin activity, stimulates DNA synthesis in cell cultures, and stimulates osteoblasts to form bone through activating a purative G, protein-coupled cation sensing system.

If humans have a requirement for aluminum, for which there is currently no evidence, it probably is much less than $1.0 \, \text{mg day}^{-1}$. Aluminum toxicity apparently is not a concern for healthy individuals. Cooking foods in aluminum cook-ware does not lead to detrimental intakes of aluminum. High dietary ingestion of aluminum probably is not a cause of Alzheimer's disease. However, high intakes of aluminum through such sources as buffered analgesics and antacids by susceptible individuals (e.g., those with impaired kidney function including the elderly and low-birthweight infants) may lead to pathological consequences and thus should be avoided. For most healthy individuals,

an aluminum intake of $125 \, \text{mg day}^{-1}$ should not lead to toxicological consequences.

Arsenic

Arsenic deprivation has been induced in chickens, hamsters, goats, pigs, and rats. In the goat, pig, and rat, the most consistent signs of deprivation were depressed growth and abnormal reproduction characterized by impaired fertility and elevated perinatal mortality. Other notable signs of deprivation in goats were depressed serum triacylglycerol concentrations and death during lactation. Myocardial damage was also present in lactating goats. Other signs of arsenic deprivation have been reported, including changes in mineral concentrations in various organs. However, listing all signs reported to be caused by arsenic deficiency may be misleading because studies with chicks, rats, and hamsters have revealed that the nature and severity of the signs are affected by a number of dietary and other factors. For example, female rats fed a diet that is conducive to kidney calcification have more severe calcification when dietary arsenic is low; kidney iron was also elevated. Male rats fed the same diet do not show these changes.

Other factors that affect the response to arsenic deprivation include methionine, arginine, choline, taurine, and guanidoacetic acid. In other words, the signs of arsenic deprivation were changed and generally enhanced by nutritional stressors that affected sulfur amino acid or labile methyl-group metabolism; this suggests that arsenic has a biochemical function that affects these substances. Further evidence for this suggestion is the finding that arsenic deprivation slightly increases liver S-adenosylhomo-cysteine (SAH) and decreases liver S-adenosyl-methionine (SAM) concentrations in animal models, thus resulting in a decreased SAM/SAH ratio; SAM and SAH are involved in methyl transfer. Additionally, arsenite can induce the isolated cell production of certain proteins known as heat shock proteins. The control of production of these proteins in response to arsenite apparently is at the transcriptional level, and involves changes in the methylation of core histones. It also has been shown that arsenic can increase the methylation of the *p53* promoter, or DNA, in human lung cells.

It has been suggested, based upon animal data, that a possible arsenic requirement for humans eating $8.37 \, \text{MJ}$ (2000 kcal) would be $12-25 \, \mu\text{g day}^{-1}$; this is near the typical daily intake shown in **Table 3**. Because of mechanisms for the homeostatic regulation of arsenic (including methylation,

Table 3 Human body content, and deficient, typical, and rich sources of intakes of ultratrace elements

Element	Apparent deficient intake (species)	Human body content	Typical human daily dietary intake	Rich sources
Aluminum	160 $\mu g \, kg^{-1}$ (goat)	30–50 mg	2–10 mg	Baked goods prepared with chemical leavening agents (e.g., baking powder), processed cheese, grains, vegetables, herbs, tea, antacids, buffered analgesics
Arsenic	<25 $\mu g \, kg^{-1}$ (chicks) <35 $\mu g \, kg^{-1}$ (goat) <15 $\mu g \, kg^{-1}$ (hamster) <30 $\mu g \, kg^{-1}$ (rat)	1–2 mg	12–60 μg	Shellfish, fish, grain, cereal products
Boron	<0.3 $mg \, kg^{-1}$ (chick) 0.25–0.35 mg per day (human) <0.3 $mg \, kg^{-1}$ (rat)	10–20 mg	0.5–3.5 mg	Food and drink of plant origin, especially noncitrus fruits, leafy vegetables, nuts, pulses, avocados, legumes, wine, cider, beer, peanut butter
Bromine	0.8 $mg \, kg^{-1}$ (goat)	200–350 mg	2–8 mg	Grain, nuts, fish
Cadmium	<5 $\mu g \, kg^{-1}$ (goat) <4 $\mu g \, kg^{-1}$ (rat)	5–20 mg	10–20 μg	Shellfish, grains – especially those grown on high-cadmium soils, leafy vegetables
Fluorine	<0.3 $mg \, kg^{-1}$ (goat) <0.45 $mg \, kg^{-1}$ (rat)	3 g	Fluoridated areas, 1–3 mg Nonfluoridated areas, 0.3–0.6 mg	Fish, tea, fluoridated water
Germanium	0.7 $mg \, kg^{-1}$ (rat)	3 mg	0.4–3.4 mg	Wheat bran, vegetables, leguminous seeds
Lead	<32 $\mu g \, kg^{-1}$ (pig) <45 $\mu g \, kg^{-1}$ (rat)	Children less than age 10 years, 2 mg Adults, 120 mg	15–100 μg	Seafood, plant foodstuffs grown under high-lead conditions
Lithium	<1.5 $mg \, kg^{-1}$ (goat) <15 $\mu g \, kg^{-1}$ (rat)	350 μg	200–600 μg	Eggs, meat, processed meat, fish, milk, milk products, potatoes, vegetables (content varies with geological origin)
Molybdenum	<25 $\mu g \, kg^{-1}$ (goat) <25 $\mu g \, day^{-1}$ (human) <30 $\mu g \, kg^{-1}$ (rat)	10 mg	50–100 μg	Milk and milk products, dried legumes, pulses, organ meats (liver and kidney), cereals, and baked goods
Nickel	<100 $\mu g \, kg^{-1}$ (goat) <20 $\mu g \, kg^{-1}$ (rat)	1–2 mg	70–260 μg	Chocolate, nuts, dried beans and peas, grains
Rubidium	180 $\mu g \, kg^{-1}$ (goat)	360 mg	1–5 mg	Coffee, black tea, fruits and vegetables (especially asparague), poultry, fish
Silicon	<2.0 $mg \, kg^{-1}$ (chick) <4.5 $mg \, kg^{-1}$ (rat)	2–3 g	20–50 mg	Unrefined grains of high fiber content, cereal products, beer, coffee
Tin	<20 $\mu g \, kg^{-1}$ (rat)	7–14 mg	1–40 mg	Canned foods
Vanadium	<10 $\mu g \, kg^{-1}$ (goat)	100 μg	10–30 μg	Shellfish, mushrooms, parsley, dill seed, black pepper, some prepared foods, grains, beer, wine

then excretion in urine), its toxicity through oral intake is relatively low; it is actually less toxic than selenium, an ultratrace element with a well-established nutritional value. Toxic quantities of inorganic arsenic generally are reported in milligrams. For example, reported estimated fatal acute doses of arsenic for humans range from 70 to 300 mg or about 1.0 to 4.0 mg per kg body weight.

Some forms of organic arsenic are virtually non-toxic; a 10 g per kg body weight dose of arsenobetaine depressed spontaneous motility and respiration in male mice, but these symptoms disappeared within 1 h. Results of numerous epidemiological studies have suggested an association between chronic overexposure to arsenic and the incidence of some forms of cancer; however, the role of arsenic in carcinogenesis remains controversial. Arsenic does not seem to act as a primary carcinogen, and is either an inactive or extremely weak mitogen. In the USA, a standard known as a reference dose (RfD; lifetime exposure that is unlikely to cause adverse health effects) of 0.3 μg per kg body weight per day, or 21 μg day^{-1} for a 70 kg human, has been suggested for inorganic arsenic. Because of safety factors in the determination, the RfD for arsenic conflicts with the possible arsenic requirement; this conflict is similar to that for some other mineral elements including zinc. These conflicts are currently being addressed by nutritionists and toxicologists.

Boron

Listing the signs of boron deficiency for animal models is difficult because most studies have used stressors to enhance the response to changes in dietary boron. Thus, the response to boron deprivation varied as the diet changed in its content of nutrients such as calcium, phosphorus, magnesium, potassium, and vitamin D. Although the nature and severity of the changes varied with dietary composition, many of the findings indicated that boron deprivation impairs calcium metabolism, brain function, and energy metabolism. Studies also suggest that boron deprivation impairs immune function and exacerbates adjuvant-induced arthritis in rats. Feeding low boron to humans (<0.3 mg day^{-1}) altered the metabolism of macrominerals, electrolytes, and nitrogen, as well as oxidative metabolism, and produces changes in erythropoiesis and hematopoiesis. Boron deprivation also altered electroencephalograms to suggest depressed behavioral activation and mental alertness, depressed psychomotor skills and cognitive processes of attention and memory, and enhanced some effects of estrogen therapy such as increases in concentrations of serum 17β-estradiol and plasma copper. Other findings suggest that boron may have an essential function. *In vitro* it competitively inhibits oxidoreductase enzymes, which require pyridine or flavin nucleotides, and enzymes such as serine proteases, which form transition state analogs with boronic acid or borate derivatives. Boron has an essential function in plants, in which it influences redox actions involved in cellular membrane transport. This latter finding supports the hypothesis that boron has a role in cell membrane function or stability such that it influences the response to hormone action, transmembrane signaling, or transmembrane movement of regulatory cations or anions. Another finding in support of this hypothesis is that boron influences the transport of extracellular calcium into and the release of intracellular calcium in rat platelets activated by thrombin.

An analysis of both human and animal data has resulted in the suggestion by a World Health Organization (WHO) publication that an acceptable safe range of population mean intakes of boron for adults could well be 1.0–13 mg day^{-1}. In other words, 1.0 mg probably covers any requirement and 13 mg will not lead to any toxicological consequences. However, the US and Canada concluded in 2002 that there was still insufficient evidence to establish a clear biological function for boron in humans, so no recommended dietary intake was set for those countries. Boron has a low order of toxicity when administered orally. Toxicity signs in animals generally occur only after dietary boron exceeds 100 μg g^{-1}. The low order of toxicity of boron for humans is shown by the use of boron as a food preservative between 1870 and 1920 without apparent harm. It was reported in 1904 that when doses equivalent to more than 0.5 g of boric acid were consumed daily, disturbances in appetite, digestion, and health occurred. It was concluded in this report that this quantity of boron per day was too much for an average person to receive regularly. The upper limit (UL) for the US and Canada has been set at 20 mg day^{-1} based on extrapolation from animal studies.

Bromine

It has been reported that a dietary deficiency of bromide results in depression of growth, fertility, hematocrit, hemoglobin, and life expectancy, and increases in milk fat and spontaneous abortions in goats. Other biological actions that suggest bromine could possibly act in an essential role include the findings that bromide alleviates growth retardation caused by hyperthyroidism in mice and chicks, and insomnia exhibited by many hemodialysis patients has been associated with bromide deficit.

If humans have a requirement for bromide, which has not yet been shown to be the case, based on deficient intakes for animals it is probably no more than $1.0\,mg\,day^{-1}$. Bromine ingested as the bromide ion has a low order of toxicity; thus bromine is not of toxicological concern in nutrition.

Cadmium

Deficiency of cadmium reportedly depresses growth of rats and goats. Other *in vitro* biochemical actions that suggest cadmium could possibly act as an essential element include the finding that it has transforming growth factor activity and stimulates growth of cells in soft agar.

If humans have a requirement for cadmium, which is still uncertain, based on deficient intakes for animals it is probably less than $5\,\mu g\,day^{-1}$. Although cadmium may be an essential element at these extremely low amounts, it is of more concern because of its toxicological properties. Cadmium has a long half-life in the body and thus high intakes can lead to accumulation, resulting in damage to some organs, especially the kidney. The toxicological aspects of cadmium have been discussed earlier (*See:* xx).

Fluorine

Reported unequivocal or specific signs of fluoride deficiency are almost nonexistent. A study with goats indicated that a fluoride deficiency decreases life expectancy and caused pathological hisrology in the kidney and endocrine organs. Most of the evidence accepted as showing a need for fluoride comes from studies in which it was orally administered in pharmacological doses. Pharmacological doses of fluoride have been shown to prevent tooth caries, improve fertility, hematopoiesis and growth in iron-deficient mice and rats, prevent phosphorus-induced nephro-calcinosis, and perhaps prevent bone loss leading to osteoporosis.

Although fluoride is not generally considered an essential element in the classical sense for humans, it still is considered a beneficial element. Because of this, in the US-Canada, the AI has been set, on the basis of reducing dental caries without adverse effects, at: $0.01\,mg\,day^{-1}$ for infants 0–6 months; 0.5 mg for 6–12 months; 0.7 mg for 1–3 years; 1 mg for 4–8 years; 2 mg for 9–13 years; 3 mg for 14–18 years; 3 mg for women and 4 mg for men. These intakes provide amounts of fluoride that will give protection against dental caries and generally not result in any consequential mottling of teeth; they should not be considered intakes that are needed to prevent a nutritional deficiency of fluoride. Chronic fluoride toxicity through excessive intake mainly through water supplies and industrial exposure has been reported in many parts of the world. Chronic toxicity resulting from the ingestion of water and food providing in excess of $2.0\,mg\,day^{-1}$ is manifested by dental fluorosis or mottled enamel ranging from barely discernible with intakes not much above $2.0\,mg\,day^{-1}$ to stained and pitted enamel with much higher amounts. Crippling skeletal fluorosis apparently occurs in people who ingest 10–25 mg day^{-1} for 7–20 years. The UL (mg per day) is 0.7 mg for 0–6 months, 0.9 mg for 7–12 months, 1.3 mg for 1–3 years, and 2.2 mg for 4–8 years, and 10 mg for all older age groups including pregnant and lactating women.

Germanium

A low germanium intake has been found to alter bone and liver mineral composition and decrease tibial DNA in rats. Germanium also reverses changes in rats caused by silicon deprivation, and is touted as having anticancer properties because some organic complexes of germanium can inhibit tumor formation in animal models.

If humans have a requirement for germanium, based on animal deprivation studies, it is probably less than $0.5\,mg\,day^{-1}$. The toxicity of germanium depends upon its form. Some organic forms of germanium are less toxic than inorganic forms. Inorganic germanium toxicity results in kidney damage. Some individuals consuming high amounts of organic germanium supplements contaminated with inorganic germanium have died from kidney failure. Although germanium has long been believed to have a low order of toxicity because of its diffusible state and rapid elimination from the body, until more knowledge is obtained about the intakes at which germanium becomes toxic, they probably should not greatly exceed those found in a typical diet. An intake of no more than $5.0\,mg\,day^{-1}$ would meet any possible need for germanium and most likely will be below the level found to have toxicological consequences.

Lead

A large number of findings have come from one source that suggests that a low dietary intake of lead is disadvantageous to pigs and rats. Apparent deficiency signs found include: depressed growth; anemia; elevated serum cholesterol, phospholipids and bile acids; disturbed iron metabolism; decreased liver glucose, triacylglycerols, LDL-cholesterol and phospholipids; increased liver cholesterol; and altered blood and liver enzymes. A beneficial action of lead ($2\,\mu g\,g^{-1}$ versus $30\,ng\,g^{-1}$ diet) is that it alleviates iron deficiency signs in young rats.

If humans have a requirement for lead, which has not yet been demonstrated to be the case, it is probably less than 30 μg day^{-1} based on animal deprivation studies. Although lead may have beneficial effects at low intakes, lead toxicity is of more concern than lead deficiency. Lead is considered one of the major environmental pollutants because of the past use of lead-based paints and the combustion of fuels containing lead additives. The toxicological aspects of lead are discussed elsewhere (*See:* xx).

Lithium

Lithium deficiency reportedly results in depressed fertility, birthweight, and life span, and altered activity of liver and blood enzymes in goats. In rats, lithium deficiency apparently depresses fertility, birthweight, litter size, and weaning weight. Other *in vitro* biochemical actions suggesting that lithium could possibly act as an essential element include the stimulation of growth of some cultured cells, and having insulinomimetic action. Lithium is best known for its pharmacological properties; it is used to treat manic-depressive psychosis. Its ability to affect mental function perhaps explains the report that incidence of violent crimes is lower in areas with high-lithium drinking water.

If humans have a requirement for lithium, based on animal deprivation studies it is probably less than 25 μg day^{-1}, which is much less than the usual dietary intake (see **Table 3**). Lithium is not a particularly toxic element, but the principal disadvantage in the use of lithium for psychiatric disorders is the narrow safety margin between therapeutic and toxic doses. About 500 mg lithium per day is needed to raise serum concentrations to be effective in these disorders; this is close to the concentration where mild toxicity signs of gastrointestinal disturbances, muscular weakness, tremor, drowsiness, and a dazed feeling begin to appear. Severe toxicity results in coma, muscle tremor, convulsions, and even death.

Molybdenum

The evidence for the essentiality of molybdenum is substantial and conclusive. Molybdenum functions as a cofactor in enzymes that catalyze the hydroxylation of various substrates. Aldehyde oxidase oxidizes and detoxifies various pyrimidines, purines, pteridines, and related compounds. Xanthine oxidase/dehydrogenase catalyzes the transformation of hypoxanthine to xanthine, and xanthine to uric acid. Sulfite oxidase catalyzes the transformation of sulfite to sulfate. Attempts to produce molybdenum deficiency signs in rats, chickens, and humans have resulted in only limited success, and no success in healthy humans.

Deficiency signs in animals are best obtained when the diet is supplemented with massive amounts of tungsten, an antagonist of molybdenum metabolism. Nonetheless, reported deficiency signs for goats and pigs are depressed food consumption and growth, impaired reproduction characterized by increased mortality in both mothers and offspring, and elevated copper concentrations in liver and brain. A molybdenum-responsive syndrome found in hatching chicks is characterized by a high incidence of late embryonic mortality, mandibular distortion, anophthalmia, and defects in leg bone and feather development. The incidence of this syndrome was particularly high in commercial flocks reared on diets containing high concentrations of copper, another molybdenum metabolism antagonist.

Examples of nutritional standards that have been set for molybdenum are the current US-Canada recommendations, which are the following: Adequate Intake for infants aged 0–0.5 years, 2 μg and aged 0.5–1 years, 3 μg; RDA for children 1–3 years, 17 μg; 4–8 years, 22 μg; 9–13 years, 34 μg; 14–18 years, 43 μg; women from 19–>70 years, 34 μg; and men aged 19–>70 years, 45 μg. The recommended intake is 50 μg day^{-1} in pregnancy and lactation. These values were set using balance data in adults with extrapolation to the other groups. Usual dietary intakes are substantially higher than these recommendations. Large oral doses are necessary to overcome the homeostatic control of molybdenum; thus, it is a relatively nontoxic nutrient. The UL for children 1–3 years is 300 μg, for 4–8 years, 600 μg, and 9–13 years, 1100 μg. For adolescents the UL is 1700 μg, and for adults, 2000 μg, including pregnant and lactating women, based on doses that caused reproductive damage in animals.

Nickel

Based on recent studies with rats and goats, nickel deprivation depresses growth, reproductive performance and plasma glucose, and alters the distribution of other elements in the body, including calcium, iron, and zinc. As with other ultratrace elements, the nature and severity of signs of nickel deprivation are affected by diet composition. For example, vitamin B$_{12}$ status affects signs of nickel deprivation in rats, and the effects suggest that vitamin B$_{12}$ must be present for optimal nickel function. The nickel function also may involve folic acid because an interaction between these two affected the vitamin B$_{12}$ and folic acid-dependent pathway of methionine synthesis from homocysteine. Nickel might function as a cofactor or structural component in specific metalloenzymes in higher organisms because such enzymes have been identified in bacteria, fungi, plants, and invertebrates. These nickel-containing enzymes include urease, hydrogenase, methylcoenzyme M reductase, and carbon monoxide dehydrogenase. Moreover, nickel can activate numerous enzymes *in vitro*.

Based on a lack of human studies, no recommended intake levels have been set for humans. Life-threatening toxicity of nickel through oral intake is unlikely. Because of excellent homeostatic regulation, nickel salts exert their toxic action mainly by gastrointestinal irritation and not by inherent toxicity. Based on extrapolation from animal studies, the UL has been set for the US and Canada at the following doses of soluble nickel salts: 1–3 years, 0.2 mg; 4–8 years, 0.3 mg; 9–13 years, 0.6 mg; and all adolescents and adults, 1 mg.

Rubidium

Rubidium deficiency in goats reportedly results in depressed food intake and life expectancy, and increased spontaneous abortions. If rubidium is required by humans, the requirement probably would be no more than a few hundred micrograms per day, based on animal data. Rubidium is a relatively nontoxic element and thus is not of toxicological concern from the nutritional point of view.

Silicon

Most of the signs of silicon deficiency in chickens and rats indicate aberrant metabolism of connective tissue and bone. For example, chicks fed a silicon-deficient diet exhibit structural abnormalities of the skull, depressed collagen content in bone, and long-bone abnormalities characterized by small, poorly formed joints and defective endochondral bone growth. Silicon deprivation can affect the response to other dietary manipulations. For example, rats fed a diet low in calcium and high in aluminum accumulated high amounts of aluminum in the brain; silicon supplements prevented the accumulation. Also, high dietary aluminum depressed brain zinc concentrations in thyroidectomized rats fed low dietary silicon; silicon supplements prevented the depression. This effect was not seen in nonthyroidectomized rats. Other biochemical actions suggest that silicon is an essential element. Silicon is consistently found in collagen, and in bone tissue culture has been found to be needed for maximal bone prolylhydroxylase activity. Silicon deficiency decreases ornithine aminotransferase, an enzyme in the collagen formation pathway, in rats. Finally, silicon is essential for some lower forms of life in which silica serves a structural role and possibly affects gene expression.

Much of the silicon found in most diets probably occurs as aluminosilicates and silica from which silicon is not readily available. Owing to lack of evidence for a biological role for silicon in humans, no recommended intakes have been set. Silicon is essentially nontoxic when taken orally. Magnesium trisilicate, an over-the-counter antacid, has been used by humans for more than 40 years without obvious deleterious effects. Other silicates are food additives used as anticaking or antifoaming agents.

Tin

A dietary deficiency of tin has been reported to depress growth, response to sound, and feed efficiency, alter the mineral composition of several organs, and cause hair loss in rats. Additionally, tin has been shown to influence heme oxygenase activity and has been associated with thymus immune and homeostatic functions.

Owing to lack of data no recommended intakes have been set for tin. Inorganic tin is relatively nontoxic. However, the routine consumption of foods packed in unlacquered tin-plated cans may result in excessive exposure to tin, which could adversely affect the metabolism of other essential trace elements including zinc and copper. Because 50 mg day^{-1} of tin was found to affect zinc and copper metabolism, routine intakes near this amount probably should be avoided.

Vanadium

Vanadium-deprived goats were found to exhibit an increased abortion rate and depressed milk production. About 40% of kids from vanadium-deprived goats died between days 7 and 91 of life with some deaths preceded by convulsions; only 8% of kids from vanadium-supplemented goats died during the same time. Also, skeletal deformations were seen in the forelegs, and forefoot tarsal joints were thickened. In rats, vanadium deprivation increases thyroid weight and decreases growth. Other biochemical actions support the suggestion that vanadium could possibly act in an essential role. *In vitro* studies with cells and pharmacological studies with animals have shown that vanadium has: insulin-mimetic properties; numerous stimulatory effects on cell proliferation and differentiation; effects on cell phosphorylation-dephosphorylation; effects on glucose and ion transport across the plasma membrane: and effects on oxidation-reduction processes. Some algae, lichens, fungi, and bacteria contain enzymes that require vanadium for activity. The enzymes include nitrogenase in bacteria, and bromoperoxidase, iodoperoxidase, and chloroperoxidase in algae, lichens, and fungi, respectively. The haloperoxidases, catalyze the oxidation of halide ions by hydrogen peroxide, thus facilitating the formation of a carbon–halogen bond. The best known haloperoxidase in animals is thyroid peroxidase. Vanadium deprivation in rats affects the response of thyroid peroxidase to changing dietary iodine concentrations. Since a functional role for vanadium has not been determined in humans no recommended intakes have been set.

Vanadium can be a relatively toxic element. Green tongue, cramps and diarrhea, and neurological effects have occurred in humans ingesting vanadium salts. Based on renal damage in animals, the UL for adults is 1.8 mg vanadium salts per day, with insufficient data to set a UL for other age groups.

Dietary Sources

The requirements for the ultratrace elements will be met if a person consumes a diet based on the dietary guidelines recommended by. For some areas of the world, especially in developing countries where traditional, monotonous diets are based primarily on a cereal (particularly rice) or tuber staple, the intake of several ultratrace elements (e.g., boron, molybdenum) could possibly be low. Reported typical dietary intakes (mostly for industrialized countries) and rich sources of the ultratrace elements are shown in Table 3.

See also: **Iodine**: Physiology, Dietary Sources and Requirements. **Selenium**.

Further Reading

Chappell WR, Abernathy CO, and Cothern CR (eds.) (1994) *Arsenic Exposure and Health*. Northwood: Science and Technology Letters.

Ciba Foundation (1986) *Silicon Biochemistry*. Chichester: John Wiley & Sons.

Editorial (1994) Health effects of boron. *Environmental Health Perspectives Supplement* **102**(supplement 7).

FAO/WHO (1996) *Trace Elements in Human Nutrition and Health*. Geneva: World Health Organization.

Frieden E (ed.) (1984) *Biochemistry of the Essential Ultratrace Elements*. New York: Plenum.

Institute of Medicine (2002) *Dietary Reference Intakes for Vitamin A, Vitamin K, Arsenic, Boron, Chromium, Copper, Iodine, Iron, Manganese, Molybdenum, Nickel, Silicon, Vanadium, and Zinc*. Washington DC: National Academy Press.

Mertz W (ed.) (1986, 1987) *Trace Elements in Human and Animal Nutrition*, vols 1 and 2. Orlando and San Diego: Academic Press.

Nielsen FH (1986) Other elements: Sb, Bs, B, Br, Cs, Ge, Rb, Ag, Sr, Sn, Ti, Zr, Be, Bi, Ga, Au, In, Nb, Sc, Te, Tl, W. In: Mertz W (ed.) *Trace Elements in Human and Animal Nutrition*, vol. 2, pp. 415–463. Orlando: Academic Press.

Nielsen FH (1994) Ultratrace minerals. In: Shils ME, Olson JA, and Shike M (eds.) *Modern Nutrition in Health and Disease*, 8th edn, vol. 1, pp. 269–286. Philadelphia: Lea & Febiger. (9th edition with updated chapter on ultratrace minerals in progress.)

Nielsen FH (1996) Other trace elements. In: Ziegler EE and Filer LJ Jr (eds.) *Present Knowledge in Nutrition*, 7th edn, pp. 353–376. Washington DC: ILSI Press.

Sigel H and Sigel A (eds.) (1995) *Metal Ions in Biological Systems*, vol. 23, Nickel and its Role in Biology. New York: Marcel Dekker.

Sigel H and Sigel A (eds.) (1995) *Metal Ions in Biological Systems*, vol. 31, Vanadium and its Role in Life. New York: Marcel Dekker.

VEGETARIAN DIETS

J Dwyer, Tufts University, Boston, MA, USA

Published by Elsevier Ltd.

Introduction

Vegetarian eating patterns are the norm in many parts of the world, while in Western countries they are the exception. Currently, about 2.5% of adults in the US and 4% of adults in Canada follow some sort of self-described vegetarian diet. This article examines the nutritional adequacy of vegetarian diets and some eating patterns and practices that affect it, focusing on Western countries.

Definitions are important in discussing vegetarian diets and nutritional adequacy since both of these terms cover a multitude of disparate characteristics.

Vegetarianism

For most vegetarians today, their investment in vegetarian eating as an all-encompassing philosophical system for organizing all of life is minimal. Food preferences, habit, and flavor take precedence over philosophy in dictating their eating choices. That is, these individuals have vegetarian eating styles but they do not subscribe to vegetarianism.

There is a smaller group of vegetarians whose eating patterns serve as badges of honor for a deeper and more encompassing set of beliefs that includes and is reflected in but is not limited to their eating patterns. This belief system is referred to as vegetarianism. Vegetarianism is a philosophy and belief system rather than simply an eating pattern. Those who subscribe to vegetarianism hold strong convictions about the moral, metaphysical, ethical, or political appropriateness of their eating choices. Often more restrictive animal food and other dietary avoidances are accompanied by the most deeply held views. In fact, it is a minority of all of those who consume vegetarian diets who subscribe to vegetarianism. Advocates of vegetarianism have become more militant in recent years. With some vegans, it remains an ethical, philosophical, or predominantly religious conviction, or a deeply rooted health concern that is privately held and the diet is practiced with great conviction. Other vegans are strongly committed to enlisting additional followers and appear to have become more militant in recent years. Some have adopted broader agendas, including that of animal rights, while others do not. In the US, animal rights organizations such as People for the Ethical Treatment of Animals (PETA), the PETA foundation, the Animal Liberation Front, and the Physicians' Committee for Responsible Medicine (PCRM) in the US are all very vocal. They finance advertizing, journal articles, and educational efforts to encourage adoption of their views. Extensive efforts are directed toward youth. Similar groups are also active in other countries.

Vegetarian Eating Patterns

The term vegetarian diet does not fully describe the variety in nutrient intakes and health status of those who follow such eating patterns. There are many different types of vegetarian eating patterns (see **Table 1**). The impact of these patterns on nutritional status and health requires more complete characterization of diet and other aspects of lifestyle than such a simple descriptor.

The terms vegetarian, lactovegetarian, and vegan focus on foods that are left after others have been omitted from the diet. From the nutritional standpoint the animal food groups (e.g., meat fish, fowl, eggs, milk, and milk products) are nutrient-dense foods. In traditional diets of usual foods, they were often rich sources of certain nutrients. Depending on the particular animal food group under consideration, these nutrients may include protein of high biological value, highly bioavailable iron, zinc, calcium, vitamins A, D, B_{12} and B_6, riboflavin, omega 3 fatty acids, and iodine. When these food groups are eliminated entirely from the diet, intakes of the nutrients these groups are rich in may fall short.

Although dietary diversity in the number of food groups consumed is less among vegetarians, diversity within food groups is often considerable and is sufficient to provide adequate amounts of nutrients.

Table 1 Common types of vegetarian dietary patterns categorized by animal food use

Pattern	Comments
Meat avoiders	Limit or avoid red meat and other flesh foods; may also restrict poultry, fish, and seafood. Diets are similar in most respects to nonvegetarian diets
Lacto-ovo vegetarians	Avoidances include all meat, poultry, and often fish, but consume milk products and eggs. Iron may be limiting and it can be obtained from iron-fortified cereals. Low-fat dairy products are preferred to keep intakes of saturated fat and total fat moderate
Lacto vegetarians	Avoid all meat, fish, poultry, and eggs. Nutrient considerations same as above
Macrobiotics	Numerous restrictions generally including avoidance of all meat, poultry, milk and eggs, but may consume fish in small amounts. Also avoid sugar and other refined sweeteners, foods that are members of the nightshade family (peppers, egg plant, tomatoes, and potatoes) and tropical fruits. Current variations of the diet are less restrictive than the versions of 30 years ago, but deficiencies of energy, iron, calcium, vitamin B_{12}, vitamin D, and other nutrients may still arise in weanlings, pregnant women, and young children if diets are nutritionally unplanned
Vegans	Avoidances include all animal products including meat, fish, poultry, eggs, and dairy products. Some vegans may also refuse to use any animal products in daily life. Without careful planning, energy, vitamins B_{12} and D, and bioavailable sources of iron may be low. Concentrated sources of energy-dense foods such as sugars and fats are helpful in increasing energy intakes. Vitamins B_{12} and D and calcium can be supplied from fortified soy milk, fortified cereals, and/or dietary supplements of these nutrients. Usually protein is adequate if a variety of protein sources is consumed
Other patterns	Raw food eaters and 'living food' eaters avoid animal foods and eat raw plant foods, including fruits, vegetables and cereals with special health foods such as wheatgrass or carrot juice. Fruitarians consume diets mostly of fruits, nuts, honey, and olive oil. Rastafarians eat a near-vegan diet and avoid alcohol, salt-preserved foods and additives. Yogic groups vary in their eating patterns but are often lacto vegetarian

Variety within food groups may even be increased on vegetarian diets. For example, among those consuming vegan diets the amount and type of legumes as well as other vegetables and fruits is often increased.

Eating patterns appear to be more closely associated with health outcomes than are nutrient intakes alone. Therefore, it is important to also consider other phytochemicals and zoochemicals in vegetarian diets that may have health effects.

Vegetarians' intakes of some of the bioactive constituents that are rich in fruits and vegetables such as the flavonoids, antioxidants, and dietary fiber may be much higher than those of omnivores. If these substances prove to have beneficial effects on health, such increased intakes may be important.

From the nutritional standpoint there are beneficial trade-offs from vegetarians' limited animal food intakes. Animal foods are major sources of dietary constituents that are in excess in Western diets, such as high amounts of calories, fat, saturated fat, cholesterol, and low amounts of dietary fiber. Consumption of fewer animal foods, especially if it leads to lesser intakes of these constituents may have positive effects on overall nutritional status. Thus, there are both nutritional benefits and risks to limiting animal foods. The exact effects on nutritional status will vary depending on the food group avoided, the degree of limitation, substitutions of other rich food sources, use of fortified foods and dietary supplements, and other changes in dietary intake that occur at the same time. The nutritional goal is to maximize the benefits and minimize the

risks by a judicious choice of the type and amount of animal foods or other sources of the nutrients they contain.

Nutritional Adequacy

In English-speaking North America, dietary reference intakes (DRI) have been issued by the Food and Nutrition Board, Institute of Medicine, National Academy of Sciences. Nutritional adequacy is defined as meeting nutrient needs such as the recommended dietary allowances (RDAs) or the adequate intakes (AI), while avoiding excess and staying below the tolerable upper levels of intakes (UL) and keeping within the macronutrient ranges specified by expert groups. Similar reference standards are available in other countries.

It is useful to screen out those vegetarians who are likely to be at high risk of dietary inadequacy by using some simple characteristics of their diets and lifestyles to determine if further dietary assessment is likely to be needed. The entire pattern of intake (including avoidances, substitutions and additions of foods, and use of dietary supplements) describes the individual vegetarian's profile of nutrient adequacy or inadequacy.

Because dietary practices among vegetarians are so variable, individual assessment of their dietary intakes is recommended. Those at special risk are those in the nutritionally vulnerable groups due to age, life stage (pregnancy, lactation) or illness, especially if they eschew many animal food groups (vegans), have numerous other food avoidances, or hold beliefs that otherwise limit their dietary intakes.

Adequate Vegetarian Diet Patterns

There are many individuals who have little or no risk of dietary inadequacy from their vegetarian eating patterns; for example, an adult male who regards himself as a vegetarian (also referred to as a meat avoider, or semi-vegetarian) but has a dietary pattern that consists solely of occasionally avoiding red meat about half of the time with no other dietary alterations. Such an individual is unlikely to need further dietary assessment.

Some characteristics of sound, adequate vegetarian diet patterns include the following:

- Use of a nutritionally sound food guide of diet planning; vegan and vegetarian food guides that conform to the latest recommendations of expert groups may help to ensure that nutrient needs will be met with balance and without excessive intakes.
- If diet alone does not meet the RDAs, regular use of appropriate vitamin mineral supplements plus use of a nutritionally sound food guide.
- Vegans and some other vegetarians sometimes have multiple food avoidances; intakes of nutrients likely to be deficient can be increased by use of rich sources of whole foods, foods fortified with the nutrients falling short, and/or vitamin or mineral supplements.
- Consumption of a wide variety of food groups and foods within each group.
- Membership of a family with a long history of adherence to healthy vegetarian eating styles.
- Avoidances are limited to a few foods or are sporadic in nature.

Signs of Possibly Inadequate Vegetarian Diet Patterns

The more of the following characteristics that apply, the higher the potential risk of inadequacy and the greater the need for further assessment.

Diet   First it is important to examine what food groups, foods, or products are avoided or de-emphasized on vegetarian diets, and then some additional characteristics of dietary patterns, personal characteristics, and belief systems that further increase risk of dietary inadequacy and other health problems:

- **Many types and extensive avoidance of animal food groups.** Assessment of the nutritional adequacy of vegetarian eating patterns begins by examining animal food groups (red meat, poultry, fish and seafood, milk and milk products, eggs) and specific foods within these that are avoided entirely or eaten only in minimal amounts. Unless other foods or food groups rich in these nutrients or nutrient-containing dietary supplements are used, problems may arise.
- **Many types and extensive avoidance of fortified foods, nutrient-containing dietary supplements, and processed foods.** Some vegetarians believe that fortified foods (highly fortified cereals, calcium fortified soy milk and/or juices, B_{12} fortified yeast), processed foods (frozen, canned, and in extreme cases cooked foods for raw food eaters), and nutrient-containing dietary supplements (vitamins, minerals, fatty acids) should be avoided for various philosophical, ideological, or religious reasons, and refuse to use them. Usage needs to be assessed since such avoidances limit options for nutrition intervention strategies.
- **Few acceptable foods and supplements.** Foods and groups that are stressed and emphasized on the vegetarian diet should be noted. If very few foods or food groups are acceptable for one reason or another, or if only special foods are permitted (organic, nonprocessed, etc.) this may further limit intakes. Some vegetarians are willing to use both fortified foods and nutrient-containing dietary supplements. Use of these may have implications for health and should be recorded. Nutrient intervention strategies for increasing intakes of nutrients falling short in diets may be limited since such individuals may refuse to use fortified foods and/or dietary supplements.
- **Many practices such as fasting, altered diet during illness, and use of special foods for medicinal purposes.** These practices may further increase risks of nutritional inadequacy. If medical care or treatment is avoided, additional risks may accrue.

Other practices   Other practices must also be considered:

- **Other lifestyle practices with beneficial potential health impacts.** Vegetarians have other health habits and lifestyles that alter risks for chronic diseases for the better, such as nonsmoking, abstinence from alcohol, and high levels of physical activity. Therefore, differences in their health outcomes are probably due to a range of factors, and not solely to differences in their diets.
- **Lack of ongoing health surveillance by a physician.** Lack of medical supervision increases the

chances that preventable or treatable health problems will be dealt with expeditiously.

Personal characteristics Among these are the following:

- **Nutritionally vulnerable because of age or physiological condition.** The very young, the old, the rapidly growing, pregnant and lactating women, pubertal children, the elderly, and the ill and frail all fall into this group. Individuals at especially high risk are those with chronic diseases and conditions that alter nutritional needs who also have inadequate dietary intakes.
- **Low weight for height.** If weight for height, as measured by body mass index, is below 18.5 or if unintentional weight loss has totaled more than about 5–7 kg (10–15 pounds), there is reason for concern.
- **Rapid weight loss.** Unintentional loss of more than 5% of weight in a month is a cause for concern.

Beliefs Ideology is also important:

- **Deeply held beliefs in alternative philosophical or religious systems that govern food choice.** Some individuals feel bound to make their diets conform to their ethical, philosophical, or religious systems. This can further constrain choice and nutrient intakes.
- **Membership of a quasi-philosophical or religious group that includes vegetarian diets that are not planned in line with nutritional recommendations by experts.** Some groups, e.g., the Seventh-Day Adventists or certain other lacto-ovo vegetarian groups, make a conscious effort to incorporate the recommendations of expert groups, such as those of the Food and Nutrition Board/Institute of Medicine and Health Canada in English-speaking North America into the regimens they recommend. In such cases, the group support provided may be of positive benefit and help to ensure nutritional adequacy. However, at times in the past other groups have insisted on regimens that did not incorporate such recommendations. For those who are active in such groups, the group's support may reinforce negative attitudes toward meeting such expert recommendations.

Using the characteristics above, it is usually possible to sort out those consuming vegetarian diets who are at low or no risk of inadequacy from those who may potentially have problems and need further assessment and counseling.

Key Nutritional Concerns for Vegetarians

Of particular concern with respect to risk of inadequacy for vegetarians are energy, vitamins B_{12} and D, riboflavin, omega 3 fatty acids, calcium, iron, zinc, and iodine. Intakes of these tend to be lower on vegan diets, and may also be low on other diets that include extensive avoidances. Vegetarians of all types can easily meet current recommendations for all nutrients if they are willing to use fortified foods and supplements. However, some vegetarians are unwilling to use these options, increasing risks of deficiency and making dietary planning more difficult.

Vegetarian and particularly vegan diets tend to be low in energy, total fat, saturated fat, cholesterol, dietary fiber, and sodium. If processed foods are avoided added sugars are also low. Current recommendations for acceptable macronutrient distribution ranges (AMDR) in the US are for fat 20–55% of calories and for protein 10–35% of calories, with added sugars no more than 25% of calories, and the remainder from other carbohydrates.

Key Nutrients for Vegetarians over the Life Cycle

Well-planned vegan and vegetarian diets can meet nutritional needs at all stages of the life cycle including pregnancy, lactation, infancy, childhood, and adolescence. There are very few longitudinal studies of those on the more restrictive vegetarian diets; an exception is a Dutch cohort of macrobiotic vegetarians who have been followed from birth to adolescence, and who continue to have some health problems. More studies are needed so that long-lasting effects of diet early in life can be better ascertained.

Some vegetarian parents feed their children diets that are inadequate. The problem is not that nutritionally adequate diets cannot be planned, but that the eater's or cook's ideologies and concerns may get in the way. Thus, actual diets, as eaten, may not conform to the recommendations of expert nutritional bodies. Under such circumstances health problems have arisen and continue to do so, especially among infants and children on vegan diets that are limited in other foods as well.

Vegan diets present more problems of micronutrient adequacy than do other vegetarian diets across the life cycle and particularly in infants and children because more food groups are eliminated, sources of vitamins B_{12} and D may be lacking and the caloric density of the diet is lower and bulk higher than that of vegetarians or omnivorous infants. They may also have diets that are limited in other foods, and thus in nutrients such as calcium and iron.

Vegetarian infants are usually breast-fed. They generally thrive until 4–6 months of age, and continue to do so if they are weaned to diets containing cows' milk-based or soy formulas and sufficient food energy. In countries where infant formulas do not provide adequate amounts of micronutrients, dietary supplements may be needed. Today, many more fortified vegan foods are widely available than in the past. They are helpful in meeting the nutrient needs of weanlings and toddlers. Also, dietary supplements are available, and for some vegans these are acceptable alternatives. Good sources of vitamin B_{12} need to be identified and also of vitamin D if exposures to sunlight are not adequate. Sources of other nutrients such as linolenic acid, the omega 3 fatty acid, should be included so that docosahexanenoic acid (DHA) intakes are satisfactory. Vegan diets may also be low in calcium, iron, and zinc, and the forms in which iron and zinc are present may not be highly bioavailable. A source of riboflavin also needs to be identified.

Vegetarian diets need to be carefully monitored when they are fed to young children. Soy milk is not appropriate under 1 year of age. When soy milk is used later in childhood, especially if the child is a vegan, it should be fortified with vitamins D and B_{12} and calcium.

For pubertal children, energy, calcium, iron, vitamins D and B_{12}, as well as iron are of particular concern with respect to dietary adequacy, but these can usually be dealt with by dietary planning.

Current Vegetarian Eating Patterns and Practices

Until about 40 years ago, in Western countries virtually all of the common vegetarian eating patterns involved avoidance of animal flesh (meat and poultry); categorization of vegetarian patterns was relatively straightforward and consisted simply of differentiating between those who ate no animal foods at all (vegan vegetarians), those who also consumed milk and milk products (lacto vegetarians), and those who ate eggs as well (lacto-ovo vegetarians). This simple categorization scheme broke down in the 1960s and 1970s as a result of greater exposure to the cuisines of other cultures, new Eastern religions and philosophical systems with a vegetarian tradition, and other influences, which led to the emergence of new patterns of vegetarianism.

Today, myriad vegetarian eating patterns exist, and they cannot be easily described by focusing on a single dimension, such as animal food intake.

Meatless and vegetarian eating patterns and life styles are growing in popularity today. They continue to be fostered by a greater availability and variety of meat alternatives and analogs for animal products. There is also a good deal of favorable publicity about phytochemicals with supposedly beneficial health effects. At the same time, concerns about the healthfulness of animal foods have been triggered by publicity on the bovine spongiform encephalopathy (BSE) epidemic in the UK, a later epidemic of hoof and mouth disease in cattle, and most recently an epidemic of SARS spread from animals to people. Worries about saturated fat/trans fat coronary artery disease links, dietary fat and cancers, food safety, and other factors probably also contributed to the increased prevalence of vegetarian eating.

At the same time, vegetarian eating patterns are much more heterogeneous today than in the past. The availability and variety of plant foods, as well as commercially available and tasty meat analogs has greatly increased. Fortified foods today include soy milks fortified with vitamins B_{12} and D and a highly bioavailable form of calcium, and highly fortified breakfast cereals. These foods and nutrient-containing dietary supplements make it easier for vegans and vegetarians to obtain nutrients that would otherwise be low or lacking.

Conformity to Nutritional Recommendations

Well-planned vegetarian diets have nutritional profiles that are in line with recent expert recommendations. A well-planned vegetarian diet pattern, if sustained throughout adulthood, may reduce risks of coronary artery and other chronic degenerative diseases associated with excessive weight. Generally, vegetarian diets tend to be low in saturated fat and cholesterol and high in complex carbohydrates, dietary fiber, magnesium, potassium, folic acid, and antioxidant nutrients such as vitamins C and E. They also tend to be relatively low in energy. Thus, the diet-related risks for a number of chronic degenerative diseases associated with intakes of these nutrients may be decreased on vegetarian diets. Some risks are clearly lower; for example, vegetarians generally tend to have lower weight for height than do nonvegetarians. Constipation tends to be less of a problem in this group, perhaps due in part to the higher intake of dietary fiber.

Conclusions

Vegetarian diets should be planned in accordance with expert nutritional recommendations. When this is followed, such diets are healthful and nutritionally adequate. When they are not planned, the nutrients that are likely to fall short usually differ somewhat from those on nonvegetarian diets. In some cases these deficits can be remedied by dietary counseling. In others differences between ideologies about diet and nutrient needs are such that acceptable dietary strategies cannot be found.

Nutrition scientists and practitioners can help vegetarians who seek their advice by monitoring the nutritional status of high-risk individuals, by identifying food sources of specific nutrients, and by suggesting dietary modifications that may be necessary to meet individual needs when intakes fall short.

See also: **Anemia**: Iron-Deficiency Anemia. **Phytochemicals**: Classification and Occurrence; Epidemiological Factors. **Supplementation**: Dietary Supplements.

Further Reading

Abrams HL (2000) Vegetarianism: another view. In: Kiple F and Connee K (eds.) *The Cambridge World History of Food*, pp. 1564–1573. Cambridge: Cambridge University Press.

American Dietetic Association and Dietitians of Canada (2003) Position of the American Dietetic Association and Dietitians of Canada: Vegetarian diets. *Canadian Journal of Diet Practice Research* **64**: 62–81.

Draper A, Lewis J, Malhotra N, and Wheeler E (1993) The energy and nutrient intakes of different types of vegetarian: a case for supplements? *British Journal of Nutrition* **70**: 812

Dwyer JT and Jacobs C (1988) Vegetarian children: appropriate and inappropriate diets. *American Journal of Clinical Nutrition* **48**: 811S–818S.

Engs R (2000) *Clean Living Movements: American Cycles of Health Reform*, pp. 1–20. Westport, CN: Praeger Publishers.

Fernandez-Armesto F (2002) *Near a Thousand Tables* New York: Free Press.

Haddad E (1994) Development of a vegetarian food guide. *American Journal of Clinical Nutrition* **59**: 1248S–1254S.

Havala S and Dwyer J (1994) Position of the American Dietetic Association: vegetarian diets. *Journal of the American Dietetic Association* **93**: 1317–1319.

Institute of Medicine (2000) *Dietary Reference Intakes: Applications in Dietary Assessment*. Washington DC: National Academy Press.

Key T, Davey G, and Appleby PN (1999) Health benefits of a vegetarian diet. *Proceedings of the Nutrition Society* **58**: 271–275.

Key T, Fraser GE, Thorogood M, Appleby PN, Beral V, Reeves G *et al.* (1998) Mortality in vegetarians and nonvegetarians: detailed findings from a collaborative analysis of 5 prospective studies. *American Journal of Clinical Nutrition* **70**: S516–S524.

Levenstein H (1993) *Paradox of Plenty: A Social History of Eating in Modern America* Oxford: Oxford University Press.

Mangels AR and Messina V (2001) Considerations in planning vegan diets: infants. *Journal of the American Dietetic Association* **101**: 670–677.

Messina V and Mangels AR (2001) Considerations in planning vegan diets: children. *Journal of the American Dietetic Association* **212**: 661–669.

Messina V and Mangels AR (2001) Considerations in planning vegan diets: children. *Journal of the American Dietetic Association* **101**: 661–669.

Messina V, Melina V, and Mangels AR (2003) A new food guide for North American Vegetarians. *Canadian Journal of Diet in Practice and Research* **64**: 82–86.

Obarzanek E, Sacks FM, Vollmer WM, Bray GA, Miller ER, Lin PH, Karanja NM, Most-Windhouser MM, Moore TJ, Swain JF, Bales CW, and Proschan MA on behalf of the DASH Research Group (2001) Effects on blood lipids of a blood pressure lowering diet: the Dietary Approaches to Stop Hypertension (DASH) Trial. *American Journal of Clinical Nutrition* **74**: 80–89.

Sanders T (1999) Essential fatty acid requirements of vegetarians in pregnancy, lactation and infancy. *American Journal of Clinical Nutrition* **70**: 555S–559S.

Van Dusseldorp M, Scheede J, Refsum H, Ueland PM, Thomas CMG, de Boer E, and Van Staveren WA (1999) Risk of persistent cobalamin deficiency in adolescents fed a macrobiotic diet in early life. *American Journal of Clinical Nutrition* **609**: 664–671.

Van Staveren W, Dhuyvetter JHM, Bons A, Zeelen M, and Hautvast JGAJ (1985) Food consumption and height/weight of Dutch preschool children on alternative diets. *Journal of the American Dietetic Association* **85**: 1579–1584.

Whorton J (2000) Vegetarianism. In: Kiple F and Connee K (eds.) *The Cambridge World History of Food*, pp. 1553–1565. Cambridge: Cambridge University Press.

VITAMIN A

Contents

Biochemistry and Physiological Role

J L Napoli, University of California, Berkeley, CA, USA

In 1913, E.V. McCollum isolated a yellow, fat-soluble substance from egg yolks that was critical for animal growth. He called it fat-soluble A, indicating the first isolated of several dietary microconstituents emerging as obligatory for vertebrate life and health. Later, fat-soluble A was renamed vitamin A, derived from the terminology 'vital amine,' coined by Casmir Funk to describe these obligatory micronutrients.

Currently, the term vitamin A refers to the specific organic compound all-*trans*-retinol (atROH). atROH, however, does not have biological activity in its own right. Rather, it serves as a circulating substrate for metabolism into the compounds that fulfill the biological functions attributed to vitamin A. These metabolites include, but may not be limited to, 11-*cis*-retinal (11cROH) and all-*trans*-retinoic acid (atRA). The term 'retinoids' describes all compounds that support vitamin A activity, both naturally occurring and synthetic, including atROH. **Figure 1** illustrates the structures of key carotenoids and retinoids.

Daily Recommended Dietary Allowance of Vitamin A

The Food and Nutrition Board of the Institute of Medicine revised the Recommended Dietary Allowance (RDA) of vitamin A in 2001 as 900 retinol activity equivalents (RAE) for men and 700 RAE for women. The RAE was introduced to avoid the ambiguity of international units (IU), which arises because 1 IU of vitamin A (0.3 µg) and 1 IU of the vitamin A precursor (provitamin A) all-*trans*-β-carotene (0.6 µg) do not have the same biological activity. Rather, 6 IU of β-carotene and 12 IU

of mixed carotenoids provide the biological activity of 1 IU of vitamin A. The RAE refers to the amounts necessary for the same degree of biological activity: 1 µg atROH = 12 µg β-carotene = 24 µg mixed carotenoids = 1 RAE.

Liver, dairy products, and saltwater fish, including herring, sardines, and tuna, serve as dietary sources of vitamin A and its esters. Cod and halibut liver oil provide especially rich sources of vitamin A, as does the liver of the polar bear, which benefits from occupying the top of the marine food chain. Carrots, yellow squash, corn, and dark-green leafy vegetables serve as dietary sources of provitamin A carotenoids. Because less than 10% of the 600 naturally occurring carotenoids generate vitamin A, vegetable color does not necessarily indicate vitamin A value. In the United States and Europe, retinol and its esters serve as the chief sources of dietary vitamin A, but elsewhere carotenoids serve as the primary source. According to the World Health Organization (WHO), the major inadequacies of dietary micronutrients involve vitamin A, iron, and iodine. Although vitamin A intake seems adequate in most populations in the United States, Canada, and Europe, this appears evolutionarily aberrant. The recurrent vitamin A-deficiency problem in Third World populations indicates that human diets in nonindustrialized countries are limited in vitamin A.

Vitamin A Status

atROH represents the quantitatively major circulating plasma retinoid in serum, but serum atROH does not reflect vitamin A status unless low (<0.35 µmol/l or 10 µg/dl) or unequivocally adequate (>1.1 µmol/l in children and >1.4 µmol/l in adults). Humans show a range of normal serum atROH values, with unknown factors contributing to the individual's normal value, and fever, infection, and/or inadequate intake of other nutrients (e.g., zinc and protein) can depress serum retinol. Liver reserves provide the most reliable measure of human vitamin A status. Noninvasive assessments of liver vitamin A reserves (the relative

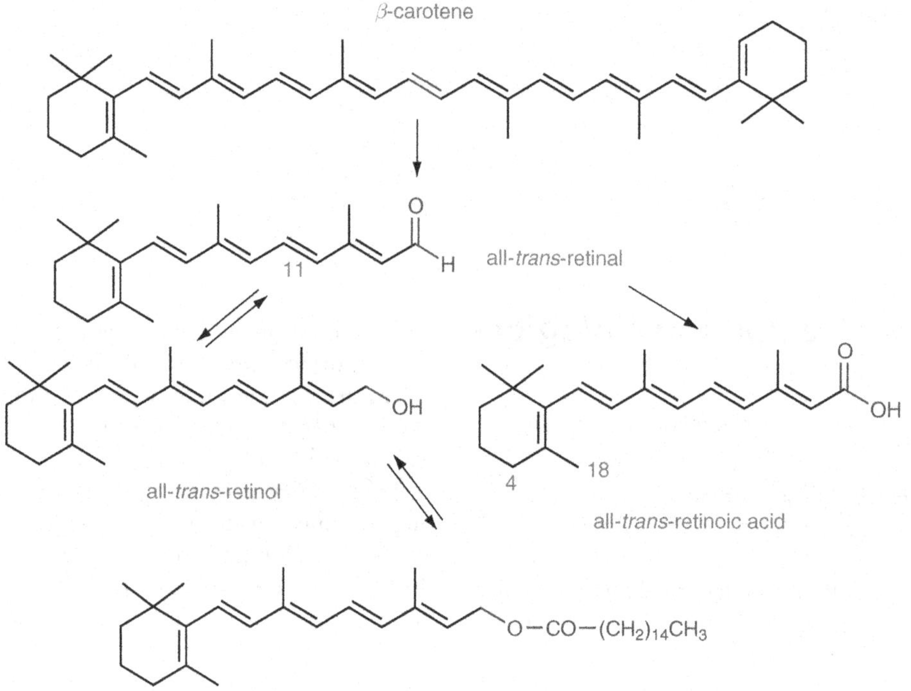

Figure 1 Structures of β-carotene and common endogenous retinoids. The numbers indicate the position of *trans* to *cis* isomerization of atRCHO (C11) and the positions of hydroxylation of atRA (C4 and C18).

dose–response and modified relative dose–response tests) measure the amount of dose in serum relative to the original plasma atROH after a small oral dose of marker vitamin A. The larger the proportion of dose that appears in serum, the lower the liver reserves.

Binding Proteins

Several high-affinity (low K_d), soluble binding proteins seem crucial to vitamin A homeostasis and/or function. Two are widely distributed throughout many tissues and cell types, whereas others have limited expression loci (**Table 1**). These binding proteins occur in all vertebrates, have highly conserved amino acid sequences among orthologs, and show high specificity for distinct retinoids. Where measured, their concentrations exceed the concentrations of their ligands. Indeed, CRBP(II) accounts for ~1% of the soluble intestinal enterocyte proteins. These qualities and experimental data indicate that retinoids exist *in vivo* bound to specific proteins. For example, purification of CRBP(I) from tissues produces predominantly holoprotein, despite the capacity of membranes to sequester more atROH than occurs physiologically and the time-consuming isolation techniques originally

used to isolate these proteins (including tissue homogenization, centrifugation, and several types of column chromatography). The locus of atROH at equilibrium would depend on both affinity for potential acceptors and acceptor capacity. Nature (*in vivo*) and the scientist (*in vitro*) provide plenty of opportunities for retinol to equilibrate between CRBP(I) and potential acceptors (membranes, lipid droplets, etc.). Evidently, the large capacity of membranes and other potential acceptors does not overcome the comparatively limited capacity of CRBP(I) to sequester retinol, consistent with tight binding.

CRBP (types I and II) and CRABP (types I and II) have molecular weights of ~15 kDa and belong to the intracellular lipid binding protein (iLBP) gene family, which includes the various fatty acid binding proteins. The family members have similar three-dimensional structures, despite low primary amino acid conservation among nonorthologous members. These proteins form globular but flattened structures of 10 antiparallel strands of β-sheets, 5 orthogonal to and above the other 5, referred to as a β-clam (**Figure 2**). The polar head group of atROH (i.e., the functional group that undergoes esterification or dehydrogenation) lies buried deep within CRBP, protected from the milieu of oxidants, nucleophiles, and enzymes.

Table 1 Examples of retinoid binding proteins

Retinoid binding protein	Ligand(s)	K_d (nM)	Adult distribution
CRBP (cellular retinol binding protein, type I)	atROH	~0.1	Nearly ubiquitous (low in intestine)
	atRCHO	10–50	
CRBP(II)	atROH	10–50	Intestine
	atRCHO	10–50	
CRABP (cellular retinoic acid binding protein, type I)	atRA	0.4	Widespread
CRABP(II)	atRA	2	Limited (e.g., skin, uterus, ovary)
CRALBP (cellular retinal binding protein)	11cROH	—	Eye, especially retinal pigment epithelium
	11cRCHO		
SRBP (serum retinol binding protein)	atROH	—	Serum

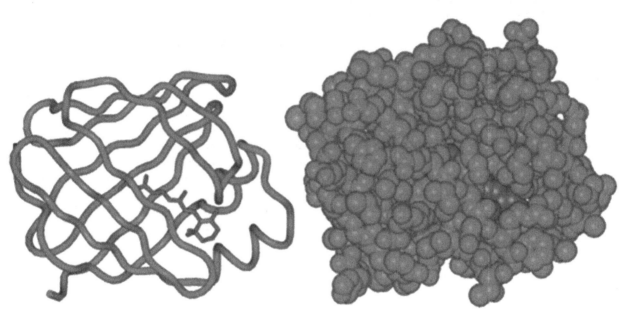

Figure 2 Ribbon (left) and space-filling (right) models of CRBP(I). (Courtesy of Marcia Newcomer (1995) Retinoid-binding proteins: Structural determinants important for function. *FASEB Journal* **9**: 229–239, Louisiana State University.)

CRBP(I) null mice are phenotypically normal until retinol depletion, but they eliminate retinol and its esters sixfold faster than wild-type mice, presumably through enhanced catabolism via enzymes that normally have limited access. In contrast, CRBP(II) null mice pups suffer 100% mortality by 24 h after birth when born to dams fed a vitamin A-marginal diet. Retinoid binding proteins apparently confer selective advantage to vertebrates by promoted sequestering, transport, and storage of vitamin A and limiting its catabolism. CRBP(III) has been detected in mouse heart and skeletal muscle, which express little or no CRBP(I) or CRBP(II), but not in other retinoid target tissues, such as liver, kidney, and brain. CRBP(III) seems to bind about equally well with atROH, 9cROH, and 13cROH (K_d ~80–110 nM). Humans express yet another CRBP, originally referred to as CRBP(III), but distinct from mouse

CRBP(III) and therefore really CRBP(IV). CRBP(IV) mRNA is much more abundant in human liver and intestine than CRBP(I) mRNA, but the mouse does not encode a complete CRBP(IV) gene. CRBP(IV) binds atROH with a K_d of ~60 nM but does not bind *cis*-isomers. The precise functions of CRBP(III) and CRBP(IV) have not been clarified: Presumably, they moderate retinol metabolism, similar to CRBP(I) and CRBP(II).

CRABP(I) and -(II) do not have well-defined physiological functions. Mice doubly null in CRABP(I) and -(II) have an approximately fourfold higher rate of death from unknown causes by 6 weeks after birth than wild-type mice, but the survivors appear essentially normal, with one exception. The doubly null mouse as well as the CRABP(II)-only null mouse respectively show 83 and 45% incidence of a small outgrowth anomaly on the postaxial side of digit five, predominantly in the forelimbs. The double mutants do not exhibit enhanced sensitivity to atRA, suggesting that CRABP do not serve primarily to protect against atRA toxicity or teratogenicity.

CRALBP (~36 kDa) belongs to a gene family that includes the α-tocopherol transfer protein (TTP). *In vitro*, CRALBP sequesters 11cROH in the retinal pigment epithelium (RPE) of the rods, driving forward the *trans* to *cis* isomerization, and also facilitates dehydrogenation of 11cROH into 11cRCHO. Mutations in human CRALBP cause night blindness and photoreceptor degeneration.

SRBP (~20 kDa) belongs to the lipocalin family, which includes apolipoprotein D, β-lactoglobulin, odorant binding protein, and androgen-dependent secretory protein. SRBP has a globular structure formed by eight antiparallel β-sheets in two orthogonal sheets that mold a β-barrel. The β-ionone ring of atROH lies deep within SRBP, whereas the hydroxyl group lies closest to the opening. atROH in serum remains bound with SRBP, despite high concentrations of a potential alternative high-capacity carrier, albumin. This illustrates the affinity of SRBP for atROH and the importance of sequestering retinoids within specific proteins. Liver is the major site of SRBP synthesis: Accordingly, liver expresses

SRBP mRNA most abundantly. Extrahepatic tissues, however, also express SRBP mRNA, including adipose and kidney, but the functions of SRBP produced extrahepatically remain unknown. Knocking out the SRBP gene produces a phenotypically normal mouse, except for impaired vision after weaning. Vision can be restored after months of feeding a vitamin A-adequate diet. Thus, the eye, which consumes (but does not store) the vast majority of vitamin A, normally relies on SRBP for retinol delivery. Retinol delivered by albumin and lipoproteins apparently supports the nonvisual functions of vitamin A, at least in the SRBP null mouse kept under laboratory conditions.

Vitamin A and the Visual Cycle

Figure 3 depicts a model of the functions of multiple proteins and forms of vitamin A that constitute the visual cycle. SRBP delivers atROH to the RPE, possibly through a plasma membrane SRBP receptor. No SRBP receptor has been isolated, however, and molecular characterization remains elusive. As in other tissues, CRBP(I) sequesters atROH and allows its esterification by the 25-kDa endoplasmic reticulum (ER) enzyme lecithin:retinol acyltransferase (LRAT). In fact, the amount of CRBP(I) may

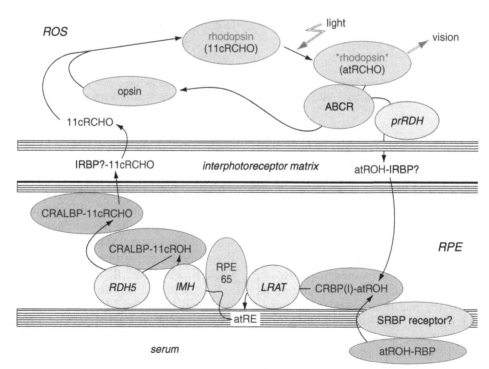

Figure 3 Model of the mammalian visual cycle. ABCR, ATP-binding cassette; atRCHO, all-*trans*-retinal; atROH, all-*trans*-retinol; atRE, all-*trans*-retinyl esters; 11cRCHO, 11-*cis*-retinal; 11cROH, 11-*cis*-retinol; CRALBP, cellular retinal binding protein; CRBP(I), cellular retinol binding protein, type I; IRBP, interphotoreceptor retinoid binding protein; IMH, isomerohydrolase; LRAT, lecithin:retinol acyltransferase; ROS, rod outer segment; RPE, retinal pigment epithelium; RPE65, RPE protein 65; SRBP, serum retinol binding protein.

represent the controlling event in the rate of atROH uptake, and uptake may be coupled to retinyl ester (RE) formation. RPE65, an ~65-kDa RPE protein, binds the highly hydrophobic atRE with a K_d of ~20 pM. This accelerates mobilization of atRE and delivery to the next step, isomerization by an isomerohydrolase (IMH). The RPE65 null mouse cannot produce 11-cis-retinoids, attesting to its importance in mobilizing atRE in the quantity and rate necessary to support the visual cycle. The IMH both hydrolyzes atRE and isomerizes the double bond at C11 to produce 11cROH. Unfortunately, little is known about the IMH: It has not been isolated or cloned. The cytosolic protein CRALBP sequesters 11cROH and also 11cRCHO produced by the ER enzyme 11-cis-retinol dehydrogenase (11cRDH), and it seems to enhance isomerization. The 11cRDH of the RPE belongs to the SDR (short-chain dehydrogenase/reductase) gene family: RDH4 and RDH5 encode the murine and human 11cRDH genes, respectively. 11cRDH also has been referred to as 9cRDH (9-cis-RDH) or cRDH, but the eye expresses 11cRDH mRNA far more intensely than other tissues, and more efficient potential 9cRDHs have been cloned and characterized, namely the SDR isozymes CRAD1 and -3 (cis-retinol/androgen dehydrogenase). Mutations in RDH5 cause the rare autosomal recessive disorder fundus albipunctatus, which is a form of night blindness characterized by delayed regeneration of photopigments in rods and cones. Enzymes in addition to RDH4/5 probably contribute to dehydrogenation of 11cROH in the RPE, which explains why the RDH5 mutation does not cause blindness.

Interphotoreceptor retinoid binding protein (IRBP) occupies the space between the RPE and the rod outer segment (ROS), the interphotoreceptor matrix, and binds both 11cROH and 11cRCHO. Retinoids do not require IRBP for transfer between the two membranes, however, because IRBP null mice show no gross abnormalities of the visual cycle, even though they have severe retinal abnormalities. Although retinoids have very limited solubility in the aqueous phase, membranes of the RPE and ROS transfer retinoids between them in the absence of IRBP.

In the ROS, 11cRCHO forms a Schiff's base adduct with a lysine residue in the protein opsin to create rhodopsin. Light isomerizes the 11cRCHO of rhodopsin into atRCHO. The isomerization straightens the retinoid side chain, changing the conformation of rhodopsin. This conformation change initiates a nerve impulse through G proteins and releases atRCHO, regenerating opsin. An ATP transporter ABCR facilitates leaching of atRCHO

from rhodopsin, and an ER enzyme, prRDH (photoreceptor retinol dehydrogenase), also an SDR, reduces atRCHO into atROH. atROH cycles back to the RPE and binds with CRBP(I).

Vitamin A Homeostasis and Activation into atRA

Intestinal absorptive cells absorb dietary carotenoids and retinol during the bile–acid-mediated process of lipid absorption. Within the enterocyte, central cleavage by a soluble 63-kDa carotene 15,15′-monooxygenase catalyzes the principal route of carotenoid metabolism (**Figure 4**). Carotene 15,15′-monooxygenase belongs to the same gene family as RPE65 (the mouse proteins have only 37% amino acid identity, however), suggesting a family of proteins/enzymes dedicated to transport/metabolism of highly hydrophobic substances. Intestine expresses the carotene 15,15′-monooxygenase mRNA, but kidney and liver show much more intense expression, and the testis curiously shows most intense expression, consistent with the ability of tissues other than the intestine to cleave carotenoids. Carotene 15,15′-monooxygenase also metabolizes carotenoids without provitamin A activity, such as lycopene, although with lower efficiency.

CRBP(II) sequesters atRCHO generated from carotenoids and allows its reduction into atROH, catalyzed by an ER retinal reductase (uncharacterized). In contrast to CRBP(I), CRBP(II) does not allow oxidation/dehydrogenation of its ligands. LRAT accesses the CRBP(II)–atROH complex and produces atRE for incorporation into chylomicrons. During conversion into remnants by lipoprotein lipase in adipose, chylomicrons retain most of their RE, as they do cholesterol esters.

Hepatocytes sequester RE and cholesteryl esters by receptor-mediated endocytosis of chylomicron remnants. Substantial RE hydrolysis apparently occurs before engulfing of the remnants by lysosomes. CRBP(I) sequesters the atROH released and allows esterification by LRAT but protects from esterification via other acyltransferases, just like CRBP(II) functions in the intestine. Ultimately, liver stellate cells accumulate most of the RE. CRBP(I) seems necessary for retinoid transfer from hepatocytes to stellate cells because the CRBP(I) null mouse does not accumulate RE in stellate cells. The mechanism of transfer, however, has not been established.

Liver senses local and extrahepatic need for atRA biosynthesis by an unknown signal (possibly atRA) and need for atROH in the visual cycle, and it responds by mobilizing RE to maintain serum

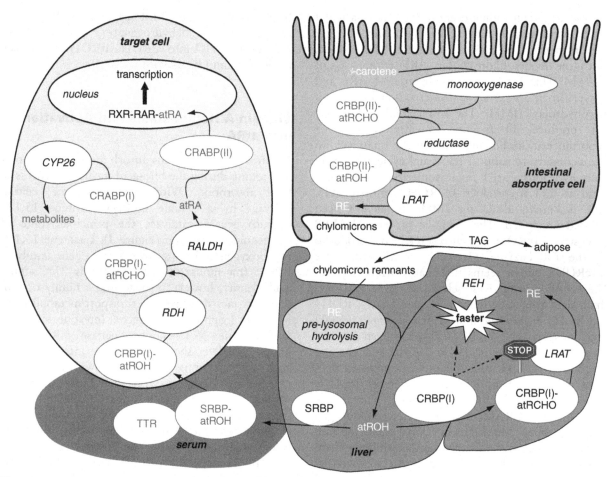

Figure 4 Model of atRA biogeneration in mammals. REH, retinyl ester hydrolase (e.g., ES4 and ES10); TTR, transthyretin; RAR-RXR, the heterodimer of retinoic acid receptors with retinoid X receptors; atRCHO, all-*trans*-retinal; atROH, all-*trans*-retinol; CRBP(I), cellular retinol binding protein, type I; LRAT, lecithin:retinol acyltransferase; SRBP, serum retinol binding protein. CRBP(I), CRABP(I), and CRABP(II) have been placed in the same cell for simplicity. This does not necessarily occur *in vivo*.

retinol levels. ES-10 and ES-4, two neutral ER-localized, bile salt-independent carboxyesterases, provide at least 94% of the RE hydrolysis activity in liver. Kidney also expresses ES-4, and kidney, testis, lung, and skin express ES-10. Either SRBP or CRBP(I) sequesters the atROH released. SRBP delivers atROH to serum, whereas CRBP(I), unlike CRBP(II), allows dehydrogenation into atRCHO to support atRA biosynthesis. (**Figure 4** shows atRA biogeneration only in target cells, but it also occurs in liver; likewise, RE storage also occurs in target cells in animals exposed to higher dietary atROH, suggesting that the liver does not initially sequester all dietary retinoids.) What keeps the CRBP(I)-bound atROH from undergoing futile cycling back to atRE? Apo-CRBP(I) stimulates endogenous microsomal RE hydrolysis and inhibits LRAT (**Figure 5**). Note that apo-CRBP(I) exerts potent effects at concentrations of ~2.5 µM—well within the range of the CRBP(I) expressed in liver. Thus,

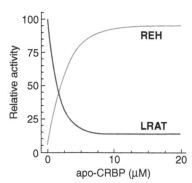

Figure 5 The effect of apo-CRBP(I) on the rates of retinol esterification (lecithin:retinol acyltransferase (LRAT)) and retinyl ester hydrolysis (REH).

the ratio apo-CRBP/holo-CRBP signals atROH status and directs atROH flux into or out of atRE.

SRBP–atROH circulates as a complex with transthyretin (TTR) that protects it from degradation.

The mechanism of atROH delivery from SRBP into cells has not been established. Some data suggest a specific SRBP membrane receptor, whereas other data indicate that CRBP(I) pulls atROH transfer from SRBP through the membrane. A third hypothesis is that an SRBP receptor is mainly in the eye, the quantitatively major site of atROH consumption.

Extrahepatic cell atROH supports atRA biosynthesis but also undergoes esterification if delivered in sufficient quantities. CRBP(I) allows dehydrogenation of atROH by an ~35-kDa ER retinol dehydrogenase (RDH) but protects atROH from dehydrogenation via other dehydrogenases. RDH (*Rdh1*) belongs to the SDR gene family. The SDR gene family consists of ~50 mammalian members that catalyze intermediary metabolism, and the metabolism of steroids and prostaglandins, in addition to retinoids.

The mechanism of atROH transfer from CRBP(I) or -(II) to RDH and LRAT has not been elucidated. Specific cross-linking of holo-CRBP(I) with both RDH1 and LRAT, however, indicates close proximity of CRBP(I) to the two enzymes. Notably, apo-CRBP(I) at concentrations of $1 \mu M$ prevents cytosolic dehydrogenation of atROH, even by soluble enzymes that access the CRBP(I)–atROH complex, while not impacting ER SDR until reaching much higher concentrations. This suggests the importance of membrane RDH, rather than soluble dehydrogenases, to atRA biosynthesis. Obviously, atRA biosynthesis *in vivo* occurs in the absence of CRBP(I), as indicated by lack of morphological pathology in the CRBP(I) null mouse. This was predicted by *in vitro* experiments that showed that neither RDH nor LRAT require presentation of atROH by CRBP(I). Rather, CRBP(I) operates as a molecular chaperone that restricts metabolism to enzymes that can access its atROH.

In the early 1950s, cytosolic alcohol dehydrogenases (ADHs) were suggested to metabolize atROH. This was an attempt to explain atRCHO generation and the controversial and poorly understood putative occurrence (at the time) of atRA in tissues, when other families of dehydrogenases remained anonymous. ADHs do recognize atROH *in vitro*, albeit only when presented free of CRBP(I) and with comparatively low efficiencies. However, enzymes have poor substrate discrimination *in vitro* and do not metabolize many of the same substrates *in vivo* because of intracellular constraints. Mice null in both ADH class I (*Adh1*) and ADH class IV (*Adh4*) show no vitamin A-deficiency phenotype, nor do mice null in ADH class III (*Adh3*). *Adh1* null mice show a decreased rate of metabolism of 50–100 mg/kg atROH, but this demonstrates only

that extraordinary high exposure can defeat physiological controls imposed by retinoid binding proteins. Vitamin A excess has not been a problem throughout evolution (mice do not usually eat polar bear or marine fish liver): No pressure forced evolution of protective mechanisms against such exposure. Natural selection exerted the opposite pressure (i.e., evolution of retinoid binding proteins to conserve vitamin A).

Retinal dehydrogenases (RALDHs) catalyze the irreversible conversion of atRCHO into atRA and can do so in the presence of CRBP(I) using atRCHO generated *in situ* from CRBP(I)–atROH and RDH. These ~54-kDa soluble enzymes belong to the ADLH gene family. RALDH1 (*Aldh1a1*), -2 (*Aldh1a2*), and -3 (*Aldh1a3*) contribute most to atRA generation, whereas RALDH4 has much more efficient activity with 9-*cis*-retinal. The RALDH1 null mouse remains fertile and healthy but may have decreased ability to produce atRA in the liver. The RALDH2 null mouse dies *in utero* by midgestation, demonstrating its unique contribution to atRA synthesis during embryogenesis. The situation may differ in the adult. RALDH1–3 show overlapping expression patterns in the adult, with RALDH1 expressed most intensely. Interestingly, atRA regulates mRNA levels of RALDH1 differently in different tissues. For example, vitamin A sufficiency increases kidney and liver RALDH1 mRNA, whereas vitamin A insufficiency increases testis RALDH1 mRNA. This may represent a mechanism to divert atROH from liver to testis for atRA production during vitamin A scarcity.

Other Active Retinoids

Discrete loci synthesize 3,4-didehydro-atRA, such as skin. 3,4-Didehydro-atRA binds RAR with high affinity, similar to atRA. The purpose of creating a signaling molecule that functions similar to atRA in specialized loci, which also biosynthesize atRA, has not been clarified.

Although 9-*cis*-RA was reported as a hormone *in vivo*, at best, its concentrations are much lower than atRA. Its putative function as a physiological ligand that controls RXR is controversial.

atRA Catabolism

atRA induces its own metabolism via cytochrome P450 (CYP) into a variety of initial catabolites, including 5,6-epoxy-atRA, 18-hydroxy-atRA, and 4-hydroxy-atRA. Metabolism of atRA limits its activity; conversely, inhibitors of atRA metabolism enhance atRA potency. CYP26A1 may catalyze the major degree of atRA catabolism, as evidenced by null mice dying in mid- to late gestation with serious morphological defects. Two other P450's, CYP26B1 and CYP26C1, also catabolize atRA, but null mice have not been reported. Several other CYPs reportedly catabolize atRA, but these candidates (CYP1A1/2, CYP2A6, CYP2C8/9, CYP2E1, and CYPP3A4/5) are not induced by atRA—in contrast to the well-established ability of atRA to induce its own metabolism as well as CYP26A1 transcription—and most have inefficient kinetics *in vitro* with atRA.

Presenting atRA to microsomes bound with CRABP(I) enhances kinetic efficiency of catabolism sevenfold. There seems to be little doubt that CRABP(I) sequesters atRA: Delivering the sequestered atRA for efficient catabolism seems to be a logical mechanism to discharge the ligand without releasing it back into the cell. Unfortunately, this insight does not reveal the primary purpose for CRABP(I) impounding atRA in the first place.

Regulation of Retinoid Homeostasis

atRA regulates retinoid homeostasis. It induces LRAT transcription ~100-fold and induces CRBP(I) transcription. These may be housekeeping functions that maintain retinol esterification and handling during vitamin A sufficiency. On the other hand, induction of CYP26A1 by atRA can be viewed both as a general mechanism of clearance and as a site-specific mechanism to maintain an environment during specific stages of development.

Several xenobiotics, including ethanol and polychlorinated biphenyls, reduce RE stores, possibly through enhancing atRA catabolism by inducing CYP. In addition, clofibrate, a ligand of PPARα (peroxisome proliferator activated receptor), causes a remarkably rapid depletion of liver retinoids and decreases TTR mRNA fourfold. In contrast, PPARγ, expressed in liver stellate cells among others, induces transcription of carotene 15,15′-monooxygenase. PPARγ also induces expression of CRBP(I), CRBP(II), LRAT, and RARβ. These actions of PPARα and -γ with retinoids reflect their effects on lipid metabolism: PPARα enhances fatty acid catabolism, whereas PPARγ enhances adipogenesis and fatty acid storage.

Mechanism of atRA Action

atRA induces transcription by binding with three ligand-activated transcription factors, RARs (retinoic acid receptors) α, β, and γ, each encoded by a distinct member of the nuclear hormone receptor gene superfamily. RARs function *in vivo* bound with three additional distinct members of the nuclear receptor gene family: RXR (retinoid X receptor) α, β, and γ. Forty-eight RXR–RAR combinations can occur because each receptor gene can express two to four protein isoforms, stemming from differential promoter use and alternative splicing. RXR in complex with RA acts 'silently' (i.e., it can function sans ligand). The RXR–RAR heterodimer recognizes several types of RARE (atRA response elements). The two most common consist of two direct repeats of (A/G)G(G/T)TCA separated by two (DR2) or five (DR5) nucleotides. This multiplicity of heterodimers and response elements suggests a mechanism for the pleiotropic functions of vitamin A.

atRA binding with RAR induces the receptor to convert from an open form to a more structured form that wraps the ligand. This conformation change leads to remodeling of coregulators bound to the RXR–RAR complex. Remodeling releases a complex array of co-corepressors and recruits a complex array of coactivators, accompanied by chromatin remodeling, histone acetylation, and recruitment of basal transcription factors, including TATA binding protein and RNA polymerase II. More than 500 genes have been reported as transcriptionally regulated by atRA either directly by this process or indirectly through events set into motion by this process.

RXR's influence extends beyond serving as an obligatory partner of RAR. RXR forms heterodimers with ~11 nuclear receptors, including the vitamin D receptor PPAR and the thyroid hormone receptors. 'The' RXR ligand, if not 9cRA, would have significant signaling impact.

CRABP(II), but not CRABP(I), delivers atRA to RAR and thereby induces transcription. The limited expression loci of CRABP(II), however, suggest that this action would be specialized rather than general.

Physiological Functions of atRA

All vertebrates require retinal for the visual cycle and atRA to support the systemic functions of vitamin A, including controlling the differentiation programs of epithelia cells and cells in nerve and bone and also the immune and reproductive systems. atRA frequently, but not always, induces terminal differentiation. atRA also regulates expression of genes in differentiated cells and genes crucial to spermatogenesis, hematopoiesis, estrus, placental development, embryogenesis, and apoptosis. atRA may also serve as a tumor suppressor.

The many RAR knockouts illustrate the physiological functions of vitamin A. Disruption of the RARα gene, the RAR with the most widespread, if not ubiquitous, expression in the embryo and adult, does not cause embryonic lethality but reduces the homozygous null population by 60% within 12–24 h after birth and by 90% within 2 months. The RARα null mice that survive 4 or 5 months have severe germinal epithelium degeneration and are sterile. RARβ gene null mice are fertile and viable and show no immediate signs of morphological abnormalities. Nevertheless, complementary data show that RARβ may mediate the antiproliferative function of atRA and as such may serve as a tumor suppressor. Moreover, RARβ null mice have virtually no hippocampal long-term potentiation or long-term depression, the forms of synaptic plasticity that provide a mechanism of short-term spatial learning and memory. This phenomenon can be reproduced by vitamin A depletion. RARγ null mice have an 86% incidence of skeletal abnormalities by embryonic day 18.5 but are born in Mendelian frequency. Postnatally, the homozygous null pups show retarded rates of growth, limiting them to 40–80% of the weight of wild-type pups. By 1–3 weeks old, 50% of RARγ null mice die; by 3 months, 80% die. Mature males also have squamous metaplasia of the seminal vesicles and prostate glands, similar to vitamin A deficiency, but other epithelia appear normal. These data reveal that even though RAR tend to express in site specific patterns in normal circumstances, they also exhibit a great degree of functional redundancy, enabling a mouse null in one receptor to (partially) compensate for the other two.

Numerous studies have correlated vitamin A insufficiency in laboratory animals with increased incidence of spontaneous and carcinogen-induced cancer. Chemopreventive trials in humans show some promise for retinoids in actinic keratoses, oral premalignant lesions, laryngeal leukoplakia, and cervical dysplasia. The US Food and Drug Administration has approved retinoids for acute promyelocytic leukemia and for non-life-threatening diseases, such as cystic acne and psoriasis. Retinoids also provide the active ingredients in agents to treat sun/age-damaged skin.

WHO recognizes vitamin A deficiency as a mortality factor for childhood measles. Two large doses (60,000 RAE each) of a water-soluble vitamin A formulation given to children on each of 2 days decrease the risk of death from measles 81% in areas of prevalent vitamin A deficiency.

See also: **Fish**.

Further Reading

Ahuja HS, Szanto A, Nagy L, and Davies PJ (2003) The retinoid X receptor and its ligands: Versatile regulators of metabolic function, cell differentiation and cell death. *Journal of Biological Regulatory and Homeostatic Agents* 17: 29–45.

Aranda A and Pascual A (2001) Nuclear hormone receptors and gene expression. *Physiological Reviews* 81: 1269–1304.

Blomhoff R, Green MH, Green JB, Berg T, and Norum KR (1991) Vitamin A metabolism: New perspectives on absorption, transport, and storage. *Physiological Reviews* 71: 951–990.

Harrison EH (1998) Lipases and carboxyesterases: Possible roles in the hepatic metabolism of retinol. *Annual Reviews of Nutrition* 18: 259–276.

Maden M (2001) Role of retinoic acid in embryonic and post-embryonic development. *Proceedings of the Nutrition Society* 59: 65–73.

Mark M, Ghyselinck NB, Wendling O *et al.* (1999) A genetic dissection of the retinoid signaling pathway in the mouse. *Proceedings of the Nutrition Society* 58: 609–613.

Napoli JL (2000) Retinoic acid: Its biosynthesis and metabolism. *Progress in Nucleic Acids Research* 63: 139–188.

Newcomer ME (1995) Retinoid-binding proteins: Structural determinants important for function. *FASEB Journal* 9: 229–239.

Olson JA (1994) Needs and sources of carotenoids and vitamin A. *Nutrition Reviews* 52: S67–S73.

Saari JC (2000) Biochemistry of visual pigment regeneration: The Friedenwald lecture. *Investigative Ophthalmology and Visual Science* 41: 337–348.

Stephensen CB (2001) Vitamin A, infection, and immune function. *Annual Reviews of Nutrition* 21: 167–192.

Sun SY and Lotan R (2002) Retinoids and their receptors in cancer development and chemoprevention. *Critical Reviews in Oncology and Hematology* 41: 41–55.

Wolf G (1984) Multiple functions of vitamin A. *Physiological Reviews* 64: 873–937.

Deficiency and Interventions

K P West Jr, Johns Hopkins University, Baltimore, MD, USA

Vitamin A (VA) deficiency is the leading cause of pediatric blindness, increases risk of severe infection, and is an underlying cause of child mortality in many developing countries. Night blindness, the mildest ocular manifestation of VA deficiency, has been recognized since antiquity, with the condition depicted in bas-relief on the Egyptian pyramid in Sakura, dating to the Middle Kingdom, and Hippocrates in the fourth century BC recognizing and treating the condition with animal liver. Corneal destruction and consequent blindness, as well as milder conjunctival lesions of xerophthalmia, were linked to dietary insufficiency in the eighteenth and nineteenth centuries, with cod liver oil emerging as recommended treatment for the various conditions of night blindness, Bitot's spots, and corneal necrosis (keratomalacia) more than a century ago. Discovery in the early twentieth century of 'fat-soluble A,' an ether-soluble factor in butter and egg yolk critical for sustaining growth, health, and vision in animals, accelerated recognition and treatment of xerophthalmia in children as well as decades of subsequent research that led to the synthesis of vitamin A and its analogues, an understanding of the vitamin's roles in the visual cycle, and discovery of the vitamin's involvement in maintaining epithelial, immune, hematopoietic, and osteoid function and multiple facets of human health.

Vitamin A Deficiency Disorders

Vitamin A is essential for maintaining normal retinal function and differentiation of rapidly dividing, bipotential cells. These regulatory roles give rise to specific manifestations of hypovitaminosis A, such as poor photoreceptor function leading to night blindness, metaplasia, and keratinization of mucosal epithelial surfaces leading to clinical abnormalities of conjunctival and corneal xerosis as well as epidermoid metaplasia and other epithelial defects throughout the respiratory, genitourinary, and gastrointestinal tracts and glandular ducts. Deficiency can also impair development or functioning of multiple arms of the immune system that can weaken host defenses against infection. Collectively, all pathophysiological consequences attributed in varying degrees to VA depletion are termed 'vitamin A deficiency disorders (VADD) (**Figure 1**).

Biochemical Depletion

Tissue depletion of vitamin A, although not a disorder per se, precedes the functional consequences of deficiency. In uncomplicated hypovitaminosis A, plasma retinol tends to be homoeostatically controlled until body (primarily liver) stores are low, after which plasma concentration declines. Plasma retinol may also decline during states of chronic inflammation and clinically significant infection, in parallel with raised circulating concentrations of acute phase proteins, likely reflecting increased tissue delivery, reduced hepatic mobilization via retinol binding protein, and increased urinary loss of vitamin A. Plasma retinol gradually normalizes during recovery from infection if there are adequate hepatic stores of the vitamin. If not, infection can

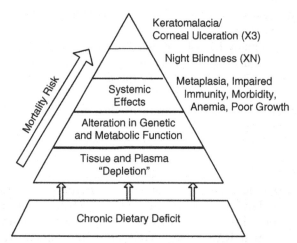

Figure 1 Concept of vitamin A deficiency disorders (VADD), due primarily to underlying chronic dietary deficit in preformed vitamin A and provitamin A carotenoids. From West KP Jr (2002) Extent of vitamin A deficiency among preschool children and women of reproductive age. *Journal of Nutrition* **132**: 2857S–2866S.

leave the host more tissue depleted and at risk. Despite nondietary influences, plasma or serum retinol measurement remains the most common biochemical index of vitamin A status. Vitamin A deficiency is generally diagnosed at a serum retinol concentration below a cutoff of 0.70 μmol/l (20 μg/dl), below which 20 to >50% of concentrations occur in a VA-deficient population compared to <3% of well-nourished societies. A serum retinol concentration of <0.35 μmol/l is indicative of severe deficiency. Decrements in serum retinol concentration below these cutoffs are associated with marked increases in risk of xerophthalmia and infection. Other indices of tissue retinol depletion include the relative dose–response, a before–after test dose difference in serum retinol that indirectly reflects hepatic retinol adequacy, breast milk retinol concentration for assessing both maternal status and intake adequacy of breast-fed infants, stable isotopic dilution to assess the total body vitamin A pool, impression cytology that detects early or mild metaplasia on the bulbar conjunctiva, and clinical stages of xerophthalmia.

Xerophthalmia

Conjunctival and corneal epithelium deprived of vitamin A undergoes keratinizing metaplasia. Columnar epithelial cells become squamous and mucus-producing goblet cells disappear, providing the histopathologic mechanisms for deficiency-induced xerotic (drying) changes to the ocular surfaces. VA deficiency is also required for rod vision in dim light. VA deficiency-induced night blindness often occurs with histopathologic changes on the ocular surface.

Table 1 WHO and IVACG classification and minimum prevalence criteria for xerophthalmia and vitamin A deficiency as a public health problem

Definition (code)	Minimum prevalence (%)	Highest risk period
Children 1–5 years of age		
Night blindness (XN)	1.0	2–6 years
Conjunctival xerosis (X1A)	—	—
Bitot's spots (X1B)	0.5	2–6 years
Cornea xerosis (X2)/corneal ulceration (X3A)/keratomalacia (X3B)	0.01	1–3 years
Xerophthalmic corneal scar (XS)	0.05	>1 year
Deficient serum retinol (<0.70 µmol/l)	15.0	<6 months; 1–5 years
Pregnant/lactating women		
Night blindness (XN) during most recent pregnancy	5.0	3rd trimester
Low serum retinol (<1.05 µmol/l)	20.0	

Adapted from Sommer A and Davidson FR (2002) Assessment and control of vitamin A deficiency: The Annecy Accords. *Journal of Nutrition*. **132**: 28455–28505.

Thus, night blindness and clinical eye signs are both listed under one xerophthalmia classification scheme (**Table 1**).

Night blindness Vitamin A, as retinaldehyde, is an essential cofactor in the generation of rhodopsin. This is a photosensitive pigment in rod photoreceptors of the retina that responds to light (it is 'bleached') by releasing vitamin A and initiating neural impulses to the brain that permit vision under conditions of low illumination. The utilization and recycling of vitamin A in this process is known as the 'visual cycle.' Hypovitaminosis A restricts rhodopsin production, which in turn raises the scotopic (low light) visual threshold. Gradually, a perceptive threshold is reached that leads to recognition of night blindness (XN), the earliest symptom of xerophthalmia. It is marked by an inability to move about in the dark. Children between 1 and 5 years of age and pregnant women appear to be at greatest risk of XN. Where endemic, there is often a local term for XN that translates into 'evening' or 'twilight' blindness or 'chicken eyes' (lacking rod cells, chickens cannot see at night), making the condition readily detectable by history. Typically, gestational night blindness resolves spontaneously with child birth and expulsion of the placenta, likely relieving maternal metabolic demands for vitamin A.

Conjunctival xerosis and Bitot's spots Early xerosis of the conjunctiva can be detected subclinically by filter paper impression cytology, showing distorted, enlarged, and noncontiguous sheaths of epithelial cells and the disappearance of goblet cells. In advanced vitamin A deficiency, xerosis appears clinically as a dry, unwetable surface of the bulbar conjunctiva (X1A). The affected areas are usually overlaid with superficial white, cheesy, or foamy patches of triangular or oval shape that consist of desquamated keratin and bacteria (often the xerosis bacillus). These are known as Bitot's spots (X1B). They are nearly always bilateral, found temporal (and, in more advanced cases, also nasal) to the corneal limbus, and more reliably diagnosed than X1A. Bitot's spots are not blinding but are reflective of chronic moderate to severe systemic depletion of vitamin A.

Corneal xerophthalmia Corneal xerophthalmia is manifested in increasingly severe stages. The earliest corneal lesions appear as superficial punctate defects, evident with a slit lamp, that with advanced deficiency become more numerous and concentrated. The cornea is considered xerotic (X2) when punctate keratopathy covers large areas of the surface, rendering a hazy, nonwetable, lusterless, and irregular appearance on handlight examination. Stromal edema may be present. In more severe cases, thick, elevated xerotic plaques may form. Usually, both eyes are affected. Corneal ulcers (X3A) can be sharply demarcated, round or oval defects that are usually shallow but may also perforate the cornea. Healed ulcers form a leukoma (scar) or adherent leukoma if the iris has plugged the perforated ulcer. Most ulcers occur peripheral to the visual axis and thus may not threaten central vision if treated promptly. Keratomalacia (X3B) refers to a full-thickness softening and necrosis of the corneal stroma that can cause protruding, opaque, yellow to gray lesions to form (**Figure 2**). These tend to collapse or slough off, leaving a descemetocele following VA treatment. Keratomalacia usually impairs vision in the involved eye, although the degree of visual loss depends on the location, thickness, and extent of corneal necrosis and resultant scar. Due to the generally malnourished and ill state of children with corneal xerophthalmia, the mortality rate of hospitalized cases is 4–25%.

Other VADD

Infection A bidirectional relationship exists between hypovitaminosis A and infection, each exacerbating the other, representing a classic 'vicious cycle.' Thus, infection may be considered both a cause of VA deficiency and, in terms of severity and sequelae, a 'disorder' as well. Cross-sectionally, xerophthalmia

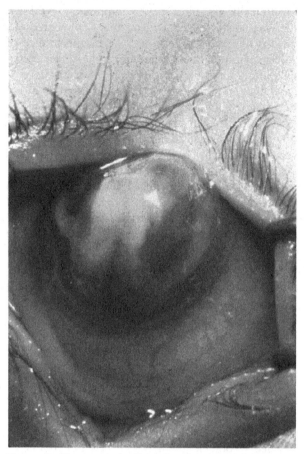

Figure 2 Keratomalacia. From Sommer A (1995) Vitamin A deficiency and its consequences. A Field Guild to detection and control. 3rd ed. Geneva, WHO.

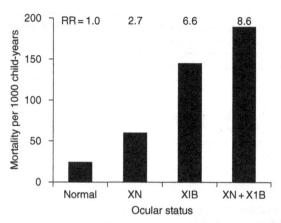

Figure 3 Risk of mortality among ~3500 Indonesian preschool children by ocular status at the outset of each 3-month interval. RR, relative risk of mortality. Adapted from Sommer A *et al.* (1983) Increased mortality in children with mild vitamin A deficiency. *Lancet* **2**: 585–588.

or severe hyporetinolemia has been consistently associated with higher frequencies of diarrhea, fever, and other infections, although directionality is difficult to parse from such evidence.

VA deficiency raises the risk of infection presumably due to compromised 'barrier' epithelial function and impaired innate, cell-mediated, and humoral immune mechanisms. VA-deficient Southeast Asian preschoolers (i.e., with mild xerophthalmia) were twice as likely to develop acute respiratory infection and (in Indonesia) three times more likely to develop diarrhea over subsequent 3- to 6-month periods. Deficient children are also more likely to die. This was so among Indonesian preschool children, whose risk of mortality increased with increased severity of mild eye signs (**Figure 3**). In Nepal, siblings of patients were more likely to develop the eye lesions but were also at a twofold higher risk of dying than children living in unaffected households, reflecting a clustering of child mortality risk within VA-deficient households.

Data from children and animals support the plausibility of these findings. VA-deficient children show increased bacterial adherence to respiratory epithelium, low lymphocyte counts and T helper to cytotoxic/suppressor cell ratios, and a weaker delayed-type hypersensitivity response compared to nonxerophthalmic children. In animals, VA deficiency produces keratinizing metaplasia of epithelial linings that may affect 'barrier' defenses. It also compromises acquired immunity, indicated by lymphoid atrophy, reduced numbers of circulating lymphocytes, impaired blast transformation responses to antigen, T cell-dependent antibody responses, and natural killer cell activity, and a greatly increased risk of infection and death.

Anemia and Poor Growth Children with xerophthalmia and night blind mothers tend to be anemic relative to peers without eye disease. VA-supplemented trials often show improvement in indicators of iron status, including reductions in anemia. Mechanisms involved in this interaction are not clear but may involve enhanced iron absorption, storage, and transport as well as direct effects on hematopoiesis in the presence of adequate iron stores.

VA deficiency decelerates growth in animals and has been associated with both stunting and wasting malnutrition in children, possibly reflecting roles for the vitamin in osteogenesis and protein metabolism. Trials, however, have shown inconsistent effects of VA supplementation on child growth, possibly due to variations in the extent of infection, seasonality in dietary protein and energy adequacy, exclusion criteria, and levels of VA status among study children. It appears that VA supplementation can influence ponderal and linear growth, as well as body composition, in children for whom VA deficiency is a 'growth limiting' nutritional deficit.

Epidemiology

The epidemiology of VA deficiency provides a basis for quantifying its extent and health consequences; describing its demographic patterns, geocultural context, and dietary causes; and with which to target interventions for treatment and prophylaxis. It is mostly understood in relation to hyporetinolemia and xerophthalmia (**Table 1**), especially the noncorneal stages involving night blindness and Bitot's spots due to conjunctival xerosis. The latter eye signs are common, specific, and likely to exhibit risks relevant to more widespread hypovitaminosis A. Importantly, although both conditions represent 'mild' non-blinding xerophthalmia, they typically occur in moderate to severe systemic VA deficiency.

Magnitude

Current estimates suggest that VA deficiency (serum retinol <0.70 μmol/l) afflicts 25% or 127 million preschool-aged children in the developing world, of whom 4–5 million have xerophthalmia. The number of potentially blinding corneal cases occurring annually is less well-known but, based on historic data, efficacy of VA interventions, and successes in controlling precipitating factors (such as measles), it is likely to be ~250,000 cases globally per year. The geographic distribution of VA deficiency, based on joint distributions of preschool xerophthalmia and hyporetinolemia, is presented in **Figure 4**. However, increasing evidence shows that VA deficiency extends beyond the preschool years. For example, in Southeast Asia, >80 million children 5–15 years of age are thought to be hyporetinolemic, 9 million of whom have mild xerophthalmia. The burden of preadolescent school-aged VA deficiency in Africa and Latin America remains unestimated due to lack of population data. Adult VA deficiency is

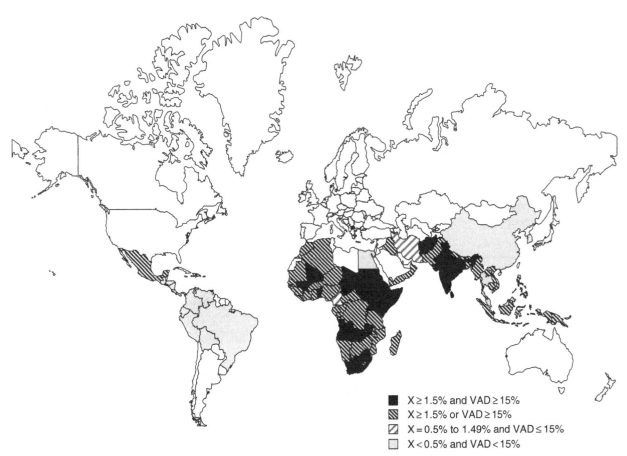

Figure 4 Global geographic distribution of xerophthalmia (X, all clinical stages) and vitamin A deficiency (VAD, serum retinol concentrations <0.70 μmol/l) in preschool-aged children. From West KP Jr (2002) Extent of vitamin A deficiency among children and women of reproductive age. *Journal of Nutrition.*

most notable in women living in undernourished conditions during and after pregnancy. Globally, approximately 20 million pregnant women have low vitamin A status (serum retinol concentration <1.05 μmol/l), of whom 7 million are thought to be deficient (serum retinol <0.70 μmol/l) and 6 million night blind, typically in the latter half of pregnancy. Regions of the world at greatest risk of VA deficiency are Southeast Asia and sub-Saharan Africa, where ~45 and 30% of all affected children and pregnant women reside, respectively.

High-Risk Groups

Preschool children and women during and following pregnancy are at highest risk for developing vitamin A deficiency and suffering its consequences. Infants in most poor populations are born with low VA status, which may predispose them to risk of blinding keratomalacia at <6 months of age. Without adequate VA from breast milk and complementary foods, VA stores can remain low to deficient throughout the first year of life and beyond. Risk of potentially blinding corneal xerophthalmia (**Figure 2**) peaks in the second through fourth years of life, typically following epidemics of acute infection such as severe measles, which can exacerbate a chronically wasted and vitamin A-deficient state. Milder stages of xerophthalmia, night blindness and Bitot's spots typically affect 1–5% of young children, with prevalence increasing from ~1 year of age through, in some cultures, the school-aged years. Boys tend to have higher rates of mild xerophthalmia than girls, possibly reflecting differences in dietary practices. In traditional societies, the increase follows weaning of children from VA-containing breast milk to a household diet chronically lacking preformed vitamin A or its carotenoid precursors.

VA deficiency persists through adolescence and into adulthood, as indicated by frequent reports of low serum retinol level (<0.70 μmol/l) in ~25% and night blindness in 5–20% of pregnant or lactating women in endemically deficient areas. Deficiency presumably results from heightened nutritional demand from late gestation through lactation superimposed on a chronic, poor dietary intake and preexisting low VA status of women. Although rarely blinding, maternal night blindness can identify high-risk women in populations in which it is associated with hyporetinolemia, anemia, wasting malnutrition, increased infant mortality, and markedly increased risks of maternal morbidity and mortality (**Figure 5**). In recent years, widespread maternal VA deficiency has been observed to coexist with HIV infection and AIDS throughout sub-Saharan Africa. However, modest, absent, or inconsistent effects of maternal VA supplementation on infant and maternal health, survival, or rates of transmission in trials suggest that VA deficiency may be more a consequence than a determinant of HIV-induced disease severity.

Geographic Clustering

Patterns of childhood hyporetinolemia or abnormal impression cytology plus xerophthalmia define the geographic risk of VA deficiency as a periequatorial nutritional problem throughout the world (**Figure 4**). Within regions, VA deficiency tends to cluster in parallel with indices of underdevelopment, low availability of food sources of vitamin A, and disease patterns. In a large study in Aceh, Indonesia, villages in which cases of xerophthalmia were detected tended to be poorer than xerophthalmia-free communities and, within a village, cases arose more frequently from households of low socioeconomic standing than did children with normal eyes (controls) (**Table 2**). Also, in multiple

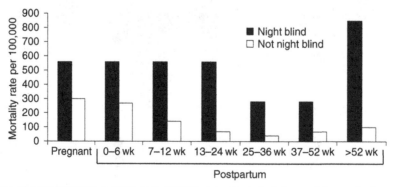

Figure 5 Mortality rates of rural Nepalese women (per 100,000 pregnancies) during and for up to 2 years following pregnancy according to whether mothers experienced night blindness (*n* = 361) or not (*n* = 3052) during pregnancy. From Christian P *et al.* (2000) Night blindness during pregnancy and subsequent mortality among women in Nepal: Effects of vitamin A and B-carotene supplementation. *American Journal of Epidemiology.*

Table 2 Household characteristics of xerophthalmia cases, controls, and the remaining Aceh study population

Household characteristic	Cases (%) (N = 466)	Village-matched controls (%) (N = 466)	Aceh study households (%) (N = 15,915)
Unprotected water source	47.5	43.8	41.1[a]
No private latrine	86.7	83.6	71.3[a]
Bamboo house walls	47.1	33.5	31.6[a]
Household head farms	57.3	55.5	53.4
Mother has <6 years of education	94.3	86.6	80.3[a]
History of child death	12.1	9.7	7.5[a]

[a]Significant linear trend in proportions ($p < 0.001$).
Adapted from Mele L et al. (1991) Nutritional and household risk factors for xerophthalmia in Aceh, Indonesia: A case-control study. American Journal of Clinical Nutrition **53**: 1460–1465.

surveys in Africa and Asia, preschool children incur an approximately twofold higher risk of having or developing xerophthalmia in villages in which at least one other child has been diagnosed compared to villages in which xerophthalmia has not been previously seen (**Table 3**). More striking is a 7- to 13-fold higher risk of xerophthalmia in siblings of cases compared to children in homes with no previous history of xerophthalmia. Maternal night blindness and childhood xerophthalmia tend to coexist at both household and community levels, reflecting the chronicity of dietary inadequacy in undernourished communities. Spatial clustering of deficiency risk seems to arise mostly from shared dietary practices in homes and villages rather than other exposures that lead to common infections. The exception to this observation is likely to be in households and communities afflicted by HIV/AIDS.

Periodicity

The occurrence of xerophthalmia can follow predictable, although not parallel, seasonal patterns in different areas of the world. Typically, a seasonal peak in VA deficiency emerges from a convergence of causal risk factors. In Southeast Asia, for example, a distinct peak in the incidence of mild xerophthalmia occurs during the late dry and early monsoon seasons (April–July). This peak follows a postharvest growth spurt in the cool dry season. It also coincides with a general scarcity of pro-vitamin A-rich vegetables and fruits and a seasonal increase in the incidence of diarrhea, respiratory infection, and measles. In this area of the world, the seasonal peak is often curbed abruptly midway through the 'mango season,' reflecting a likely impact of widespread consumption of this β-carotene-rich fruit. Periodicity, where it exists, can help identify causes and target prevention to specific times of the year.

Causes

Breast-feeding and diet Dietary risk in children refers to inadequate breast-feeding combined with low intakes of VA-rich foods from the household diet. A low dietary fat intake (e.g., $\leq 5\%$ of calories) may restrict absorption of pro-vitamin A carotenoids from vegetables and fruits and thus also predispose children to deficiency.

Breast milk is the most important initial dietary source of vitamin A for an infant. Commonly, breast milk from marginally nourished mothers in developing countries contains $\sim 500 \mu g$ of retinol activity equivalents (RAE) per liter, delivering $325 \mu g$ RAE per day to infants consuming a typical intake of ~ 650 ml per day. In the absence of a recommended dietary allowance for vitamin A, an 'adequate intake' of $400-500 \mu g$ RAE has been set as a guide for infants in their first year, making infant VA intakes from breast milk marginal and, beyond infancy, marginally above an estimated deficient threshold thereafter (i.e., $210 \mu g$ RAE). Decrements

Table 3 Age-adjusted village and household odds ratios for risk of xerophthalmia among preschool children[a]

	Malawi		Zambia		Indonesia		Nepal	
	n	OR[b]	n	OR	n	OR	n	OR
Village	50	1.2 (1.0–1.5)[c]	110	1.7 (0.9–3.2)	460	1.8 (1.4–2.2)	40	2.3 (1.6–3.4)
Household	2899	7.3 (3.2–16.7)	2449	7.9 (3.5–17.8)	16,337	10.5 (7.0–15.7)	2909	13.2 (6.0–29.0)

[a]Numbers of children <6 years of age in each country: Malawi, $n = 5441$; Zambia, $n = 4316$; Indonesia, $n = 28,586$; and Nepal, $n = 4764$.
[b]Pairwise odds ratio based on alternating logistic regression.
[c]95% confidence intervals in parentheses.
Adapted from Katz J et al. (1993) Clustering of xerophthalmia within households and villages. International Journal of Epidemiology **22**: 709–715.

in intake or concentration below this minimum increasingly place breast-fed children at risk, with greatest risk for those fully weaned and lacking a nutritious home diet. Studies in Asia and Africa show that breast-fed infants and toddlers are 65–90% less likely to have or develop xerophthalmia than non-breast-fed peers of the same age. Xerophthalmic children have been shown to begin weaning earlier (by ~1 month) and to be weaned ~6 months earlier than nonxerophthalmic children. Even when breast-fed, the more frequent the daily feeds, the greater the reduction in risk of xerophthalmia, reflecting the potential benefit achieved by promoting breast-feeding. However, the nutritional margin is still evident in the protective effects of vitamin A in reducing mortality in late infancy and early childhood, even where breast-feeding is ubiquitous for the first 2 or 3 years of life.

Complementary feeding affects childhood risk of VA deficiency. Indonesian preschoolers were at a two- to sixfold higher risk of xerophthalmia if food sources of vitamin A, such as dark green leaves, mango or papaya, egg, meat or fish with liver, and milk and other dairy products, were not routinely given during the first year of complementary feeding, instilling a pattern that may place children at risk throughout their first several years of life. Across undernourished regions of the world, studies reveal less frequent dietary intakes of foods rich in preformed vitamin A and carotenoid precursors by preschool-aged children with a history of xerophthalmia than children who remain free from the eye disease (**Figure 6**). Similar dietary differences are evident among women with versus those without a history of maternal night blindness.

Infection As noted previously, a vicious cycle exists between VA deficiency and infection; thus, infection

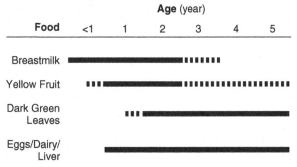

Figure 6 Foods that protect against hypovitaminosis A (xerophthalmia), based on numerous studies. Dark line, strong evidence; dashed line, suggestive evidence. From Sommer A and West KP Jr (1996) Vitamin A Deficiency: Health, Survival and Vision. New York: Oxford University Press.

can be viewed as a cause of deficiency. Prospective studies show that severe infections, such as measles, chicken pox, diarrhea, and acute respiratory illness, decrease serum as well as apparent hepatic levels of retinol and increase the risk of xerophthalmia. In some settings, measles has been observed to increase the risk of children developing corneal xerophthalmia by >13-fold. In Indonesia, young children with diarrhea and acute respiratory infections were also twice as likely to develop mild xerophthalmia (XN or X1B) than apparently disease-free children. Similar patterns have been observed in undernourished populations of women, whereby maternal infection early in gestation raises the risk of becoming night blind later in pregnancy. Explanations for a role of infection as a cause of VA deficiency include decreased absorption of vitamin A, increased metabolic requirements, impaired retinol transport, greatly increased renal excretion during the acute phase response, and slow normalization of these mechanisms coupled with a chronically decreased dietary VA intake during extended recovery or repeated illness.

Impact of Interventions

VA deficiency can be prevented through direct supplementation, fortification of commonly eaten food items, or other food-based interventions that include home gardening, nutrition education, and agronomic approaches. Most evaluations have assessed the impact of direct supplementation and, occasionally, fortification on vitamin A status, xerophthalmia, survival, and other health outcomes. Data on the efficacy of dietary regimens are limited to change in vitamin A status.

Vitamin A Status

The impact of vitamin A prophylaxis on status varies by indicator, dosage and mode of delivery of the supplement, level of initial deficiency, and other risk factors. A single, high-potency supplement (210 μmol, 60 mg retinol activity equivalents or 200,000 IU) has been shown to elevate serum retinol in deficiency-prone populations for periods of 1–6 months, with most data suggesting protection from hyporetinolemia for only a few months. Continuous intake of 50–100% of the recommended allowance of vitamin A through fortified foods gradually improves and sustains adequate serum and breast milk retinol concentrations or, when assessed by indirect means, hepatic retinol adequacy. Regular consumption of pro-vitamin A food sources (dark green leaves and yellow vegetables and fruits) has variable, although generally positive, effects on vitamin A status. Dietary carotenoid intake appears most efficacious in raising serum retinol from deficient concentrations to minimally adequate levels in children and women but often fails to optimize vitamin A status. Variations in food matrix, methods of storage and preparation, amounts of preformed vitamin A and fat in the diet, gut integrity and function, protein energy and VA status of the host, and other factors may affect dietary efficacy. Among these, food matrix factors may be most important in determining bioavailability of pro-vitamin A carotenoid for uptake, conversion, and absorption. The belief has long been held that β-carotene, the most ubiquitous provitamin A carotenoid in the diet, can be converted from dietary sources to vitamin A in the body at a ratio of 6:1, but it is now recognized that conversion is far less efficient, conservatively set at 12:1 and 24:1 for other pro-vitamin A carotenoids (e.g., α-carotene and β-cryptoxanthin) for a mixed vegetarian diet. The change effectively reduces by half previous estimates of vitamin A activity in the developing world's nonanimal food supply and begins to address persistent questions of how VA deficiency can coexist amid at least a seasonal abundance of vegetables and fruits.

Xerophthalmia

Practically any intervention that delivers adequate amounts of VA will control VA deficiency. High-potency vitamin A delivered to preschool children every 4–6 months is ~90% efficacious in preventing both corneal and noncorneal xerophthalmia. Prophylactic failure (~10%) may reflect inadequacy of dosage for some children who are severely VA deficient or become ill. Xerophthalmia, on the other hand, virtually disappears in child populations consuming adequate amounts of vitamin A-fortified foods. There is less experience with regard to preventing night blindness in women, other than in large trials that suggest supplementation at recommended dietary levels may be insufficient to prevent all xerophthalmia, depending on background severity. Supervised dietary treatment has been reported to cure or improve noncorneal xerophthalmia; however, population trials to assess the impact of dietary change in preventing xerophthalmia have yet to be carried out.

Mortality

There has been extensive investigation into the effects of VA on mortality during the past two decades in preschool-aged children and, more recently, in young infants and women of reproductive age. The impact of vitamin A supplementation on preschool child mortality has been firmly established through eight controlled community trials performed in the 1980s and early 1990s involving ~160,000 children on three subcontinents (**Table 4**). In six trials, children 6 months to 6 years of age were supplemented every 4–6 months with an oral dose of vitamin A containing 60 mg retinol equivalents (RE) (or 200,000 IU). Half this dosage was provided to children <12 months of age. One study, in India, provided a small weekly dose to children and the other, in Indonesia, supplied half of a recommended allowance of vitamin A to children in treatment villages through a routinely marketed fortified mono-sodium glutamate product (a meal flavor enhancer). Rates of mortality in supplemented groups were compared to rates among children in concurrent control groups. Six of the eight trials showed reductions of 19–54% in preschool child mortality beyond either 6 or 12 months of age. Meta-analyses of data from these trials have estimated the reduction in mortality to range from 23 to 34%, with the latter value likely applicable to Southeast Asia. The estimates are remarkably consistent given differences in study designs and analytic approaches. Cumulative mortality curves from trials with positive results show a characteristic departure in mortality experience from control groups soon after initiation of vitamin A supplementation (**Figure 7**). Notably, the largest mortality impacts occurred in the two trials that mimicked a normal dietary intake of vitamin A compared to its periodic delivery as a bolus. Investigations of illnesses and events prior to death suggest that vitamin A reduced mortality associated with measles, diarrhea, and acute wasting malnutrition. A lack of apparent impact on mortality attributable to acute respiratory infection has been a perplexing, although consistent, finding across these and other trials. In contrast, administration of vitamin A, in the community prior to measles epidemics or on hospital admission as treatment for severe measles infection, has been shown to lower case fatality by ~50%.

High-potency VA (50,000–100,000 IU) may also substantially reduce early infant mortality, but this appears to depend almost entirely on the timing or age of supplement receipt. That is, in several trials involving infants of various ages through 6 months, during 4- to 6-monthly community dosing, or at the times of DPT vaccinations (typically at 6, 10, and 14 weeks of age), little or no effect in reducing mortality has been shown. However, two trials to date, in Indonesia and India, have reported 64 and 22% reductions, respectively, in mortality for infants <6 months of age when they were dosed at or soon after birth with 45,000–50,000 IU of VA (**Table 4**). In the trial reported from India, the effect was restricted to low-birth-weight infants (<2500 g), suggesting an impact on growth-restricted or preterm newborns. Explanations include plausible maturational effects

Table 4 Vitamin A mortality prevention trials

Location/target group	Vitamin A dosage[a]	N	% change[b]
Infants <1 month			
Bandung Indonesia	15 mg RAE at birth	2067	↓64*
Madurai, India	7.2 mg RAE at birth	11,619[c]	↓22*
Sarlahi, Nepal	15 mg RAE ~1–3 weeks of age	1621	↑7
Infants 1–5 months			
Sarlahi, Nepal	30 mg RAE	4617	↑4
Jumla, Nepal	15 mg RAE	1058	↑1
Infants <6 months			
Sarlahi, Nepal	7 mg RAE/week to mothers	15,987	↑4
Children 6–72 months			
Aceh, Indonesia	60 mg RAE/6 months	29,236	↓34*
West Java, Indonesia	0.81 mg RAE/day	11,220	↓46*
Tamil Nadu, India	2.5 mg RAE/week	15,419	↓54*
Hyderabad, India	60 mg RAE/6 months	15,775	↓6
Sarlahi, Nepal	60 mg RAE/4 months	28,640	↓30*
Jumla, Nepal	60 mg RAE/5 months	7197	↓29*
Khartoum, Sudan	60 mg RE/6 months	29,615	↑6
Northern Ghana	60 mg RE/4 months	21,906	↓19*
Pregnant/lactating women			
Sarlahi, Nepal	7 mg RAE/week	22,189[d]	↓44

[a]RAE, Retinol activity equivalents; trials providing 60 mg RE gave a half dose to infants <12 months.
[b]Percentage change in mortality rate among vitamin A recipients compared to controls of similar age or lifestage for all trials.
[c]Child-years of observation.
[d]Number of pregnancies.
*Indicates statistically significant differences (p < 0.05).
From Sommer and West (1996) Vitamin A Deficiency: Health, Survival and Vision. New York: Oxford University Press and West (2003) Vitamin A Deficiency Disorders in Children and Women Food and Nutrition Bulletin. **24**: S78–S90.

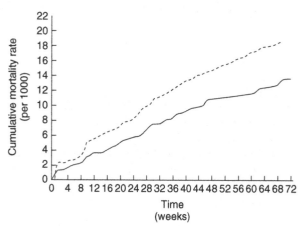

Figure 7 Cumulative mortality of children randomized to 4-monthly placebo control (dashed line) versus 200,000 IU of vitamin A (solid line) during a large community trial in Sarlahi District, rural Nepal. From Sommer A and West KP Jr (1996) Vitamin A Deficiency: Health, Survival and Vision. New York: Oxford University Press.

on an immature immune system, gut, and airway that may enhance resistance to infection months later. Additional confirmatory trials are under way in Southeast Asia and sub-Saharan Africa.

Finally, improving intake of VA, either preformed or as pro-vitamin A β-carotene in amounts approximating a recommended dietary intake, may reduce the risk of pregnancy-related death where maternal mortality is high and deficiency evident by widespread night blindness during pregnancy. In rural Nepal, supplementing women with VA lowered mortality related to pregnancy from 704 to 385 deaths per 100,000 pregnancies (44%), likely due to less severe infection, eclampsia, anemia, and possibly other obstetric causes. Malnourished women (e.g., those with night blindness) may likely benefit most from supplemental VA intake. Additional trials addressing this question are under way in Bangladesh and Ghana.

Morbidity

Direct effects of VA on morbidity have been difficult to establish, possibly due to variation in disease sensitivity to VA and inherent problems in measuring the incidence, duration, and severity of morbidity in community studies. Vitamin A interventions exert modest, if any, impact on the prevalence of common childhood morbidities typically obtained by history. In contrast, VA appears to reduce the severity of potentially fatal infections, such as measles, persistent diarrhea, dysentery, and falciparum malaria, especially in the presence of wasting malnutrition. The protective effect becomes stronger with episode severity. Thus, febrile illnesses appear to be more responsive to vitamin A than nonfebrile events. Illnesses for which care is sought show a response to VA. In a large trial in Ghana, VA supplementation decreased childhood clinic visits for illness (RR = 0.88), hospitalization rates for severe disease (RR = 0.62), and severity of illness among children admitted for diarrhea compared to placebo recipients. In Brazil, prior VA receipt had no effect on children's diarrheal episodes of 1 or 2 days' duration (RR = 0.97) but was increasingly protective against episodes lasting ≥3 days with four or more stools per day (RR = 0.91) and episodes of ≥3 days with five or more stools per day (RR = 0.80). Vitamin A treatment of measles has led to fewer and less severe complications and enhanced immunologic and clinical recovery. However, multiple treatment trials report little effect of vitamin A on recovery from childhood pneumonia. This remains a paradox given decades of experimental animal evidence linking VA deficiency to extensive metaplasia and keratinization and, presumably, greater susceptibility to pathogen invasion and infection of the respiratory tract.

Management

Treatment

Children with xerophthalmia and measles should be treated immediately with oral, high-potency vitamin A (200,000 IU) according to WHO and IVACG guidelines (**Table 5**) and provided other supportive nutritional and medical therapy as indicated. Corneal lesions should be topically treated with a suitable antibiotic (e.g., tetracycline or chloramphenicol) to prevent bacterial infection. Corneal xerophthalmia typically improves with VA treatment within 1 week, with complete resolution within 4 weeks,

depending on the size, thickness, and location of the lesion and nutritional and health status of the patient. Night blindness is typically cured within 24 h of VA treatment. Most Bitot's spots begin to respond within 2–5 days and disappear within 2 weeks, although some may persist, particularly in older children. High-potency vitamin A is indicated for women of reproductive age with corneal disease. For milder lesions, smaller daily (10,000 IU) or weekly (25,000 IU) doses are recommended for at least 3 months. Children presenting with severe wasting malnutrition should be given a single large oral dose (200,000 IU). It is also judicious to give cases of severe diarrhea, dysentery, respiratory infection, and exanthematous infections the same single, large oral dose of vitamin A.

Prevention

Hypovitaminosis A is prevented by increasing intakes of preformed vitamin A or pro-vitamin A carotenoids to levels that maintain adequate status. This can be done through direct supplementation of targeted risk groups, food fortification, or a number of dietary approaches that protect breast-feeding and improve the quality of the home diet.

Administration of high-potency, oral vitamin A (200,000 IU), adjusted for age (**Table 5**), on a 4- to 6-monthly basis is a common preventive approach in many developing countries. Half a dose is dispensed to infants 6–11 months and a quarter dose is given to younger infants to minimize risk of toxicity in high-risk areas. The intervention is based on the principle that a large dose of vitamin A is stored primarily in the liver, from where it is mobilized as needed. Beyond treatment, supplements can be provided during routine health care (e.g., for growth monitoring, immunization, other extension services) or more extensively and systematically in targeted populations on a regular basis (e.g., semiannual or every 4 months). Scaling up semiannual delivery of high-

Table 5 Vitamin A treatment and prevention schedules

Age	Treatment at diagnosis[a]	Prevention	
		Dosage (IU)	Frequency
<6 months	50,000 IU	50,000	With each of 3 doses of DPT/polio vaccine
6–11 months	100,000 IU	100,000	Every 4–6 months
12–59 months	200,000 IU	200,000	Every 4–6 months
Women	By severity of eye signs[b]	200,000	2 doses 24 h apart ≤6 weeks after delivery

[a]Treat all cases of xerophthalmia and measles on days 1 and 2; give an additional dose for xerophthalmia on day 14. For severe malnutrition give one dose on day 1.
[b]For women of reproductive age, give 200,000 IU only for corneal xerophthalmia on days 1, 2 and 14; for night blindness or Bitot's spots, give 10,000 IU per day or 25,000 IU per week for ≥3 months.
Based on Ross D (2002) Recommendations for vitamin A Supplementation. *Journal of Nutrition* **131**: 2902S–2906S.

potency VA through national campaigns, such as National Immunization Days, and other mechanisms that have routinely achieved 80% or greater coverage has probably been decisive in reducing preventable, VA deficiency-induced child deaths annually from an estimated 1.7 million in 1991 to approximately 0.7 million in 2002. With accelerated immunization nearing completion, momentum established for periodic VA delivery has, in many countries, been transferred to campaigns such as National Child Health Days that, in early reports, are achieving comparable rates of coverage. Nearly four decades of distributing billions of high-potency VA supplements for population prophylaxis attests to the acceptance, effectiveness, and safety of this approach. However, it is essential to adequately inform the health and lay communities of potential benefits and risks, the latter including a 2–4% rate of (mild and self-limiting) bulging fontanel in young infants and ~5% rate of nausea, vomiting, irritability, or diarrhea following high-potency VA receipt.

Providing mothers two sequential doses of 200,000 IU each as soon after birth as possible, but always within 6 weeks to avoid excessive risk of periconceptional exposure, is a safe and effective way to improve vitamin A status of mothers and their breast-fed infants. Otherwise, supplements of up to 10,000 IU per day or 25,000 IU per week offer safe prophylactic regimens to women against VA deficiency during reproductive years.

Increasingly, developing countries are fortifying staple food items with a quarter to a full day's recommended allowance of VA to prevent deficiency in high-risk populations. Potential food vehicles should be technically fortifiable at required concentrations and consumed within a range that may be both effective in target groups and safe in the entire population. Fortification has been effectively carried out on a scaled-up basis with a limited number of products in a limited number of countries, including nonfat milk powder and vegetable oils in food assistance programs and sugar in Central America. Other food carriers have been successfully demonstrated, including monosodium glutamate (flavor enhancer) in Indonesia and the Philippines, nonrefrigerated margarine and wheat flour in the Philippines, and a powdered beverage in Tanzania. Additional foods are being fortified with VA each year. This trend will likely continue with increased use of processed foods and as the food industry becomes engaged in solving VA and other micronutrient deficiency problems.

Dietary diversification is widely held to be the most culturally appropriate and potentially sustainable approach to preventing VA deficiency. Although pilot trials show efficacy of a variety of dietary approaches for improving VA intake and status, data on the effectiveness and cost of population food-based interventions are generally lacking. Dietary intakes can be improved through home and school gardening initiatives, nutrition education, and social marketing of locally available food sources of vitamin A. However, effective dietary change requires a thorough understanding of local cultural, food system, and behavioral factors that increase the risk of VA deficiency.

See also: **Anemia**: Iron-Deficiency Anemia.

Further Reading

Beaton GH, Martorell R, Aronson KJ et al. (1993) *Effectiveness of Vitamin A Supplementation in the Control of Young Child Morbidity and Mortality in Developing Countries*, ACC/SCN State of the Art Series Nutrition Policy Discussion Paper No. 13. Geneva: World Health Organization.

Christian P, West KP Jr, Khatry SK et al. (1998) Night blindness of pregnancy in rural Nepal—Nutritional and health risks. *International Journal of Epidemiology* 27: 231–237.

Christian P, West KP Jr, Khatry SK et al. (2000) Night blindness during pregnancy and subsequent mortality among women in Nepal: Effects of vitamin A and β-carotene supplementation. *American Journal of Epidemiology* 152: 542–547.

De Benoist B, Martines J, and Goodman T (eds.) (2001) Special issue on vitamin A supplementation and the control of vitamin A deficiency. *Food and Nutrition Bulletin Supplement* 22(3): 213–340.

Gillespie S and Mason J (1994) *Controlling Vitamin A Deficiency. A Report Based on the ACC/SCN Consultative Group Meeting on Strategies for the Control of Vitamin A Deficiency*. Geneva: United Nations Administrative Committee on Coordination, Subcommittee on Nutrition.

Institute of Medicine (2001) Vitamin A. In *Dietary Reference Intakes*, pp. 82–161. Washington, DC: National Academy of Medicine.

Sommer A (1995) *Vitamin A Deficiency and Its Consequences: A Field Guide to Detection and Control*, 3rd edn. Geneva: World Health Organization.

Sommer A and West KP Jr (1996) *Vitamin A Deficiency: Health, Survival and Vision*. New York: Oxford University Press.

West KP Jr (2003) Public health impact of preventing vitamin A deficiency in the first six months of life. In: Delange FM and West KP Jr (eds.) *Micronutrient Deficiencies in the First Months of Life*, Nestle Nutrition Workshop Series Pediatric Program, vol. 52, pp. 103–127. Vevey/Basel: Nestec/Karger.

West KP Jr and Sommer A (1987) *Delivery of Oral Doses of Vitamin A to Prevent Vitamin A Deficiency and Nutritional Blindness. A State-of-the-Art Review*, Nutrition Policy Discussion Paper No. 2. Rome: United Nations Administrative Committee on Coordination, Subcommittee on Nutrition.

WHO/UNICEF/IVACG (1997) *Vitamin A Supplements: A Guide to Their Use in the Treatment and Prevention of Vitamin A Deficiency and Xerophthalmia*, 2nd edn. Geneva: World Health Organization.

Physiology

A C Ross, The Pennsylvania State University, University Park, PA, USA

Introduction

Vitamin A is a fat-soluble micronutrient that is required by all vertebrates to maintain vision, epithelial tissues, immune functions, reproduction, and for life itself. It was discovered in 1913 as a minor component in eggs, butter, whole milk, and fish liver oils. It soon became apparent that vitamin A exists in two chemically distinct yet structurally related forms. The first form to be characterized was retinol, a lipid alcohol that is present only in foods of animal origin. Retinol is also known as 'preformed vitamin A' because it can be metabolized directly into compounds that exert the biological effects of vitamin A. A second form of vitamin A, present in deep-yellow vegetables, was characterized as β-carotene, which is synthesized only by plants but can be converted to retinol during absorption in the small intestines. These carotenoids are sometimes referred to as 'provitamin A.' The nutritional requirement for vitamin A can be met by preformed retinol, provitamin A carotenoids, or a mixture, and therefore it is possible to obtain a sufficient intake of vitamin A from carnivorous, herbivorous, or omnivorous diets.

Neither retinol nor the provitamin A carotenoids are directly bioactive. Retinol must be activated in a series of oxidative reactions, while the provitamin A carotenoids must first be cleaved to produce retinol. Of numerous metabolites of vitamin A, two are well recognized as crucial to its physiological functions. 11-*cis*-retinaldehyde (retinal) is a component of the visual pigment required for vision, rhodopsin. Retinoic acid, an acidic derivative, is required for the regulation of gene expression in essentially all tissues.

Besides the natural forms of vitamin A, a large number of structurally related analogs of vitamin A have been synthesized as potential therapeutic agents. The term 'retinoid' applies to both natural dietary forms of vitamin A, its metabolites, and those synthetic analogs that possess some, but usually not all, of the biological activities of vitamin A.

Chemistry

Vitamin A and its metabolites comprise a group of more than a dozen molecules that differ in isomeric form, oxidation state, and whether they are unesterified (free), esterified with a fatty acid, or conjugated.

All-*trans*-Retinol (Vitamin A Alcohol)

Retinol, the parent molecule of the vitamin A family, is a fat-soluble lipid alcohol ($C_{20}H_{30}0$, molecular mass 286.4) composed of a methyl substituted cyclohexenyl (β-ionone) ring, an 11-carbon conjugated tetraene side chain, and a terminal hydroxyl group (**Figure 1A, R_1**). Most of the double bonds can exist in either *trans* or *cis* conformation. All-*trans*-retinol is the most stable and most prevalent form in foods and tissues, but small amounts of other geometric isomers such as 9-*cis*- and 13-*cis*-retinol are found in some cells. The terminal hydroxyl group of retinol can be free or esterified with a

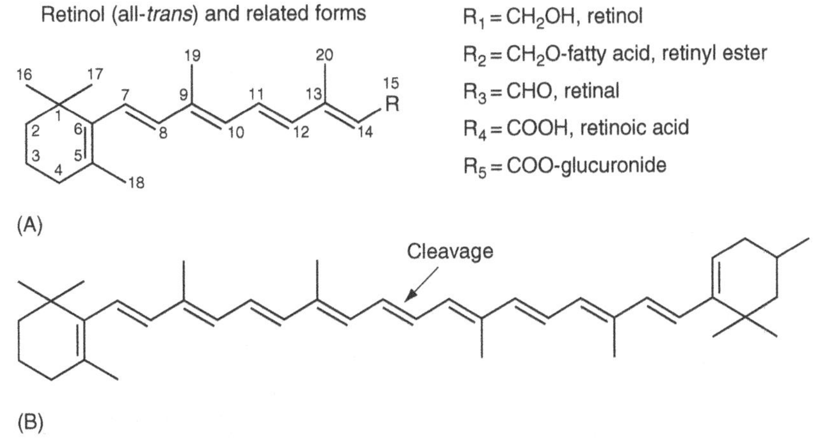

Retinol (all-*trans*) and related forms

$R_1 = CH_2OH$, retinol

$R_2 = CH_2O$-fatty acid, retinyl ester

$R_3 = CHO$, retinal

$R_4 = COOH$, retinoic acid

$R_5 = COO$-glucuronide

Figure 1 (A) Structure of all-*trans*-retinol and several related forms. (B) Beta-carotene (all-*trans*) showing the position of 15,15′ double bond that through cleavage yields retinal, which can be reduced to form retinal, giving rise to all of the structures indicated in **Figure 1A**.

fatty acid. Esterification reduces the susceptibility of retinol to oxidation and changes its physical state from a crystalline lipid to an oil. Fatty acid esters of retinol (**Figure 1A**, R_2) are the predominant form of vitamin A in most tissues. In some pharmaceutical products, retinol is present as retinyl acetate. Variant forms of vitamin A are present in some foods and human tissues. For example, vitamin A_2, (3,4-didehydroretinol) is present in freshwater fish, and is also a product of retinol metabolism in human skin.

Oxidized Metabolites of Retinol

Figure 2 illustrates key steps in the metabolism of vitamin A. Retinol is oxidized within cells to generate retinal (**Figure 1A**, R_3) and retinoic acid (**Figure 1A**, R_4). 11-*cis*-Retinal, the isomer of retinal critical for vision, absorbs light maximally at ~365 nm when in organic solvent, but when coupled with a protein, such as opsin, its peak absorptivity is shifted into the visible range of the electromagnetic spectrum (see 'Vision'). In its all-*trans* isomeric form, retinal is a transient intermediate in the bioconversion of retinol to retinoic acid. Retinoic acid exists in several isomeric forms, two of which (all-*trans*-retinoic acid and 9-*cis*-retinoic acid) interact specifically with nuclear receptor proteins.

Numerous metabolites of retinol or retinoic acid are more polar than retinol or retinoic acid due to additional oxidation of the cyclohexenyl ring, often on carbon 4. Some retinoids, particularly retinoic acid and 4-keto-retinoic acid, may be conjugated with glucuronic acid, forming retinyl- or retinoyl-β-glucuronide (R_5); these metabolites are water-soluble and therefore readily excreted. While some polar and water-soluble retinoids possess bioactivity, most show reduced, or no, activity compared to their precursors.

Carotenoids

Carotenoids are produced only by plants and a few microalgae. In plants, they function as accessory light-gathering pigments that enhance the efficiency of photosynthesis. Of the 600 or so carotenoids found in nature, only β-carotene, α-carotene, and β-cryptoxanthin have the structural features necessary for vitamin A activity. Beta-carotene is a hydrocarbon ($C_{40}H_{56}$, molecular mass 536) with two β-ionone rings, a polyene chain, and structural symmetry around the central 15,15' double bond (**Figure 1B**). The oxidative cleavage of this bond releases two molecules of retinal, which can be reduced to form vitamin A (retinol). Other isomers of β-carotene with potential nutritional activity include 9-*cis*-β-carotene produced by certain microalgae. Other common carotenoids found in fruits and vegetables, such as lycopene, lutein, and zeaxanthin, are absorbable but they lack structural features essential for vitamin A activity.

Dietary Sources and Nutritional Equivalency

Preformed vitamin A is present at highest concentration in liver and fish oils, and at lower concentrations in nonorgan meats. Food sources of preformed vitamin A and provitamin A are provided in **Table 1**. In 1990, 39% of the vitamin A (including carotenes) in the diets of Americans came from fruits and vegetables. Meats and dairy products each supplied about 20% of the vitamin A consumed. Foods that contain small amounts of vitamin A can still contribute significant amounts of vitamin A to an individual's diet if they are consumed often or in large amounts.

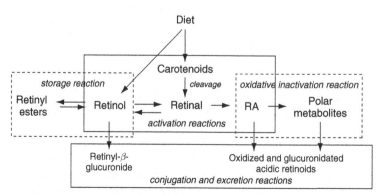

Figure 2 Schematic of principal reactions of vitamin A metabolism.

Table 1 Food sources of vitamin A

Food	%DV*
Animal sources of preformed vitamin A	
Liver, beef, cooked, 3 oz	610
Liver, chicken, cooked, 3 oz	280
Fat-free milk, fortified with vitamin A, 1 cup	10
Cheese pizza, 1/8 of a 12-inch diameter pie	8
Milk, whole (3.25% fat;), 1 cup	6
Cheddar cheese, 1 oz	6
Whole egg, 1 medium	6
Plant sources of β -carotene and other provitamin A carotenoids	
Carrot, 1 raw (7.5 inches long)	410
Carrots, boiled, 1/2 cup, slices	380
Carrot juice, canned, 1/2 cup	260
Sweet potatoes, canned, drained solids, 1/2 cup	140
Spinach, frozen, boiled, 1/2 cup	150
Mango, raw, 1 cup, sliced	130
Vegetable soup, canned, chunky, ready-to-serve, 1 cup	115
Cantaloupe, raw, 1 cup	100
Kale, frozen, boiled, 1/2 cup	80
Spinach, raw, 1 cup	40
Apricot nectar, canned, 1/2 cup	35
Oatmeal, instant, fortified, plain, water, 1 packet	30
Tomato juice, canned, 6 oz	20
Apricots, with skin, juice pack, 2 halves	10
Pepper, sweet, red, raw, 1 ring, 3-inch diam. 1/4-inch thick	10
Peas, frozen, boiled, 1/2 cup	10
Peach, raw, 1 medium	10
Peaches, canned, water pack, 1/2 cup halves or sliced	10
Papaya, raw, 1 cup, cubes	8

*% DV = Daily Value. %DVs are reference numbers based on the Recommended Dietary Allowance (RDA). Percent DVs are based on a 2000 calorie diet. They were developed to help consumers determine if a food contains a lot or a little of a specific nutrient. The DV for vitamin A is 5 000 IU (1 500 micrograms retinol which is 1500 μg RAE). Most food labels do not list a food's vitamin A content. The %DV listed in **Table 1** refer to the vitamin A provided in one serving. Data from Clinical Nutritional Service (2003) *Facts about Dietry Supplements*. Maryland, USA: Warren Grant Magnuson Clinical Center.

Units of Nutritional Activity

Owing to the multiple forms of vitamin A in most diets and the lower efficiency of utilization of carotenoids compared to preformed vitamin A, the total amount of vitamin A (bioactivity) in foods or in the total diet must be expressed in equivalents. Over the years, several equivalency units and conversion factors have been adopted. Most recently, the retinol activity equivalent was adopted by the Institute of Medicine (IOM) in 2001 to replace older units of bioactivity because new information indicated that the conversion of carotenoids is less efficient than previously thought. One microgram of retinol activity equivalent (RAE) is equivalent in terms of activity to 1 μg of all-*trans*-retinol or 2 μg of β-carotene in oily solution. One microgram of RAE is also equivalent to higher amounts of other provitamin A carotenoids in foods because they are less bioavailable than β-carotene in oil. On average, carotenoids must be ingested in the following amounts to provide the equivalent nutritional value of 1 μg of all-*trans*-retinol:

- 2 μg of supplemental β-carotene (in an oily, easily absorbed solution);
- 12 μg of β-carotene in fruits and vegetables (due to association with food matrices); and
- 24 μg of α-carotene or β-cryptoxanthin (due to food matrices and structure of compounds).

Prior to 2001, the retinol equivalent (RE) was used and this unit is still found in most food composition tables. While similar in theory to the RAE, the RE is based on older conversion factors for carotenoids in foods. Using RAE, the vitamin A activity of the provitamin A carotenoids in foods is half that using RE. An older unit, the international unit (IU or USP), which should eventually be replaced by these newer units, is still used in food tables and on some supplement labels. One IU is equal to 0.3 μg of all-*trans*-retinol. Finally, another indicator of nutritional value, % daily value (%DV), is a less quantitative but more convenient means for consumers to compare foods and select those with a substantial portion of a given nutrient. The %DV does not require extensive knowledge of nutritional units; this value appears on food package labels in the US. Besides its application in food labeling, the %DV is a useful value for quickly comparing the vitamin A contents of various common foods.

Transport and Metabolism

Few retinoids are appreciably soluble in water or aqueous body fluids. They gain solubility through association with specific proteins.

Retinol-Binding Protein

Plasma retinol is transported by a specific 21-kDa transport protein, retinal binding protein (RBP). Most RBP is produced in the liver, but some extrahepatic organs also synthesize it. Each molecule of RBP binds one molecule of all-*trans*-retinol noncovalently. In plasma, the retinol-RBP complex (holo-RBP) forms a larger complex with a cotransport protein, transthyretin (TTR), which also binds the hormone thyroxine.

Cellular Retinoid-Binding Proteins

Cellular retinoid-binding proteins (CRBP) are present in the cytoplasm of many types of cells. These proteins are similar in structure and size (~14.6 kDa), and each contains a single binding site that preferentially binds a particular form of retinoid (retinol, retinal, or retinoic acid), often preferring a specific isomer. Four cellular retinol-binding proteins (CRBP-I, -II, -III, and -IV) and two cellular retinoic acid-binding proteins (CRABP-I and -II) are expressed in many cells, yet each has a different tissue distribution. These proteins function as chaperones that confer aqueous solubility on otherwise insoluble retinoids while directing them to specific enzymes that then catalyze their further metabolism. These binding proteins may also play a role, although it is not yet well defined, in the delivery of retinoids (RA) to the nucleus for binding to nuclear retinoid receptors, which are discussed later.

Intestinal Metabolism

Dietary retinyl esters must be hydrolyzed in the lumen of the small intestine before retinol is absorbed, while carotenoids must be absorbed into the intestinal mucosa before being cleaved intracellularly. Several enzymes with retinyl ester hydrolase (REH) activity are present in pancreatic juice or on the brush border of duodenal and jujenal enterocytes (**Figure 3**). Retinol and carotenoids must be solubilized in the lumen in mixed micelles composed of bile acids and products of lipid digestion prior to their uptake into enterocytes. These processes require the release of an adequate amount of bile salts and a minimal quantity of dietary fat (approximately 5%), which must be consumed concomitantly. The retinol thus liberated diffuses into the enterocyte, is bound by CRBP-II, and is then esterified. The newly formed retinyl esters are incorporated into the lipid core of chylomicra, lipoproteins that transport dietary fat into the lymphatic system for absorption. The overall efficiency of retinol absorption is quite high, about 70–90%, and is not significantly downregulated as vitamin A consumption increases.

The efficiency of absorption of β-carotene is considerably lower (9–22%) and more variable than that of retinol. In fact, in controlled studies some subjects have absorbed little, if any, of a test dose of β-carotene. In individuals who do absorb dietary carotenoids, the efficiency of absorption tends to fall as intake increases. The type of carotenoid and its physical form in the ingested foodstuff also affect the efficiency of carotene absorption. Pure β-carotene in an oily solution or supplements is absorbed more efficiently than an equivalent amount of β-carotene in foods. Much of the carotenoid present in foods is bound within a matrix of polysaccharides, fibers, and phenolic compounds that is incompletely digested. Although the absorption of provitamin A carotenoids from fruits is generally better than from fibrous vegetables, it is still low as compared to β-carotene in oil (see section on Units).

Once in the enterocyte, provitamin A carotenoids are cleaved by one or more carotene monooxygenases, and the product (initially retinal) is metabolized to form retinol and, subsequently, retinyl esters (see **Figure 2**). In humans about one-third of ingested β-carotene escapes cleavage and, instead, is incorporated intact into chylomicrons.

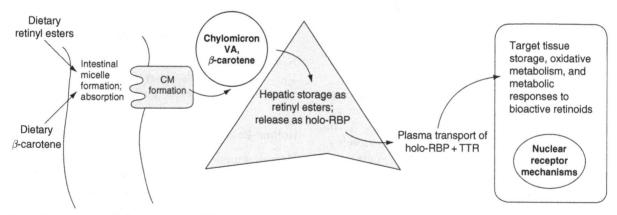

Figure 3 Absorption of dietary vitamin A (VA) via chylomicrons (CM), vitamin A storage in liver, and the release of retinal to plasma as holo-retinol-binding protein (RBP), which combines with transthyretin (TTR), to deliver retinal to organs that produce retinal (eyes) or retinoic acid (essentially all tissues) for the biological functions attributed to vitamin A.

A small fraction of intestinal β-carotene is oxidized to retinoic acid and absorbed into portal blood. It is speculated that the cleavage of dietary 9-*cis*-β-carotene and its subsequent oxidative metabolism may be a significant source of 9-*cis*-retinoic acid.

Hepatic Vitamin A Uptake, Storage and Release

Once chylomicra enter lymph and plasma, chylomicron remnants are formed rapidly by lipolysis. The majority of chylomicron remnants, still containing vitamin A, are quickly cleared into liver parenchymal cells (hepatocytes) by receptor-mediated endocytosis. Adipose and other tissues, including the mammary glands during lactation, also take up small amounts of newly absorbed vitamin A during the lipolysis of chylomicra. Within a few hours of chylomicron remnant clearance by hepatocytes, most of these newly absorbed retinyl esters are hydrolyzed and the retinol component is re-esterified, forming new retinyl esters. Newly formed retinyl palmitate and stearate are deposited in lipid droplets in vitamin A-storing stellate cells. In the vitamin A adequate state, more than 90% of total body vitamin A is stored in liver stellate cells. Small numbers of similar stellate cells have been described in extrahepatic tissues, suggesting the presence of a network of vitamin A-storing cells throughout the body.

As retinol is needed, stellate cell retinyl esters are hydrolyzed by one or more REHs and retinol is transferred back to hepatocytes for combination with newly synthesized RBP. The holo-RBP complex then passes through the Golgi secretory apparatus and binds noncovalently with a tetramer of TTR. The larger size of this transport complex ($\sim$75 kDa) compared to holo-RBP alone ($\sim$21 kDa) helps to prevent the rapid loss of retinol and RBP during renal glomerular filtration.

Plasma Concentrations

In normal plasma in the fasting state, more than 95% of retinol is bound to RBP. Retinyl esters also are present during the absorption of vitamin A-rich meals, but they are bound to plasma lipoproteins.

Although there is a significant relationship between plasma retinol and liver vitamin A storage (considered a 'gold standard' for assessing vitamin A status), the relationship is by no means linear. In fact, plasma retinol is nearly constant over a rather wide range of liver vitamin A concentrations, all consistent with vitamin A adequacy. The constancy of plasma retinol reflects its close homeostatic regulation. Plasma retinol levels in normal adults show only minor day-to-day variations, staying close to $\sim$2 and 1.7 μmol l^{-1} in males and females, respectively. The molar concentration of RBP (1.9–2.4 μmol l^{-1}) is slightly higher and thus RBP is normally 80–90% saturated. A small proportion of circulating RBP is apo-RBP (RBP without retinol). Owing to its reduced affinity for TTR, apo-RBP is readily filtered in the kidneys and catabolized.

When liver vitamin A reserves fall below about 20–30 μg retinol g liver, the secretion of holo-RBP is compromised due to inadequate retinol. Plasma retinol levels begin to fall and, if liver vitamin A continues to decline, plasma levels will fall into the deficient range and will be inadequate to supply retinol to tissues. Essentially all of the vitamin A in liver can be mobilized when it is needed to meet the needs of peripheral tissues. But ultimately, vitamin A intake must increase to bring plasma retinol levels back to the normal range.

Conversely, when vitamin A is consumed in excess of needs, its concentration in liver can increase markedly. When the concentration rises above about 300 μg g^{-1}, as occurs in hypervitaminosis A (see later section), the levels of plasma retinol and RBP remain almost normal but total vitamin A increases due to retinyl esters bound to plasma lipoproteins.

Plasma Vitamin A Kinetics

Both RBP and TTR have a relatively short half-life ($\sim$0.5 and 2–3 days, respectively) and, therefore, they must be synthesized continuously to maintain normal plasma levels. Plasma retinol, RBP, and TTR are reduced in states of impaired protein synthesis, which may be due to an inadequate intake of protein or energy or to impairments in metabolism. Plasma RBP and TTR are sometimes used as clinical indicators of visceral protein synthesis. During infection and/or inflammation, plasma retinol, RBP, and TTR fall transiently, even though liver vitamin A reserves are adequate, due to altered protein synthesis during the acute-phase response. Because multiple nutritional and metabolic disturbances can lead to a similar decrease in plasma retinol, RBP, and TTR, laboratory values must be interpreted with caution.

Studies using computer-based compartmental modeling to analyze plasma retinol kinetics have shown that each molecule of retinol circulates through the plasma compartment several times before it is irreversibly degraded (see 'Tissue Retinoid Metabolism'). In a young man who consumed

105 μmol of retinyl palmitate in a test meal, 50 μmol of retinol passed through his plasma per day, while only 4 μmol day^{-1} was degraded. Unlike retinol, RBP is not recycled, implying that RBP is synthesized in extrahepatic tissues for the release and continued recycling of retinol. Some extrahepatic tissues, such as kidney and adipose, contain RBP mRNA at a level ~5–10% of that in liver. The kidneys evidently play a very significant role in the recycling and conservation of retinol after the glomerular filtration of holo-RBP. Cell culture studies have shown that holo-RBP can bind to renal epithelial cells and cross the epithelium by transcytosis, suggesting a mechanism for the recovery of retinol lost by filtration.

Overall, the body is efficient at conserving retinol, but relatively inefficient in degrading and eliminating excess retinoids. These differences seem to explain the propensity for retinyl esters to accumulate in tissues when vitamin A is consumed in amounts that substantially exceed requirements.

Carotenoids

Carotenoids circulate in plasma in association with low-density and high-density lipoproteins. The level of β-carotene reflects its recent intake, but it also is higher when plasma lipoprotein levels are elevated. Beta-carotene is stored at relatively low concentrations in liver and fatty tissues. A prolonged slow rate of postabsorptive conversion to retinol has been observed in volunteers in isotope kinetic studies.

Tissue Retinoid Metabolism

Tissues obtain retinol from holo-RBP throughout the day, and retinyl esters from chylomicrons and chylomicron remnants after consumption of vitamin A-containing meals. Although the majority of the body's vitamin A is stored in the liver, many organs contain small reserves of retinyl esters. These small local supplies are believed to be critical for the generation of bioactive retinoids, formed through oxidative metabolism (**Figure 2**). Retinol that is liberated by the hydrolysis of retinyl esters is oxidized to retinoic acid in a two-step process in which retinal is an obligate intermediate. The oxidation of retinol to retinal has been attributed to several enzymes of the alcohol dehydrogenase and the short-chain dehydrogenase/reductase gene families. Both of these types of enzymes also oxidize other substrates and the specifics of retinol oxidation in various tissues have been difficult to define. It is likely that the CRBP proteins function as chaperones for retinol during its oxidative metabolism. Since retinal can be reduced to form retinol, the retinal that is generated from the metabolism of carotenoids can give rise to retinyl esters and all of the other metabolites of retinol (see **Figure 2**). In the second oxidative step, which is irreversible, retinal is converted to retinoic acid. This step also may be catalyzed by several enzymes. Retinoic acid is present, sometimes in several isomeric forms, at nanomolar concentrations in many tissues. Its half-life is very short, a few hours or less, which implies that it is produced continuously to maintain tissue retinoic acid levels.

The β-ionone ring of retinol and retinoic acid also can be oxidized, usually at carbon 4 to form 4-hydroxy and 4-oxo metabolites. The metabolism of retinoic acid is, in part, autoregulated due to the ability of retinoic acid to induce the expression of cytochrome P450 enzymes that form 4-oxo derivatives of retinoic acid. At this time, although limited evidence suggests that ring-oxidized retinoids still possess bioactivity, most evidence supports the thinking that they are metabolites in a catabolic pathway, destined for excretion. Ring-oxidized metabolites, which are normally present in plasma in low concentrations, are readily removed by the liver and conjugated with glucuronic acid, which makes them soluble in water. Glucuronides comprise a substantial fraction of the total retinoid excreted in bile and eliminated by the fecal route.

Production and oxidation both serve to maintain normal tissue retinoid levels. Nonetheless, these physiological processes can be overwhelmed by an excess of dietary vitamin A, resulting in excessive vitamin A in tissues and plasma, or by the use of synthetic retinoids that lead to substantial elevations in tissue bioactive retinoids (see the article section 'Hypervitaminosis A and Vitamin A Toxicity').

Physiological Actions

Vision

The retinal pigment epithelium cells (RPE) of the retina form an epithelial cell layer that takes up retinol from choroid capillaries and stores it as retinyl esters, to be used as substrate for the generation of 11-*cis*-retinal. In the layer of rod and cone photoreceptor cells adjacent to the RPE, 11-*cis*-retinal combines covalently with the protein opsin to generate the visual pigment rhodopsin in rods and, similarly, iodopsin in cones. Each rod outer segment is densely packed with some 10^8 molecules of rhodopsin per cell. The small quantity of vitamin A stored in the retina would be inadequate to maintain vision were it not for the visual cycle, a process in which 11-*cis*-retinal is regenerated after photobleaching. The absorption of light by rhodopsin catalyzes the photoisomerization of the 11-*cis*-retinal moiety of rhodopsin to all-*trans*-retinal (resulting in bleaching), which induces the release of all-*trans*-retinal from opsin. The change in retinal's isomeric configuration is crucial for initiating a signal transduction cascade from the rods to nearby retinal ganglion cells, and thereafter to the optic nerve for transmission to the brain's visual cortex. For vision to continue, 11-*cis*-retinal must be regenerated. This is accomplished in a series of biochemical reactions constituting the visual cycle, some of which take place in the rod cell outer segment and others in the RPE. The regeneration of 11-*cis*-retinal (dark adaptation) is slow (on the order of minutes) compared to the photoisomerization (fractions of a second). However, normal vision continues without a period of blindness as long as retinol can be drawn from retinyl esters stored in the RPE, rapidly isomerized to 11-*cis*-retinol, re-oxidized to 11-*cis*-retinal, and passed to the rod cell outer membrane where rhodopsin is regenerated. When the supply of retinyl esters in the RPE is not adequate, there is significant slowing of the visual cycle, resulting in the condition known as night blindness, a loss of the ability to quickly dark adapt after exposure to bright light. Night blindness is often the first-detected clinical sign of vitamin A deficiency (see the article section 'Hypervitaminosis A and Vitamin A Toxicity').

Cornea The cornea, an avascular tissue, requires retinoic acid for the normal differentiation of the corneal and conjunctival epithelium. Holo-RBP, which is present in the lacrimal glands and tears, is likely to provide the substrate for the local biogenesis of retinoic acid. Retinoid deficiency results first in a loss of goblet secretory cells, which can be detected histologically. Corneal xerosis and Bitôt's spots (foamy deposits) are strong signs of prolonged vitamin A deficiency (see 'Hypervitaminosis A and Vitamin A Toxicity'). Vitamin A must be administered immediately to prevent the progression of corneal xerosis to corneal ulceration, which causes life-long blindness.

Cell Morphology and Differentiation

Soon after the discovery of vitamin A, a light microscopic investigation of the tissues of vitamin A-deficient rats revealed marked abnormalities in many epithelial tissues. It is now recognized that essentially all organ systems require retinoids. Some epithelial tissues (skin, respiratory tract, the immune system, the reproductive organs, etc.) are especially sensitive to a lack, as well as an excess, of vitamin A.

The systemic effects of vitamin A deficiency include dryness of the skin (follicular hyperkarotosis), loss of mucus-secreting goblet cells in the trachea and respiratory tract, and a generalized flattening of epithelia (squamous metaplasia, sometimes with keratinization) throughout the body. The hematopoietic system is also affected, as are reproductive organs. In the testes, spermatogenesis is inhibited by vitamin A deficiency. Although a lack or an excess of retinoids is recognized to affect many organ systems, the developing embryo and the functions of the immune system have been studied most intensively. Essentially all of the functions of vitamin A other than those involving the retina are mediated by its active metabolite, RA, in conjunction with nuclear retinoid receptors.

Nuclear Retinoid Receptors

The nuclear retinoid receptor proteins are synthesized in the cytoplasm but reside in the nucleus where they form dimers capable of binding to specific sequences of DNA in target genes (retinoid response elements, RAREs). The family consists of six retinoid receptors (RARα, β and □, and RXR□□ and □) that belong to the superfamily of steroid hormone receptors. The RAR and RXR function as ligand-activated transcription factors to either activate or repress the transcription of hormone-responsive genes. Two isomers of retinoic acid, all-*trans*-retinoic acid and 9-*cis*-retinoic acid, function as the major ligands for the RAR and RXR subfamilies, respectively. The binding of all-*trans*-retinoic acid to the RAR induces a conformational change in the receptor dimer pair, bound to its response elements (RARE) in the regulatory region of the DNA of target genes. This conformational change, in turn, promotes the interaction of the retinoid receptor dimer with other transcriptional regulators. Ligand binding may promote the dissociation of corepressor molecules and the binding of coactivator molecules, leading to gene activation when the basal transcriptional complex is recruited. This multiprotein complex then functions enzymatically to transcribe the DNA template into messenger RNA. Additionally, some receptor functions appear to be ligand independent. Similarly to all-*trans*-retinoic acid, 9-*cis*-retinoic acid has been shown to bind to nuclear receptors of the RXR family. However, the physiological role of 9-*cis*-retinoic acid *in vivo* is currently unclear and, moreover, other ligands besides 9-*cis*-RA (such as polyunsaturated fatty acids) may also activate the RXR. Besides forming dimers with the RAR, the RXR bind in a similar manner with the nuclear receptors for vitamin D, thyroid hormone, and several other lipophilic hormones and xenobiotic agents.

Embryonic Development

Vitamin A is essential in appropriate amounts for normal embryogenesis. Retinoids are required from the early, postgastrulation stage of embryonic development. The requirement for retinoids has been deduced from molecular developmental studies in mice, and other species. These studies have consistently shown a highly regulated pattern of expression of the genes for nuclear retinoid receptors, retinoid-binding proteins, and enzymes of retinoid production and catabolism. It is likely, based on the expression of retinoid biosynthetic enzymes, that maternally derived retinol is metabolized by the embryo to produce retinoic acid at specific times in specific cells, and that retinoic acid is also catabolized in a highly regulated, tissue-specific manner. Retinoic acid has been proposed to be an essential morphogen whose concentration, or concentration gradient, is a key determinant of the expression of one or more families of genes, particularly the *Hox* gene family. This gene family is crucial in determining the formation of the anterior-posterior body axis. Some of these key genes contain a RARE.

In animals, both vitamin A deficiency and an excess of dietary vitamin A or retinoid analogs, at specific critical periods of development, can result in severe developmental defects, and may be lethal to the embryo. The differentiation of cells in the neural crest and the development of the head and sensory organs, nervous system, heart, limbs, and skeletomuscular system are often affected. Birth defects of a similar nature have occurred in women exposed to excessive dietary vitamin A, or to pharmacologic retinoids for treatment of skin diseases, in early pregnancy.

Immunity

Impaired immunity was one of the earliest effects described for vitamin A deficiency. Numerous abnormalities have been described. A dysregulation of T cell functions has been implicated in many abnormal immune responses, as vitamin A-deficient animals often have reduced T cell counts and an altered pattern of differentiation markers on T cell subsets. The response of T cells to antigens and mitogens tends to be low. Similarly, the functional capacity of cytotoxic cells, such as cytotoxic T cells and natural killer cells, and macrophages is often low. Numerous alterations have been documented in the production of cytokines that regulate T cell

immunity and antibody production by B cells. Because the immune response elicited by pathogens, vaccines, or other experimental treatments can differ significantly depending on the type of stimuli, it is not surprising that the effect of vitamin A status has also varied depending on the type of natural infection or experimental challenge. Consistently, however, the administration of vitamin A, or therapeutic doses of retinoic acid, has restored a more normal pattern of T cell-dependent immune responses, often quite rapidly, to previously vitamin A-deficient hosts.

In children at risk of vitamin A deficiency, vitamin A supplementation, given prophylactically or as therapy during illness, has significantly reduced the severity of measles and measles-related mortality (see 'Hypervitaminosis A and Vitamin A Toxicity').

Recommended Dietary Allowances and Tolerable Upper Intake Levels for Vitamin A

Recommended dietary allowances (RDA) for the US and Canada were recently revised by the Institute of Medicine (IOM). Owing to the serious, potentially irreversible, effects caused by an excess of vitamin A, guidelines were also established for a tolerable upper intake level (UL), defined as the highest intake of a nutrient that is likely to pose no risk of adverse health effects in nearly all healthy individuals. The 2001 RDA and UL for vitamin A for various life stages are listed in **Table 2**.

Infancy and Childhood

Recommendations for an adequate intake (AI) of vitamin A for children 0–6 and 7–12 months of age are based on the vitamin A content of human breast milk and on usual milk intakes for these age groups. The vitamin A content of breast milk from well-nourished women was estimated to be $1.7\,\mu\text{mol}\,\text{l}^{-1}$; therefore, it provides approximately 400 µg RAE day^{-1} to 0- to 6-month-old infants. This value was used by the IOM as the AI for infants in this age group. The AI is 500 µg RAE day^{-1} for 7- to 12-month-old infants, who are assumed to also consume complementary foods.

Physiological studies have shown that the placental transfer of vitamin A is limited in most mammals. Thus, it is normal for the liver and plasma vitamin A levels of newborns to be much lower than those in adults. In humans, premature infants often have lower plasma retinol levels than full-term infants. The period of breastfeeding is important for the accrual of vitamin A reserves as shown by

Table 2 Recommended dietary allowances (RDA) for vitamin A in micrograms (µg), retinol activity equivalents (RAE) and international units (IU), and tolerable upper intake levels (UL, µg retinol day^{-1}) for children and adults

Age (years)	Children	Men	Women	Pregnancy	Lactation
RDA (µg RAE day^{-1})					
1–3	300 µg or 1000 IU				
4–8	400 µg or 1333 IU				
9–13	600 µg or 2000 IU				
14–18		900 µg or 3000 IU	700 µg or 2330 IU	750 µg or 2500 IU	1200 µg or 4000 IU
19+		900 µg or 3000 IU	700 µg or 2330 IU	770 µg or 2565 IU	1300 µg or 4335 IU
UL (µg retinol day^{-1})					
1–3	600 µg				
4–8	900 µg				
9–13	1700 µg				
14–18		3000 µg	2800 µg	2800 µg	2800 µg
19+		3000 µg	3000 µg	3000 µg	3000 µg

animal studies in which liver vitamin A stores have increased rapidly in the suckling young of well-nourished healthy mothers. The importance of the neonatal period for establishing vitamin A reserves in young children is well recognized, and programs to promote maternal nutrition and breast feeding have become an integral component of public health programs to improve the vitamin A status of women and children worldwide.

For infants born prematurely, vitamin A (provided in enteral feeds or intramuscularly) is now recognized as an important component of medical care, and as a significant factor in reducing the risk of bronchopulmonary dysplasia and chronic lung disease.

Childhood and Adolescence

Little information specific to this age group is available, and recommendations are based on adult values, scaled down based on body weight.

Adulthood

Adults require a maintenance level of vitamin A. The RDA is based on maintaining an adequate level of vitamin A in liver while meeting normal tissue demands. In animals fed a normal vitamin A adequate diet, retinyl esters tend to accumulate as the animal ages, such that it becomes very difficult to induce vitamin A deficiency in adult animals, even by feeding them a diet free of vitamin A. These data imply that tissue reserves readily make up for lapses in the day-to-day intake of vitamin A. As is evident from **Table 1**, some foods contain an amount of vitamin A well in excess of 100% of the daily value (%DV).

Pregnancy and Lactation

The requirement for vitamin A is increased during pregnancy and lactation, but only to the extent needed for growth of maternal and fetal tissues. Nearly all of the vitamin A in breast milk is in the form of retinyl esters. Milk vitamin A concentration is influenced by recent maternal vitamin A intake. Physiological studies have shown that the lactating mammary glands derive retinol from holo-RBP and from the metabolism of chylomicra. As chylomicron vitamin A increases, milk vitamin A also increases. The RDA for lactation (**Table 2**) is calculated to provide sufficient vitamin A for the mother's needs and for the secretion of vitamin A in breast milk.

Upper Levels

There are three major adverse effects of hypervitaminosis A:

- birth defects;
- liver abnormalities; and
- reduced bone mineral density, which may result in osteoporosis.

The critical adverse effects used to establish the upper level (UL) were risk of teratogenicity for women of reproductive age, and liver abnormalities for all other life stage groups. For vitamin A, the UL applies specifically to chronic intakes of preformed vitamin A (not carotenoids) obtained from foods, fortified foods, and supplements. The UL is not meant to apply to individuals taking vitamin A under medical supervision. For several life stage groups, the UL are less than three times the RDA (**Table 2**). Based on epidemiological studies of vitamin A intakes and birth outcomes in pregnant women, and on the well-documented teratogenic effects of excessive vitamin A in experimental animals, the UL for women of reproductive age is 2800–3000 µg day^{-1}. The UL based on risk of damage to the liver, although calculated in a different way to that for teratogenicity, has the same value of 2800–3000 µg day^{-1}. Like the

RDA, the UL for younger age groups was scaled down based on body weight.

Risk of reduced bone mineral density was also considered in setting the UL, but dose-response data were insufficient to estimate a UL based on this effect. Nonetheless, there is increasing concern that bone health may be adversely affected by intakes of vitamin A not very much higher than the RDA. Epidemiological studies in Swedish men and women, and similar studies in the US, have provided evidence that a chronic intake of preformed vitamin A on the order of 2–3 times the recommended levels (near the UL) may increase the loss of bone mineral density and incidence of hip fracture. Although more research is needed, an upper intake of 2800–3000 μg preformed vitamin A per day also appears to be a prudent guideline for maintaining bone health.

Users of supplements that contain retinol or a retinyl ester should evaluate their average combined intake from diet (especially liver, milk, dairy products), fortified foods (including breakfast cereals), and all dietary supplements to ensure that it does not exceed the UL. Children's vitamin supplements should be checked to make sure that the amount of vitamin A is suitable for the child's age.

Hypervitaminosis A and Vitamin A Toxicity

Hypervitaminosis A is a rare but serious, sometimes fatal, condition. Hypervitaminosis A refers to high storage levels of vitamin A in the body that can lead to toxic symptoms. Toxic symptoms can arise after consuming very large amounts of preformed vitamin A over a short period of time, or they may develop slowly (chronic toxicity), depending on the duration and dose of vitamin A (retinol) consumed. Case reports of vitamin A toxicity include cases of excessive intakes of foods high in retinol such as liver (see **Table 1**), but most cases of vitamin A toxicity result from an excess intake of vitamin A in supplements. Symptoms resembling hypervitaminosis A have been reported in a few patients taking prescription retinoids for therapy. The clinical hallmarks of vitamin A toxicity include nausea and vomiting, headache, dizziness, blurred vision, muscular uncoordination, abnormal liver functions, and pain in weight-bearing bones and joints.

Besides eliminating intake of vitamin A, or retinoids, there is little that can be done, and no antidote, to treat hypervitaminosis A. Tissue retinoid levels fall gradually, but due to the body's tendency to conserve vitamin A, the loss is very slow. Thus, care should be exercised to avoid overconsumption

or supplementation with preformed vitamin A (see 'Upper Levels', **Table 2**).

Excessive Consumption of β-Carotene

Beta-carotene and other carotenoids in foods, even when consumed at high levels, are believed to be nontoxic, and therefore no UL was established for β-carotene. Nonetheless, a 'safe range' of intracellular β-carotene has yet to be determined. Individuals who have consumed large amounts of carotenoid-rich foods, juices, or extracts containing a large amount of β-carotene over a prolonged period of time may show signs of carotene accumulation in fatty tissues, to the point where yellowing of the skin (carotenodermia) is apparent. This condition is not known to be harmful and the color subsides over time after carotene intake is reduced to normal levels. Nonetheless, epidemiological evidence suggests that the use of high-dose β-carotene as a dietary supplement should not be regarded as safe because the current knowledge of the metabolism of high doses is inadequate, and some epidemiological studies have indicated that high doses of β-carotene, at least in smokers, may be detrimental (see 00045).

See also: **Carotenoids**: Chemistry, Sources and Physiology; Epidemiology of Health Effects. **Vitamin A**: Biochemistry and Physiological Role.

Further Reading

Altucci L and Gronemeyer H (2001) Nuclear receptors in cell life and death. *Trends in Endocrinology and Metabolism* 12: 460–468.

Collins MD and Mao GE (1999) Teratology of retinoids. *Annual Reviews of Pharmacology and Toxicology* 39: 399–430.

De Luca LM, Kosa K, and Andreola F (1997) The role of vitamin A in differentiation and skin carcinogenesis. *Journal of Nutritional Biochemistry* 8: 426–437.

Harrison EH and Hussain MM (2001) Mechanisms involved in the intestinal digestion and absorption of dietary vitamin A. *Journal of Nutrition* 131: 1405–1408.

Li E and Tso P (2003) Vitamin A uptake from foods. *Current Opinions in Lipidology* 14: 241–247.

Institute of Medicine (2000) *Dietary Reference Intakes for Vitamin C, Vitamin E, Selenium, and Carotenoids*, ch. 8. Washington: National Academy Press.

Noy N (2000) Retinoid-binding proteins: mediators of retinoid action. *Biochemical Journal* 348: 481–495.

Institute of Medicine (2001) *Dietary Reference Intakes for Vitamin A, Vitamin K, Arsenic, Boron, Chromium, Copper, Iodine, Iron, Manganese, Molybdenum, Nickel, Silicon, Vanadium, and Zinc*, ch. 4. Washington: National Academy Press.

Ross AC (1996) Vitamin A deficiency and retinoid repletion regulate the antibody response to bacterial antigens and the maintenance of natural killer cells. *Clinical Immunology and Immunopathology* 80(supplement): S36–S72.

Ross AC (1999) Vitamin A and retinoids. In: Shils ME, Olson JA, Shike M *et al.* (eds.) *Modern Nutrition in Health and Disease*, 9th edn, pp. 305–327. Baltimore: William & Wilkins.

Ross AC (2003) Retinoid production and catabolism: Role of diet in regulating retinol esterification and retinoic acid oxidation. *Journal of Nutrition* 133(suppl): 291S–296S.

Ross AC, Zolfaghari R, and Weisz J (2001) Vitamin A: recent advances in the biotransformation, transport, and metabolism of retinoids. *Current Opinions in Gastroenterology* 17: 184–192.

Olson JA (1984) Serum level of vitamin A and carotenoids as reflectors of nutritional status. *Journal of the National Cancer Institute* 73: 1439–1444.

Saari JC (2000) Biochemistry of visual pigment regeneration: the Friedenwald lecture. *Investigative Ophthalmology and Visual Science* 41: 337–348.

Sommer A and West KP Jr (1996) *Vitamin A Deficiency: Health, Survival, and Vision* New York: Oxford University Press.

Soprano DR and Blaner WS (1994) Plasma retinol-binding protein. In: Sporn MB, Roberts AB, and Goodman DS (eds.) *The Retinoids: Biology, Chemistry and Medicine*, 2nd edn., pp. 257–281. New York: Raven Press.

Stephensen CB (2001) Vitamin A, infection, and immune function. *Annual Reviews of Nutrition* 21: 167–192.

Stoltzfus RJ and Humphrey JH (2002) Vitamin A and the nursing mother-infant dyad: evidence for intervention. *Advances in Experimental Medicine and Biology* 503: 39–47.

Tanumihardjo SA (2002) Influencing the conversion of carotenoids to retinol: bioavailability to bioconversion to bioefficacy. *International Journal of Vitamin and Nutrition Research* 72: 40–45.

Underwood BA and Smitasiri S (1999) Micronutrient malnutrition: Policies and programs for control and their implications. *Annual Reviews of Nutrition* 19: 303–324.

van het Hof KH, West CE, Weststrate JA *et al.* (2000) Dietary factors that affect the bioavailability of carotenoids. *Journal of Nutrition* 130: 503–506.

Von Reinersdorff D, Green MH, and Green JB (1998) Development of a compartmental model describing the dynamics of vitamin A metabolism in men. *Advances in Experimental Medicine and Biology* 445: 207–223.

VITAMIN B$_6$

D A Bender, University College London, London, UK

Vitamin B$_6$ has a central role in amino acid metabolism as the coenzyme for a variety of reactions, including transamination and decarboxylation. It is also the coenzyme of glycogen phosphorylase and acts to modulate the activity of steroid and other hormones (including retinoids and vitamin D) that act by regulation of gene expression.

Severe deficiency disease has only been reported in a single outbreak in infants fed overheated formula. However, a significant proportion of people in developed countries have marginal vitamin B$_6$ status, and this may be associated with enhanced responsiveness to steroid hormone action and may be a factor in the development of hormone-dependent cancer of the breast, uterus, and prostate. A number of drugs have antivitamin activity, and prolonged use may lead to secondary development of pellagra, as a result of impaired tryptophan metabolism.

Estrogens do not cause vitamin B$_6$ deficiency. However, there is evidence that high doses of vitamin B$_6$ may overcome some of the side effects of estrogenic steroids used in contraceptives and as menopausal hormone replacement therapy. At very high levels of intake, supplements may cause sensory nerve damage.

Absorption and Metabolism

The main form of vitamin B$_6$ in foods is pyridoxal phosphate, bound as a Schiff base to lysine in dietary proteins. There is also a small amount of pyridoxamine phosphate. In plant foods a significant amount of the vitamin is present as pyridoxine, and a number of plants contain pyridoxine glycosides, which have limited availability. Heating foods can lead to the formation of (phospho)pyridoxyllysine, which has antivitamin activity.

Pyridoxal phosphate bound to proteins is released on digestion of the protein. The phosphorylated vitamers are dephosphorylated by membrane-bound alkaline phosphatase in the intestinal mucosa; all three vitamers are absorbed by carrier-mediated diffusion, followed by oxidation and phosphorylation, so there is accumulation of pyridoxal phosphate, which does not cross cell membranes, by metabolic trapping.

Both pyridoxal and the phosphate circulate in the bloodstream; the phosphate is dephosphorylated by extracellular alkaline phosphatase, and tissues take up pyridoxal by carrier-mediated diffusion, followed by metabolic trapping as phosphate esters. Pyridoxine and pyridoxamine phosphates are oxidized to pyridoxal phosphate (**Figure 1**).

Tissue concentrations of pyridoxal phosphate are controlled by the balance between phosphorylation and dephosphorylation. The activity of the phosphatases is greater than that of the kinase in most tissues so that pyridoxal phosphate that is not bound to enzymes will be dephosphorylated. Free pyridoxal either leaves the cell or is oxidized to 4-pyridoxic acid by aldehyde dehydrogenase, which is present in all tissues, and also by hepatic and renal aldehyde oxidase. 4-Pyridoxic acid is the main excretory product.

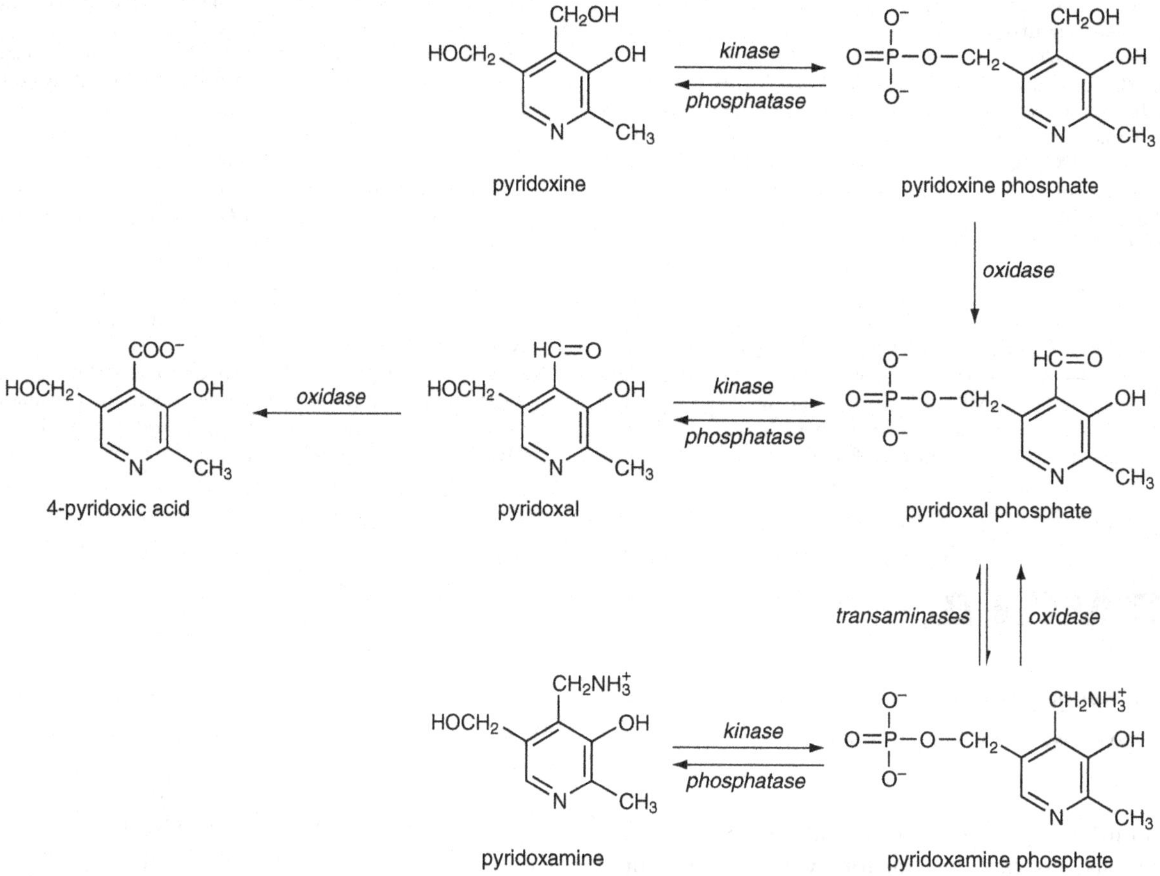

Figure 1 Metabolism of vitamin B₆.

Approximately 80% of total body vitamin B₆ is in muscle, associated with glycogen phosphorylase. This does not seem to function as a true reserve of the vitamin and is not released from muscle in times of deficiency.

Metabolic Functions of Vitamin B₆

The metabolically active vitamer is pyridoxal phosphate, which is involved in many reactions of amino acid metabolism, where the carbonyl group is the reactive moiety, in glycogen phosphorylase, where it is the phosphate group that is important in catalysis, and in the release of hormone receptors from tight nuclear binding, where again it is the carbonyl group that is important.

The Role of Pyridoxal Phosphate in Amino Acid Metabolism

The various reactions of pyridoxal phosphate in amino acid metabolism (**Figure 2**) all depend on the same chemical principle—the ability to stabilize amino acid carbanions, and hence to weaken bonds about the α-carbon of the substrate. This is achieved by reaction

of the α-amino group with the carbonyl group of the coenzyme to form a Schiff base (aldimine).

Pyridoxal phosphate is bound to enzymes, in the absence of the substrate, by the formation of an internal Schiff base to the ε-amino group of a lysine residue at the active site. Thus the first reaction between the substrate and the coenzyme is transfer of the aldimine linkage from this ε-amino group to the α-amino group of the substrate.

The ring nitrogen of pyridoxal phosphate exerts a strong electron-withdrawing effect on the aldimine, and this leads to weakening of all three bonds about the α-carbon of the substrate. In nonenzymic model systems, all the possible pyridoxal-catalyzed reactions are observed: α-decarboxylation, aminotransfer, racemization, and side chain elimination and replacement reactions. By contrast, enzymes show specificity for the reaction pathway followed; which bond is cleaved will depend on the orientation of the Schiff base relative to reactive groups of the catalytic site.

α-**Decarboxylation** If the electron-withdrawing effect of the ring nitrogen is primarily centered on the α-carbon–carboxyl bond, the result is

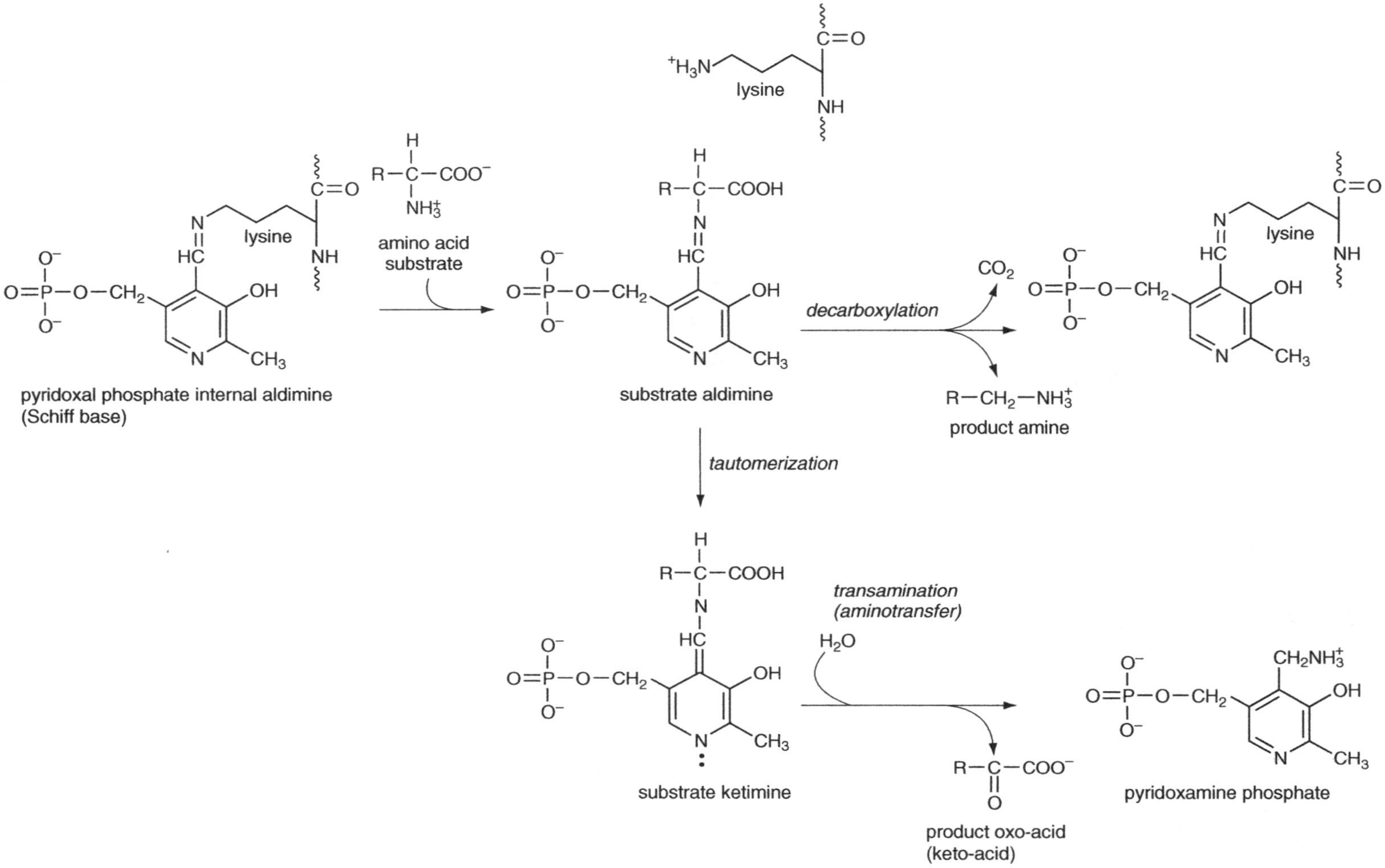

Figure 2 Roles of vitamin B_6 in amino acid metabolism.

decarboxylation of the amino acid with the release of carbon dioxide. The resultant carbanion is then protonated, and the primary amine corresponding to the amino acid is displaced by the lysine residue at the active site, with reformation of the internal Schiff base.

A number of the products of the decarboxylation of amino acids are important as neurotransmitters and hormones—5-hydroxytryptamine, the catecholamines dopamine, noradrenaline, and adrenaline, and histamine and γ-aminobutyrate (GABA)—and as the diamines and polyamines involved in the regulation of DNA metabolism. The decarboxylation of phosphatidylserine to phosphatidylethanolamine is important in phospholipid metabolism.

Racemization of amino acids Deprotonation of the α-carbon of the amino acid leads to tautomerization of the Schiff base to yield a quinonoid ketimine. The simplest reaction that the ketimine can undergo is reprotonation at the now symmetrical α-carbon. Displacement of the substrate by the reactive lysine residue results in the racemic mixture of D- and L-amino acid.

Amino acid racemases have long been known to be important in bacterial metabolism since several D-amino acids are required for the synthesis of cell wall mucopolysaccharides. D-Serine is found in relatively large amounts in mammalian brain, where it acts as an agonist of the N-methyl-D-aspartate (NMDA) type of glutamate receptor. Serine racemase has been purified from rat brain and cloned from human brain.

Transamination Hydrolysis of the α-carbon–amino bond of the ketimine formed by deprotonation of the α-carbon of the amino acid results in the release of the 2-oxo-acid corresponding to the amino acid substrate and leaves pyridoxamine phosphate at the catalytic site of the enzyme. This is the half-reaction of transamination. The process is completed by reaction of pyridoxamine phosphate with a second oxo-acid substrate, forming an intermediate ketimine, followed by the reverse of the reaction sequence shown in **Figure 3**, releasing the amino acid corresponding to this second substrate after displacement from the aldimine by the reactive lysine residue to reform the internal Schiff base.

Transamination is of central importance in amino acid metabolism, providing pathways for catabolism of most amino acids as well as the synthesis of those amino acids for which there is a source of the oxo-acid other than from the amino acid itself—the nonessential amino acids.

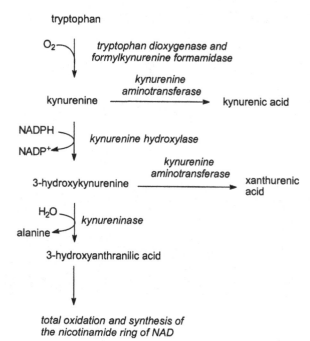

Figure 3 Tryptophan metabolism, the basis of the tryptophan load test for vitamin B₆ status.

The Role of Pyridoxal Phosphate in Steroid Hormone Action

Pyridoxal phosphate has a role in controlling the action of hormones that act by binding to a nuclear receptor protein and modulating gene expression. Such hormones include androgens, estrogens, progesterone, glucocorticoids, calcitriol (the active metabolite of vitamin D), retinoic acid and other retinoids, and thyroid hormone. Pyridoxal phosphate reacts with a lysine residue in the receptor protein and displaces the hormone–receptor complex from DNA binding, so terminating the hormone action.

In experimental animals, vitamin B₆ deficiency results in increased and prolonged nuclear uptake and retention of steroid hormones in target tissues, and there is enhanced sensitivity to hormone action. In a variety of cells in culture that have been transfected with a glucocorticoid, estrogen or progesterone response element linked to a reporter gene, acute vitamin B₆ depletion (by incubation with 4-deoxypyridoxine) leads to a 2-fold increase in expression of the reporter gene in response to hormone action. Conversely, incubation of these cells with high concentrations of pyridoxal, leading to a high intracellular concentration of pyridoxal phosphate, results in a halving of the expression of the reporter gene in response to hormone stimulation.

Assessment of Vitamin B₆ Nutritional Status

The fasting plasma concentration of either total vitamin B_6 or, more specifically, pyridoxal phosphate is widely used as an index of vitamin B_6 nutritional status, as is the urinary excretion of 4-pyridoxic acid. The generally accepted criteria of adequacy are shown in **Table 1**.

Various pyridoxal phosphate dependent enzymes compete with each other for the available pool of coenzyme. Thus the extent to which an enzyme is saturated with its coenzyme provides a means of assessing the adequacy of the body pool of coenzyme. This can be determined by measuring the activity of the enzyme before and after the activation of any apoenzyme present in the sample by incubation with pyridoxal phosphate added *in vitro*. Erythrocyte aspartate and alanine transaminases are both commonly used; the results are usually expressed as an activation coefficient—the ratio of activity with added coenzyme to that without.

It seems to be normal for a proportion of pyridoxal phosphate-dependent enzymes to be present as inactive apoenzyme, without coenzyme. This may be a mechanism for metabolic regulation. It is possible that increasing the intake of vitamin B_6, so as to

Table 1 Indices of vitamin B₆ nutritional status

Index	Adequate status
Plasma total vitamin B₆	>40 nmol (10 µg)/l
Plasma pyridoxal phosphate	>30 nmol (7.5 µg)/l
Erythrocyte alanine aminotransferase activation coefficient	<1.25
Erythrocyte aspartate aminotransferase activation coefficient	<1.80
Erythrocyte aspartate aminotransferase	>0.13 units (8.4 µkat)/l
Urine 4-pyridoxic acid	>3.0 µmol/24 h >1.3 mmol/mol creatinine
Urine total vitamin B₆	>0.5 µmol/24 h >0.2 mmol/mol creatinine
Urine xanthurenic acid after 2 g tryptophan load	<65 µmol/24 h increase
Urine cystathionine after 3 g methionine load	<350 µmol/24 h increase

Data from Bitsch R (1993) Vitamin B₆. *International Journal of Vitamin and Nutrition Research* **63**: 278–282; Leklem JE (1990) Vitamin B-6: A status report. *Journal of Nutrition* **120**(supplement 11): 1503–1507; McChrisley B, Thye FW, McNair HM and Driskell JA (1988) Plasma B₆ vitamer and 4-pyridoxic acid concentrations of men fed controlled diets. *Journal of Chromatography* **428**: 35–42.

ensure complete saturation of pyridoxal phosphate-dependent enzymes, may not be desirable.

Tryptophan Load Test

The oxidative pathway of tryptophan metabolism is shown in **Figure 3**. Kynureninase is a pyridoxal phosphate-dependent enzyme, and in deficiency its activity is lower than that of tryptophan dioxygenase, so that there is an accumulation of hydroxykynurenine and kynurenine, resulting in greater metabolic flux through kynurenine transaminase and increased formation of kynurenic and xanthurenic acids. Kynureninase is exquisitely sensitive to vitamin B_6 deficiency because it undergoes a slow inactivation as a result of catalysing the half-reaction of transamination instead of its normal reaction. The resultant enzyme with pyridoxamine phosphate at the catalytic site is catalytically inactive and can only be reactivated if there is an adequate concentration of pyridoxal phosphate to displace the pyridoxamine phosphate.

The ability to metabolise a test dose of tryptophan has been widely adopted as a convenient and sensitive index of vitamin B_6 nutritional status. However, induction of tryptophan dioxygenase by glucocorticoid hormones will result in a greater rate of formation of kynurenine and hydroxykynurenine than the capacity of kynureninase, and will thus lead to increased formation of kynurenic and xanthurenic acids—an effect similar to that seen in vitamin B_6 deficiency. Such results may be erroneously interpreted as indicating vitamin B_6 deficiency in a variety of subjects whose problem is increased glucocorticoid secretion as a result of stress or illness, not vitamin B_6 deficiency.

Inhibition of kynureninase (e.g., by estrogen metabolites) also results in accumulation of kynurenine and hydroxykynurenine, and hence increased formation of kynurenic and xanthurenic acids, again giving results which falsely suggest vitamin B_6 deficiency. This has been widely, but incorrectly, interpreted as estrogen-induced vitamin B_6 deficiency: it is in fact simple competitive inhibition of the enzyme that is the basis of the tryptophan load test by estrogen metabolites.

While the tryptophan load test is a useful index of status in controlled depletion/repletion studies to determine vitamin B_6 requirements, it is not an appropriate index of status in population studies.

Methionine Loading Test

The metabolism of methionine, shown in **Figure 4**, includes two pyridoxal phosphate-dependent steps, catalysed by cystathionine synthetase and

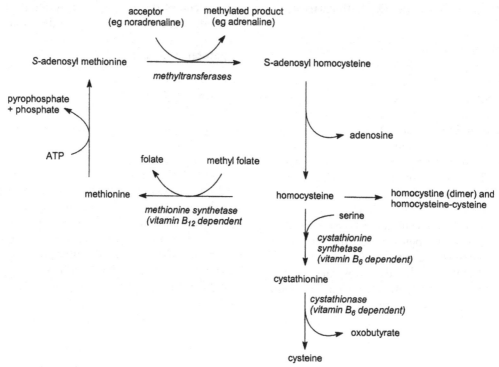

Figure 4 Methionine metabolism, the basis of the methionine load test for vitamin B₆ status.

cystathionase. In vitamin B₆ deficiency there is an increase in the plasma concentration of homocysteine, and increased urinary excretion of cystathionine and homocysteine, both after a loading dose of methionine and under basal conditions. The ability to metabolize a test dose of methionine therefore provides an index of vitamin B₆ nutritional status.

Some 10–25% of the population have a genetic predisposition to hyperhomocysteinemia, which is a risk factor for atherosclerosis and coronary heart disease, as a result of polymorphisms in the gene for methylenetetrahydrofolate reductase. There is no evidence that supplements of vitamin B₆ reduce fasting plasma homocysteine in these subjects, and like the tryptophan load test, the methionine load test may be an appropriate index of status in controlled depletion/repletion studies to determine vitamin B₆ requirements, but not in population studies.

Requirements and Reference Intakes

The total body pool of vitamin B₆ is of the order of 15 μmol (3.7 mg) per kilogram body weight. Isotope tracer studies suggest there is turnover of about 0.13% per day, and hence a minimum requirement for replacement of 0.02 μmol (5 μg) per kilogram body weight—some 350 μg per day for a 70 kg adult. However, depletion/repletion studies suggest that requirements are higher than this.

Most studies of vitamin B₆ requirements have followed the development of abnormalities of tryptophan (and sometimes also methionine) metabolism during depletion and normalization during repletion with graded intakes of the vitamin.

Although some 80% of the total body pool of vitamin B₆ is associated with muscle glycogen phosphorylase, this pool turns over relatively slowly. The major metabolic role of the remaining 20% of total body vitamin B₆, which turns over considerably more rapidly, is in amino acid metabolism. Therefore, a priori, it seems likely that protein intake will affect vitamin B₆ requirements. People maintained on (experimental) vitamin B₆-deficient diets develop abnormalities of tryptophan and methionine metabolism faster, and their blood vitamin B₆ falls more rapidly, when their protein intake is high. Similarly, during repletion of deficient subjects, tryptophan and methionine metabolism and blood vitamin B₆ are normalized faster at low than at high levels of protein intake.

These studies suggest a mean requirement of 13 μg of vitamin B₆ per gram of dietary protein; reference intakes are based on 15–16 μg per gram of protein. At average intakes of about 100 g of protein per day, this gives an RDA of 1.4–1.6 mg of vitamin B₆. More recent depletion/repletion studies, using more sensitive indices of status, in which subjects were repleted with either a constant intake of vitamin B₆ and varying amounts of protein or a constant amount of protein and varying amounts of vitamin B_6, have shown average requirements of 15–16 µg/g of dietary protein, suggesting a reference intake of 18–20 µg/g protein.

In 1998 the reference intake in the United States and Canada was reduced from the previous RDA of 2 mg/day for men and 1.6 mg/day for women to 1.3 mg/day for both, compared with the UK RNI of 1.2 mg for women and 1.4 mg for men. The report cites six studies that demonstrated that this level of intake would maintain a plasma concentration of pyridoxal phosphate at least 20 nmol/l, although, as shown in **Table 1**, the more generally accepted criterion of adequacy is 30 nmol/l.

Possible Benefits of Higher Levels of Intake

The identification of hyperhomocysteinaemia as an independent risk factor in atherosclerosis and coronary heart disease has led to suggestions that higher intakes of vitamin B_6 may be beneficial. As shown in **Figure 4**, homocysteine may undergo either of two metabolic fates: remethylation to methionine (a reaction that is dependent on vitamin B_{12} and folate) or vitamin B_6-dependent trans-sulfuration to yield cysteine.

A number of studies have shown that while folate supplements lower fasting homocysteine in moderately hyperhomocysteinemic subjects, 10 mg/day vitamin B_6 has no effect, although they do reduce the peak plasma concentration of homocysteine following a test dose of methionine.

Vitamin B₆ Requirements of Infants

Estimation of the RDA for vitamin B_6 of infants presents a problem, and there is a clear need for further research to achieve a realistic estimate of infants' requirements. Human milk, which must be assumed to be adequate for infant nutrition, provides only some 40–100 µg per liter, or 3–8 µg of vitamin B_6 per gram of protein—very much lower than the apparent requirement for adults. There is no reason why infants should have a lower requirement than adults, and indeed since they must increase their total body pool of the vitamin as they grow, they might be expected to have a proportionally higher requirement than adults.

A first approximation of the vitamin B_6 needs of infants came from studies of those who convulsed as a result of gross deficiency caused by overheated infant milk formula in the 1950s. At intakes of 60 µg per day there was an incidence of convulsions of 0.3%. Provision of 260 µg per day prevented or cured convulsions, but 300 µg per day was required to normalize

tryptophan metabolism. This is almost certainly a considerable overestimate of requirements since pyridoxyllysine, formed by heating the vitamin with proteins, has antivitamin activity, and would therefore result in a higher apparent requirement.

Based on the body content of 15 µmol (3.7 mg) of vitamin B_6 per kilogram body weight, and the rate of weight gain, the minimum requirement for infants over the first 6 months of life would appear to be 100 µg (417 nmol) per day to establish tissue reserves.

Pharmacological Uses and Toxicity of Vitamin B₆ Supplements

Supplements of vitamin B_6 ranging from 25 to 500 mg/day, and sometimes higher, have been recommended for treatment of a variety of conditions in which there is an underlying physiological or biochemical mechanism to justify the use of supplements, although in most cases there is little evidence of efficacy. Such conditions include postnatal depression, depression and other side effects associated with oral contraceptives, hyperemesis of pregnancy, and the premenstrual syndrome.

Supplements have also been used empirically, with little or no rational basis, and little or no evidence of efficacy, in the treatment of a variety of conditions, including acute alcohol intoxication, atopic dermatitis, autism, carpal tunnel syndrome, dental caries, diabetic neuropathy, Down's syndrome, Huntington's chorea, schizophrenia, and steroid-dependent asthma.

Doses of 50–200 mg per day have an antiemetic effect, and the vitamin is widely used, alone or in conjunction with other antiemetics, to minimize the nausea associated with radiotherapy and to treat pregnancy sickness. There is no evidence that vitamin B_6 has any beneficial effect in pregnancy sickness, nor that women who suffer from morning sickness have lower vitamin B_6 nutritional status than other pregnant women.

Vitamin B₆ and the Side Effects of Oral Contraceptives

Although oestrogens do not cause vitamin B_6 deficiency, the administration of vitamin B_6 supplements has beneficial effects on some of the side effects of both administered and endogenous oestrogens. The supplements act in two main areas: in normalizing glucose tolerance and as an antidepressant.

Impairment of glucose tolerance is common in pregnancy and may indeed be severe enough to be classified as gestational diabetes mellitus, which generally resolves at parturition, although in some subjects it may persist. High-estrogen oral contraceptives may also cause impaired glucose tolerance. This seems to be the result of increased tissue and blood concentrations of xanthurenic acid, because of the inhibition of kynureninase by estrogen metabolites. Xanthurenic acid forms a complex with insulin which has little or no hormonal activity. Vitamin B₆ supplements may have a beneficial effect by activating apokynureninase or kynureninase that has been inactivated by undergoing transamination.

One of the relatively common side effects of oestrogenic oral contraceptives is depression, affecting about 6% of women in some studies. This frequently responds well to the administration of relatively large amounts of vitamin B₆ (generally in excess of 40 mg per day). Postnatal depression also responds to similar supplements in some studies.

Again, this does not seem to be due to correction of vitamin B₆ deficiency, but rather to a direct effect of pyridoxal phosphate on the metabolism of tryptophan. High concentrations of pyridoxal phosphate attenuate the response to glucocorticoid hormones; tryptophan dioxygenase is a glucocorticoid-induced enzyme, and thus its synthesis and activity will be reduced by high intakes of vitamin B₆. This reduces the oxidative metabolism of tryptophan and increases the amount available for synthesis of 5-hydroxytryptamine in the brain.

Vitamin B₆ in the Premenstrual Syndrome

The studies showing a beneficial action of vitamin B₆ in overcoming depression associated with oral contraceptives have led to the use of the vitamin in depression and other pathology associated with endogenous estrogens in the premenstrual syndrome. There is no evidence of poorer vitamin B₆ nutritional status in women who suffer from the premenstrual syndrome.

There are few well-controlled studies of the effects of vitamin B₆ in premenstrual syndrome. In general, those that have been properly controlled report little benefit from doses between 50 and 200 mg per day compared with placebo, although some studies do claim a beneficial effect. Interestingly, meta-analysis of controlled crossover trials shows that whichever treatment is used second, active vitamin or placebo, is (marginally) more effective. There is no obvious explanation for this observation.

Despite the lack of evidence of efficacy, vitamin B₆ is widely prescribed (and self-prescribed) for the treatment of premenstrual syndrome.

Vitamin B₆ for Prevention of the Complications of Diabetes Mellitus

A number of studies have suggested that vitamin B₆ (and specifically pyridoxamine) may be effective in preventing the adverse effects of poor glycemic control that lead to the development of the complications of diabetes mellitus, many of which are mediated by nonenzymic glycation of proteins. Pyridoxamine is a potent inhibitor of the rearrangement of the immediate product of protein glycation to the 'advanced glycation end-product.'

Toxicity of Vitamin B₆

Animal studies have demonstrated the development of signs of peripheral neuropathy, with ataxia, muscle weakness, and loss of balance, in dogs given 200 mg pyridoxine per kilogram body weight for 40–75 days, and the development of a swaying gait and ataxia within 9 days at a dose of 300 mg per kilogram body weight. At a dose of 50 mg per kilogram body weight, there are no clinical signs of toxicity, but histologically there is a loss of myelin in dorsal nerve roots. At higher doses there is more widespread neuronal damage, with loss of myelin and degeneration of sensory fibers in peripheral nerves, the dorsal columns of the spinal cord, and the descending spinal tract of the trigeminal nerve. The clinical signs of vitamin B₆ toxicity in animals regress after withdrawal of these massive doses, but sensory nerve conduction velocity, which decreases during the development of the neuropathy, does not recover fully. The mechanism of the neurotoxic action of vitamin B₆ is unknown.

The development of sensory neuropathy has been reported in patients taking 2–7 g of pyridoxine per day. Although there was residual damage in some patients, withdrawal of these extremely high doses resulted in a considerable recovery of sensory nerve function.

There is little evidence that intakes of up 200 mg vitamin B₆ per day for prolonged periods are associated with any adverse effects. The US Food and Nutrition Board set a tolerable upper level for adults of 100 mg/day; the EU Scientific Committee on Food set 25 mg/day.

Vitamin B₆ Deficiency

Gross clinical deficiency of vitamin B₆ is more or less unknown. The vitamin is widely distributed in foods, and intestinal flora synthesize relatively large amounts, at least some of which is believed to be absorbed.

In vitamin B$_6$-deficient experimental animals there are more or less specific skin lesions (e.g., acrodynia in the rat) and fissures or ulceration at the corners of the mouth and over the tongue, as well as a number of endocrine abnormalities, defects in the metabolism of tryptophan, methionine, and other amino acids, hypochromic microcytic anemia (the first step of heme biosynthesis is a pyridoxal phosphate-dependent reaction), changes in leucocyte count and activity, a tendency to epileptiform convulsions, and peripheral nervous system damage resulting in ataxia and sensory neuropathy.

Much of our knowledge of human vitamin B$_6$ deficiency is derived from an outbreak in the early 1950s, which resulted from an infant milk preparation which had undergone severe heating in manufacture. The probable result of this was the formation of pyridoxyllysine by reaction between pyridoxal phosphate and the ϵ-amino groups of lysine in proteins. In addition to a number of metabolic abnormalities, many of the affected infants convulsed. They responded to the administration of vitamin B$_6$ supplements.

Investigation of the neurochemical basis of the convulsions in vitamin B$_6$ deficiency helped to elucidate the role of GABA as a neurotransmitter; GABA is synthesized by the decarboxylation of glutamate. More recent studies have suggested that the accumulation of hydroxykynurenine in the brain may be the critical factor precipitating convulsions in deficiency; GABA is depleted in the brains of deficient adult and neonate animals, while hydroxykynurenine accumulation is considerably more marked in neonates than adults—only neonates convulse in vitamin B$_6$ deficiency. GABA depletion may be a necessary but not sufficient condition for convulsions in vitamin B$_6$ deficiency.

Groups at Risk of Deficiency

A number of studies have shown that between 10 and 20% of the apparently healthy population have low plasma concentrations of pyridoxal phosphate or abnormal erythrocyte transaminase activation coefficient, suggesting vitamin B$_6$ inadequacy or deficiency. In most studies, only one of these indices of vitamin B$_6$ nutritional status has been assessed. Where both have been assessed, while each shows some 10% of the population apparently inadequately provided with vitamin B$_6$, few of the subjects show inadequacy by both criteria.

There is a decrease in the plasma concentration of vitamin B$_6$ with increasing age, and some studies have shown a high prevalence of abnormal transaminase activation coefficient in elderly subjects, suggesting that the elderly may be at risk of vitamin B$_6$ deficiency. It is not known whether this reflects an inadequate intake, a greater requirement, or changes in the tissue distribution and metabolism of the vitamin with increasing age.

Drug-Induced Vitamin B₆ Deficiency

A number of drugs that react with carbonyl compounds are capable of causing vitamin B$_6$ deficiency on prolonged use. These include the antituberculosis drug isoniazid (iso-nicotinic acid hydrazide), penicillamine, and the anti-Parkinsonian drugs, benserazide and carbidopa. In general, the main effect is impairment of tryptophan metabolism by inhibition of kynureninase, and hence the development of the niacin-deficiency disease, pellagra. The condition therefore responds to the administration of either vitamin B$_6$ or niacin.

See also: **Niacin**.

Further Reading

Bender DA (1987) Oestrogens and vitamin B$_6$—Actions and interactions. *World Review of Nutrition and Dietetics* 51: 140–188.

Bender DA (1989) Vitamin B$_6$ requirements and recommendations. *European Journal of Clinical Nutrition* 43: 289–309.

Bender DA (1999) Non-nutritional uses of vitamin B$_6$. *British Journal of Nutrition* 81: 7–20.

Bender DA (2003) In *Nutritional Biochemistry of the Vitamins*, 2nd edn, pp. 232–269. New York: Cambridge University Press.

Coburn SP (1994) A critical review of minimal vitamin B$_6$ requirements for growth in various species with a proposed method of calculation. *Vitamins and Hormones* 48: 259–300.

Coburn SP (1996) Modelling vitamin B$_6$ metabolism. *Advances in Food and Nutrition Research* 40: 107–132.

Fasella PM (1967) Pyridoxal phosphate. *Annual Review of Biochemistry* 36: 185–210.

Ink SL and Henderson LM (1984) Vitamin B$_6$ metabolism. *Annual Review of Nutrition* 4: 455–470.

Kruger WD (2000) Vitamins and homocysteine metabolism. *Vitamins and Hormones* 60: 333–352.

Oka T (2001) Modulation of gene expression by vitamin B$_6$. *Nutrition Research Reviews* 14: 257–265.

Wiss O and Weber F (1964) Biochemical pathology of vitamin B$_6$ deficiency. *Vitamins and Hormones* 22: 495–501.

VITAMIN D

Contents

Physiology, Dietary Sources and Requirements

M F Holick, Boston University Medical Center, Boston, MA, USA

Introduction

Vitamin D is a fat-soluble vitamin that is recognized for its importance for bone health. Vitamin D is neither a vitamin nor a nutrient because exposure to sunlight can provide the body's requirement for vitamin D. We take vitamin D for granted because it is casual exposure to sunlight that provides most humans with their vitamin D requirement. This recognition and the fortification of milk and other foods including some margarines, cereals, and orange juice with vitamin D has eradicated vitamin D deficiency rickets as a significant health problem for children in the US and countries that practice this fortification process. However, it is now recognized that both children and adults are at risk for developing vitamin D deficiency. The recommended adequate dietary intake for vitamin D is $200\,IU\,day^{-1}$ for children and adults <50 years old, $400\,IU\,day^{-1}$ for adults 51–70 years, and $600\,IU\,day^{-1}$ for those >70 years. However, without adequate sun exposure, $1000\,IU\,day^{-1}$ is needed. Once vitamin D is formed in the skin or ingested in the diet, it enters the bloodstream and travels to the liver and kidney where it is hydroxylated on carbons 25 and 1 to form 25-hydroxyvitamin D (25(OH)D) and 1,25-dihydroxyvitamin D (1,25(OH)D), respectively. 25-Hydroxyvitamin D is the major circulating form of the vitamin that is measured to determine the vitamin D status of patients. 1,25-Dihydroxyvitamin D is the biologically active form of vitamin D that is responsible for maintaining calcium homeostasis and bone health. It is now recognized that vitamin D deficiency increases the risk of many chronic diseases including cancers of the breast, prostate, and colon, type 1 diabetes mellitus, multiple sclerosis, rheumatoid arthritis, and heart disease.

Origin and Structure of Vitamin D

As the industrial revolution began to take hold in Northern Europe in the 17th century, it was quickly associated with a new disease that caused severe growth retardation and bony deformities in young children (**Figure 1**). This disease was commonly known as rickets or 'English disease' and plagued the children of the industrialized cities in Europe and North America for more than 250 years. Although Sniadecki in 1822 and Palm in 1890 both recognized that it was lack of exposure to sunlight that was the likely cause of rickets in children, Huldschinsky, in 1919, was the first to prove that exposure of the skin to ultraviolet radiation could cure rickets. Within 2 years, Hess and Unger reported that exposure of several rachitic children to sunlight was adequate for curing this bone-deforming disease.

Steenbock and Black and Hess independently recognized that exposure of animals and their food to ultraviolet radiation imparted antirachitic activity. This led to the recommendation for the ultraviolet irradiation of foods as a means of fortifying them with vitamin D. This resulted in the addition of provitamin D to milk followed by ultraviolet irradiation. As soon as it was possible to commercially synthesize vitamin D in large quantities, it was added directly to milk and other foods.

The first vitamin D was isolated from the irradiation of the yeast sterol ergosterol (**Figure 2**). This vitamin D was thought to be identical to that produced in the skin of animals and humans. However, studies revealed that when vitamin D produced from yeast was fed to chickens, they were unable to utilize it and developed rickets. When chickens were fed natural vitamin D from fish liver oil, rickets was prevented. This led to the conclusion that vitamin D originating from yeast was different from that in fish liver oil and animal and human skin. In 1937, this mystery was solved when the structure of provitamin D from pig skin was determined. A structural analysis revealed that provitamin D derived from ergosterol differed from that derived from pig skin. The provitamin D (ergosterol; provitamin D_2) that came from yeast had a double bond between carbons 22 and 23 and a methyl group on carbon 24.

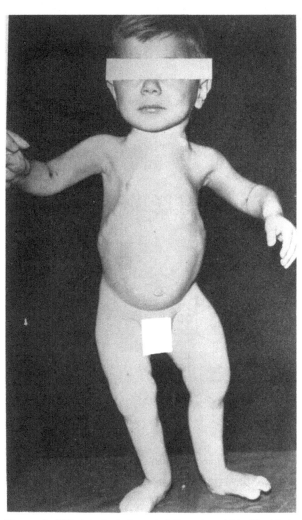

Figure 1 This is a typical presentation of a child with rickets. The child is suffering from severe muscle weakness, has bony deformities including bowed legs, and knob-like projects in the middle of his ribcage called the rachitic rosary. (Reproduced with permission from Fraser D and Scriver CR (1979) Disorders associated with hereditary or acquired abnormalities of vitamin D function: hereditary disorders associated with vitamin D resistance or defective phosphate metabolism. In: De Groot LJ *et al.* (eds.) *Endocrinology*, pp. 797–808. New York: Grune and Stratton.)

The provitamin D in animal skin had a side-chain that was identical to cholesterol, i.e., it did not contain either a double bond or methyl group on carbons 22–23 and 24, respectively, and was identified as 7-dehydrocholesterol (provitamin D_3) (**Figure 2**). The vitamin Ds generated from ergosterol and 7-dehydrocholesterol were called ergocalciferol (vitamin D_2) and cholecalciferol (vitamin D_3), respectively.

Production of Vitamin D in the Skin

During exposure to sunlight, the ultraviolet B photons with energies between 290 and 315 nm are absorbed by provitamin D_3 (7-dehydrocholesterol) in the skin. This absorption results in a photolysis of the B-ring of provitamin D_3 resulting in the formation of previtamin D_3 (**Figure 3**). However, since previtamin D_3 is thermodynamically unstable, it quickly undergoes an isomerization (rearrangement) of its triple bond system to form vitamin D_3. This isomerization process is enhanced in skin cells because the previtamin D_3 is synthesized in the cell membrane, which restricts its movement thereby accelerating the transformation of previtamin D_3 to vitamin D_3. Once vitamin D_3 is formed in the skin cell membrane, it is no longer restricted in its movement and freely translocates into the extracellular space to find its way into the dermal capillary bloodstream where it is bound to a specific vitamin D-binding protein (**Figure 3**).

An increase in skin pigmentation and zenith angle of the sun (change in latitude, season, and time of day) and the topical application of a sunscreen can markedly diminish or even prevent the production of vitamin D_3 in the skin. Over the age of ~65 years, there is a three- to fourfold decline in the synthetic capacity of the skin to produce vitamin D_3. Excessive exposure to sunlight cannot cause vitamin D_3 intoxication because once previtamin D_3 and vitamin D_3 are made in the skin, excessive quantities are rapidly destroyed by sunlight (**Figure 3**).

Absorption, Metabolism, and Excretion of Vitamin D

Vitamin D (vitamin D without a subscript represents either vitamin D_2 or D_3) is fat soluble and, therefore, once ingested vitamin D_2 and vitamin D_3 are incorporated into the chylomicron fraction and absorbed in the small intestine into the lymphatic system. Both dietary vitamin D_2 and vitamin D_3, and cutaneous vitamin D_3 enter the circulation and are bound to a specific α_1-globulin known as the vitamin D-binding protein. It is believed that this protein acts as a buffering system whereby it helps maintain circulating concentrations of 25(OH)D so that the free unbound form of 25(OH)D can enter into the renal tubular cells to be metabolized.

Neither vitamin D_2 nor vitamin D_3 possess any intrinsic biologic activity on calcium metabolism. They both require a hydroxylation on carbon 25 to form 25(OH)D (**Figure 4**). 25(OH)D is the major circulating form of vitamin D and at physiologic concentrations it has little biologic activity on calcium metabolism. It must undergo a hydroxylation

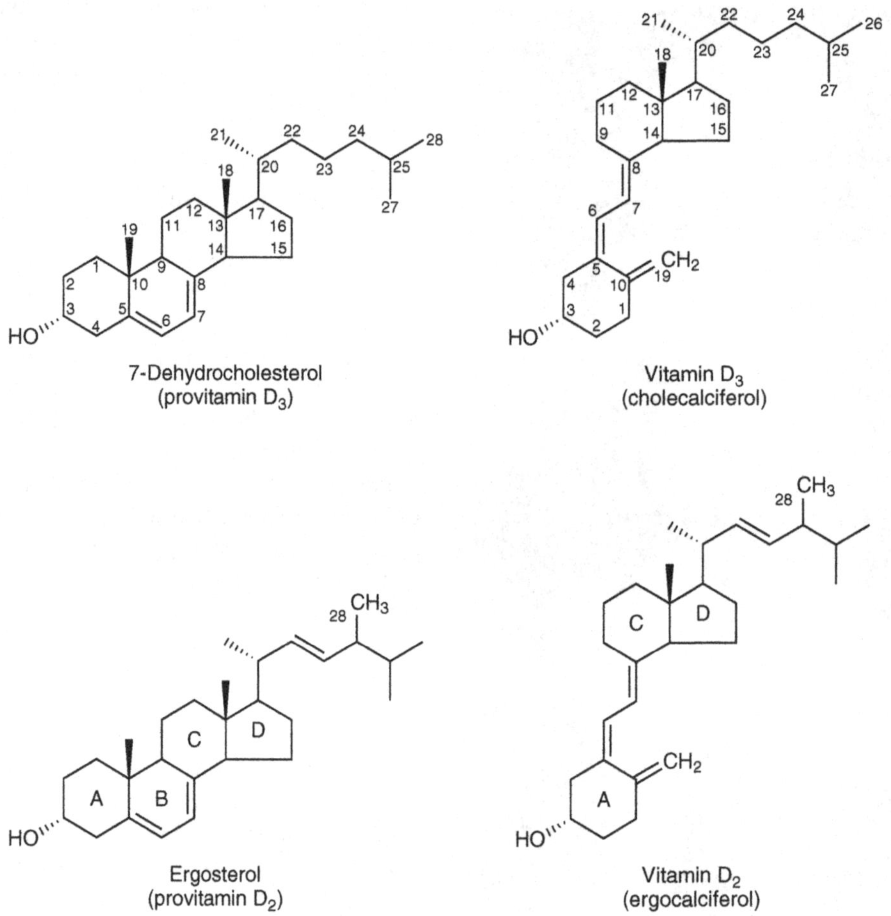

Figure 2 Structures for 7-dehydrocholesterol (provitamin D_3), ergosterol (provitamin D_2), vitamin D_3 (cholecalciferol), and vitamin D_2 (ergocalciferol). The carbons are numbered and the ring systems are labeled.

on carbon 1 in the kidney to form $1,25(OH)_2D$, the biologically active form of vitamin D (**Figure 4**). The metabolism of $25(OH)D$ to $1,25(OH)_2D$ is tightly regulated by parathyroid hormone (PTH) and serum phosphorus levels (**Figure 5**). PTH and low serum phosphorus levels increase the production of $1,25(OH)_2D$.

$25(OH)D$ and $1,25(OH)_2D$ act as substrate for a 24-hydroxylase (an enzyme that attaches an hydroxyl on carbon-24), which is found in the kidney and other target tissues for $1,25(OH)_2D$. Once $1,25(OH)_2D$ is hydroxylated on carbon 24, this is the first step in its degradation to a water-soluble acid, calcitroic acid (**Figure 4**). Whereas, vitamin D is excreted in the bile, calcitroic acid is excreted by the kidney.

There continues to be speculation and controversy as to whether the 24-hydroxylation of $25(OH)D$ and $1,25(OH)_2D$ to 24, 25-dihydroxyvitamin D and 1,24,25-trihydroxyvitamin D, respectively, has important physiologic functions other than simply initiating the degradation of both metabolites.

Biologic Functions of Vitamin D on Calcium Metabolism

$1,25(OH)_2D$ interacts with a specific nuclear receptor that is commonly known as the vitamin D receptor (VDR) and is one of the many members of the super family of steroid hormone receptors that includes retinoic acid, thyroid hormone, glucocorticoids, and sex steroids. Once $1,25(OH)_2D$ interacts with the VDR, the complex forms a heterodimer with retinoic acid X receptor (RXR) (**Figure 6**). This new complex sits on specific segments of vitamin D responsive genes known as vitamin D responsive elements (VDREs) to either increase or decrease transcriptional activity of the vitamin D-sensitive genes such as osteocalcin, calcium binding protein (calbindin), PTH, and osteonectin (**Figure 6**).

In the intestine, $1,25(OH)_2D$ enhances the absorption of dietary calcium and phosphorus across the microvilli of the small intestinal absorptive cells (**Figure 5**). $1,25(OH)_2D$ also interacts with monocytic stem cells in the bone marrow to initiate

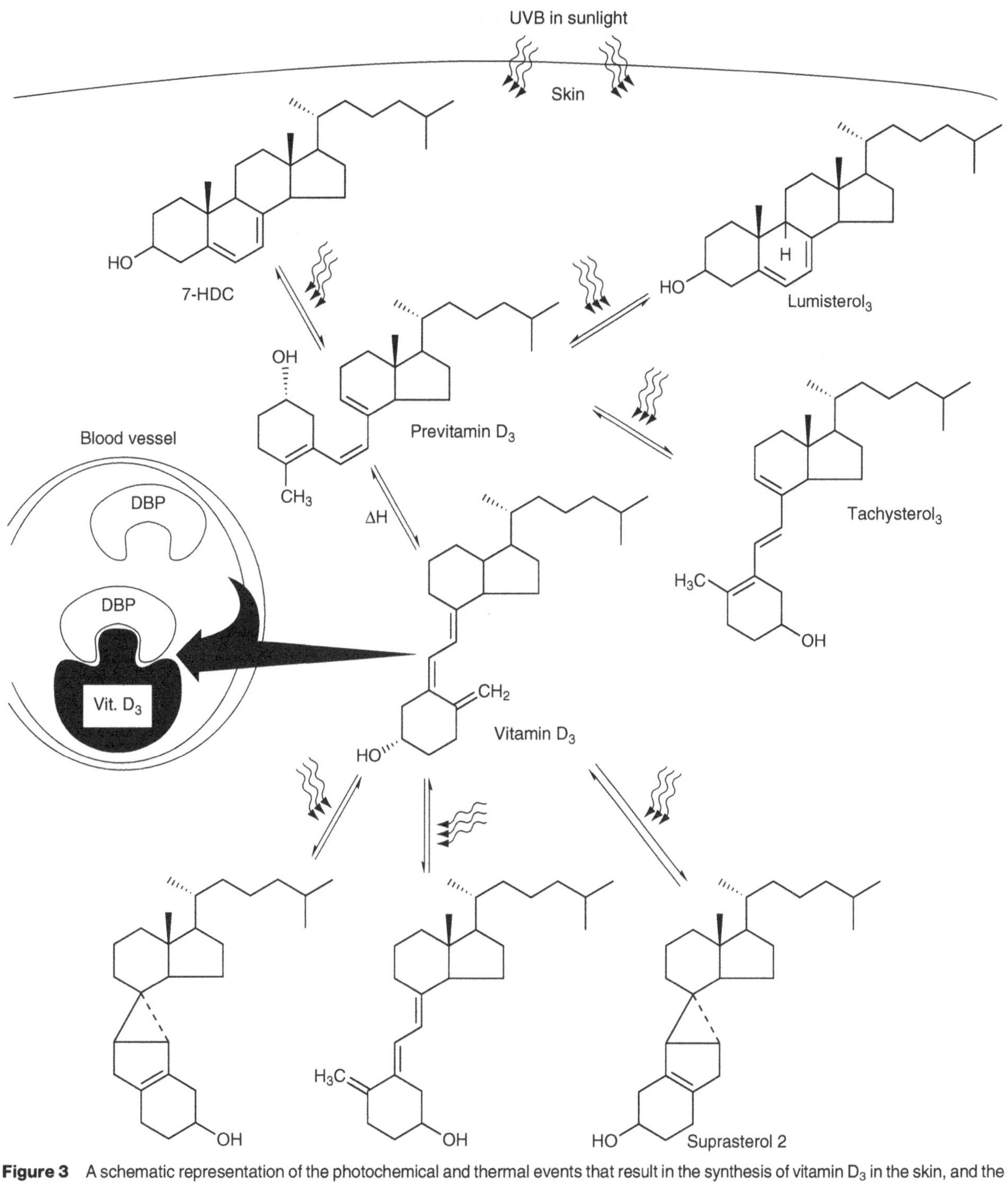

Figure 3 A schematic representation of the photochemical and thermal events that result in the synthesis of vitamin D_3 in the skin, and the photodegradation of previtamin D_3 and vitamin D_3 to biologically inert photoproducts. 7-Dehydrocholesterol (7-DHC) in the skin is converted to previtamin D_3 by the action of solar ultraviolet B radiation. Once formed, previtamin D_3 is transformed into vitamin D_3 by a heat-dependent (ΔH) process. Vitamin D_3 exits the skin into the dermal capillary blood system and is bound to a specific vitamin D-binding protein (DBP). When previtamin D_3 and vitamin D_3 are exposed to solar ultraviolet B radiation, they are converted to a variety of photoproducts that have little or no activity on calcium metabolism. (Reproduced with permission from Holick MF (1995) Vitamin D: Photobiology, Metabolism, and Clinical Applications. In: DeGroot LJ et al. (eds.) Endocrinology, 3rd edn, pp. 990–1013. Philadelphia: W.B. Saunders.)

their transformation into mature osteoclasts (**Figure** 5). Thus, $1,25(OH)_2D_3$ regulates serum calcium levels by enhancing the efficiency of intestinal calcium absorption and stimulating resorption of calcium from the bone. It remains controversial as to whether $1,25(OH)_2D$ has any

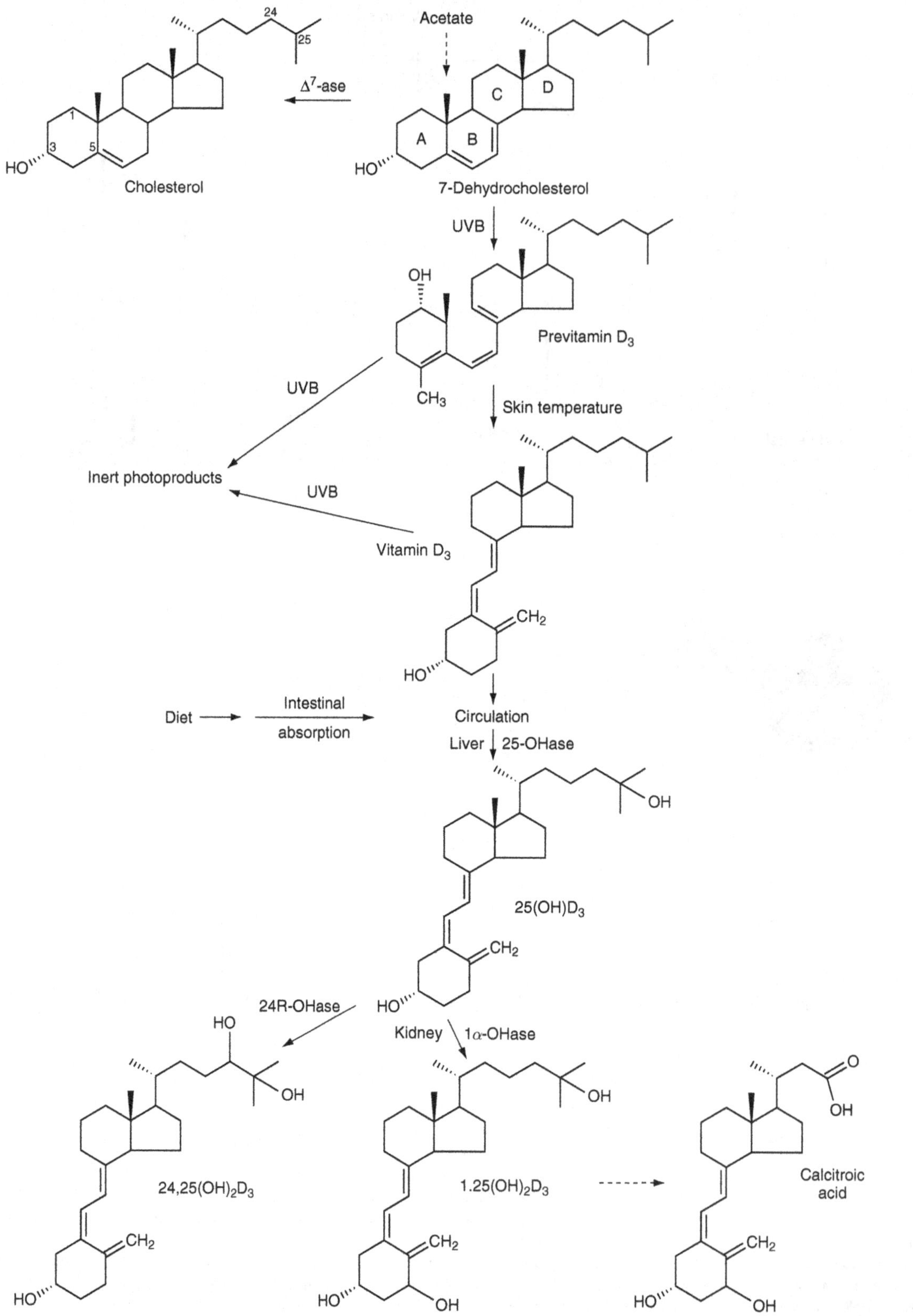

Figure 4   A schematic representation of the origin of vitamin D_3 and its metabolism in the liver by the hepatic vitamin D-25-hydroxylase. Once formed, the 25-hydroxyvitamin D_3 ($25(OH)D_3$) is metabolized by either a $25(OH)D$-1α-hydroxylase or a $25(OH)D$-24-hydroxylase. 1,25-Dihydroxyvitamin D_3 ($1,25(OH)_2D_3$) can either go to its target tissues to carry out its biologic function(s), or it can be metabolized in its side-chain and degraded to calcitroic acid. (Reproduced with permission from Holick MF (1995) Vitamin D: Photobiology, Metabolism, and Clinical Applications. In: DeGroot LJ *et al.* (eds.) *Endocrinology*, 3rd edn, pp. 990–1013. Philadelphia: W.B. Saunders.)

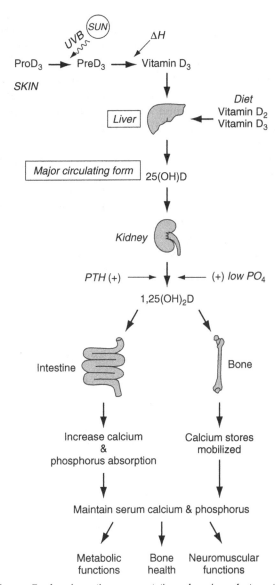

Figure 5 A schematic representation of various factors that regulate the metabolism of vitamin D to 1,25-dihydroxyvitamin D₃. (Copyright Michael F Holick (2004) Vitamin D: Importance in the prevention of cancers, type 1 diabetes, heart disease, and osteoporosis. *American Journal of Clinical Nutrition* **79**: 362–371, used with permission.)

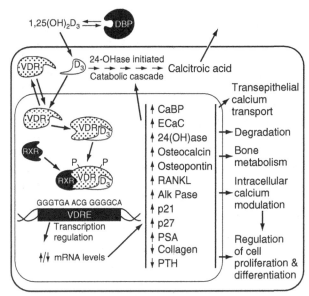

Figure 6 A schematic representation of the mechanism of action of 1,25(OH)₂D in various target cells resulting in a variety of biological responses. The free form of 1,25(OH)₂D₃ enters the target cell and interacts with its nuclear vitamin D receptor (VDR), which is phosphorylated (Pi). The 1,25(OH)₂D–VDR complex combines with the retinoic acid X receptor (RXR) to form a heterodimer, which, in turn, interacts with the vitamin D responsive element (VDRE), causing an enhancement or inhibition of transcription of vitamin D-responsive genes including calcium-binding protein (CaBP), ECaC, 24-OHase, RANKL, alkaline phosphatase (alk Pase), prostate-specific antigen (PSA), and PTH.

now routinely used for the treatment of the hyperproliferative skin disorder psoriasis.

Evaluation for and Consequences of Vitamin D Deficiency

Vitamin D deficiency in young children causes rickets. As a child becomes vitamin D deficient, this results in a decrease in the efficiency of intestinal calcium absorption. There is a decline in blood-ionized calcium, which causes the parathyroid glands to produce and secrete more parathyroid hormone (PTH). PTH tries to conserve calcium by enhancing tubular reabsorption of calcium in the kidney. However, in the face of developing hypocalcemia, which could disturb neuromuscular function and a wide variety of metabolic and cellular processes, the body calls upon 1,25(OH)₂D and PTH to mobilize stem cells to become functional osteoclasts, which, in turn, mobilize calcium from the skeleton. In addition, PTH causes a loss of phosphorus into the urine causing hypophosphatemia. Thus, in early vitamin D deficiency the serum calcium is normal; it is the low serum phosphorus that causes the extracellular CaXPO₄ to be too low for normal mineralization of

direct action on the renal handling of either calcium or phosphorus.

There are a variety of other tissues including the brain, gonads, pancreas, stomach, activated T and B lymphocytes, monocytes, and skin that have nuclear VDR. Although the exact physiologic function of 1,25(OH)₂D's interaction with these VDRs is not well understood, it is known that *in vivo* and *in vitro* 1,25(OH)₂D₃ can inhibit proliferation and induce terminal differentiation of various normal and tumor cells including normal human keratinocytes. This is the reason why activated vitamin D compounds are bone matrix. This causes a disruption in the orderly sequence of events in the differentiation of hypertrophied chondrocytes in the epiphyseal plates resulting in their disorganization causing a widening of the epiphyseal plates (end of long bones), demineralization of the skeleton, and bony deformities (**Figure 1**).

Once the epiphyseal plates are closed later in adolescence, vitamin D deficiency can no longer cause bone deformities. Instead, there is an inability to mineralize newly deposited bone matrix leading to wide osteoid seams within the trabecular and cortical bone causing the bone disease commonly known as osteomalacia. In addition, the secondary hyperparathyroidism that results from vitamin D deficiency results in the mobilization of precious calcium stores from the bone thereby exacerbating bone loss and causing osteoporosis. This can increase a person's risk for fracture.

The hallmark for determining the vitamin D status is the measurement of the circulating concentration of 25(OH)D. The 25(OH)D is low or undetectable in vitamin D deficiency and markedly elevated in vitamin D intoxication. Measurement of 1,25(OH)$_2$D is of little value for determining the vitamin D nutritional status because its synthesis is tightly regulated. Indeed, as a person becomes vitamin D deficient, there is an increase in the secretion of PTH which, in turn, increases the production of 1,25(OH)$_2$D. Thus, early in vitamin D deficiency one can see a normal fasting serum calcium, low-normal to low phosphorus, low 25(OH)D, and elevated PTH, 1,25(OH)$_2$D and alkaline phosphatase. In chronic vitamin D deficiency, all the above are seen with the exception that 1,25(OH)$_2$D is low-normal or low.

Nonskeletal Consequences of Vitamin D Deficiency

As early as 1941, it was appreciated that if you lived at higher latitudes in the US you were at higher risk of dying of cancer. A multitude of epidemiologic studies clearly show that if you live at higher latitudes and are more prone to vitamin D deficiency then you are at higher risk of dying of colon, prostate, breast, ovarian, and a variety of other cancers. It is also known that living at higher latitudes increases risk of having high blood pressure and heart disease as well as autoimmune diseases including multiple sclerosis and type I diabetes.

Essentially every cell and organ in the body requires vitamin D, i.e., they all have a VDR. It is also known that most tissues in the body can activate vitamin D. Thus, maintaining adequate levels of 25(OH)D in the circulation of at least 20 ng ml^{-1} and preferably 30 ng ml^{-1} is necessary for various organs including colon, breast, and prostate to convert it to 1,25(OH)$_2$D, which in turn can help regulate various genes responsible for cell growth and differentiation. This could be the explanation for how vitamin D sufficiency is protective against most common cancers. The immune cells also recognize 1,25(OH)$_2$D$_3$. This may explain why children who at 1 year of age had received 2000 IU of vitamin D a day decreased their risk of developing type I diabetes by 80%. Increasing intake of vitamin D and sun exposure has now been associated with decreased risk of developing multiple sclerosis, rheumatoid arthritis, and even Crohn's disease.

The relationship of vitamin D to cardiovascular disease is finally being understood. 1,25(OH)$_2$D inhibits the production of the blood pressure hormone renin. It also alters cardiomyocyte growth and modulates the inflammatory response of atherosclerosis (**Figure 7**).

Recommended Dietary Intake of Vitamin D

Vitamin D is very rare in foods naturally, with the exception of fatty fish and some fish liver oils. Although milk in the US is fortified with 400 IU of vitamin D/quart, several surveys during the past decade have demonstrated that approximately 80% of milk in the US contained less than 300 IU/quart. Fifty pecent of the milk samples contained less than 200 IU/quart and 15% had no detectable vitamin D. Some orange juice and other juice products are fortified with calcium and 100 IU of vitamin D$_3$/8 oz. Multivitamin preparations that contain vitamin D are a good source of vitamin D as are pharmaceutical preparations.

In 1997, the Institute of Medicine and the National Academy of Sciences reviewed the recommended dietary intake for several nutrients and vitamins including vitamin D. The recommended dietary allowance (RDA) was defined as the daily intake level that is sufficient to meet nutrient requirements for nearly all (97–98%) individuals in life-stage and gender group. The RDA was meant to apply to individuals and not groups. When sufficient scientific evidence was not available to calculate an estimated average requirement (EAR), i.e., a nutrient value that was estimated to meet the requirement defined by a specified indicator of adequacy in 50% of individuals in a life-stage and gender group, the Committee recommended using an adequate intake (AI). The AI is based on the observation of experimentally determined approximations of average nutrient intake by a defined population or subgroup that appears to sustain a defined nutritional state

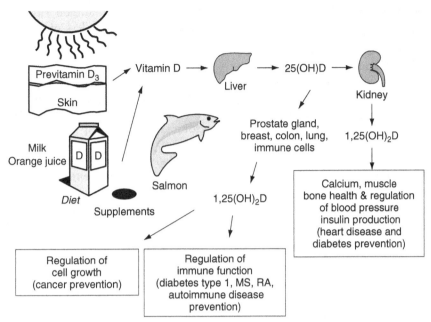

Figure 7 Photoproduction and sources of vitamin D. Vitamin D is metabolized in the liver to 25-hydroxyvitamin D [25(OH)D], which is responsible for maintaining calcium homeostasis. 25(OH)D is also converted to 1,25(OH)₂ D in a variety of other cells and tissues for the purpose of regulating cell growth, immune function, as well as a variety of other physiologic processes that are important for the prevention of many chronic diseases. MS, multiple sclerosis; RA, rheumatoid arthritis. (Copyright Michael F Holick (2004) Vitamin D: Importance in the prevention of cancers, type 1 diabetes, heart disease, and osteoporosis. *American Journal of Clinical Nutrition* **79**: 362–371, used with permission.)

such as normal circulation nutrient values or growth. Because sunlight played such an important role in providing humans with their vitamin D requirement and, therefore, was a variable that was difficult to quantify in most studies that were reviewed by the Committee, it was concluded that an AI rather than an RDA should be used for vitamin D (**Table 1**).

Adequate Intake for Ages 0–6 Months

It is well documented that human and cows' milk has very little vitamin D naturally. Human milk contains on average between 10 and 50 IU l⁻¹ (0.25–1.25 μg). This is dependent on the mother's exposure to sunlight and her vitamin D intake. Several studies have suggested that infant intakes of vitamin D of between 8.5

and 15 μg day⁻¹ would provide the maximum effect on their linear growth. A study in infants from Northern China (40–47 °N) found that vitamin D supplements of 2.5, 5, or 10 μg day⁻¹ resulted in 36, 29, and 2% of the infants being vitamin D deficient with 25(OH)D levels of less than 25 nmol l⁻¹ (10 ng ml⁻¹). None of the infants, however, had manifestations of rickets. Chinese infants from two southern cities (22 °N and 30 °N) maintained normal vitamin D status on as little as 2.5 μg day⁻¹ of vitamin D.

There was a seasonal variation of vitamin D status of infants when they were fed human milk only and did not receive vitamin D supplements; their 25(OH)D levels decreased in the winter due to less exposure to sunlight. However, this decrease did not occur in infants receiving a vitamin D supplement of 10 μg/day beginning at 3 weeks of age.

Therefore, based on the available literature, it was concluded that a minimum intake of 2.5 μg day⁻¹ of vitamin D was adequate to prevent rickets. However, at this intake and in the absence of sunlight, infants are at risk for developing vitamin D insufficiency; therefore, it was recommended that an AI of 5 μg day⁻¹ (200 IU) was prudent. 10 μg day⁻¹ (400 IU), the current amount in 1 l of standard infant formula or one quart of commercial cows' milk, was not considered to be excessive.

Table 1 Adequate Intake (AI) and Tolerable Upper Limit (UL) for Vitamin D

Age	AI μg (IU)/d	UL μg (IU)/d
0–6 m	5 (200 IU)	25 (1000 IU)
6 m–12 yr	5 (200 IU)	25 (1000 IU)
1 yr–18 yr	5 (200 IU)	50 (2000 IU)
19 yr–50 yr	5 (200 IU)	50 (2000 IU)
51 yr–70 yr	10 (400 IU)	50 (2000 IU)
71+ yr	15 (600 IU)	50 (2000 IU)

Adequate Intake for Ages 6–12 Months

Infants between 6 and 12 months of age who were fed human milk and exposed to an average of 35 min day^{-1} of sunshine had similar 25(OH)D concentrations at 1 year of age whether the infants received 400 IU of vitamin D or no vitamin D supplementation. However, in Norway, in the winter, older infants who received an average of 5 μg day^{-1} of vitamin D had normal 25(OH)D levels that were intermediate between those of infants studied at the end of the summer and formula-fed infants.

Therefore, in the absence of any sunlight exposure, an AI of 5 μg day^{-1} was recommended. However, an intake of 10 μg day^{-1} was not considered to be excessive.

Adequate Intake for Ages 1–18 Years

There are no studies in the scientific literature that systematically evaluated the influence of different amounts of vitamin D on either serum 25(OH)D or bone mineral content in this age group. Sunlight exposure is very important for this age group to obtain its required vitamin D. In South Africa, children aged 1–8 years of mixed race showed no evidence of vitamin D deficiency. A longitudinal study in Norway, where sun exposure was presumed to vary widely over a year, an intake of vitamin D of about 2.5 μg day^{-1} from fortified margarine in children aged 8–18 years was adequate to prevent vitamin D deficiency.

During puberty, there is a need to increase the efficiency of dietary calcium absorption in order to satisfy the rapid growth of the skeleton. As a result, there is an increase in the metabolism of 25(OH)D to 1,25(OH)$_2$D. Because the blood levels of 1,25(OH)$_2$D are approximately 1000 times less than 25(OH)D, this increase in metabolism does not appear to increase the requirement of vitamin D for either boys or girls between the ages of 8 and 18 years. An average daily intake of 2.5 μg day^{-1} prevented any evidence of vitamin D deficiency in Scandinavian children in this age group. However, intakes less than 2.5 μg day^{-1} in Turkish children aged 12–17 years resulted in a decrease in 25(OH)D levels consistent with vitamin D deficiency.

Therefore, based on the available literature, it appears that children between 1 and 18 years obtain most of their vitamin D from exposure to sunlight and do not normally need to ingest vitamin D. However, for children who live in far northern and southern latitudes, vitamin D supplementation may be necessary. An AI of 5 μg day^{-1} (200 IU) was recommended to maintain vitamin D sufficiency in this age group regardless of exposure to sunlight.

Adequate Intake for Ages 19–50 Years

There is only sparse literature regarding the role that sunlight and diet play in maintaining an adequate vitamin D status for men and women in this age group. This age group depends on sunlight for most of its vitamin D requirement. Regardless of exposure to sunlight, it was estimated that an AI of 5 μg day^{-1} is sufficient for preventing vitamin D deficiency in this age group.

Adequate Intake for Ages 51–70 Years

The Committee recommended a doubling of the dietary intake of vitamin D for this age group. This was based on several studies that demonstrated the importance of increasing dietary intakes of vitamin D to maximize bone health. An evaluation of 333 ambulatory Caucasian women (mean age 58 ± 6 years) found that serum PTH concentrations were elevated in the winter (between March and May) in women consuming less than 5.5 μg (220 IU) day^{-1} of vitamin D. There was no seasonal variation in serum PTH concentrations when vitamin D intakes were greater than 5.5 μg (220 IU) day^{-1}. When bone loss was evaluated between seasons in women (62 ± 0.5 years) who had a usual vitamin D intake of 2.5 μg day^{-1}, a dietary supplement of 10 μg day^{-1} decreased spinal and hip-bone density loss.

Thus, since this age group does not obtain as much of its vitamin D from exposure to sunlight, it is at more risk for developing vitamin D deficiency. Therefore, in the absence of exposure to sunlight, there appears to be an increased requirement for vitamin D in this age group and an AI of 10 μg (400 IU) day^{-1} was recommended. This is twice the previous RDA for this age group.

Adequate Intake for Ages Greater Than 70 Years

There was strong evidence-based literature that demonstrated a decrease in the circulating concentration of 25(OH)D, and an increase in the PTH level correlated with an increased risk of skeletal fractures in both the hip and spine in this age group. Studies in both men and women supplemented with 10–25 μg day^{-1} of vitamin D demonstrated reduced bone resorption, increased bone mineral content, and a decrease in vertebral and nonvertebral fractures. Therefore, because this age group is even less likely to receive an adequate amount of exposure to sunlight than adults aged 50–70 years and because they have a reduced capacity to produce vitamin D in their skin, it was recommended that men and women in this age group, regardless of exposure to sunlight, have an AI of 15 µg (600 IU) day^{-1}, which is three times the previous RDA for vitamin D for this age group.

Adequate Intake for Pregnancy and Lactation

Although there is an increase in the metabolism of 25(OH)D to 1,25(OH)$_2$D during the last trimester of pregnancy and during lactation there is nothing in the evidence-based literature to suggest that there is an increased vitamin D requirement for pregnant and lactating women. Therefore, it was recommended that the AI of vitamin D for pregnancy and lactation follow that recommended for their age group, i.e., 5 µg (200 IU)/day^{-1}. However, the 400 IU of vitamin D found in prenatal supplements was not considered to be excessive.

Healthy Vitamin D Intakes

Since the publication of these recommendations there have been a multitude of studies that suggest that the AIs for vitamin D are inadequate if there is no exposure to sunlight. In the absence of sunlight, children above 1 year and all adults need 1000 IU of vitamin D to maintain a healthy level of 25(OH)D (above 20 ng ml^{-1}) in their circulation.

Tolerable Upper Intake Levels and Vitamin D Intoxication

An excessive intake of vitamin D can lead to vitamin D intoxication. This is characterized by a marked increase in serum 25(OH)D that is usually greater than 375 nmol l^{-1} (150 ng ml^{-1}), and is associated with hypercalciuria and hypercalcemia. This can lead to soft tissue calcification and increased risk of kidney stones. The safe upper limit for vitamin D, as recommended by the Committee, is found in **Table 1**.

Vitamin D intoxication usually occurs when a person ingests more than 5000 IU of vitamin D daily for several months. A person does not need to be concerned about becoming vitamin D intoxicated if they take a multivitamin that contains 400 IU of vitamin D, drink a quart of milk that contains 400 IU of vitamin D, and are exposed to sunlight.

See also: **Calcium**. **Vitamin D**: Rickets and Osteomalacia.

Further Reading

Aksnes L and Aarskog D (1982) Plasma concentrations of vitamin D metabolites in puberty: effect of sexual maturation and implications for growth. *Journal of Clinical Endocrinology and Metabolism* 55: 94–101.

Apperly FL (1941) The relation of solar radiation to cancer mortality in North America. *Cancer Research* 1: 191–195.

Bouillon R, Okamura WH, and Norman AW (1995) Structure-function relationships in the vitamin D endocrine system. *Endocrine Reviews* 16: 200–257.

Chapuy MC, Arlot M, Duboeuf F *et al.* (1992) Vitamin D$_3$ and calcium to prevent hip fractures in elderly women. *New England Journal of Medicine* 327: 1637–1642.

Darwish H and DeLuca HF (1993) Vitamin D-regulated gene expression. *Critical Reviews in Eukaryotic Gene Expression* 3: 89–116.

DeLuca H (1988) The vitamin D story: A collaborative effort of basic science and clinical medicine. *Federal Proceedings of the American Society of Experimental Biology* 2: 224–236.

Fieser LD and Fieser M (1959) Vitamin D. In: Fieser LD and Fieser M (eds) *Steroids*, pp. 90–168. New York: Reinhold.

Grant WB (2002) An estimate of premature cancer mortality in the U.S. due to inadequate doses of solar ultraviolet-B radiation. *Cancer* 70: 2861–2869.

Heaney RP, Dowell MS, Hale CA, and Bendich A (2003) Calcium absorption varies within the reference range for serum 25-hydroxyvitamin D. *Journal of American College of Nutrition* 22(2): 142–146.

Holick MF (1994) Vitamin D: new horizons for the 21st century. *American Journal of Clinical Nutrition* 60: 619–630.

Holick MF (2003) Vitamin D: photobiology, metabolism, mechanism of action, and clinical application. In: Favus MJ (ed.) *Primer on the Metabolic Bone Diseases and Disorders of Mineral Metabolism*, 5th edn, pp. 129–137. Washington DC: American Society for Bone and Mineral Research.

Holick MF (2004) Vitamin D: Importance in the prevention of cancers, type 1 diabetes, heart disease, and osteoporosis. *American Journal of Clinical Nutrition* 79: 362–371.

Holick MF and Jenkins M (2004) *The UV Advantage* New York: iBooks.

Hypponen E, Laara E, Jarvelin M-R, and Virtanen SM (2001) Intake of vitamin D and risk of type 1 diabetes: a birth-cohort study. *Lancet* 358: 1500–1503.

Krall E, Sahyoun N, Tannenbaum S, Dallal G, and Dawson-Hughes B (1989) Effect of vitamin D intake on seasonal variations in parathyroid hormone secretion in postmenopausal women. *New England Journal of Medicine* 321: 1777–1783.

Luscombe CJ, Fryer AA, French ME, Liu S, Saxby MF, and Jones PW (2001) Exposure to ultraviolet radiation: association with susceptibility and age at presentation with prostate cancer. *Lancet* 192: 145–149.

Malabanan A, Veronikis IE, and Holick MF (1998) Redefining vitamin D insufficiency. *Lancet* 351: 805–806.

Markestad T and Elzouki AY (1991) Vitamin D deficiency rickets in northern Europe and Libya. In: Glorieux FH (ed.) *Rickets Nestle Nutrition Workshop Series*, vol. 21, pp. 203–213. New York: Raven Press.

Specker BL, Valanis B, Hertzberg V, Edwards N, and Tsang (1985) Sunshine exposure and serum 25-hydroxyvitamin D concentrations in exclusively breast-fed infants. *Journal of Pediatrics* 107: 372–376.

Rickets and Osteomalacia

J J B Anderson, University of North Carolina, Chapel Hill, NC, USA

Introduction

Rickets and osteomalacia, diseases of impaired mineralization of bone tissue that occur among infants/young children or during adulthood, result from nutritional deficiencies of vitamin D (cholecalciferol) and/or calcium. Rickets has more severe deformities of bones because of the continued growth of the skeleton, but osteomalacia, especially less severe disease, commonly coexists with osteoporosis in many older adults. The latter comorbidities have been increasing, at least in part, as a result of both low dietary intakes of vitamin D and calcium and insufficient skin production of vitamin D because of limited skin exposure to ultraviolet (UV) light. This problem is likely to be more widespread than currently acknowledged because of behavioral changes in technologically advanced societies.

The last few years have witnessed a resurgence of rickets and osteomalacia in the US and possibly in other technologically advanced nations. The prevalence of rickets in the US has occurred primarily among young children of color, i.e., African-Americans and Hispanics, after cessation of breast-feeding and the failure to provide adequate amounts of vitamin D-fortified milk. The prevalence of osteomalacia has been suspected to be increasing because of low serum 25-hydroxycholecalciferol (25HCC) measurements in several studies of adults. In addition, new recommendations for healthy 25-hydroxyvitamin D (25(OH)D$_3$) concentrations have emerged from interpretation of the results of studies assessing the sufficiency of vitamin D to meet requirements across the life cycle.

The terminology of the vitamin D metabolites has not changed, and relatively little new resulted from basic research on vitamin D or cholecalciferol skin biosynthesis and subsequent biotransformations in the liver and kidney (**Figure 1**). Understandings of the role of the hormonal form of vitamin D, 1,25-dihydroxyvitamin D (1,25(OH)$_2$D$_3$), in intestinal absorbing cells have been expanded. In addition, new information suggests that the consumption of dietary calcium at adequate levels may reduce the critical need for vitamin D for the maintenance of serum calcium concentration. New information is also emerging on the role of vitamin D in patients with chronic renal failure and in the prevention of colon cancer.

This article reviews vitamin D status and highlights new research findings on vitamin D.

Dietary Vitamin D Intakes and Low Vitamin D Status in the US

Vitamin D intakes have not been assessed in national surveys and only rarely in research investigations involving smaller sample sizes. The few

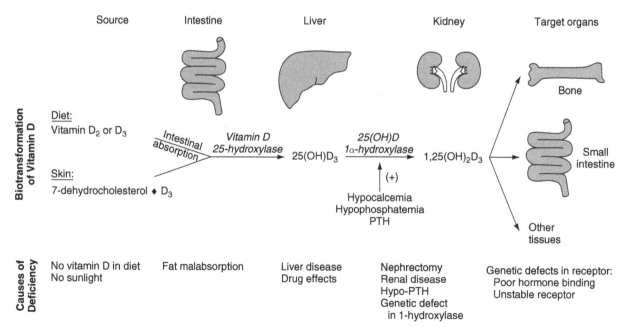

Figure 1   Causes of vitamin D deficiency. PTH, parathyroid hormone.

studies that have estimated vitamin D intakes typically find them to be below recommended amounts, especially among the elderly and, more recently, among adults. In the US, at least, most experts think that both intakes are too low and exposures of skin to sunlight are inadequate.

Role of the Diet in Providing Vitamin D

The few sources of vitamin D consumed in the diets of North Americans are fortified milks, fortified ready-to-eat breakfast cereals, and fish. For infants and young children who develop rickets, it has been established that they consume little milk and fish, but some cereals. No supplements containing calcium and vitamin D are ingested. For adults and the elderly, similar low consumption patterns of vitamin D-rich foods exist. Therefore, evidence strongly supports low intake of vitamin D as a major determinant of rickets and osteomalacia.

Role of Skin Biosynthesis of Vitamin D

The other major determinant is poor skin exposure to sunlight, mainly to UV-B that is responsible for the conversion of 7-dehydrocholesterol to $25(OH)D_3$ in the dermis layer of the skin. In the US, inadequate exposure has become a major contributor over the last few decades because of concerns about skin cancer and because of increased indoor activities, including television and computers. (This poor dietary consumption and poor skin production of vitamin D seems to be paralleling the increase in overweight.) Because it is even more difficult to assess skin exposure for vitamin D synthesis, it has been extremely difficult to estimate with accuracy the additional need for dietary vitamin D. Seasonal variations yield wide swings or oscillations in skin production, depending on the position of the sun. For example, in the northern hemisphere, the highest skin production rates occur in the late spring, summer, and early autumn months (May to October), whereas in the southern hemisphere, November to April are the months of the highest vitamin D production. Living near the equator extends these periods of optimal production. It is the winter months when low or even zero skin production occurs that are most problematic for the development of rickets or osteomalcia and, in the elderly, osteoporosis.

Vitamin D Recommendations

The current recommendations for consumption of vitamin D in the US are given in **Table 1**. The recommendations are defined as adequate intakes

Table 1 Recommended adequate intakes (AIs) of vitamin D in the US

Life stage group	Age, years	AI, mcg/day
Infants and Children	0–8	5
Males, Females	9–50	5
	51–70	10
	>70	15
Pregnancy	–	5
Lactation	–	5

From: Institute of Medicine, Food and Nutrition Board (1997) *Dietary Reference Intakes for Calcium, Phosphorus, Magnesium, Vitamin D, and Fluoride.* Washington, DC: National Academy Press.

(AIs) rather than as recommended dietary allowances (RDAs) because insufficient data have been accumulated to determine estimated average requirements (EARs) across the life cycle. The AIs listed in **Table 1** are totally independent of skin production of vitamin D. Because of the uncertainty of knowing the amount of endogenous vitamin D, it is very difficult to determine, with accuracy, the amounts needed from the diet (see below).

Primary Causes and Abnormalities of Rickets and Osteomalacia

The primary cause of rickets and osteomalacia is vitamin D deficiency and the clinical characteristics of these diseases depend on age at onset. The biochemical patterns of too low a serum concentration of $25(OH)D_3$, however, remain quite similar (**Table 2**) even though the structural effects on the skeleton differ. One common microscopic feature of the skeleton is that both rickets and osteomalacia

Table 2 Characteristic clinical features and blood serum measurements in rickets and osteomalacia

Age	Clinical features	Blood serum measurements
Children	Skeletal deformations (rickets) Impaired growth Undermineralized bone	Hypocalcemia Hypophosphatemia Secondary hyperparathyroidism Low 25-hydroxyvitamin D Elevated alkaline phosphatase
Adults	Undermineralized bone (osteomalacia) Fractures	Hypocalcemia Hypophosphatemia Low 25-hydroxyvitamin D Elevated alkaline phosphatase Elevated osteocalcin[a]

[a]This finding has not been consistently reported.

have unmineralized bone matrix (osteoid), also known as widened osteoid seams.

In rare cases, e.g., in central Nigeria, rickets may occur despite elevated serum $25(OH)D_3$ concentrations. The rickets in these cases results from severely inadequate dietary calcium. It is likely that most cases of rickets result from a combination of insufficient skin biosynthesis and inadequate dietary intake of vitamin D.

Other biochemical changes include depressed serum concentrations of calcium and inorganic phosphate, largely because of insufficient intestinal absorption directly relating to too little of these ions in the usual diet. Serum alkaline phosphatase, especially bone-specific alkaline phosphatase, is elevated because of osteoblastic cell overproduction when these cells attempt to form new bone tissue.

Radiographic changes, the primary diagnostic evidence for many years, show widened growth plates of the long bones and reduced bone density (translucence) in rickets. In osteomalacia, unmineralization is evident and pseudofractures may be visible in nonweight-bearing bones.

Secondary Causes and Abnormalities of Rickets and Osteomalacia

The secondary causes of rickets and osteomalacia that result from vitamin D deficiency are illustrated in **Figure 1**. For example, in liver disease, serum concentrations of $25(OH)D_3$ are invariably too low, and in renal disease too little of the hormonal form of vitamin D, $1,25(OH)_2D_3$, is produced. Other causes relate to reduced cell receptor responsiveness to the hormone because of genetic mutations and, hence, inappropriate adaptations that normally contribute to conservation of calcium and/or phosphate ions.

Public Health Consequences of Vitamin D Deficiency

Despite the earlier belief that these classical deficiency diseases had been eliminated, the surprising increase in incidence of rickets and osteomalacia places the burden on society to be ever more vigilant in assessing for vitamin D deficits. Two obvious explanations exist for the rise in vitamin D deficiency in the US: reduced consumption of vitamin D-fortified milks and reduced skin exposures to sunlight because of greater indoor activities. The deficit in vitamin D has possibly even greater consequences as the average age at death is extending in our populations. Low vitamin D intakes in later life, often

coexisting with low dietary calcium, may increase the risk of osteoporotic fractures.

Supplements of vitamin D (400 IU or greater) are recommended for the elderly by health professionals in order to ensure adequate intakes, but even higher amounts are considered safe. The tolerable upper level of safety (UL) established in the US by the Institute of Medicine has been set at $50\,mg\,day^{-1}$ (equivalent to $2000\,IU\,day^{-1}$). Supplemental vitamin D becomes increasingly important as skin biosynthesis capability declines with age. Oral capsules of vitamin D containing up to 100 000 IU have been found to be safe and effective in reducing fractures. An alternative approach is injection of a depot of vitamin D ($\sim$200 000 IU) in the late autumn for slow release over the winter months when sunlight, especially UV-B, is limited or unavailable.

Rising Prevalence of Rickets

The increase in rickets in the US is occurring primarily in African-American and Hispanic children who have gone off breast-feeding and are not getting sufficient calcium and vitamin D in their diets. This problem has been more common in the southern US despite greater availability of sunlight. In large part, rickets is an educational issue that requires input from both medical and public health professionals.

Rising Prevalence of Osteomalacia

The increase in low serum $25(OH)D_3$ found in so-called ordinary adults in a hospital survey of surgical patients in Massachusetts opened the eyes of health authorities who did not expect to find such low blood concentrations, which indicate future osteomalacia and also osteoporosis. This evidence suggests that many adults in the US are not consuming adequate amounts of vitamin D and calcium in their usual patterns of food selection and that supplementation of these two nutrients is probably inadequate among adults. Low intakes among the elderly result from the same type of eating pattern, but typically with even lower caloric consumption (see below).

Life Cycle Changes in Vitamin D Production and Metabolism

Production of vitamin D by the skin typically declines during late adulthood or the early elderly period because of changes in the skin *per se*, i.e., reduction in thickness, reduction in circulating 7-dehydrocholesterol, and decline in the rate of conversion of 7-dehydrocholesterol to cholecalciferol. When these physiological decrements are combined with less direct exposure to sun by the elderly, even in Florida, they have little opportunity to make the vitamin in their skin. Sun-screens and broad-brimmed hats and other protective clothing complete this scenario, which is aimed at preventing skin cancer.

Special Populations at Risk of Low Vitamin D Intakes and Low Status

Several at-risk subpopulations for poor vitamin D status have been identified. Except for migrant populations, these groups have already been mentioned previously.

The Elderly

Elderly individuals prefer to stay indoors and many are actually 'shut-ins' who have little opportunity for direct sun exposure (UV-B does not penetrate glass windows in rooms or solaria). The shut-ins are most likely to be deficient in vitamin D and calcium and at increased risk for fractures of the hip, especially with increasing age. They need supplementation on a daily basis with a calcium salt ($\sim$1000 mg of elemental calcium) plus vitamin D (400 IU or more) to counter not only hypovitaminosis D but also secondary hyperparathyroidism and possibly osteoporosis. Two large prospective trials have demonstrated efficacy of such therapy in reducing hip and other nonverteabral fractures.

Vegetarians

Vegans are at risk of low serum 25(OH)D$_3$ and the pathologic changes mentioned above for the elderly unless they consume a supplement of vitamin D and calcium because plant foods are typically low in each nutrient. Fortification of plant foods, such as of soy milk, may overcome this concern.

Long-Term Breast-Fed Infants and Young Children of Dark Skin

Although breast-feeding is strongly recommended and lauded, the switching of infants from breast-milk to other beverages does not always include cows' milk or other calcium-rich drinks. In the southern US, this switching has led to a modest epidemic of rickets, which should not occur with our established knowledge about causation. Dark pigmentation reduces the efficiency of the skin to produce vitamin D and because many children with such skin coloration do not tolerate milk (lactose) well, they consume too little vitamin D and calcium. Supplementation and/or alternate food sources should easily correct these nutrient deficits.

Migrant Populations

Migration of dark-skinned people, especially Muslims, from the Middle East and other Asian nations to the UK and other Northern European nations has led to decreased skin production of vitamin D, especially in the winter months, and to reported cases of rickets and osteomalacia. Cultural practices, i.e., limited food selections and clothing that covers the bodies of women and children, contribute to the etiology of these diseases. Supplementation with calcium and vitamin D should prove effective in promoting bone health of affected individuals.

Excessive Consumption of Vitamin D and Toxic Effects

Because the hormonal form of vitamin D, 1,25DHCC, acts on the DNA in the genome, high intakes or excessive drug dosages of the vitamin lead to synthetic overexpression of proteins that contribute to toxic effects. In recent years, the amounts of vitamin D needed to cause toxic effects has been found to be considerably higher than previously thought; but caution is needed via monitoring of serum 25HCC to ensure that blood concentrations do not get too high. Concern is expressed here that excessive treatment of those with rickets or osteomalacia with high doses of vitamin D may result in toxicity.

Summary

The continuing discovery of low serum 25(OH)D$_3$ concentrations among adults suggests that under-recognition of osteomalacia among adults and the elderly exists in the US and possibly in other technologically advanced nations. The hidden nature of the disease has resulted from poor diagnostic criteria; new criteria with lower cut-off points are under review. The surprising resurgence of rickets in the southern US has resulted from too little guidance by health professionals, poor nutrition knowledge of mothers, or other aspects, such as poverty. Correction of both rickets and osteomalacia can be simply achieved with vitamin D and calcium supplements and increased numbers of servings of calcium-rich foods. Public health agencies need to become more active in this regard.

See also: **Calcium**. **Vegetarian Diets**. **Vitamin D**: Physiology, Dietary Sources and Requirements.

Further Reading

Anderson JJB (1999) Plant-based diets and bone health: nutritional implications. *American Journal of Clinical Nutrition* 70(supplement): 539S–542S.

Chapuy MC, Arlot ME, Delmas PD, and Meunier PJ (1994) Effect of calcium and cholecalciferol treatment for three years on hip fractures in elderly women. *British Medical Journal* 308: 1081–1082.

Chapuy MC, Arlot ME, Duboeuf F *et al.* (1992) Vitamin D3 and calcium to prevent hip fractures in elderly women. *New England Journal of Medicine* 327: 1637–1642.

Chapuy MC, Pamphile R, Paris E *et al.* (2002) Combined calcium and vitamin D3 supplementation in elderly women: confirmation of reversal of secondary hyperparathyroidism and hip fracture risk: The Decalyos II Stusy. *Osteoporosis International* 13: 257–264.

Cheng S, Tylavsky F, Kroger H *et al.* (2003) Association of low 25-hydroxyvitamin D concentrations with elevated parathyroid hormone concentrations and low cortical bone density in early pubertal and prepubertal Finnish girls. *American Journal of Clinical Nutrition* 78: 485–492.

Dawson-Hughes B, Harris SS, and Dallal GE (1997) Plasma calcidiol, season, and serum parathyroid hormone concentrations in healthy elderly men and women. *American Journal of Clinical Nutrition* 65: 65–71.

Delucia MC, Mitnick ME, and Carpenter TO (2003) Nutritional rickets with normal circulating 25-hydroxyvitamin D: a call for reexamining the role of dietary calcium intake in North American infants. *Journal of Clinical Endocrinology and Metabolism* 88: 3539–3545.

Gartner LM and Greer FR (2003) Prevention of rickets and vitamin D deficiency; new guidelines for vitamin D intake. *Pediatrics* 111: 908–910.

Gloth FM III, Gundberg CM, Hollis BW *et al.* (1995) Vitamin D deficiency in homebound elderly persons. *Journal of the American Medical Association* 274: 1683–1686.

Heaney RP (1999) Lessons for nutritional science from vitamin D. *American Journal of Clinical Nutrition* 69: 825–826.

Heaney RP, Davies KM, Chen TC *et al.* (2003) Human serum 25-hydroxycholecalciferol response to extended oral dosing with cholecalciferol. *American Journal of Clinical Nutrition* 77: 204–210.

Henry A and Bowyer L (2003) Fracture of the neck of the femur and osteomalacia in pregnancy. *BJOG: An International Journal of Obstetrics and Gynaecology* 110: 329–330.

Holick MF (1995) Vitamin D and bone health. *Journal of Nutrition* 126: 1159S–1164S.

Holick MF (2001) Sunlight "D"ilemma: risk of skin cancer or bone disease and muscle weakness. *Lancet* 357: 4–6.

Institute of Medicine, Food and Nutrition Board (1997) *Dietary Reference Intakes for Calcium, Phosphorus, Magnesium, Vitamin D, and Fluoride.* Washington, DC: National Academy Press.

Jacques PF, Felson DT, Tucker KL *et al.* (1997) Plasma 25-hydroxyvitamin D and its determinants in an elderly population. *American Journal of Clinical Nutrition* 66: 929–936.

Kreiter SR, Schwartz RP, Kirkman HN Jr *et al.* (2000) Nutritional rickets in African American breast-fed infants. *Journal of Pediatrics* 137: 153–157.

Lamberg-Allardt C, Karkkainen M, Seppanen R, and Bistrom H (1993) Low serum 25-hydroxyvitamin D concentrations and secondary hyperparathyroidism in middle-aged white strict vegetarians. *American Journal of Clinical Nutrition* 58: 684–689.

Norman AW (2001) Vitamin D. In: Bowman BA and Russell RM (eds.) *Present Knowledge in Nutrition*, 8th edn, pp. 146–155. Washington DC: ILSI Press.

Oginni LM, Sharp CA, Worsfold M *et al.* (1999) Healing of rickets after calcium supplementation. *Lancet* 353: 296–297.

Okonofua F, Gill DS, Alabi ZO *et al.* (1991) Rickets in Nigerian children: a consequence of calcium malnutrition. *Metabolism* 40: 209–213.

Panunzio MF, Pisano A, Telesfor P, and Tomaiuolo P (2003) Diet can increase 25-hydroxyvitamin-D3 plasma levels in the elderly: a dietary intervention trial. *Nutrition Research* 23: 1177–1181.

Thomas MK, Lloyd-Jones DM, Thadani RM *et al.* (1998) Hypovitaminosis D in medical inpatients. *New England Journal of Medicine* 338: 777–783.

Trivedi DP, Doll R, and Khaw KT (2003) Effect of four monthly oral vitamin D3 (cholecalciferol) supplementation on fractures and mortality in men and women living in the community: randomized double blind controlled trial. *British Medical Journal* 326: 469–474.

Utiger RD (1998) The need for more vitamin D. *New England Journal of Medicine* 338: 828–829.

Vieth R, Chan PCR, and MacFarlane GD (2001) Efficacy and safety of vitamin D3 input exceeding the lowest observed adverse effect concentration. *American Journal of Clinical Nutrition* 73: 288–294.

Webb AR, Kline L, and Holick MF (1988) Influence of season and latitude on the cutaneous synthesis of vitamin D3: exposure to winter sunlight in Boston and Edmonton will not promote vitamin D3 synthesis in human skin. *Journal of Clinical Endocrinology and Metabolism* 67: 373–378.

VITAMIN E

Contents
Metabolism and Requirements
Physiology and Health Effects

Metabolism and Requirements

M G Traber, Oregon State University, Corvallis, OR, USA

Introduction

Vitamin E is the most potent fat-soluble antioxidant in human plasma. Although vitamin E was first discovered in 1922, its metabolic function remains an enigma. There are eight different molecular forms with vitamin E antioxidant activity, yet the body preferentially retains α-tocopherol. This preference for α-tocopherol has led the Food and Nutrition Board in its 2000 Dietary Reference Intakes (DRIs) for vitamin E to recommend that only α-tocopherol, not the other forms, meets human requirements for vitamin E. Moreover, only α-tocopherol is recognized by the hepatic α-tocopherol transfer protein (α-TTP). This protein regulates plasma α-tocopherol concentrations and genetic abnormalities in the protein (or its absence) leads to vitamin E deficiency in humans.

General Description and Scientific Name

Dietary components with vitamin E antioxidant activity include α-, β-, γ-, and δ-tocopherols and α-, β-, γ-, and δ-tocotrienols. These compounds all have a chromanol ring with a phytyl tail (tocopherols) or an unsaturated tail (tocotrienols) (**Figure 1**) and vary in the number of methyl groups on the chromanol ring: α-tocopherol or α-tocotrienol has three methyl groups, β- or γ- have two, and δ- tocopherol and δ-tocotrienol have one.

The naturally occurring form of α-tocopherol is called RRR-α-tocopherol; on labels it is called d-α-tocopherol and it is more formally known as 2,5,7,8-tetramethyl-$2R$-($4'R$,$8'R$,12 trimethyltridecyl)-6-chromanol. At positions 2, 4', and 8'of α-tocopherol are chiral carbon centers that are in the R-conformation in naturally occurring α-tocopherol, but theoretically can take on either the R- or the S-conformation. Position 2 is the most important for biologic activity. Therefore, the DRIs for vitamin E are given in milligrams of $2R$-α-tocopherol (**Table 1** see below for discussion).

The chemical synthesis of α-tocopherol results in an equal mixture of eight different stereoisomers (RRR, RSR, RRS, RSS, SRR, SSR, SRS, SSS) or, more formally, 2,5,7,8-tetramethyl-$2RS$-($4'RS$,$8'RS$,12 trimethyltridecyl)-6-chromanol. To indicate that synthetic α-tocopherol is a racemic mixture, it is called all-rac-α-tocopherol, or on labels, dl-α-tocopherol. The first letter of the three-letter combination is the 2 position; therefore, only half of the synthetic α-tocopherol is in the 'active' $2R$-α-tocopherol conformation. **Table 2** lists the factors used to convert international units (IU) to milligrams. For example, if a vitamin E supplement is labeled 400 IU and it is dl-α-tocopheryl acetate, then 400 times 0.45 equals 180 mg $2R$-α-tocopherol, but if it is labeled d-α-tocopheryl acetate, then 400 times 0.67 equals 268 mg $2R$-α-tocopherol.

Vitamin E Supplements

Most vitamin E supplements and food fortificants contain all rac-α-tocopherol, but can contain mixtures of tocopherols or tocotrienols. Supplements often are sold as esters, which protect α-tocopherol from oxidation. These can be acetates, succinates, or nicotinates of α-tocopherol. Either the natural stereoisomer (RRR-α-tocopherol) or the synthetic (all rac-α-tocopherol) can be sold as an ester, e.g., d- or dl-α-tocopheryl acetate, respectively.

Dietary Vitamin E

Vitamin E can be readily obtained from food. Generally, the richest sources are vegetable oils. Wheat germ oil, safflower oil, and sunflower oil contain predominantly α-tocopherol, while soy and corn oils contain predominantly γ-tocopherol. All of these oils are polyunsaturated. Good sources of monounsaturated oils, such as olive or canola oils, also contain predominantly α-tocopherol. Whole grains and nuts are also good sources of vitamin E. Fruits and vegetables, although rich in water-soluble antioxidants, are not good sources of vitamin E.

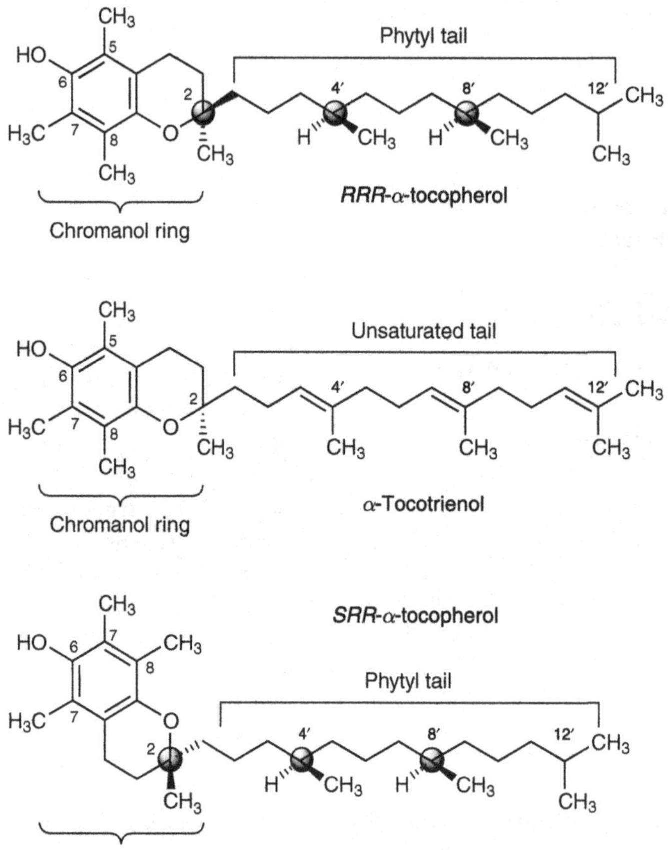

Figure 1 Structures of *RRR*-α-tocopherol, α-tocotrienol, and *SRR*-α-tocopherol.

Table 1 Estimated average requirements (EARs), recommended dietary allowances (RDAs), and average intakes (AIs) ($mg\,day^{-1}$) for α-tocopherol in adults and children

Lifestage	EAR	RDA	AI
0–6 months			4
7–12 months			6
1–3 years	5	6	
4–8 years	6	7	
9–13 years	9	11	
14–18 years	12	15	
Adult (male or female)	12	15	
Pregnant	12	15	
Lactation	16	19	

Adapted from Food and Nutrition Board and Institute of Medicine (2000) *Dietary Reference Intakes for Vitamin C, Vitamin E, Selenium, and Carotenoids*. Washington, DC: National Academy Press.

Table 2 Factors to convert international units (IU) of vitamin E to milligrams of 2*R*-α-tocopherol

	mg/IU[a]
***all rac*-α-Tocopherol and esters**	
dl-α-Tocopheryl acetate	0.45
dl-α-Tocopheryl succinate	0.45
dl-α-Tocopherol	0.45
***RRR*-α-Tocopherol and esters**	
d-α-Tocopheryl acetate	0.67
d-α-Tocopheryl succinate	0.67
d-α-Tocopherol	0.67

[a]Multiply the IU in foods or supplements times the indicated factor to obtain the milligrams of active vitamin E.
Adapted from Food and Nutrition Board and Institute of Medicine (2000) *Dietary Reference Intakes for Vitamin C, Vitamin E, Selenium, and Carotenoids*. Washington, DC: National Academy Press.

α-Tocopherol equivalents

It is often assumed for the purpose of calculating vitamin E intakes from food in α-tocopherol equivalents (α-TEs) that γ-tocopherol can substitute for α-tocopherol with an efficiency of 10%. However, functionally γ-tocopherol is not equivalent to α-tocopherol and some caution should be used in applying α-TEs to estimates of α-tocopherol intakes when corn or soybean oils (hydrogenated vegetable oils) represent the major oils present in foods. These oils have high γ-tocopherol contents and if food tables reporting α-TEs are used to estimate dietary α-tocopherol, α-tocopherol intakes are overestimated. α-TEs are no longer recommended in the Food and Nutrition Board of the Institute of Medicine, National Academy of Sciences 2000 DRIs; only milligrams of α-tocopherol and 2R-α-tocopherol (for synthetic vitamin E) should be included in estimates of vitamin E intakes.

Vitamin E Actions and Metabolism

Antioxidant Activity

Vitamin E is the most potent, lipid-soluble antioxidant in human plasma and tissues. Thus, vitamin E protects polyunsaturated fatty acids within membrane phospholipids and plasma lipoproteins. When a peroxyl radical forms in a membrane, it is 1000 times more likely to attack a vitamin E molecule than a polyunsaturated fatty acid (**Figure 2**). The hydroxyl group on the chromanol ring of vitamin E reacts with the peroxyl radical to form the corresponding lipid hydroperoxide and tocopheroxyl radical. Thus, vitamin E acts as a chain-breaking antioxidant, preventing further auto-oxidation of lipids.

The tocopheroxyl radical has a number of possible fates. It can react with another radical to form nonreactive products. Alternatively, it can be further oxidized to the tocopheryl quinone, a two-electron oxidation product. Another possibility is 'vitamin E recycling,' where the tocopheroxyl radical is restored to its unoxidized form by other antioxidants such as vitamin C, ubiquinol, or thiols, such as glutathione. This process will deplete these other antioxidants. For this reason, it is important to maintain a good intake of other dietary antioxidants.

Biologic Activity

Biologic activity is a term that has been used historically to indicate a disconnection between vitamin E antioxidant activities and *in vivo* activities.

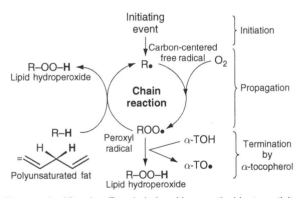

Figure 2 Vitamin E: chain-breaking antioxidant activity. Adapted from Burton GW and Traber MG (1990) Vitamin E: antioxidant activity, biokinetics, and bioavailability. *Annu Rev Nutr* **10**: 357–382.

Observations in rodent experiments carried out in the 1930s formed the basis for determining the 'biologic activity' of vitamin E. Although the various vitamin E forms had somewhat similar structures and antioxidant activities, they differed in their abilities to prevent or reverse specific vitamin E deficiency symptoms (e.g., fetal resorption, muscular dystrophy, and encephalomalacia). α-Tocopherol with three methyl groups and a free hydroxyl group on the chromanol ring with the phytyl tail meeting the ring in the R-orientation (**Figure 1**) had the highest biological activity. This specific structural requirement for biological, but not chemical, activity is now known to be dependent upon the hepatic α-tocopherol transfer protein (α-TTP), as discussed below. α-TTP maintains plasma and, indirectly, tissue α-tocopherol concentrations.

Molecular Function

In addition to antioxidant activity, there are specific α-tocopherol-dependent functions that normalize cellular functions in a variety of cells. α-Tocopherol plays a critical role through its ability to inhibit the activity of protein kinase C, a central player in many signal transduction pathways. Specifically, it modulates pathways of platelet aggregation, endothelial cell nitric oxide production, monocyte/macrophage superoxide production, and smooth muscle cell proliferation. Regulation of adhesion molecule expression and inflammatory cell cytokine production by α-tocopherol has also been reported. However, most of the information in this area has been obtained from *in vitro* studies. More studies in humans are needed to relate α-tocopherol intakes and tissue concentrations to optimal tissue responses.

Vitamin E metabolism

α- and γ-tocopherols, as well as α-and γ-tocotrienols, are metabolized to α- and γ-CEHCs (2,5,7,8-tetramethyl-and 2,7,8-trimethyl-2-(2′ carboxyethyl)-6-hydroxychromans), respectively. About 1% of a dose of α-tocopherol or tocotrienol, or 5% of a dose of γ-tocopherol or tocotrienol is excreted in the urine as CEHCs. The importance of vitamin E metabolism in the regulation of vitamin E status is unknown.

Recommended Intake Levels

In 2000, the Food and Nutrition Board of the Institute of Medicine, National Academy of Sciences published the DRIs for vitamin C, vitamin E, selenium, and the carotenoids. Their recommendations for vitamin E appear in **Table 1**.

The requirements for vitamin E intakes are based primarily on long-term (5–7 years) depletion and repletion studies in humans. Serum α-tocopherol concentrations and corresponding hydrogen peroxide-induced erythrocyte hemolysis were determined at various intervals. Serum concentrations necessary to prevent *in vitro* erythrocyte hemolysis in response known levels of vitamin E intake in subjects who had undergone experimentally induced vitamin E deficiency were used to determine estimated average requirements (EARs) for vitamin E. The recommended dietary allowances (RDAs) are levels that represent the daily α-tocopherol intakes required to ensure adequate nutrition in 95–97.5% of the population and are an overestimation of the level needed for most people in any given group.

Vitamin E Units

According to the US Pharmacopoeia (USP), 1 IU of vitamin E equals 1 mg *all rac* α-tocopheryl acetate, 0.67 mg *RRR*-α-tocopherol, or 0.74 mg *RRR*-α-tocopheryl acetate. These conversions were estimated on the relative 'biologic activities' of the various forms when tested in the rat assay for vitamin E deficiency, the fetal resorption assay. These USP IUs are currently used in labeling vitamin E supplements and food fortificants. It should be noted that the current RDA does not use vitamin E USP units but rather the recommendation for adults is set at 15 mg of *RRR*-α-tocopherol or 2R-α-tocopherols. Most foods contain *RRR*-α-tocopherol naturally, but foods that have been fortified with vitamin E contain the synthetic form, e.g., fortified breakfast cereals. If the amount of vitamin E on the label is given in international units, then this must be multiplied by the factors given in **Table 2** to obtain the amount of 2R-β-tocopherol.

Overdosage

In 2000 the Food and Nutrition Board of the Institute of Medicine, National Academy of Sciences recommended 1000 mg as an upper limit (UL) of all forms of α-tocopherol in supplements taken by adults 19 years and older, including pregnant and lactating women. ULs were set for children and adolescents by adjusting the adult limit on the basis of relative body weight. **Table 3** gives the α-tocopherol UL by age group. No UL was set for infants due to lack of adequate data. In 2000 the Food and Nutrition Board did recommend that food be the only source of vitamin E for infants. However, a UL of 21 mg day^{-1} was suggested for premature infants with birth weights of 1.5 kg, based on the adult UL.

The vitamin E UL was set for supplements because it is almost impossible to consume enough α-tocopherol-containing foods to achieve a daily 1000 mg intake for prolonged periods of time. The

Table 3 Upper limits (UL) for α-tocopherol intakes

Age (years)	UL (mg day^{-1})
1–3	200
4–8	300
9–13	600
14–18	800
>19	1000

Adapted from Food and Nutrition Board and Institute of Medicine (2000) *Dietary Reference Intakes for Vitamin C, Vitamin E, Selenium, and Carotenoids.* Washington, DC: National Academy Press.

UL was defined for all forms of α-tocopherol, not just the 2R forms, because all of the forms in *all rac*-α-tocopherol are absorbed and delivered to the liver. The appropriate conversion factors are different from those shown in **Table 2**, and necessary to estimate the UL for supplements containing either *RRR*- or *all rac*-α-tocopherol supplements. The ULs given in IU are shown in **Table 4**. The UL for *RRR*-α-tocopherol is apparently higher because each capsule contains less α-tocopherol than those containing *all rac*-α-tocopherol.

Precautions and Adverse Reactions

High vitamin E intakes are associated with an increased tendency to bleed. It is not known if this is a result of decreased platelet aggregation caused by an inhibition of protein kinase C by α-tocopherol, some other platelet-related mechanism, or decreased clotting due to a vitamin K and E interaction causing abnormal blood clotting.

Individuals who are deficient in vitamin K or who are on anticoagulant therapy are at increased risk of uncontrolled bleeding. Patients on anticoagulant therapy should be monitored when taking vitamin E supplements to ensure adequate vitamin K intakes.

Table 4 Upper limits (UL) reported in IU for α-tocopherol-containing supplements

	Number of IU that equal the UL
all rac-α-Tocopherol and esters	
dl-α-Tocopheryl acetate	1100
dl-α-Tocopheryl succinate	1100
dl-α-Tocopherol	1100
RRR-α-Tocopherol and esters	
d-α-Tocopheryl acetate	1500
d-α-Tocopheryl succinate	1500
d-α-Tocopherol	1500

Adapted from Food and Nutrition Board and Institute of Medicine (2000) *Dietary Reference Intakes for Vitamin C, Vitamin E, Selenium, and Carotenoids.* Washington, DC: National Academy Press.

Adverse Effects of Drugs on Vitamin E Status

Drugs intended to promote weight loss by impairing fat absorption, such as Orlistat or sucrose polyester, can also impair vitamin E and other fat-soluble vitamin absorption. Therefore, multivitamin supplementation is recommended with these drugs. Vitamin supplements should be taken with meals at times other than when these drugs are taken to allow adequate absorption of the fat-soluble vitamins.

Vitamin E Bioavailability

Absorption and Plasma Transport

Intestinal absorption of vitamin E is dependent upon normal processes of fat absorption. Specifically, both biliary and pancreatic secretions are necessary for solubilization of vitamin E in mixed micelles containing bile acids, fatty acids, and monoglycerides (**Figure 3**). α-Tocopheryl acetates (or other esters) from vitamin E supplements are hydrolyzed by pancreatic esterases to α-tocopherol prior to absorption. Following micellar uptake by enterocytes, vitamin E is incorporated into chylomicrons and secreted into the lymph. Once in the circulation, chylomicron triglycerides are hydrolyzed by lipoprotein lipase. During chylomicron catabolism in the circulation, vitamin E is nonspecifically transferred both to tissues and to other circulating lipoproteins.

It is not until the vitamin E-containing chylomicrons reach the liver that discrimination between the various dietary vitamin E forms occurs. The hepatic α-TTP preferentially facilitates secretion of α-tocopherol, specifically $2R$-α-tocopherols, and not other tocopherols or tocotrienols from the liver into the plasma in very low-density lipoproteins (VLDLs). In the circulation, VLDLs are catabolized to low-density lipoproteins (LDL are also known as the 'bad cholesterol' because high LDL levels are associated with increased risk of heart disease). During this lipolytic process, all of the circulating lipoproteins become enriched with α-tocopherol.

There is no evidence that vitamin E is transported in the plasma by a specific carrier protein, but rather it is nonspecifically transported in lipoproteins. An advantage of vitamin E transport in lipoproteins is that easily oxidizable lipids are protected by the simultaneous transport of this lipid-soluble antioxidant. Similarly, delivery of vitamin E to tissues is dependent upon lipid and lipoprotein metabolism. Thus, as peroxidizable lipids are taken up by tissue, the tissues simultaneously acquire a lipid-soluble antioxidant.

Plasma Concentrations, Kinetics, and Tissue Delivery

Plasma α-tocopherol concentrations in normal humans range from 11 to 37 μmol l^{-1}. When plasma lipids are taken into account the lower limits of normal are 1.6 μmol α-tocopherol/mmol lipid or 2.5 μmol α-tocopherol/mmol cholesterol. α-Tocopherol is transported in plasma lipoproteins, so if lipid concentrations are extraordinarily high or low, then correction for lipid levels are helpful to determine adequacy of vitamin E status. Additionally, α-tocopherol concentrations in erythrocytes, adipose tissue, or even peripheral nerves have been used to assess vitamin E status.

The apparent half-life of RRR-α-tocopherol in plasma of normal subjects is approximately 48 h, while that of SRR-α-tocopherol or γ-tocopherol is only 15 h.

Vitamin E is delivered to tissues by three mechanisms: transfer from triglyceride-rich lipoproteins during lipolysis; as a result of tissue lipoprotein uptake by various receptors that mediate lipoprotein uptake; and as a result of vitamin E exchange between lipoproteins or tissues. The regulation of tissue vitamin E is not well understood, but α-tocopherol is the predominant form in tissues as a result of its dominance in plasma.

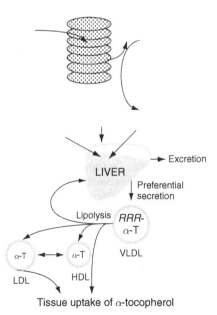

Figure 3 Intestinal vitamin E absorption and plasma lipoprotein transport. (Adapted from Traber MG (1998) Vitamin E. In: Shils ME, Olson JA, Shike M, and Ross AC (eds.) *Modern Nutrition in Health and Disease,* pp. 347–362. Baltimore: Williams & Wilkins.)

Human Vitamin E Deficiency

Vitamin E deficiency was first described in children with fat malabsorption syndromes, principally abetalipoproteinemia, cystic fibrosis, and cholestatic liver disease. Subsequently, humans with severe vitamin E deficiency with no known defect in lipid or lipoprotein metabolism were described to have a defect in the α-TTP gene.

Erythrocyte fragility, hemolysis, and anemia were described as vitamin E deficiency symptoms in various animals fed diets devoid of vitamin E. Additionally, studies in experimental animals have shown that a deficiency of both selenium (a required component of glutathione peroxidases) and vitamin E causes a more rapid and severe onset of debilitating deficiency symptoms. Hypothetically, a deficiency of both vitamins E and C should also cause more severe antioxidant deficiency symptoms, but most animals make their own vitamin C, so this interaction has not been unequivocally demonstrated in humans or animals.

In contrast to experimental vitamin E deficiency in rodents, in humans the major vitamin E deficiency symptom is a peripheral neuropathy characterized by the degeneration of the large caliber axons in the sensory neurons.

Vitamin E deficiency occurs only rarely in humans and almost never as a result of inadequate vitamin E intakes, therefore, interactions with other nutrients have not been well studied. There have been reports of vitamin E deficiency symptoms in persons with protein-calorie malnutrition. Vitamin E deficiency does occur as a result of genetic abnormalities in α-TTP and as a result of various fat malabsorption syndromes. Vitamin E supplementation halts the progression of the neurologic abnormalities caused by inadequate nerve tissue α-tocopherol and, in some cases, has reversed them.

Patients with these disorders require daily pharmacologic vitamin E doses for life to overcome the mechanisms leading to deficiency. Generally, patients with 'ataxia with vitamin E deficiency' are advised to consume 1000 mg RRR-α-tocopherol per day in divided doses, patients with abetalipoproteinemia 100 mg per kg body weight, and cystic fibrosis sufferers 400 mg day^{-1}. However, patients with fat malabsorption due to impaired biliary secretion generally do not absorb orally administered vitamin E. These patients are treated with special forms of vitamin E, such as α-tocopheryl polyethylene glycol succinate, that spontaneously form micelles, obviating the need for bile acids.

Chronic Disease Prevention

The frequency of human vitamin E deficiency is very rare. In individuals at risk, it is clear that vitamin E supplements should be recommended to prevent deficiency symptoms. What about vitamin E supplement use in normal individuals? Dietary changes such as decreasing fat intakes, substituting fat-free foods for fat-containing ones, and increased reliance on meals away from the home have resulted in decreased consumption of α-tocopherol-containing foods. Therefore, intakes of the vitamin E RDA of 15 mg α-tocopherol, may be difficult. Special attention to consuming nuts, seeds, and whole grains will improve α-tocopherol intakes; alternatively, multivitamin pills can be consumed.

Importantly, vitamin E's potential role in preventing or ameliorating chronic diseases associated with oxidative stress leads us to ask whether vitamin E supplements might be beneficial. For many vitamins, when 'excess' amounts are consumed, they are excreted and provide no added benefits. Antioxidant nutrients may, however, be different. Heart disease and stroke, cancer, chronic inflammation, impaired immune function, Alzheimer's disease – a case can be made for the role of oxygen free radicals in the etiology of all of these disorders, and even in aging itself. Do antioxidant nutrients counteract the effects of free radicals and thereby ameliorate these disorders? And, if so, do large antioxidant supplements have beneficial effects beyond 'required' amounts? The 2000 Food and Nutrition Board and Institute of Medicine DRI Report on Vitamin C, Vitamin E, Selenium, and Carotenoids stated that there was insufficient proof to warrant advocating supplementation with antioxidants. But, they also stated that the hypothesis that antioxidant supplements might have beneficial effects was promising. This remains a very controversial area in vitamin E research.

See also: **Antioxidants**: Diet and Antioxidant Defense; Observational Studies; Intervention Studies. **Ascorbic Acid**: Physiology, Dietary Sources and Requirements. **Vitamin E**: Physiology and Health Effects.

Further Reading

Food and Nutrition Board and Institute of Medicine (2000) *Dietary Reference Intakes for Vitamin C, Vitamin E, Selenium, and Carotenoids*. Washington, DC: National Academy Press.

Keaney JF Jr, Simon DI, and Freedman JE (1999) Vitamin E and vascular homeostasis: implications for atherosclerosis. *FASEB Journal* **13**: 965–975.

Ouahchi K, Arita M, Kayden H, Hentati F, Ben Hamida M, Sokol R, Arai H, Inoue K, Mandel JL, and Koenig M (1995) Ataxia with isolated vitamin E deficiency is caused by mutations in the alpha-tocopherol transfer protein. *Nature Genetics* 9: 141–145.

Pryor WA (2000) Vitamin E and heart disease: basic science to clinical intervention trials. *Free Radical Biology and Medicine* 28: 141–164.

Traber MG Vitamin E. In: Shils ME, Olson JA, Shike M, and Ross AC (eds.) *Modern Nutrition in Health and Disease*, vol. 10. Baltimore: Williams & Wilkins (in press).

Physiology and Health Effects

P A Morrissey and M Kiely, University College Cork, Cork, Ireland

In 1922, Evans and Bishop discovered a fat-soluble dietary constituent that was essential for the prevention of fetal death and sterility in rats accidentally fed a diet containing rancid lard. This was originally called 'factor X' and 'antisterility factor' but was later named vitamin E. Subsequently, the multiple nature of the vitamin began to appear when two compounds with vitamin E activity were isolated and characterized from wheat germ oil. These compounds were designated α- and β-tocopherol, derived from the Greek 'tokos' for childbirth, 'phorein' meaning to bring forth, and 'ol' for the alcohol portion of the molecule. Later, two additional tocopherols, γ- and δ-tocopherol, as well as four tocotrienols were isolated from edible plant oils. After the initial discovery, more than 40 years passed before it was proved that vitamin E deficiency could cause disease in humans and was associated with antioxidant functions in cellular systems. It took another 25 years before the non-antioxidant properties of the vitamin were highlighted.

This article reviews the chemistry of the tocopherols; their dietary sources, absorption, transport, and storage; and their metabolic function. In addition, the potential role of dietary or supplemental tocopherol intake in the prevention of chronic disease and possible mechanisms for observed protective effects are discussed. Finally, a summary of the assessment of tocopherol status in humans, intake requirements, and an overview of the safety of high intakes is provided.

Chemistry

The chemistry of vitamin E is rather complex because there are eight structurally related forms—four tocopherols (α, β, γ, and δ) and four tocotrienols (α, β, γ, and δ)—that are synthesized from homogentisic acid and isopentenyl diphosphate in the plastid envelope of plants. The structures of α-, β-, γ-, and δ-tocopherols are shown in **Figure 1**. α-Tocopherol is methylated at C5, C7, and C8 on the chromanol ring, whereas the other homologs (β, γ, and δ) have different degrees of methylation (**Figure 1**). Tocopherols have a saturated phytyl side chain attached at C2 and have three chiral centers that are in the R configuration at positions C2, $C4^1$, and $C8^1$ in the naturally occurring forms, which are given the prefix 2R, 4^1R, and 8^1R (designated RRR). The members of the tocotrienols are unsaturated at $C3^1$, $C7^1$, and $C11^1$ in the isoprenoid side chain and possess one chiral center at C2 in addition

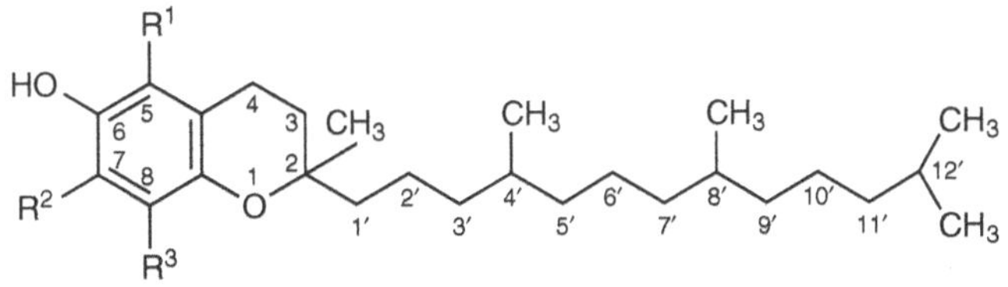

Compound	R^1	R^2	R^3
α-Tocopherol	CH_3	CH_3	CH_3
β-Tocopherol	CH_3	H	CH_3
γ-Tocopherol	H	CH_3	CH_3
δ-Tocopherol	H	H	CH_3

Figure 1 The four major forms of vitamin E (α-, β-, γ-, and δ-tocopherols) differ by the number and positions of methyl groups on the chromonol ring. In α-tocopherol, the most biologically active form, the chromonol ring is fully methylated. In β- and γ-tocopherols, the ring contains two methyl groups, whereas δ-tocopherol is methylated in one position. The corresponding tocotrienols have the same structural arrangement except for the presence of double bonds on the isoprenoid side chain of $C3^1$, $C7^1$, and $C11^1$.

to two sites of geometric isomerism at C3[1] and C7[1]. Vitamin E biological activity is expressed as mg RRR-α-tocopherol equivalents (α-TE) whenever possible. The activity of RRR-α-tocopherol is 1. The activities of RRR-β-, RRR-γ-, and RRR-δ-tocopherol are 0.5, 0.1, and 0.03, respectively.

Dietary Sources

The composition and content of the different tocopherol components in plant tissue vary considerably, ranging from extremely low levels found in potato tubers to high levels found in oil seeds. α-Tocopherol is the predominant form in photosynthetic tissues and is mainly localized in plastids. The particular enrichment in the chloroplast membranes is probably related to the ability of tocopherols to quench or to scavenge reactive oxygen species and lipid peroxy radicals by physical or chemical means. In this way, the photosynthetic apparatus can be protected from oxygen toxicity and lipid peroxidation. In nonphotosynthetic tissues, γ-tocopherol frequently predominates and can be involved in the prevention of autoxidation of polyunsaturated fatty acids.

Most of the tocopherol content of wheat germ, sunflower, safflower, and canola and olive oils is in the form of α-tocopherol, and these oils contain approximately 1700, 500, 350, 200, and 120 mg α-TE kg^{-1}, respectively. Vegetable oils (e.g., corn, cottonseed, palm, soybean, and sesame) and nuts (e.g., Brazil nuts, pecans, and peanuts) are rich sources of γ-tocopherol. Corn and soybean oils contain 5–10 times as much γ-tocopherol as α-tocopherol-rich sources of γ-tocopherol, and each contains approximately 200 mg α-TE kg^{-1}. Because of the widespread use of these plant products, γ-tocopherol is considered to represent $\sim$70% of the vitamin E consumed in the typical US diet. The level of vitamin E in nuts ranges from 7 mg α-TE kg^{-1} in coconuts to 450 mg α-TE kg^{-1} in almonds. Cereals are moderate sources of vitamin E, providing between 6 (barley) and 23 mg α-TE kg^{-1} (rye). Fresh fruit and vegetables generally contain approximately 1–10 mg α-TE kg^{-1}. The concentration of vitamin E (α-tocopherol is the predominant form) in animal products is usually low, but these may be significant dietary sources because of their high consumption.

Mean dietary intakes of 6.3–13.0 mg α-TE per day have been reported in various European and US population studies. Data from the Third National Health and Nutrition Examination Survey (NHANES III) (1988–1994) in the United States indicate a median total intake (including supplements) of α-TE of 12.9 mg day^{-1} and a median intake from food only of 11.7 mg day^{-1} in men aged 31–50 years. In women in this age range, the median total intake (including supplements) of α-TE was 9.1 mg day^{-1} and the median intake from food only was 8.0 mg day^{-1}. In the United States, fats and oils used in spreads, etc. contribute 20.2% of the total vitamin E intake; vegetables, 15.1%; meat, poultry, and fish, 12.6%; desserts, 9.9%; breakfast cereals, 9.3%; fruit, 5.3%; bread and grain products, 5.3%; dairy products, 4.5%; and mixed main dishes, 4.0%.

The North/South Ireland Food Consumption Survey, published in 2001, reported that the median daily intake of vitamin E from all sources was 6.3 mg in men and 6.0 mg in women aged 18–64 years. The largest contributors of vitamin E to the diet were vegetables and vegetable dishes (18.9%) and potatoes and potato products (12.4%), most likely as a result of the oils used in composite dishes. Nutritional supplements contributed 5.5% of the vitamin E intake in men and 11.9% in women overall. In the subgroup that regularly consumed nutritional supplements (23% of total), vitamin E was the nutrient most frequently obtained in supplemental form in men (78%) and women (73%). In these people, supplements made a larger contribution to total vitamin E intakes than did food.

Absorption Metabolism and Excretion

Because of its hydrophobicity, vitamin E requires special transport mechanisms in the aqueous environment of plasma, body fluids, and cells. In humans, vitamin E is taken up in the proximal part of the intestine depending on the amount of food lipids, bile, and pancreatic esterases that are present. It is emulsified together with the fat-soluble components of food. Lipolysis and emulsification of the formed lipid droplets then lead to the spontaneous formation of mixed micelles, which are absorbed at the brush border membrane of the mucosa by passive diffusion. Both α- and γ-tocopherol and dietary fat are taken up without preference by the intestine and secreted in chylomicron particles together with triacylglycerol and cholesterol (**Figure 2**). The nearly identical incorporation of α- and γ-tocopherol in chylomicrons after supplementation with equal amounts of the two tocopherols indicates that their absorption is not selective (**Figure 2**). The chylomicrons are stored as secretory granula and eventually excreted by exocytosis to the lymphatic compartment, from which they reach the bloodstream via the *ductus thoracicus*. The exchange between the apolipoproteins of the chylomicrons (types AI, AII, and B$_{48}$) and high-density lipoprotein (HDL) (types C and E) triggers the intravascular degradation of the chylomicrons to remnants by the

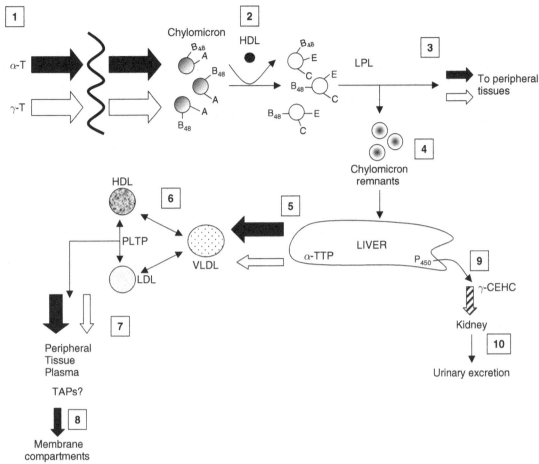

Figure 2 Absorption, transport, and metabolism of α-tocopherol (α-T) and γ-tocopherol (γ-T) in peripheral tissues. 1: Both α-T and γ-T are absorbed without preference by the intestine along with lipid and reassembled into chylomicrons. 2: Exchange between apolipoproteins of the chylomicrons (types AI, AII, and B$_{48}$) and high-density lipoprotein (HDL) (types C and E) occurs. 3: Chylomicrons are degraded to remnants by lipoprotein lipase (LPL) and some α-T and γ-T are transported to peripheral tissues. 4: The resulting chylomicron remnants are then taken up by the liver. 5: In the liver, most of the remaining α-T, but only a small fraction of γ-T, is reincorporated in nascent very low-density lipoproteins (VLDLs) by α-tocopherol transfer protein (α-TTP). 6: Plasma phospholipid transfer protein (PLTP) facilitates the exchange of tocopherol between HDL and LDL for delivery to tissues. 7: Plasma tocopherols are delivered to tissues by LDL and HDL. 8: Tocopherol-associated proteins (TAPs) probably facilitate intracellular tocopherol transfer between membrane compartments. 9: Substantial amounts of γ-T are degraded by a cytochrome P450-mediated reaction to 2,7,8-trimethyl-2-(β-carboxyethyl-6-hydroxychroman (γ-CEHC). 10: γ-CEHC is excreted into urine. Adapted from Azzi A and Stocker A (2000) Vitamin E: Non-antioxidant roles. *Progress in Lipid Research* **39**: 231–255; and from Jiang Q, Christen S, Shigenaga MK and Ames BN (2001) γ-Tocopherol, the major form of vitamin E in the US diet, deserves more attention. *American Journal of Clinical Nutrition* **74**: 714–722.

endothelial lipoprotein lipase (LPL) and is a prerequisite for the hepatic uptake of tocopherols (**Figure 2**). During LPL-mediated catabolism of chylomicron particles, some of the chylomicron-bound vitamin E appears to be transported and transferred to peripheral tissues, such as muscle, adipose, and brain (**Figure 2**). The formation of remnants favors the rapid uptake of the tocopherols via the hepatic receptors for apo-E and apo-B.

The chylomicron remnants are subsequently taken up by the liver, where α-tocopherol is preferentially incorporated into nascent very low-density lipoprotein (VLDL) by a specific 32-kDa α-tocopherol

transfer protein (α-TTP), which enables further distribution of α-tocopherol to peripheral cells (**Figure 2**). α-TTP is mainly expressed in the liver, in some parts of the brain, in the retina, in low amounts in fibroblasts, and in the placenta. α-TTP possesses stereospecificity as well as regiospecificity toward the most abundant isomer of vitamin E, (RRR)-α-tocopherol. The sorting process does not tolerate alteration at C2. As a consequence of the selective transfer mechanism, major parts of the natural homologs and nonnatural isomers of α-tocopherol are excluded from the plasma and secreted with the bile. Relative affinities of tocopherols for α-TTP are as follows: α-tocopherol, 100; β-tocopherol, 38; γ-tocopherol, 9; and δ-tocopherol, 2. A 75-kDa plasma phospholipid transfer protein (PLTP), which is known to catalyze the exchange of phospholipids and other amphipatic compounds between lipid structures, has been shown to facilitate the exchange of α-tocopherol from VLDL to HDL and LDL for further delivery to tissues (**Figure 2**).

A family of cellular tocopherol-associated proteins (TAPs) with the ability to bind and redistribute α-tocopherol has been identified. TAPs bind to α-tocopherol but not to other isomers of tocopherol. Present in all cells, TAPs may be specifically involved in intracellular α-tocopherol movement, for example, between membrane compartments and plasma membranes, or in optimizing the α-tocopherol content of membranes.

γ-Tocopherol appears to be mainly degraded to its hydrophilic 3'-carboxychromanol metabolite, 2,7,8-trimethyl-2-(β-carboxyethyl)-6-hydroxychroman (γ-CEHC) (**Figure 3**), and excreted in the urine. The mechanism of γ-tocopherol metabolism involves terminal cytochrome P450 (CYP)-mediated ω-hydroxylation of the tocopherol phytyl side chain, oxidation to the corresponding terminal carboxylic acid, and sequential removal of two- or three-carbon moieties by β-oxidation, ultimately yielding the hydrophilic 3'-carboxychromanol metabolite of the parent tocopherol that is excreted in the urine. Functional analysis of several recombinant human liver P450 enzymes revealed that tocopherol ω-hydroxylase activity was associated only with the cytochrome P450 isoform 4F2 (CYP4F2). Kinetic

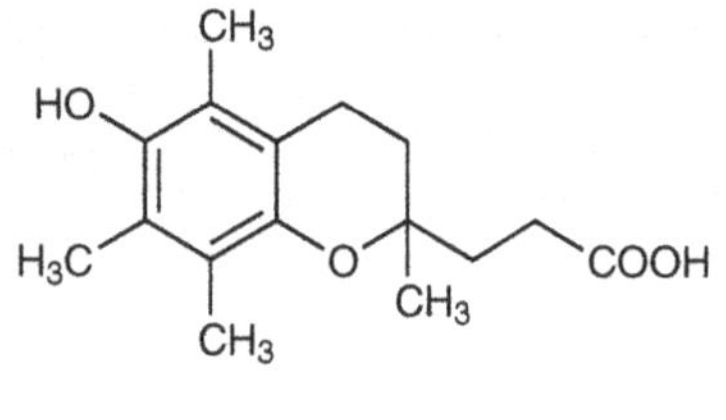

analysis of the tocopherol ω-hydroxylase activity in recombinant human CYP4F2 microsomal systems revealed similar K_m values (37 and 21 μM) but notably different V_{max} values (1.99 vs 0.16 nmol/nmol of P450/min) for γ- and α-tocopherol, respectively. The data suggest a role for the CYP-mediated ω-hydroxylase pathway in the preferential physiological retention of α-tocopherol and elimination of γ-tocopherol. In nonsupplemented individuals, a substantial proportion of the estimated daily intake of γ-tocopherol is excreted in human urine as its γ-CEHC metabolite, but a much smaller proportion of α-tocopherol is excreted as 2,5,7,8-tetramethyl-2-(β-carboxyethyl)-6-hydroxychroman (α-CEHC) (**Figure 3**). α-CEHC is excreted in large amounts only when the daily intake of α-tocopherol exceeds 150 mg or plasma concentrations of α-tocopherol are above a threshold of 30–40 μmol l^{-1}. Even then, urinary excretion of α-CEHC is lower than that of γ-CEHC.

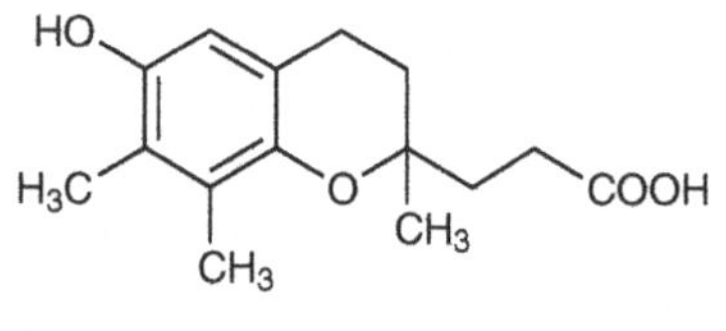

It is likely that it is the capacity of α-TTP rather than the plasma α-tocopherol concentration that determines α-tocopherol degradation. Overall, hepatic catabolism of γ-tocopherol appears to be responsible for the relatively low preservation of γ-tocopherol in plasma and tissues, whereas α-TTP-mediated α-tocopherol transfer plays a key role in the preferential enrichment of α-tocopherol in most tissues. Supplementation with α-tocopherol depletes plasma and tissue γ-tocopherol levels. This is likely due to the preferential affinity of α-TTP for α-tocopherol. However, the depletion of γ-tocopherol may also occur because an increase in α-tocopherol may further reduce the incorporation of γ-tocopherol into VLDL, which leaves more γ-tocopherol to be degraded by CYP. On the other hand, γ-tocopherol supplementation may spare α-tocopherol from being degraded.

Plasma (RRR)-α-tocopherol incorporation is a saturable process. Plasma concentrations of α-tocopherol reach a threshold of 30–40 μmol l^{-1} despite supplementation with high levels (400 mg or greater) of (RRR)-α-tocopherol. Dose–response studies showed that the limitation in plasma α-tocopherol concentration appears to be a result of rapid replacement of circulating with newly absorbed α-tocopherol. Kinetic analysis has shown that the entire plasma pool of α-tocopherol is replaced daily. The highest concentrations of α-tocopherol in the body are in adipose tissues and adrenal glands. Adipose tissues are also a major store of the vitamin, followed by liver and skeletal muscle. The rate of uptake and turnover of α-tocopherol by different tissues varies greatly. Uptake is most rapid into lungs, liver, spleen, kidney, and red cells (in rats, $t_{1/2} < 15$ days) and slowest in brain, adipose tissues, and spinal cord ($t_{1/2} < 30$

Figure 3 Chemical structures of 2,5,7,8-tetramethyl-2-(β-carboxyethyl)-6-hydroxychroman(α-CEHC) and 2,7,8-trimethyl-2-(β-carboxyethyl)-6-hydroxychroman (γ-CEHC).

days). Likewise, depletion of α-tocopherol from plasma and liver during times of dietary deficiency is rapid, whereas adipose tissue, brain, spinal cord, and neural tissues are much more difficult to deplete.

The major route for the elimination of tocopherol from the body is via the feces. Fecal tocopherol arises from incomplete absorption, secretion from mucosal cells, and biliary excretion. Excess α-tocopherol as well as forms of vitamin E not preferentially used, such as synthetic racemic isomer mixtures, or γ-tocopherol are eliminated during the process of nascent VLDL secretion in the liver and are probably excreted into bile. In addition to the urinary excretion of γ-tocopherol as γ-CEHC, biliary excretion is an alternative route for elimination of excess γ-tocopherol. This is confirmed by the fact that the ratio of γ- to α-tocopherol in bile is sevenfold higher than in plasma.

Tocopherols as Antioxidants

Under normal physiological conditions, cellular systems are incessantly challenged by stressors arising from both internal and external sources. The most important potential stressors are reduced derivatives of oxygen, which are classified as reactive oxygen species (ROS), and include the superoxide anion ($O_2^{\cdot-}$), hydroxyl radical ($^{\cdot}OH$), and oxygen-centered radicals of organic compounds (peroxyl ($ROO^{\cdot}$) and alkoxyl ($RO^{\cdot}$)) together with other nonradical reactive compounds, such as hydrogen peroxide (H_2O_2). In addition, reactive nitrogen species such as nitric oxide ($NO^{\cdot}$), nitrogen dioxide ($NO_2^{\cdot}$), peroxynitrite ($ONOO^-$), and hypochlorous acid are involved.

Cellular systems have evolved a powerful and complex antioxidant defence system to limit inappropriate exposure to these stressors. α-Tocopherol is quantitatively the most important chain-breaking antioxidant in plasma and biological membranes. The antioxidant activities of chain-breaking antioxidants are determined primarily by how rapidly they scavenge peroxyl radicals, thereby preventing the propagation of free radical reactions. When the chromanol phenolic group of α-tocopherol (TOH) encounters a $ROO^{\cdot}$ it forms hydroperoxide (ROOH), and in the process a tocopheroxyl radical ($TO^{\cdot}$) is formed:

$$TOH + ROO^{\cdot} \xrightarrow{k_1} ROOH + TO^{\cdot}$$

The rate constant (k_1) for hydrogen abstraction from α-tocopherol is $2.35 \times 10^6 \, M^{-1} s^{-1}$, which is higher than that for the other tocopherols and related phenols. Because the rate constant (k_2) for the chain propagation reaction between $ROO^{\cdot}$ and an unsaturated fatty acid (RH) ($ROO^{\cdot} + RH \rightarrow ROOH$) is much lower than k_1, at approximately $10^2 \, M^{-1} s^{-1}$ α-tocopherol outcompetes the propagation reaction and scavenges the $ROO^{\cdot}$ ~10^4 times faster than RH reacts with $ROO^{\cdot}$. Thus, the kinetic properties of antioxidants, in particular α-tocopherol, require that only relatively small concentrations are required for them to be effective. The concentration of α-tocopherol in biological membranes is approximately 1 mol per 1000–2000 mol phospholipids (i.e., ~$1:10^3$). Ascorbic acid can reduce the tocopheroxyl radical ($TO^{\cdot}$) to its native state, and it has been concluded that part of the reason why low concentrations of α-tocopherol are such efficient antioxidants in biological systems is because of this capacity to be regenerated by intracellular reductants such as ascorbic acid.

The heterocyclic chromanol ring of α-tocopherol has an optimised structure for resonance stabilization of the unpaired electron of the α-tocopheroxyl radical, and the electron-donating substituents (e.g., the three methyl groups) increase this effect. Because γ-tocopherol lacks one of the electron-donating methyl groups on the chromanol ring, it is somewhat less potent in donating electrons than α-tocopherol and is thus a slightly less powerful antioxidant. However, the unsubstituted C5 position on γ-tocopherol allows it to trap lipophilic electrophiles such as peroxynitrite, thereby protecting macromolecules from oxidation.

Vitamin E Deficiency

Vitamin E deficiency is seen rarely in humans. However, there may be a risk of vitamin E deficiency in premature infants because the placenta does not transfer α-tocopherol to the fetus in adequate amounts. When it occurs in older children and adults, it is usually a result of lipoprotein deficiencies or a lipid malabsorption syndrome. These include patients with abetalipoproteinemia or homozygous hypobetalipoproteinemia, those with cholestatic disease, and patients receiving total parenteral nutrition. There is also an extremely rare disorder in which primary vitamin E deficiency occurs in the absence of lipid malabsorption. This disorder is a rare autosomal recessive neurodegenerative disease caused by mutations in the gene for α-TTP. This disorder is known as ataxia with vitamin E deficiency (AVED). Patients with AVED have extraordinary low plasma vitamin E concentrations ($<5 \, \mu g \, ml^{-1}$) and have an onset between 4 and 18 years, with progressive development of peripheral neuropathy, spinocerebellar ataxia, dysarthria, the absence of deep tendon reflexes, and vibratory and proprioceptive sensory loss. Patients with an α-TTP defect have enhanced urinary excretion of α-CEHC despite having much lower plasma α-tocopherol concentrations than healthy subjects. Therapeutic and prophylactic vitamin E supplementation (up to 2000 mg day^{-1}) prevents the onset of the disease before irreversible neurological damage develops.

Tocopherols and Low-Density Lipoprotein Modification

The hypothesis that oxidative stress plays an important role in the pathogenesis of atherosclerosis is generally accepted. Substantial *in vitro* evidence indicates that oxidized LDL is the component central to the initiation and/or progression of atherogenesis at the molecular and cellular level. The typical LDL particle is not only rich in cholesterol but also contains approximately 1300 molecules of RH, which are very sensitive to oxidation. Vitamin E, mainly α-tocopherol, is quantitatively the most important lipophilic antioxidant present in LDL particles. On average, each LDL particle is protected by $\sim$6 mol α-tocopherol (range, 3–15 mol), 1 mol of γ-tocopherol, and small amounts of carotenoids.

All major cells of the artery wall, such as monocyte macrophages, endothelial cells, and smooth muscle cells, can modify LDL oxidatively *in vitro*. Monocytes have been shown to induce peroxidation of lipids such as those in LDL by the generation of reactive species, including superoxide anion, hydrogen peroxide, and hydroxyl radicals. Other oxidants have been implicated, including 15-lipoxygenase, myeloperoxidase-generated hypochlorous acid, and reactive nitrogen species such as peroxynitrite. *In vivo*, oxidized LDL particles are recognized by macrophage scavenger receptors and taken up by macrophages, forming lipid-laden foam cells in the fatty streak lesions. The free radical oxidation of LDL results in numerous structural changes that all depend on a common event—the peroxidation of polyunsaturated fatty acids in the LDL particle.

In vitro studies have indicated that increasing the vitamin E content of LDL particles increases their resistance to oxidation and decreases their uptake by macrophages. Vitamin E supplementation has also been reported to suppress macrophage uptake of oxidized LDL in human arterial lesions and decrease urinary F$_2$-isoprostane (a 'footprint' of free radical-mediated oxidation of arachidonic acid) concentrations. Reactive nitrogen species are also implicated in aortic oxidation of LDL and therefore potentially in atherosclerosis.

Because of the nonsubstituted 5-position, γ-tocopherol reacts with peroxynitrite and other electrophilic mutagens generated during inflammation and forms a stable carbon-centered adduct, 5-nitro-γ-tocopherol. This mechanism of protecting LDL may be significant when γ-tocopherol constitutes a major portion of vitamin E in the diet. It is worth noting that the ability of γ-tocopherol to attenuate oxidative damage produced by these reactive species may prevent or delay the progression of other diseases as well as cardiovascular disease (CVD), in which inflammation plays a role, such as cancer, rheumatoid arthritis, inflammatory bowel disease, and neurodegenerative disorders. In addition, γ-CEHC has natriuretic activity and functions in the kidney to control sodium excretion, and it regulates the body's extracellular fluid volume, an important determinant in hypertension and congestive heart failure.

Tocopherols and Other Metabolic Functions

Vitamin E, in addition to having a protective role in the oxidative modification of LDL, may affect or limit the progression of atherosclerosis and a number of other conditions in ways that are unrelated to its antioxidant activity. Some of these effects appear to stem from the ability of α-tocopherol, at physiological concentrations of vitamin E, to activate protein phosphatase 2A, which inhibits the activity of protein kinase C (PKC), a biological indicator of inflammation, by dephosphorylating the protein. PKC is an important element in the signal transduction cascade mediated by growth factors, such as platelet-derived growth factors, which are necessary for the progression and completion of the cell proliferation cycle.

The cellular effects of α-tocopherol-mediated inhibition of PKC depend on the cell type in question, but the cumulative effect is highly protective against the progression of atherosclerosis. PKC inhibition results in reduced smooth muscle cell proliferation, inhibition of platelet aggregation, and thus delayed intra-arterial thrombus formation. Endothelial cell function is preserved by the downregulation of adhesion molecule (ICAM-1 and VCAM-1) expression (possibly by downregulation of nuclear factor-κB) and hence prevention of monocyte and neutrophil adhesion, which is an important early event in the initiation of fatty streak formation and atherogenesis. In addition, PKC inhibition in monocytes reduces the production of reactive oxygen species by impairment of NADPH-oxidase assembly, which may help to reduce LDL oxidation.

The release of proinflammatory cytokines in monocytes, such as interleukin-1β and tumour necrosis factor-α, is impeded by α-tocopherol-mediated inhibition of the 5-lipoxygenase pathway, and production of eicosanoids, such as prostaglandin E_2 and thromboxane A_2, is impeded by γ-tocopherol-mediated inhibition of the cycloxygenase pathway. Lower circulating levels of inflammatory mediators, which are aggregatory and vasoconstrictive, as well as inhibition of monocyte chemoattractant protein-1 (MCP-1) production, reduces the attraction of monocytes to inflammatory sites at the arterial wall and prevents the formation of foam cells. Furthermore, α-tocopherol increases production of prostacyclin, which has anti-aggregatory and vasodilatory properties, thereby reducing the risk of a coronary event. There is evidence that in a formed atherosclerotic plaque, vitamin E may have a stabilizing effect and prevent its rupture and subsequent clot formation. This may be an important contributor to the prevention of heart disease because plaque types that are most subject to rupture present the greatest threat.

Nitric oxide (NO) produced by NO synthase in the endothelium is important in the maintenance of vascular tone; it suppresses the expression of proinflammatory cytokines, adhesion molecules, and MCP-1. It also inhibits platelet adhesion, maintains the integrity of the arterial wall, and acts as an antioxidant. Vitamin E can reduce the inhibition of NO synthase by reactive oxygen species, thus maintaining NO production, either through its antioxidant activity or perhaps by suppressing PKC activity in smooth muscle.

Tocopherols and Cardiovascular Disease—Epidemiological Evidence

The effects of dietary vitamin E have been examined in several studies, many of which have reported a clear association between the reduction in the relative risk of CVD and high intake or supplement of vitamin E, although some have shown no such association. The Vitamin Substudy of the WHO/MONICA Project showed that in European populations whose classical risk factors for CVD were very similar, the 7-fold differences in CVD mortality could be explained at least to approximately 60% by differences in the plasma levels of vitamin E and up to 90% by the combination of vitamins E, A, and C. The Edinburgh Case Control Study and Basel Prospective Study consistently revealed an increased risk of ischemic heart disease and stroke for low plasma levels of vitamin E.

However, other European population studies have not found an association between blood levels of vitamin E and end points of CVD. In the EURAMIC study, the adipose levels of vitamin E did not correlate with the relative risk of myocardial infarction.

A number of prospective studies have examined the association between vitamin E intake and risk of CHD. The Nurses' Health Study, conducted on 87 245 women, showed a 34% reduction in CHD in women who had consumed vitamin E supplements containing more than 67 mg α-TE daily for more than 2 years. However, there was no significant effect of vitamin E obtained from food sources. The Established Populations for Epidemiolodic Studies of the Elderly (EPESE) trials showed that the use of vitamin E supplements significantly decreased risks for all-cause-mortality and mortality from heart disease. Another prospective study, performed in Canada, reported a consistent inverse association between CVD and vitamin E supplement usage. The Health Professionals Study, conducted on 39 910 men aged 40–75 years, also showed that dietary intakes of vitamin E were not significantly correlated with reduced risk of CHD or death. A protective effect was seen in those who took 67–160 mg supplemental α-TE daily for more than 2 years. In contrast, the Iowa Women's Health Study reported that dietary vitamin E (mainly γ-tocopherol) was inversely associated with the risk of death from CVD. This association was particularly striking in the subgroup of women who did not consume vitamin supplements. There was little evidence that the intake of vitamin E from supplements (mainly α-tocopherol) was associated with a decreased risk of death from CVD. The reasons for the differences between dietary and supplemental vitamin E are not clear. However, some epidemiological studies point to the potential importance of γ-tocopherol in preventing heart disease. High dietary intake of nuts, an excellent source of γ-tocopherol, lowered serum cholesterol, improved plasma lipid profiles, and was inversely associated with the risk of death from heart disease.

The ability of α-tocopherol supplementation to prevent cardiovascular events in different populations was tested in four larger prospective clinical trials: The α-Tocopherol, β-Carotene Cancer Prevention (ATBC) study, the Cambridge Heart Antioxidant Study (CHAOS), the Gruppo Italiano per lo studio della Sopravvivenza nell'Infarto Miocardito (GISSI) trial, and the Heart Outcome Prevention Evaluation (HOPE) study. In addition, at least two smaller prospective clinical trials have been completed: the Secondary Prevention with

Antioxidants of Cardiovascular Disease in Endstage Renal Disease (SPACE) study and the Antioxidant Supplementation in Atherosclerosis Prevention Study (ASAP).

In the ATBC study, the subjects who were supplemented with 50 mg *all rac*-α-tocopheryl acetate day^{-1} for 5–8 years had only a moderately lower incidence (4%) of angina pectoris than did the control subjects, and among male smokers, cardiovascular mortality did not differ significantly between those who received supplementation and those who did not. However, subjects who received supplementation had a significantly higher incidence of haemorrhagic stroke than did the control subjects. Note that the ATBC study was not designed to investigate cardiovascular disease development. The results of the CHAOS trial, the first prospective trial with cardiovascular disease as an end point, were encouraging. The risks of nonfatal myocardial infarction declined 77% and total (fatal plus nonfatal) myocardial infarction declined 47% when patients with established coronary artery disease were treated with 268 or 536 mg α-TE daily for approximately 500 days. The GISSI study showed that feeding 211 mg α-TE day^{-1} for 3.5 years did not significantly reduce the rate of all-cause death, nonfatal myocardial infarction, or nonfatal stroke. However, in a later four-way reanalysis in which each individual variable was considered as an end point, there were significantly fewer (20%) cardiovascular deaths in the α-tocopherol group than in the control group. The HOPE study reported that vitamin E (400 IU (268 mg) day^{-1} RRR-α-tocopherol) treatment of CVD patients had no effect on reducing the primary end points, which included nonfatal myocardial infarction, stroke, and cardiovascular death. In the SPACE trial, haemodialysis patients with preexisting cardiovascular disease received 536 mg (RRR)-α-tocopherol or placebo day^{-1}. Patients who received vitamin E had a striking 54% reduction in cardiac events compared with control subjects.

In the ASAP study, men and women (all subjects had hypercholesterolemia at entry) were given vitamin E (91 mg twice daily), slow-release vitamin C (250 mg twice daily), a combination of both, or placebo for 3 years. The progression of atherosclerosis (the mean intima-media thickness of the common carotid artery measured) was significantly retarded only in the men who smoked and took both vitamins. It is important to note that, in general, women develop fewer cardiovascular events than do men. Thus, women may profit less from vitamin E treatment than men. In studies in which many women are enrolled, the low incidence of CVD may weaken the statistical power of the overall trial.

Tocopherols and Cancer—Epidemiological Evidence

Clinical and epidemiological data, together with evidence from experimental models, support a role for the involvement of free radicals throughout the cancer process. Attempts to prevent cancer using vitamin E are based on the rationale that oncogenesis results from free radicals attacking DNA. As an antioxidant, vitamin E may inhibit cancer formation by scavenging reactive oxygen or nitrogen species. Several studies of oral, pharyngeal, and cervical cancer found a relationship between vitamin E status and cancer risk. The evidence for stomach and pancreatic cancers has not been consistent, and no association with breast cancer has been found.

The Linxian, China, intervention trial provided evidence that nutritional supplementation may lower the risk of certain cancers. A modest but significant reduction in cancer mortality was observed in a general population trial in those receiving daily (for 5.25 years) a combination of β-carotene (15 mg), vitamin E (30 mg), and selenium (50 μg). The subjects who received this mixture had a 13% lower incidence of cancer and a 10% lower mortality from stomach and oesophageal cancer than did the subjects who did not receive the mixture. In the ATBC study, male smokers who took vitamin E supplements had a 34% lower incidence of prostate cancer and 41% lower mortality from prostate cancer than did those who did not take the supplements. In the United States, in a nested case–control study conducted to examine the association of α-tocopherol, γ-tocopherol, and selenium with the incidence of prostate cancer, a striking fivefold reduction in risk was observed for the men in the highest quintile of γ-tocopherol compared with those in the lowest. Overall, evidence for the protection from cancer by vitamin E is not compelling.

Tocopherols and Other Diseases—Epidemiological Evidence

Vitamin E appears to act as an immunosuppressant due to its ability to suppress both humoral and cellular immune responses. Tocopherol supplementation significantly enhances lymphocyte proliferation, interleukin-2 production, and delayed-type hypersensitivity skin response and decreases prostaglandin E$_2$ production by inhibiting cyclooxygenase activity. There appears to be compelling evidence that intervention with dietary antioxidants, such as vitamin E, may help maintain the well-preserved immune function of 'very healthy' elderly, restore the age-related decrease in immune function, and reduce the risk of several age-associated chronic diseases. Epidemiological evidence suggests an association between the incidence of cataract and vitamin E status. In a prospective study, the sum of serum α- and γ-tocopherol, but neither tocopherol alone, was inversely associated with the incidence of age-related nuclear cataracts.

Among the most common neurologic diseases are neurodegenerative disorders such as Alzheimer's and Parkinson's disease, which may be caused by oxidative stress and mitochondrial dysfunction leading to progressive neural death. An increasing number of studies show that antioxidants (vitamin E and polyphenols) can block neuronal death *in vitro*. In a 2-year, double-blind, placebo-controlled, randomised trial of patients with moderately severe impairment from Alzheimer's disease, treatment with $1340\,\mathrm{mg\,day^{-1}}$ α-TE significantly slowed the progression of the disease. Clinical treatment of Alzheimer's patients with large doses of vitamin E ($670\,\mathrm{mg}$ α-TE twice daily) is one of the key therapeutic guidelines of the American Academy of Neurology. In a multicentre, double-blind trial, vitamin E ($1340\,\mathrm{mg}$ α-TE day^{-1}) was not beneficial in slowing functional decline or ameliorating the clinical features of Parkinson's disease. Administration of vitamin E significantly relieved symptoms in patients suffering from several types of acute or chronic inflammatory conditions, such as acute arthritis, rheumatoid arthritis, and osteoarthritis.

Vitamin E Status and Requirements

Interest in the role of vitamin E in disease prevention has encouraged the search for reliable indices of vitamin E status. Most studies in human subjects make use of static biomarkers of status, usually α-tocopherol concentrations in plasma, serum, erythrocytes, lymphocytes, platelets, lipoproteins, adipose tissues, buccal mucosal cells, and LDL, and the α-tocopherol:γ-tocopherol ratio in serum or plasma. Other markers of vitamin E status include susceptibility of erythrocyte or plasma LDL to oxidation, breath hydrocarbon exhalation, and the concentration of α-tocopherol quinone in cerebrospinal fluid. There is no consensus as to the threshold concentration of plasma or serum α-tocopherol at which a person can be defined as having inadequate tocopherol status, but values of <11.6, 11.6–16.2, and $>16.2\,\mu\mathrm{mol^{-1}}$ are normally regarded as indicating a deficient, low, and acceptable vitamin E status, respectively. It is recommended that plasma or serum α-tocopherol concentrations be lipid-corrected (i.e., expressed relative to either the sum of cholesterol and triacylglycerol or cholesterol alone). For convenience, α-tocopherol:cholesterol is the simplest to obtain and probably the most useful, with values below $2.2\,\mu\mathrm{mol}$ α-tocopherol/mmol cholesterol indicating a risk or deficiency and an optimal value >5.2. It has been estimated that an average daily dietary intake of 15–$30\,\mathrm{mg}$ α-tocopherol would be required to maintain this plasma level, an amount that could be obtained from dietary sources if a concerted effort were made to eat foods rich in vitamin E.

The US Institute of Medicine Food and Nutrition Board set an estimated average requirement (EAR) of $12\,\mathrm{mg}$ α-tocopherol for adults $>19\,\mathrm{years}$ on the criterion of vitamin E intakes that were sufficient to prevent hydrogen peroxide-induced hemolysis in men. The same value was set for men and women on the basis that although body weight is smaller on average in women than men, fat mass as a percentage of body weight is higher on average in women. Because information is not available on the standard deviation of the requirement for vitamin E, the recommended dietary allowance (RDA) was established for men and women as the EAR ($12\,\mathrm{mg}$) plus twice the coefficient of variation (assumed to be 10%), rounded up, giving a value of $15\,\mathrm{mg\,day^{-1}}$. In Europe, the Scientific Committee for Food did not set a population reference intake (PRI) for vitamin E on the basis that there is no evidence for deficiency from low intakes, and the frequency of distribution of intakes is skewed to the right, making it difficult to set a PRI that is not inappropriately high, especially for those with a low consumption of polyunsaturated fatty acid (PUFA), whose requirements are lower than those with a high consumption of PUFA.

It has been suggested that the optimum concentration of α-tocopherol in plasma for protection against cardiovascular disease and cancer is $>30\,\mu\mathrm{mol\,l^{-1}}$, given normal plasma lipid levels and in conjunction with a plasma vitamin C concentration $>50\,\mu\mathrm{mol\,l^{-1}}$ and a β-carotene level $>0.4\,\mu\mathrm{mol\,l^{-1}}$. This has not been proven in large-scale human intervention trials, but even in the absence of conclusive evidence for a prophylactic effect of vitamin E on chronic disease prevention, some experts believe that a recommendation of a daily intake of 87–$100\,\mathrm{mg}$ α-tocopherol is justifiable based on current evidence. Realistically, these levels can be achieved only by using nutritional supplements. The tolerable upper intake level for vitamin E is $1000\,\mathrm{mg\,day^{-1}}$, based on studies showing hemorrhagic toxicity in rats, in the absence of human dose–response data.

See also: **Antioxidants**: Diet and Antioxidant Defense.
Fatty Acids: Omega-3 Polyunsaturated; Omega-6
Polyunsaturated.

Further Reading

Azzi A and Stocker A (2002) Vitamin E: Non-antioxidant roles. *Progress in Lipid Research* **39**: 231–255.

Brigeluis-Flohe R, Kelly FJ, Salonen JT *et al.* (2002) The European perspective on vitamin E: Current knowledge and future research. *American Journal of Clinical Nutrition* **76**: 703–716.

Esposito E, Rotilio D, Di Matteo V *et al.* (2002) A review of specific dietary antioxidants and the effects on biochemical mechanisms related to neurodegenerative processes. *Neurobiology of Ageing* **23**: 719–735.

Frei B (1994) In *Natural Antioxidants in Human Health and Disease*. London: Academic Press.

Halliwell B (1996) Antioxidants in human health and disease. *Annual Review of Nutrition* **16**: 33–50.

Institute of Medicine (2000) *Dietary Reference Intakes for Vitamin C, Vitamin E, Selenium and Carotenoids*. Washington, DC: National Academy Press.

Jiang Q, Christen S, Shigenaga MK, and Ames BN (2001) γ-Tocopherol, the major form of vitamin E in the US diet, deserves move attention. *American Journal of Clinical Nutrition* **74**: 712–722.

Machlin LJ (1984) Vitamin E. In: Machlin LJ (ed.) *Handbook of Vitamins: Nutritional Biochemical and Clinical Aspects*, pp. 99–145. New York: Marcel Dekker.

Morrissey PA and Kiely M (2002) Vitamin E, nutritional significance. In: Roginski H, Fuguay JW, and Fox PF (eds.) *Encyclopedia of Dairy Science*, pp. 2670–2677. London: Elsevier.

Neuzil J, Weber C, and Kontush A (2001) The role of vitamin E in atherogenesis: Linking the chemical, biological and clinical aspects to the disease. *Atherosclerosis* **157**: 257–283.

Packer L and Fuchs J (eds.) (1993) *Vitamin E in Health and Disease*. New York: Marcel Dekker.

Pryor WA (2000) Vitamin E and heart disease: Basic science to clinical intervention trials. *Free Radical Biology and Medicine* **28**: 141–164.

Rimbach G, Minihane AM, Majewicz J *et al.* (2002) Regulation of cell signalling by vitamin E. *Proceedings of the Nutrition Society* **61**: 415–425.

Thomas SR and Stocker R (2000) Molecular action of vitamin E in lipoprotein oxidation: Implications for atherosclerosis. *Free Radical Biology and Medicine* **28**: 1795–1805.

Traber MG and Sies H (1996) Vitamin E in humans: Demand and delivery. *Annual Review of Nutrition* **16**: 321–347.

VITAMIN K

C J Bates, MRC Human Nutrition Research, Cambridge, UK

The discovery of vitamin K as an essential nutrient arose in the late 1920s from Henrik Dam's studies of sterol metabolism. He observed that chicks fed a fat-free diet developed subcutaneous hemorrhages and anemia. A lipid extract of liver or of certain plant tissues was curative, and by 1935 he claimed discovery of a new vitamin in these extracts that he named 'vitamin K' from the German *Koagulation*. By the late 1930s, two chemically similar forms of the vitamin from different sources were recognized, namely phylloquinone or K_1 and menaquinone or K_2, which had been isolated from alfalfa and from putrefied fish meal, respectively (**Figure 1**). Phylloquinone, with its saturated phytyl side chain, is now understood to be the sole representative of vitamin K that occurs in plant tissues, especially in green leafy ones, where it acts as a component of the electron transport chain. The menaquinones, or MK-n, by contrast, comprise a broad family of representatives that have a variable length, unsaturated side chain, and are composed of one or more

(sequential) isoprene units in place of the saturated phytyl side chain. These menaquinones can be produced by certain types of bacteria, both in the large bowel of animals and at other locations where they may contribute to human food sources of menaquinones. Germ-free rats become vitamin K deficient more readily than their conventional counterparts, and they can develop very low hepatic MK-4 levels. The specific menaquinone with the same side chain length as phylloquinone is called menatetranone, or MK-4, and this is produced commercially for human medication, especially in Japan. There is evidence that phylloquinone can be converted to MK-4 in animals and humans. Most bacterially synthesized menaquinones have longer side chains, typically 7–9 isoprene units and up to 13, which are indicated by 'n' in the MK-n shorthand notation. A synthetic homolog of phylloquinone, $K_{1(25)}$, is not found in nature and can therefore be used as an internal standard in the chromatographic separation and quantitation of vitamin K. Menadione, a water-soluble form of the vitamin that has a single methyl group in place of the side chain, has vitamin K activity (it can be converted to menatetranone *in vivo*) and is used in animal feeds, but it is not used in humans because of its toxicity at high doses.

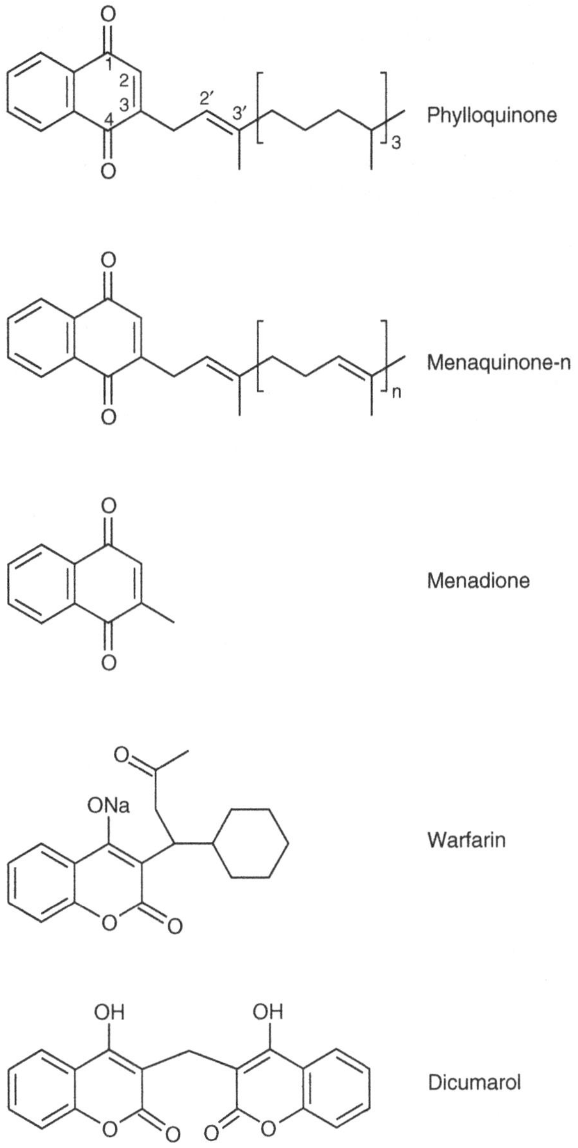

Figure 1 Chemical structures of phylloquinone, menaquinones, menadione, warfarin, and dicumarol.

Table 1 Mean estimate food contents of phylloquinone and selected menaquinones

Food item	$\mu g/100\,g$ wet weight or $\mu g/100\,ml^a$				
	Phylloquinone (vitamin K_1)	MK-4	MK-7	MK-8	MK-9
Kale	817	—	—	—	—
Spinach	387	—	—	—	—
Broccoli	156	—	—	—	—
Peas	36	—	—	—	—
Apples	3.0	—	—	—	—
Chicken	—	8.9	—	—	—
Pork	0.3	2.1	—	0.5	1.1
Luncheon meat	3.9	7.7	—	—	—
Mackerel	2.2	0.4	—	—	—
Plaice	—	0.2	0.1	1.6	
Milk	0.5	0.8	—	—	—
Hard cheese	10.4	4.7	1.3	16.9	51.1
Soft cheese	5	4	1	10	40
Natto^b	34.7	—	998	84.1	
Olive oil	53.7	—	—	—	—
Margarine	93.2	—	—	—	—
Butter	14.9	15.0	—	—	—
Corn oil	2.9	—	—	—	—
Bread	1.1	—	—	—	—

^{a}A dashed line means not detectable. Values obtained for MK-5 and MK-6 are omitted from this summary. The data demonstrate clearly (i) the huge difference in vitamin K contents between different foods and (ii) the preponderance of phylloquinone in some foods and of menaquinones (of several different chain lengths) in others.
^{b}A Japanese food made from fermented soya bean curd.
Data from Schurgers LJ and Vermeer C (2000) Determination of phylloquinone and menaqunones in food. Haemostasis **30**: 298–307, **Table 2**.

Food Sources, Absorption, Distribution, and Turnover

Food sources of phylloquinone for man (**Table 1**) include green leafy vegetables as the major quantitative source; however, its availability for absorption from these foods is thought to be relatively poor. Certain plant-derived oils, notably soya and canola oils, are also rich in the vitamin, which is probably much more readily available from such sources than it is from leaves. Menaquinones are typically obtained from foods, such as cheeses or Japanese 'natto' (fermented bean curd), in which bacterial fermentation has occurred. Smaller amounts of both phylloquinones and menaquinones are obtained from liver and other animal-derived foods.

Phylloquinone is highly lipophilic; however, at low concentrations it is transported by a saturable, energy-dependent transport system across the gut wall, mainly in the upper small intestine. Phylloquinone in foods consisting of plant tissues is much less readily bioavailable for absorption than the pure vitamin since it is tightly bound to the thylakoid membranes of the chloroplasts, and the absorption of vitamin K from plant foods is considerably improved by including additional fat in the meal. Its absorption also depends on the stimulation of bile salt and pancreatic lipase secretions. The long-chain menaquinones, which are even more lipophilic, are only passively absorbed and are much less bioavailable for absorption than phylloquinone. However, if given by injection (e.g., intracardially), they can be even more functionally active than phylloquinone.

The relative bioavailability and bioactivity of the different forms and food sources of vitamin K need more research. Preliminary studies with deuterium-labeled broccoli suggest that the bioavailability of endogenous vitamin K can be studied in humans by intrinsic stable isotope-labeling procedures.

Once absorbed, vitamin K is transported to the liver in the chylomicrons, where it becomes distributed among the triglyceride-rich chylomicron remnants (ca. 50%) and the low-density lipoprotein and high-density lipoprotein fractions of plasma (ca. 25% each). Plasma vitamin K concentrations, which are typically in the low nanomolar range in humans, are much lower than for the other fat-soluble vitamins (A, D, and E), and they are strongly correlated with the triglyceride content of the plasma. Indeed, some authorities prefer to express plasma vitamin K as a ratio to triglycerides instead of as a simple concentration. Differences between the apoE lipoprotein genetic variants affect plasma vitamin K, according to their different triglyceride clearance profiles. There is evidence for a major diurnal cycle of plasma vitamin K, with peak concentrations of both vitamin K and its associated triglycerides occurring in late evening and with lowest values in the morning. A kinetic study using radioactive vitamin K indicated that the turnover time of the exchangeable pool of the vitamin is quite short, approximately 1.5 days, and the first and second exponential decay curves had half-lives of 0.5–1 and 25–78 h, respectively. The exchangeable body pool size was only approximately 1 µg/kg body weight. The liver is an important repository of the vitamin for both plant-derived phylloquinone and the bacterially derived menaquinones. Depletion studies have indicated that the hepatic phylloquinone stores seem much more labile than the menaquinone stores, and that a functional deficiency accompanies the loss of the phylloquinone, which the remaining nondepleted menaquinones cannot prevent. Despite this, if menaquinones are given exogenously, they can be curative. Different tissues have different relative avidities for phylloquinone and menaquinones, and it has been suggested that they may have a different spectrum of functions from each other. Thus, in humans, phylloquinone is concentrated in liver, heart, and pancreas. The longer chain menaquinones, MK-6 to -11, are found mainly in liver with traces in heart and pancreas, but MK-4 is found especially in brain and kidney, where it exceeds phylloquinone concentrations. The tissue distribution in humans is similar to that in the rat.

The turnover of phylloquinone results in ca. 40–50% of the exchangeable body pool being transferred via the bile into the feces and 20% being excreted into the urine, the latter including the excretion of oxidized products that become conjugated as glucuronides.

Physiological Functions of Vitamin K: Interaction with Antagonists

Blood Coagulation Proteins

The principal physiological function that led to the discovery of vitamin K, and its confirmation as an essential vitamin for higher vertebrates, was its unique role in the blood clotting cascade. This cascade comprises a complex series of linked proenzyme-to-enzyme conversions, which leads eventually to a fibrin clot (**Figure 2**). Central to this process is the activation by calcium of gamma-carboxylated glutamyl (Gla) residues in some of the members of the cascade series: factors VII, IX, and X and factor II (prothrombin). In addition, there is an inhibitory level of control by proteins C, S, and possibly Z. All seven of these Gla proteins have Gla clusters that interact specifically with calcium so as to alter their polypeptide conformations and to permit their interaction with other members of the coagulation cascade (by exposing a phospholipid-binding domain) and hence leading either to activation or to inhibition of individual components. The Gla moieties of these and indeed all the vitamin K-dependent Gla proteins are formed by a post-translational carboxylation reaction catalyzed by the single enzyme, 'carboxylase,' at the endoplasmic reticulum sites of Gla protein synthesis. In the case of the blood coagulation proteins, the sole site of synthesis is the liver. Each carboxylated protein has a C-terminal 'propeptide' sequence that binds the carboxylase enzyme, and directs a coordinated series of carboxylations of the recipient glutamyl residues, before the propeptide is removed and the fully carboxylated protein is then secreted into the extracellular space for transport into the plasma.

Vitamin K acts as the essential recycling cofactor (or cosubstrate) for all protein carboxylation, Gla-forming reactions (**Figure 3**). In its dihydro or quinol form, the vitamin reacts with molecular oxygen, thereby creating a highly reactive, high-energy carbanion at the Glu site for insertion of carbon dioxide, creating a new Gla residue. This vitamin K quinol oxidation step provides the essential energy for the endothermic carboxylation step. The other product of the reaction is the epoxide of vitamin K, comprising a three-membered carbon–oxygen ring. Since the oxidized vitamin needs to be recycled back to the quinol form before the next protein carboxylation cycle, a two-stage reduction process ensues, forming first vitamin K quinone and then the original quinol

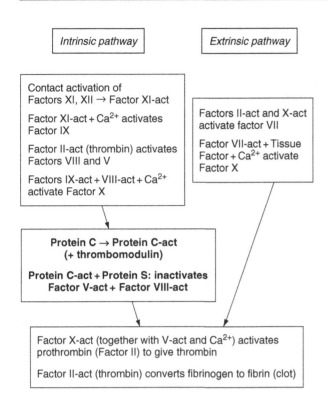

Figure 2 Vitamin K-dependent clotting factors. Factors II (prothrombin), VII, IX, and X and proteins C and S are all Gla proteins. The functions of proteins C and S, shown in bold, are inhibitory to the clotting cascade, whereas the other factors all form part of the cascade mechanism.

(Figure 3). Both of these reduction steps can be catalyzed by the enzyme vitamin K epoxide reductase, which is linked to a dithiol–disulfide reducing couple and which is highly sensitive to inhibition by the coumarin class of drugs, of which warfarin (Figure 1) is the best known and most commonly used member. The reduction of the intermediate vitamin K quinone to its quinol form can also be catalyzed by another, NAD(P)H-dependent, quinone reductase that is warfarin resistant, and for this reason the inhibition of carboxylation by warfarin can be reversed or antagonized by large doses of vitamin K provided exogenously in its normal quinone form. A severe deficiency of vitamin K, or treatment with coumarin drugs (for the control of excessive blood clotting tendency in humans), results in prolonged clotting times that can be detected by the standardized 'one stage prothrombin time' test, in which citrated or oxalated (i.e., calcium-complexed) blood is treated with tissue factor plus additional calcium so as to initiate the clotting process. However, a much more sensitive test for mild vitamin K deficiency is the PIVKA test (Proteins Induced by Vitamin K Absence or Antagonism), which is an immunological enzyme-linked immunosorbent assay (ELISA) test that specifically

recognizes undercarboxylated blood clotting proteins and particularly des-gamma-carboxy prothrombin.

Proteins C and S, and possibly also Z, function differently from the other Gla-containing blood clotting factors that are an integral part of the fibrin-forming cascade. Protein C has a regulatory role, inactivating factors V and VIII, and in conjunction with protein S it also acts as a cofactor to enhance the rate of fibrinolysis of blood clots in locations where they are unwanted and potentially harmful. The exact function of protein Z remains unresolved, although interactions with thrombin and factor X have been reported. Clearly, there is a delicate balance of pro- and anti-clot formation and removal activities among the vitamin K-dependent Gla proteins of the cascade, although the net effect of a deficiency of the vitamin or of its antagonism by drugs appears to be a reduction of the clotting tendency.

Bone Gla proteins

Protein S together with two other Gla proteins, osteocalcin (OC; or bone Gla protein) and matrix Gla protein (MGP), play a variety of only partly understood roles in bone and other mineralized tissues. Of these proteins, only OC is produced solely and specifically by mineralized tissue, whereas the other two (or at least their mRNA templates) are more widespread and occur also in soft tissues.

OC is synthesized specifically by osteoblasts and odontoblasts, and it accounts for ca. 15–20% of the noncollagen protein of the bone matrix. Approximately 20% is secreted into blood plasma, where it has no obvious function, but it has frequently been measured as an index of bone-forming (osteblastic) activity, and is present in increased amounts in plasma of people with certain bone diseases and of young infants. It is a small protein, MW 5700, with just three Gla residues. Unlike the blood coagulation Gla proteins, which in most people not severely vitamin K deficient and not vitamin K antagonist treated are almost completely carboxylated, circulating OC is at least 5–10% undercarboxylated in many population groups, as measured by assays that depend on the affinity of the undercarboxylated form for hydroxyapatite or a specific ELISA assay for the undercarboxylated form. Since vitamin K supplements can reduce its degree of undercarboxylation in many people, it has been proposed as a new and highly sensitive functional test of vitamin K status in man.

Despite the growing level of interest in its practical use as a status index, our understanding of the essential function of OC remains incomplete. Its affinity for calcium is less strong than that of the larger Gla proteins, but it binds avidly to hydroxyapatite and is chemotactic for osteoclasts

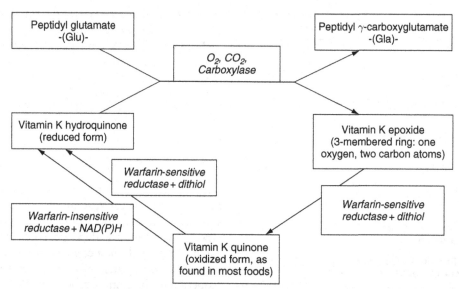

Figure 3 Vitamin K oxidation–reduction cycle during Gla formation. Oxidation of vitamin K hydroquinone (reduced vitamin) to vitamin K epoxide by molecular oxygen provides the energy needed to drive the carboxylation of peptidyl-Glu to peptidyl-Gla (i.e., gamma-carboxy glutamate). The vitamin K epoxide is then recycled by reduction with dithiols in two stages. The first stage requires a reductase enzyme that is coumarin drug (e.g., warfarin) inhibitable. The second stage can be catalyzed by either of two reductases, one of which is NAD(P)H dependent and is not warfarin inhibited.

and their progenitors. Moreover, it can enhance the differentiation of osteoclast progenitor cells in culture, which has been interpreted as implying a possible role in bone resorption. Transgenic mice that lack the gene for OC have increased bone mass, despite an increased number of osteoclasts. In humans, however, underhydroxylation of OC especially in postmenopausal women has been linked to low vitamin K intakes, reduced bone mineral density, and increased risk of fracture. Intervention with high-dose MK-4, mainly in Japan, has been reported to improve bone mineral density and decrease fracture risk. Although a single study in the United Kingdom suggested that a combination of vitamin K_1 and vitamin D supplements may benefit bone mineral density in postmenopausal women, considerably more research is needed in this area. The separate roles of OC and other vitamin K-dependent proteins also need to be clarified.

The second vitamin K-dependent Gla protein in bone, MGP, has a MW of 9600 and five Gla residues and is highly insoluble. Unlike OC, it is also found in cartilage, and, significantly, its mRNA occurs in several soft tissues including artery walls. Its synthesis is modulated by 1,25-dihydroxy vitamin D and by retinoic acid. Mice lacking the gene for MGP quickly developed calcified arteries and died of aortic rupture before 2 months of age. For this reason, MGP is believed to antagonize the pathological calcification of soft tissues and thus to

protect them. The absence of MGP also led to inappropriate calcification of growth plate cartilage, reduced growth, osteopenia, and fracture in the MGP gene knockout mice. In humans, defects in the MGP gene are associated with Keutel's syndrome and chondroplasia punctata, in which cartilage calcification is abnormal. Similar abnormalities have been observed in infants whose mothers were treated with warfarin during the first trimester of pregnancy. In one study, low vitamin K intake was associated with atherosclerotic calcification of the aorta in postmenopausal women. Also, circulating MGP levels were found to be raised in severe atherosclerosis and in type 1 diabetes in humans. A specific immunoassay for MGP has been developed that should assist further research on this potentially important regulatory protein.

The third bone-associated Gla protein, protein S, is also involved with blood clotting. It is synthesized by osteoblast-like and osteblastoma cells in culture, and it has been detected in bone matrix. It is also synthesized by hepatocytes, megakaryocytes, and endothelial cells. Children with an inborn deficiency of it developed osteopenia and bone lesions; however, its precise functional role is unknown.

All three bone Gla proteins (and probably most other Gla proteins) have 'leader' or 'pre'-peptides when first formed on the endoplasmic reticulum (ER) that are required for translocation across the ER and are removed during this process. OC, protein S, and most other Gla proteins also have a pro-peptide sequence that is removed during secretion and that directs the action of the carboxylase enzyme before secretion. MGP differs from the other Gla proteins in that its carboxylase recognition sequence is not removed; instead, only a short (five-residue) carboxy-terminal sequence is removed from it. All known mammalian Gla proteins contain the characteristic amino acid sequence Gla-X-X-X-Gla-X-Cys, where X represents an undefined amino acid. If vitamin K is in short supply or antagonized, certain Gla residues escape gamma-glutamyl formation more than others. Thus, in a study of OC, the Glu residue at position 17 was typically only 67% carboxylated, that at position 21 was 88% carboxylated, and that at position 24 was 93% carboxylated.

Surprisingly, in a meta-analysis of studies on warfarin-treated adult patients, no evidence of any increase in bone disorders was found.

Gas6 and Other Vitamin K-Requiring Gla Proteins

A Gla protein that is associated with the central nervous system, rather than with liver or bone, was discovered in 1993. In tissue culture models it had the properties of a growth arrest-specific (GAS) cell-signalling gene product. It acts as a ligand for a number of receptor protein kinases; it potentiates the growth of vascular smooth muscle cells, Schwann cells, and the neurons that synthesize gonadotropin-releasing hormones; and it can prevent apoptotic cell death. Knockout mice in which three Gas6 receptors are mutated had major neurological and spermatogenic abnormalities. There is interest in potential roles for Gas6 in Alzheimer's disease and Parkinson's disease. Clearly, these properties and emerging roles have helped to confirm the growing suspicion that vitamin K-dependent Gla proteins possess key functions beyond blood clotting and even bone remodelling. Gas6 has a MW of 75,000 with 11 or 12 Gla residues, and its structure is partly homologous with protein S.

Even less well characterized are several other Gla proteins from a variety of tissues. Kidney contains 'nephrocalcin,' with just two or three Gla residues, which may be involved in renal calcium transport (another important function that may be impaired by vitamin K deficiency in man). Atherocalcin, or plaque Gla protein, may be related or even identical to MGP. Proline-rich Gla proteins PRGP-1 and PRGP-2 are found predominantly in the spinal cord and thyroid gland, respectively, but their functions are unknown. Gla proteins occur in most vertebrates and also in molluscs, so their evolutionary appearance in the animal kingdom is probably quite ancient in origin.

Other, Probably Non-Gla Functions of Vitamin K

Vitamin K is thought to be involved in sphingolipid metabolism in certain bacteria by modulating serine palmitoyl transferase, and warfarin treatment decreased brain levels of sulfatides and galactocerebroside sulfotransferase activity in animals, which was reversible by vitamin K (either K_1 or MK-4). Therefore, it is now thought that vitamin K may be involved in sphingolipid metabolism, and this in turn has implications for its action as a second messenger as well as being a structural component. There are several functions of MK-4 that are shared by the isolated geranyl-geraniol side chain, which involve the induction of apoptosis of osteoclasts and of certain cancer cells in culture. Depriving certain tumours of vitamin K, both *in vitro* and *in vivo*, seemed to inhibit their growth and metastasis. Patients receiving warfarin for cardiovascular disease seem to have a reduced incidence of tumors, and warfarin may also suppress delayed-type hypersensitivity reactions.

Recent studies have suggested that MK-4, in particular, has a transcriptional regulatory function, for example, in osteosarcoma cell cultures, in which it binds to and activates the SXR steroid and xenobiotic receptor. This in turn increases mRNA levels for osteoblast markers: bone alkaline phosphatase, osteoprotogerin, osteopontin, and MGP. MK-4 and its isolated geranyl-geraniol side chain was also able to suppress the synthesis of prostaglandin E_2, which is a potent bone resorption catalyst. These observations have led to speculation (i) that some of the menaquinones may possess some functions that are not shared by phylloquinone, and (ii) that there may be implications for cell proliferation and for cancer risk from variations in the supply of vitamin K and in its speciation.

Population Groups at Risk of Vitamin K Deficiency

Because of the minimal extent of transfer of vitamin K across the placenta, the fetus and newborn infant have much lower circulating vitamin K than adults (typically 30-fold lower). In addition, human milk has a lower concentration of the vitamin than that of most other mammalian species. Although low vitamin K levels have not been found to affect the developing fetus in a functionally deleterious way, it is clear that the newborn, and especially the solely breast-fed infant, is at higher risk of functional deficiency than older infants and adults. In a minority of cases, this can lead to life-threatening or long-term damage associated with intracranial bleeding. Hemorrhagic disease of the newborn (HDN) is classified as early (first 24 h of life), classic (days 1–7), or late (2–12 weeks). Of these, the third category is most likely to involve dangerous intracranial bleeding. Risk factors for HDN include intestinal fat malabsorption and hepatic disease. In Western countries, since the 1950s, it has been routine practice to give prophylactic phylloquinone in a 1 or 2 mg dose at birth, and this has been found to considerably reduce the risk of HDN. An intramuscular depot dose was found to be highly effective; however, a study in the United Kingdom in the 1990s suggested a possible link with childhood cancer. Despite little subsequent support for this contraindication, the adverse publicity led to a shift in practice toward oral dosing. An oral micellar preparation containing glycholate and lecithin has been developed that has improved absorption characteristics. Another approach toward the avoidance of late HDN is vitamin K supplementation of breast-feeding mothers since breast milk vitamin K levels can be increased substantially by dosage to the mother. Modern commercial formula feeds typically contain 50–125 μg phylloquinone/l.

Antibiotic-treated patients may be at increased risk of developing vitamin K deficiency. Some antibiotics may reduce the production of usable menaquinones by gut bacteria; others, such as cephalosporin, may exert vitamin K epoxide reductase inhibitory effects. Vitamins A and E in large doses may increase the risk of vitamin K deficiency and/or its sequelae in susceptible people. Thus, in one study, patients receiving anti-coagulant drugs exhibited a further reduction of pro-thrombin levels if they were given 400 IU α-tocopherol per day for 4 weeks. The microsomal vitamin K-dependent carboxylase enzyme was found to be inhibited by α-tocopheryl quinone and, to a lesser extent, by α-tocopherol. It is also inhibited by other oxygen free radical antagonists. Control of blood clotting with warfarin-type drugs thus requires control of intakes of vitamins A and E as well as vitamin K so as to achieve consistent results.

As noted previously, some older people, especially postmenopausal women, seem to be at increased risk of developing marginal vitamin K deficiency, which manifests itself, for instance, by an increased percentage of undercarboxylated osteocalcin (ucOC) in the circulation. The sequelae of such marginal deficiency, and in particular its implications for bone health, are currently the subject of considerable research effort (**Table 2**). Several epidemiological cross-sectional studies have noted an association between higher vitamin K intakes and higher bone mineral density or lower fracture risk. One study reported that a subgroup of postmenopausal women who were 'fast losers' of calcium responded to vitamin K supplements by reduced

Table 2 Studies (1985–2001) linking vitamin K intake, status, or effects of supplementation with bone health in humans

Nature of evidence	No. of studies
Serum vitamin K positively correlated with BMD	4
Serum vitamin K lower in people with hip or vertebral fractures	3
Vitamin K intake directly correlated with BMD	2
ucOC directly correlated with risk of hip fracture	5
ucOC inversely correlated with velocity of ultrasound (a measure of bone quality)	1
ucOC inversely correlated with BMD	2
Supplementation with phylloquinone increased carboxylation of osteocalcin	7
Supplementation with phylloquinone or menaquinone reduced calcium loss	3
Supplementation with phylloquinone increased markers of bone formation and reduced markers of bone resorption	1
Supplementation with phylloquinone (+vitamin D) increased BMD	1
Supplementation with menaquinone (+vitamin D) increased BMD	2
Supplementation with menaquinone alone increased BMD and/or decreased bone loss	6
Supplementation with menaquinone reduced fracture risk	2

BMD, bone mineral density; ucOC, undercarboxylated osteocalcin. Data from Weber P (2001) Vitamin K and bone health. *Nutrition* **17**: 880–887, and S. Karger AG, Basel.

calcium and hydroxyproline excretion. Although vitamins D and K have distinct functions in calcium absorption, and its distribution, deposition, and excretion, there is evidence that synergistic interactions can occur between them, and that both can affect the same cell-signalling pathways. Osteocalcin and MGP synthesis is stimulated by 1,25-dihydroxy vitamin D in cell culture.

MK-4 in large doses has been used for prophylaxis and treatment of osteoporosis, especially in Japan. A study in The Netherlands reported reduced bone loss after 2 years of treatment of postmenopausal women with amounts of phylloquinone that are achievable from dietary sources. More long-term intervention trials are needed.

Status, Requirements, and Recommended Intakes

Vitamin K status can be measured either by its concentration in plasma or by its efficacy in ensuring optimal carboxylase function, as indicated by specific carboxylated plasma proteins. Accurate assay of the very low concentrations of vitamin K that are present in plasma was a considerable analytical challenge, which was eventually solved by high-performance liquid chromatography (HPLC) followed by high-sensitivity coulometric or fluorometric detection. A popular method uses organic solvent extraction, a cartridge cleanup step, an HPLC separation followed by postcolumn reduction of the vitamin K quinone to the reduced quinol form by metallic zinc or other reductant, and finally fluorometric quantitation of the fluorescent quinol. A useful internal standard, not found in nature, is the homolog of phylloquinone, vitamin $K_{1(25)}$. With modern detectors, analysis is possible with only 0.25 ml plasma. A published 'normal' range in the United States is 0.25–2.7 nmol/l, corresponding to approximate average daily intakes of 100 μg/day in men and 80 μg/day in women. As noted earlier, the phylloquinone content of plasma has a short half-life and is strongly correlated with plasma triglycerides. It is therefore not ideal as a long-term index of status. Alternatives include functional indices such as plasma prothrombin time (increased only by severe vitamin K deficiency), PIVKA, (which is more sensitive to marginal deficiency), and ucOC (which is the most sensitive functional indicator). These functional indices are not totally specific for vitamin K deficiency, although ucOC (for which monoclonal antibodies now exist) does appear to possess reasonably good specificity. Unfortunately, the different commercial kit assays measure different epitopes of OC, which makes harmonization difficult. Urinary total Gla is sensitive to vitamin K status, but it varies with age and has not yet proved to be very useful as a status indicator. Functional indices that are based on impaired carboxylase activity affecting other Gla proteins may be developed in the future.

Most estimates of the amount of phylloquinone needed to correct clotting changes suggest that adult human requirements are between 0.5 and 1 μg/kg/day. There are no reference nutrient intakes defined for vitamin K in the United Kingdom, although a 'safe intake' for adults was set in 1991 at 1 μg/kg/day and for infants 10 μg/day. In the United States, the Food and Nutrition Board of the National Academy of Sciences has defined an Adequate Intake (AI) of phylloquinone of 90 μg/day for adult women and 120 μg/day for adult men, with proportionately smaller values for children. For infants aged 0–6 months, the AI is only 2 μg/day, and it is 2.5 μg/day at 7–12 months, thus creating a larger proportional difference between infants and older age groups than for most micronutrients.

Both phylloquinone and the menaquinones appear to be nontoxic, even in multimilligram amounts. However, menadione, the water-soluble form of vitamin K, was found to cause hemolytic anemia, hyperbilirubinemia, and kernicturus in infants when >5 mg was given. Therefore, it is not currently used for human prophylaxis or treatment.

Since vitamin K is thought to have a wide range of functions in the body in addition to blood clotting, and some of these may have long-term health implications, research on requirements and optimal intakes, with multiple end points, is needed. Metabolic and health-related differences between the menaquinones and phylloquinone also need to be defined.

See also: **Vitamin A**: Biochemistry and Physiological Role. **Vitamin E**: Physiology and Health Effects.

Further Reading

Binkley NC and Suttie JW (1995) Vitamin K nutrition and osteoporosis. *Journal of Nutrition* **125**: 1812–1821.

Bugel S (2003) Vitamin K and bone health. *Proceedings of the Nutrition Society* **62**: 839–843.

Ferland G (1998) The vitamin K-dependent proteins: An update. *Nutrition Review* **56**: 223–230.

Greer FR (1999) Vitamin K status of lactating mothers and their infants. *Acta Paediatrica Supplement* **430**: 95–103.

Nelsestuen GL, Shah AM, and Harvey SB (2000) Vitamin K-dependent proteins. *Vitamins and Hormones* **58**: 355–389.

Saxena SP, Israels ED, and Israels LG (2001) Novel vitamin K-dependent pathways regulating cell survival. *Apoptosis* **6**: 57–68.

Shearer MJ (1997) The roles of vitamins D and K in bone health and osteoporosis prevention. *Proceedings of the Nutrition Society* **56**: 915–937.

Shearer MJ (2000) Role of vitamin K and Gla proteins in the pathophysiology of osteoporosis and vascular calcification. *Current Opinion in Clinical Nutrition and Metabolic Care* **3**: 433–438.

Suttie JW (1992) Vitamin K and human nutrition. *Journal of the American Dietetic Association* **92**: 585–590.

Suttie JW (1995) The importance of menaquinones in human nutrition. *Annual Review of Nutrition* **15**: 399–417.

Tsaioun KI (1999) Vitamin K-dependent proteins in the developing and aging nervous system. *Nutrition Review* **57**: 231–240.

Vermeer C, Jie K-SG, and Knapen MHJ (1995) Role of vitamin K in bone metabolism. *Annual Review of Nutrition* **15**: 1–22.

Vermeer C and Schurgers LJ (2000) A comprehensive review of vitamin K and vitamin K antagonists. *Hematology/Oncology Clinics of North America* **14**: 339–353.

Weber P (2001) Vitamin K and bone health. *Nutrition* **17**: 880–887.

WHOLE GRAINS

R Lang, University of Teeside, Middlesbrough, UK
S A Jebb, MRC Human Nutrition Research, Cambridge, UK

Introduction

There is growing interest in the benefits of traditional dietary patterns with an emphasis on unrefined, plant-based foods. Whole-grain foods are rich in dietary fiber, antioxidants, and a range of other nutrients that may offer health benefits. This chapter will review the epidemiological analyses showing a reduced risk of premature death and decreases in the incidence of cardiovascular disease (CVD), type 2 diabetes, and cancer. However since whole-grain consumption is frequently linked to other positive dietary and life style behaviors (including increased consumption of fruit and vegetables and increased physical activity) more randomized controlled intervention studies are required to support these association studies. Moreover, further research is required to confirm putative mechanistic hypotheses, which include the positive effects of dietary fiber on lipid metabolism, improved glucose homeostasis as a consequence of a reduced glycemic response, or the antioxidant properties of these foods, which may have beneficial effects on vascular reactivity and inflammation.

What are Whole Grains?

Cereal grains are the seeds of the plant and they house the embryo and the necessary food reserves required for germination. Forming the dietary staples in many countries, the major grains in the human diet are wheat, rice, and corn (maize). Consumption of oats, millet, barley, sorghum, and rye are more limited.

The basic structure of the grain (regardless of plant type) is shown in **Figure 1**. There are essentially three layers, the endosperm, bran, and germ layers, each of which have a unique role within germination, but which also contain essential nutrients and phytochemicals important within the human diet and linked to health benefits.

The Bran Layer

The bran layer is the outer thick-walled structure of the grain. It is rich in B vitamins and phytonutrients such as flavonoids and indoles plus a small amount of protein. It also contains antioxidant compounds including phytoestrogens such as lignans and isoflavones. These hormonally active compounds, similar to estrogen, may influence sex hormone metabolism and may impact on hormone-related disease. The bran also contains factors that may decrease bioavailability of nutrients such as phytic acid, tannins, and enzyme inhibitors. It is also where the bulk of insoluble fiber is found. The insoluble fiber contained within the bran layer has long been recognized to play an important role in intestinal health, by optimizing bowel transit time and increasing fecal weight. But some of the health benefits associated with a high-fiber diet may come from other components, and not just from the fiber itself. For example, the oligosaccharides found within the starchy endosperm layer behave in a similar manner to soluble nonstarch polysaccharides (NSP) and may therefore be useful in controlling blood lipid profiles and blood glucose. In addition, oligosaccharides are natural prebiotics, which encourage the proliferation of healthy microflora within the gut. Colonization of specific bacteria within the colon, such as bifidobacteria, has been implicated in benefits to the immune system, cholesterol lowering, and reducing the risk of colon cancer through the fermentation of these carbohydrates into short-chain fatty acids.

The Germ Layer

This is the plant embryo and it contains a concentrated source of minerals such as iron and zinc plus vitamin E. These and other antioxidants provide defense systems against reactive oxygen species not

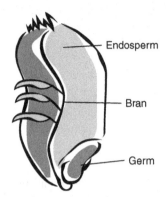

Figure 1 A grain of wheat. (Reproduced with kind permission from the British Nutrition Foundation: http://www.nutrition.org.uk)

only for the plant, but also for those who consume the grain. Indeed, the pH conditions of the stomach have been shown to cause a dramatic increase in the activity of these antioxidants. Whole grains contain a greater concentration of antioxidants than many fruits and vegetables.

The Endosperm

This makes up about 80% of the grain and is the starchy component comprising mainly carbohydrates including resistant starch and oligosaccharides such as fructans, inulin, and oligofructose. These behave in a similar manner to soluble NSP within the gut. The endosperm also contains B vitamins, in particular riboflavin and pantothenic acid, and some protein.

Definition of Whole Grain

Whole grains are defined as those that are used in their entirety in the food production process, so that all three layers are present within the product. This distinguishes them from refined grains. Regardless of how much of the grain is used, the milling process determines particle size and hence has an impact on handling within the body. Many whole and refined grains are processed in some way to enhance flavor, texture, color, and shelf life. As long as the whole of the grain is used in the process, the food is described as whole grain. However, there is some debate as to whether the disruption of the intact grain modulates the health impact. Certainly, it tends to increase the glycemic index of the food, which may have implications for the risk of metabolic disease, especially type 2 diabetes.

The vast majority of grains consumed within Western countries are refined, and the outer germ and bran layers are removed to leave only the starchy

endosperm. The refining process may reduce some nutrients such as zinc, selenium, and vitamin E by as much as 90%. In some cases vitamins and minerals are reintroduced through fortification and restoration, but the bioavailability and relative health effects of these nutrients when consumed in their natural state compared to artificial methods of fortification is not known.

At present there is no uniform definition of a whole-grain food, but for the purposes of health claims the proportion of whole-grain cereal used within a food product is critical. In 1999 the Food and Drug Administration in the US approved a health claim for use on packing to help consumers choose foods that contained a significant amount of the whole grain. Products must contain at least 51% whole grain by weight, i.e., must be the largest component of the product, to be entitled to carry the health claim. This allows a clear distinction between the refined and partially or nonrefined products available to the consumer. For example, a product made of 100% whole wheat could be labeled as whole grain, but a multigrain loaf containing 75% white flour and 25% wholemeal flour could not. In the UK, the Joint Health Claims Initiative has adopted a similar definition.

Consumption of Whole Grains

Recent studies have shown low levels of consumption of whole-grain foods in the general population of the most affluent countries. In the US data was collected from over 9000 US citizens aged 20 years or over who participated in the 1994–96 USDA's continuing survey of food intakes. Using an interview technique and serving sizes defined by the Food Guide Pyramid, food consumption over 2 nonconsecutive days was examined. It was found that 29% of the sample were nonconsumers of whole grains and the average number of daily servings was less than 1 per day. The proportion of the sample reaching the recommended 3 servings per day was 8%.

Intakes are similarly low in the UK. Using data from two nationally representative surveys wholegrain consumption was assessed: the Diet and Nutritional Survey of British Adults 1986–87 included over 2000 adults aged between 16 and 64 years, and the National Diet and Nutrition Survey of people aged 65 years and over included over 1000 free-living adults (from a total of over 2000 participants which included free-living and institutionalized individuals) during 1994–95. Dietary data was collected using a 7-day diary recording weighed food in 1986–87, and a 4-day weighed food diary in 1994–95. Whole-grain foods were identified as those having at least 51%

whole-grain ingredients by weight and a serving was defined as each occasion the food appeared within the recording period. Both surveys showed that approximately 30% of individuals did not consume any whole-grain foods during the survey period (29% in 1986–87 and 33.5% in 1994–95), and over 97% of adults did not meet the US recommendation of 3 servings per day. Median consumption was less than 1 serving per day.

In comparison to the US and the UK, whole-grain foods are consumed in greater quantities in Scandinavian countries. In Finland, rye bread has always been a staple and consequently whole-grain intakes have always been high. In Norway, food disappearance data suggest that consumption of whole-grain foods is four times that seen in the US, but is lower than that seen in Finland. In the Scandinavian studies, however, estimation of consumption of whole grain was not based on number of servings but utilized measures such as a bread score based on number of slices of bread consumed multiplied by the proportion of whole-grain flour; 24-h recall techniques of whole-grain foods consumed; and simply the number of slices of bread consumed. These differing techniques make it difficult to directly compare findings in Scandinavia with the UK and US.

However, within populations the consumption of whole grains is influenced by a number of social and demographic factors. Most surveys have found an increase in whole grain consumption with age. For example, in the UK, there was a median of 1 serving per week in the 16–24-year-olds rising to 3 servings per week in the 35–64-year-olds (1986–87 survey).

Consumption in the survey of people aged 65 years and over showed higher intakes of 5 servings per week (1994–95 survey) but it is not clear whether this reflects a secular trend or a continuing effect of age. In general, men consume more whole-grain foods than women. This may reflect a greater food intake overall, rather than a specific preference for whole-grain varieties. In the US, white adults consume more whole-grain foods than black Americans, and Mexican Americans consume the least whole grains.

In the US and UK, income and level of education are also positively associated with whole-grain consumption, but in Finland, the highest intakes of rye bread are observed in the lower socioeconomic groups. In the US and UK, whole-grain consumers are less likely to smoke, tend to be regular exercisers and consume more fruits and vegetables. These findings suggest an association of whole-grain consumption with other positive life style traits.

Whole Grains and Health

Epidemiological evidence suggests an inverse relationship between the consumption of whole-grain foods and the relative risk of a number of chronic diseases. Studies have found that habitual consumption of whole-grain foods is associated with reductions in premature mortality, risk of coronary heart disease, ischemic stroke, and type 2 diabetes.

All Cause Mortality

Three large prospective epidemiological studies have considered the relationship between whole-grain consumption and all cause mortality (Table 1). Using a variety of measures to assess whole-grain consumption, all three studies concluded that the more whole-grain foods were consumed, the lower the risk of death from a number of chronic diseases. Women in the Iowa Women's Study were followed over a 9-year period. The population was divided into quintiles of whole grain intake using a food frequency questionnaire (FFQ). Intakes varied

Table 1 Effect of whole-grain consumption on all cause mortality

Cohort	Measure of WG consumption	Reported association	Reference
Iowa Women	FFQ	40% ↓ with at least 1 serving per day Refined grains ↑ mortality with ↑ consumption	Jacobs et al. (1999) Is whole grain intake associated with reduced total and cause-specific death rates in older women? The Iowa Women's Health Study. *American Journal of Public Health* **89**: 322–329.
Norwegian County Study	Bread score (slices × %WG)	HRR graded and inverse with ↑ consumption	Jacobs et al. (2001) Reduced mortality among whole grain bread eaters in men and women in the Norwegian County Study. *European Journal of Clinical Nutrition* **55**: 137–143.
Physician's Health Study	Breakfast cereal FFQ (WG classified as 25% w/w)	HRR ↓ with ↑ consumption	Liu et al. (2003) Is intake of breakfast cereals related to total and cause-specific mortality in men? *American Journal of Clinical Nutrition* **77**: 594–599.

considerably from 1.5 servings per week in the lowest quintile and 22.5 servings per week in the highest, yet an inverse association between whole-grain intake and the risk of death was observed across quintiles, with a 40% reduction in total mortality ($P < 0.0001$) in those consuming at least one serving of whole-grain foods per day. Even when adjusted for confounders such as age, energy intake, hypertension, heart disease, diabetes, cancer, body mass index (BMI), waist–hip ratio (WHR), physical activity, alcohol intake, smoking, positive dietary habits such as fruit and vegetable consumption, fat intake, and red meat and fish consumption, the significant inverse relationship remained ($P = 0.005$). In contrast, refined grain intake was associated with increased mortality for those in the quintile of highest refined grain intake compared to those in the quintile of lowest intake (**Figure 2**).

Similarly in over 47 000 men and women in Norway aged 35–56 years studied over 9 years, hazard rate ratios (HRR) for total mortality were inverse and graded across whole-grain bread score categories in men and women between the highest and lowest bread score after adjustment for a range of dietary and lifestyle factors. The bread score was calculated using number of slices consumed per day and the proportion of whole-grain flour used. The analysis found that both components of the whole grain scoring system contributed to these inverse trends (% deaths between highest and lowest scores categories: 7% versus 10% for men and 2.7% versus 4.6% for women).

In the Physicians' Health Study, breakfast cereal consumption was used as an indicator of whole-grain intake in over 86 000 US male physicians aged 40–84 years studied over 5.5 years. Breakfast cereal consumption was assessed using a semiquantitative FFQ where men had to report the amount, frequency, brand, and type of cereal consumed over the previous year. Whole-grain cereals were classified as those with >25% whole grain or bran by weight; all others were considered to be refined grains. Whole-grain breakfast cereal consumption was inversely associated with total mortality independent of a range of dietary and lifestyle considerations.

The use of bread and cereal intakes as a measure of total whole-grain consumption is of some concern, as the extent to which they correlate with overall whole-grain consumption is uncertain. Indeed, such studies also fail to distinguish whether it is in fact something within the whole-grain package that is of benefit, or something else entirely.

Cardiovascular Disease

Cardiovascular diseases are responsible for over a third of all deaths and are the biggest contributor to the global burden of disease. There are a number of studies to suggest that individuals who consume a diet rich in whole-grain foods have a lower incidence of heart disease, although the mechanism is still unclear (see **Table 2**).

Increases in the consumption of whole grains have been shown to decrease CHD deaths and the risk of stroke and heart disease in some, but not all, epidemiological analyses. In the study of postmenopausal Iowan women there was a reduction in relative risk (RR) of ischemic heart disease of about a third in those consuming at least 1 serving of whole-grain foods per day. This relationship was attributable to differences in the consumption of dark breads and whole-grain breakfast cereals while less common whole-grain foods such as popcorn, brown rice, and oatmeal showed no relationship with CVD. A significant inverse relationship between increasing whole-grain intake and risk was also observed for CHD and total CVD, but not stroke alone (**Figure 3**).

Similar results were obtained in the Nurses' Health Study of 75 000 women aged 38–63 years who were free from existing diabetes, angina, myocardial infarction, stroke, or other CVDs at baseline. Here, a significant inverse relationship was observed between CHD and whole-grain consumption even after multivariate adjustment for known confounders such as age, smoking, BMI, alcohol, and other dietary and lifestyle factors. For each additional serving of whole-grain food per day, the authors found

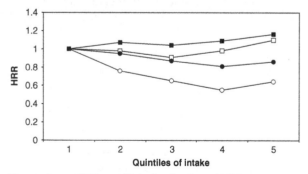

Multivariate adjusted Hazard Rate Ratios across quintiles of refined and whole grain intakes for all cause mortality

Figure 2 ○ (WG) and □ (refined) adjusted HRR for age and total energy intake. ● (WG) and □ (refined) adjusted for age, energy intake, marital status, education, high blood pressure, diabetes, heart disease, cancer, BMI, WHR, physical activity, smoking, alcohol intake, use of vitamin supplements, HRT, total fat, saturated fat, intake of fruits and vegetables, intake of meat and intake of fish and seafood.

Table 2 Summary of the evidence relating a reduced risk of CVD to increased whole-grain consumption

Evidence for a reduced risk of:	Cohort	Reported association	Reference
CHD	Californian Seventh Day Adventists	Lower RR for preference of whole grain bread	Fraser *et al.* (1999) Associations between diet and cancer, ischemic heart disease, and all-cause mortality in non-Hispanic white California Seventh-day Adventists. *American Journal of Clinical Nutrition* **70**: 532S–538S.
IHD	Iowa Women's Health Study	Lower RR for increasing whole grain consumption	Jacobs *et al.* (1998a) Whole grain intake may reduce the risk of ischaemic heart disease in postmenopausal women: The Iowa Women's Health Study. American *Journal of Clinical Nutrition* **68**: 248–257.
CHD and CVD	Iowa Women's Health Study	Lower RR for increasing whole grain consumption (except for stroke after adjustment)	Jacobs *et al.* (1999) Is whole grain intake associated with reduced total and cause-specific death rates in older women? The Iowa Women's Health Study. *American Journal of Public Health* **89**: 322–329.
CHD	Nurse's Health Study	Lower RR for increasing whole grain consumption	Liu *et al.* (1999) Whole grain consumption and risk of coronary heart disease: results from the Nurses' Health Study. *American Journal of Clinical Nutrition*. **70**: 412–419.
Ischemic stroke	Nurse's Health Study	Lower RR for increasing whole grain consumption (total stroke cases)	Liu *et al.* (2000) Whole grain consumption and risk of ischemic stroke in women: A prospective study. *JAMA* **284**: 1534–1540.

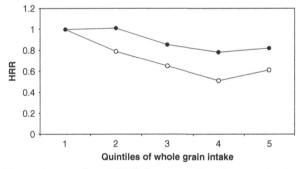

Multivariate adjusted hazard rate ratios across quintiles of whole grain intake for cardiovascular disease

Figure 3 ○ adjusted HRR for age and total energy intake. ● adjusted for age, energy intake, marital status, education, high blood pressure, diabetes, heart disease, cancer, BMI, WHR, physical activity, smoking, alcohol intake, use of vitamin supplements, HRT, total fat, saturated fat, intake of fruits and vegetables, intake of meat and intake of fish and seafood.

a relative risk of 0.91 (95% confidence interval (CI) 0.85, 0.97) for CHD risk.

In this study there was also a significant inverse relationship between whole-grain intake and risk of ischemic stroke. After adjustment for smoking and other known CVD risk factors, the relationship was attenuated but remained significant. However, after further adjustment for assorted dietary variables (folate, vitamin E, fiber, magnesium, and potassium), the effect was no longer significant. Unlike previous studies, the authors defined the different categories of stroke and found that although risk

of hemorrhagic stroke or incident fatal strokes did not appear to be influenced by whole-grain consumption, total stroke risk was inversely related to consumption of whole-grain foods.

It is notable that in many studies subjects with the highest intake of whole-grain foods also had the healthiest lifestyles and the relationship with whole-grain foods is attenuated after adjustment for other diet and lifestyle variables. The exact mechanisms of protection are unclear. Diets rich in whole-grain foods tend to reduce serum LDL-cholesterol and TAG levels whilst increasing HDL-cholesterol concentrations and blood pressure is lower. This may be due in part to the dietary fiber, but the effect usually persists after adjustment for fiber intake. Whole grains also contain a number of specific components that may have heart health benefits, including antioxidants (vitamin E and selenium), B vitamins, flavonoids, and indoles. These may reduce oxidative stress and homocysteine levels, and the isoflavone content of these grains may positively influence vascular reactivity and the inflammatory state.

Type 2 Diabetes

The prevalence of type 2 diabetes has reached epidemic proportions with over 150 million cases diagnosed worldwide; this number is expected to double by 2025. The concurrent rise in obesity has been directly linked to insulin resistance and compensatory hyperinsulinemia and eventual type 2 diabetes, with over 80% of diagnosed type 2 diabetes being the result of excess body fat. Public health recommendations to reduce fat intake, especially saturated fat, have led to a rise in the proportion of carbohydrates (particularly refined carbohydrates) in the diet with consequences for postprandial glucose and insulin metabolism. The source of carbohydrate is also important. Whole-grain foods commonly have a low glycemic index because whole-grain foods with an intact bran and germ layer have a much smaller impact on blood glucose than refined carbohydrate foods because of their larger particle size, slowing the rate of enzymic attack. The level of soluble fiber within whole grains has also been identified as a possible protector and the higher amylose content is also thought to be beneficial. Slower rates of digestion are observed when foods have more compact granules, contain high levels of viscous soluble fiber, and have a higher amylose to amylopectin ratio.

The relationship between whole grains and diabetes has been studied in five large cohorts as highlighted in **Table 3**. All of the studies have found an inverse relationship between consumption of whole grains or cereal fiber and disease reduction despite slight variations in methodology.

As a proxy measure of whole-grain consumption, the relationship between the intake of total and specific sources of dietary fiber, dietary glycemic index, and glycemic load in the Nurses' Health Study and the Health Professional's Study was examined. Among the 65 173 women who participated during 1986–1992, women in the highest quintile of cereal fiber intake had a 28% lower risk of diabetes than those in the lowest quintile of intake (RR 0.72; 95% CI 0.58, 0.90; $P = 0.001$), a significant reduction that was not observed with fruit or vegetable fiber intakes. In men there was an inverse relationship between cereal fiber intake and risk of type 2 diabetes: a reduction in risk of 30% following adjustment for confounders. Again, no significant relationship of fruit or vegetable fiber to diabetes risk was observed.

The fiber content of whole grains has been suggested as a possible explanation for the inverse relationship between total and whole-grain intakes and risk of type 2 diabetes observed in a 10-year follow-up of Finnish men ($n = 2286$) and women ($n = 2030$). When the highest and lowest quartiles of whole-grain consumption were compared there was an over 30% reduction in risk following adjustment for age, sex, geographic area, and energy intake. Cereal fiber, but not that from fruits and

Table 3 Summary of the evidence relating a reduced risk of type 2 diabetes to increased whole grain consumption, including studies where cereal or dietary fiber intake is taken as a surrogate marker for whole-grain intakes

Evidence for a reduced risk of:	Cohort	Reported Association	Reference
Epidemiological			
Type 2 diabetes	Nurse's Health Study	Lower RR with increased dietary fiber	Salmeron et al. (1997a) Dietary fiber, glycemic load, and risk of non-insulin-dependent diabetes mellitus in women. *JAMA* **277**: 472–477.
Type 2 diabetes	Health Professionals Follow-up Study	Lower RR with increased dietary fiber	Salmeron et al. (1997b) Dietary fiber, glycemic load, and risk of NIDDM in men. *Diabetes Care* **20**: 545–550.
Type 2 diabetes	Finnish Mobile Clinic Health Examination Survey	Lower RR with increased whole grains	Montonen et al. (2003) Whole-grain and fiber intake and the incidence of type 2 diabetes *American Journal of Clinical Nutrition* **77**: 622–629.
Type 2 diabetes	Health Professionals Follow-up Study	Lower RR with increased whole grains	Fung et al. (2003) Whole-grain intake and the risk of type 2 diabetes: a prospective study in men. *American Journal of Clinical Nutrition* **76**: 535–540.
Type 2 diabetes	Nurse's Health Study	Lower RR with increased whole grains	Liu et al. (2000) A prospective study of whole-grain intake and risk of type 2 diabetes mellitus in US women. *American Journal of Public Health* **90**: 1409–1415.
Risk factors for type 2 diabetes and CVD	Framingham Offspring Study	Reduction in fasting insulin with increasing whole-grain intake	McKeown et al. (2002) Whole grain intake is favourably associated with metabolic risk factors for type 2 diabetes and cardiovascular disease in the Framingham Offspring Study. *American Journal of Clinical Nutrition* **76**: 390–398.
Intervention			
Insulin sensitivity	11 hyperinsulinemic overweight patients	Reduction in fasting insulin following diet rich in whole grains	Pereira et al. (2002) Effect of whole grains on insulin sensitivity in overweight hyperinsulinaemic adults. *American Journal of Clinical Nutrition* **75**: 848–855.

vegetables, was inversely related to risk of type 2 diabetes even after adjustment for a number of confounders. Adjustment for cereal fiber considerably weakened the association between whole-grain consumption and risk of type 2 diabetes, suggesting that this may be a significant component of the whole-grain package.

The effect of whole-grain consumption specifically, rather than fiber intakes, on incidence of type 2 diabetes was examined in the Health Professional's Follow-up Study. Over a 12-year follow-up period, intakes of whole and refined grains were analyzed using a validated semiquantitative FFQ. Despite no baseline history of diabetes or CVD, 1197 cases of incident type 2 diabetes were identified in this male cohort. Following adjustment for dietary and life style confounders including age, smoking, physical activity, and fruit and vegetable intake, there was a reduced risk of type 2 diabetes of almost 40% in those with the highest quintile compared with the lowest quintile of whole-grain intakes. The results were attenuated after adjustment for BMI, although the relationship remained significant. In those with a BMI $>30\,\mathrm{kg\,m^{-2}}$ the association between whole grain and type 2 diabetes was weak, whereas in those men with a BMI $<30\,\mathrm{kg\,m^{-2}}$ a 50% risk reduction was observed in those who consumed the most whole grains. However, after adjusting for components of the whole-grain package such as cereal fiber, magnesium, and glycemic load, the statistical significance was lost (**Figure 4**).

These findings in men were similar to those observed by Liu *et al.* (2000) when they looked specifically at whole and refined grain intakes in the women participating in the Nurses' Health

Study. During the 10-year follow-up, 1879 cases of incident type 2 diabetes were confirmed. Although the women with the highest intake of whole grain had other beneficial dietary and lifestyle factors, whole-grain intake was inversely related to risk. There was a significant inverse association between the highest and lowest quintiles of whole-grain intake after adjustment for age and energy intake. Although attenuated after adjustment for BMI and other lifestyle factors, the relationship remained significant. Again BMI appeared to be the strongest confounding factor. Women in the lowest quintile of intake ratio (those with low whole grain or large refined grain intakes) had a 57% greater risk of type 2 diabetes than women in the highest quintile.

In a cross-sectional assessment of 2941 subjects in the Framingham Offspring Study the effect of whole-grain intake on metabolic risk factors for type 2 diabetes and CVD was examined. Dietary intake was assessed using a semiquantitative FFQ in the participants who were free from diabetes or high cholesterol. Breakfast cereal type was used to quantify whole-grain intakes based on a whole-grain content of over 25%. Other foods identified as whole grain were dark breads, popcorn, and oatmeal. Whole-grain intakes were similar between men and women (mean 8.3 and 8.8 servings per week, respectively) but refined grain intakes were much higher (22.0 and 18.5 servings per week, respectively). Similar to other studies, those in the highest quintile of whole-grain intakes (20.5 servings per week) had lower BMI, were less likely to smoke or drink, and dietary habits were better. Following adjustment for a host of confounding factors, whole-grain consumption in the highest quintile was associated with a significant reduction in fasting insulin in comparison to those in the lowest quintile of intake. Even after further adjustment for BMI and dietary factors such as vegetable and fat intakes, this relationship remained significant, but was no longer significant after further adjustment for magnesium, and insoluble and soluble fibers. The association between whole grain and fasting insulin was most striking in those with a BMI $>30\,\mathrm{kg\,m^{-2}}$ with the highest fasting insulin levels being observed in those with the highest BMI and the lowest intake of whole-grain foods.

Prospective epidemiological studies are generally stronger than cross-sectional associations. In the CARDIA study by Pereira and coworkers, a significant inverse relationship was observed between whole-grain foods and fasting insulin levels among over 3500 black and white young Americans aged 18–30 years. A dietary history was collected at baseline and 7 years later, while insulin measurements were collected at 10 years follow-up. After

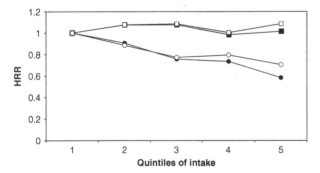

Relative risks of cumulative average whole and refined grain intakes on risk of type 2 diabetes in men by quintiles of grain intake

Figure 4 ○ adjusted for age, period, physical activity, energy intake, missing FFQ data, smoking, family history of diabetes, alcohol intake, fruit intake and vegetable intake. ● additionally adjusted for BMI <30kg/m² and >30kg/m².

adjustment for a number of dietary and lifestyle factors an inverse and graded response was observed between whole-grain intake at 7 years and the insulin measurements collected at 10 years follow-up, although the relationship was not significant in black women.

There is only one small intervention study that examines the impact of increasing wholegrain consumption. In this study, it was found that after 6 weeks there was a 10% reduction in fasting insulin compared to results observed following the refined grain diet ($141 \pm 3.9 \, \text{pmol} \, 1^{-1}$ versus $156 \pm 3.9 \, \text{pmol} \, 1^{-1}$; $P < 0.01$). This relationship remained even after adjustment for body weight changes (nonsignificant change of $-0.7 \, \text{kg}$ on whole-grain diet) and physical activity.

As for other diseases the mechanism of the effect of wholegrain on insulin sensitivity is not entirely clear and may in part be mediated through effects on body weight. Cereal fiber and possibly certain micronutrients such as magnesium may also be important since the wholegrain effect is attenuated after adjustment for these variables.

Cancer

Dietary factors are thought to account for about 35% of all cancers but the role of any specific dietary factor or dietary regime has only been established for certain types of cancer. Only a few studies have looked at the links between wholegrain intake and cancer. In the Iowa Women's Study there was a 30% reduction in cancer deaths when comparing those with the highest quintile of whole-grain intake to those in the lowest quintile, after adjustment for age and energy intake. However, once other dietary and lifestyle factors were included within the multivariate analysis this relationship was attenuated and lost its statistical significance. Similar findings were observed in the Norwegian County Study with a 28% reduction in cancer deaths from the highest to lowest quintile of wholegrain when adjusted for age and energy intake. However, the effect was no longer significant after further adjustment for other dietary and lifestyle factors.

A number of studies have used case–control designs to investigate the relationship between whole-grain consumption and cancer incidence, although these suffer from the inherent flaws of such study designs, especially those involving recall of past dietary habits. In an analysis of 40 case–control studies, 90% of the studies included had an odds ratio (OR) <1, of which 55% reached statistical significance in favor of a benefit of wholegrain. The pooled OR for high versus low intakes of whole-grain foods was 0.66 (95% CI 0.60, 0.72). Most data pertain to the link with cancers of the digestive tract. The majority of pooled-odds ratios for specific cancers were between 0.5 and 0.8, except for breast and prostate cancers, which were 0.86 and 0.90, respectively. The differing types of dietary data collection impacted on the findings. Where only whole-grain frequency was recorded the pooled OR was 0.82 in those who ate whole grains infrequently and 0.59 among habitual consumers ($P < 0.0001$ for trend). Similar results were found in those studies reporting intake by tertiles (OR 0.81 and 0.62 for the second and third tertiles, respectively; $P = 0.0001$) and those reporting actual quantities of intake found a downward trend in ORs as the dose increases, although the trend is not strong ($P = 0.18$) suggesting that the dose-response relationship between whole grain and cancer types may only be modest.

The whole-grain package contains a number of components that have been identified as having beneficial effects on cancer risk, including antioxidants and flavonoids, isoflavones, fermentable carbohydrates, and resistant starch. Although many studies have been conducted looking at the effect of individual components that can be found within the whole-grain package on cancer risk, few studies have looked specifically at whole grains *per se*. Although a relationship has been observed between whole-grain consumption and cancer deaths, studies of cancer incidence and whole-grain consumption are not significant after adjustment for potential confounders. This is a good example of how consumption of whole-grain foods appears to be a marker of dietary habits associated with a reduction in risk, and they are not necessarily specifically important in their own right.

Dietary Recommendations

The epidemiological data suggest that health benefits can be obtained at relatively low levels of whole-grain consumption, typically 1–3 servings per day. In most studies, there was no clear dose–response relationship and a suggestion of a threshold effect as benefits were seen at the third quintile of wholegrain intakes with no further reduction in risk as intakes increased. However, assessment of intakes in different countries show that this threshold level of intake is not being achieved.

International dietary Guidelines recommend increased grain consumption. At present, the USA is the only nation to specify exact quantities of whole grain foods, and it is only within the last few years that whole grains have been considered seperately from total grain foods.

The recommendations for grains have evolved over time to reflect changes in research and to simplify and clarify consumer messages. The latest American Dietary Guidelines (2005) now state a recommendation of 3 or more ounce-equivalent portions of whole-grain foods daily, with a further recommendation that at least half of grain consumption should be whole-grain.

This recommendation of three servings per day was also specifically incorporated in the Department of Health and Health Services nutrition objectives for 2010 (US Department of Health and Human Services, 2000).

In the UK, the Food Standards Agency explicitly encourages consumers to select whole-grain varieties in their healthy eating advice, although no exact quantities are given. Many other European countries also tend to place emphasis on only cereals and fiber, without necessarily specifically highlighting whole grains.

Using data compiled from focus groups and consumer interviews in the US, a number of reasons as to why consumption of whole-grain foods may be low have been indentified. Consumers report difficulties in identifying whole-grain foods and express limited knowledge about the preparation and cooking of whole-grain foods. Adolescents in particular reported that whole-grain foods were bland and have a dry taste. While breakfast cereals appear to be well received in this age group, whole-grain breads were described as dry and bitter. Furthermore, whole-grain varieties of bread, pasta, and rice tend to be more expensive and this may deter those in low income and vulnerable groups.

In a UK intervention study to increase whole-grain consumption, 25–40-year-olds were encouraged to increase whole-grain food consumption over a period of 2 weeks by gradually increasing servings from 1 to 5 servings per day. Volunteers were given positive health messages about eating more whole-grain foods, were helped in identifying such food products, and were also given advice on how to incorporate them easily into their existing diet. In post study focus groups, participants were positive about the changes made and were happy to continue consuming whole-grain foods but at lower levels than that prescribed during the study period. Similar to findings in the US, breakfast was found to be a good meal to change habit and breakfast cereals and bread type was deemed the easiest way of incorporating whole-grain foods.

Consumer research suggests that few people are aware of the health benefits of whole-grain foods. Although other food groups, such as fruits and vegetables, have been identified as possessing health benefits, the association between whole-grain foods and a reduced risk of a number of chronic diseases is not recognized among the general population or indeed health professionals. Recent health claims in the US and UK may help to address this knowledge gap. In addition, consumer initiatives such as the 'Whole Grain for Health' campaign in the UK, and 'Go Grains' in Australia provide ongoing education relating to the benefits of including whole-grain products within the diet.

See also: **Dietary Fiber**: Physiological Effects and Effects on Absorption; Potential Role in Etiology of Disease; Role in Nutritional Management of Disease.

Further Reading

Anderson JW (2002) Whole-grains intake and risk for coronary heart disease. In: Marquart L, Slavin JL, and Fulcher RG (eds.) *Whole-grain Foods in Health and Disease*, pp. 155–185. Minnesota: American Association of Cereal Chemists, Inc.

Fung TT, Hu FB, Pereira MA, Liu S, Stampfer MJ, Colditz GA, and Willett WC (2002) Whole grain intake and the risk of type 2 diabetes in men: a prospective study in men. *American Journal of Clinical Nutrition* 76: 535–540.

Jacobs DR Jr, Marquart L, Slavin J, and Kushi LH (1998b) Whole-grain intake and cancer: an expanded review and meta-analysis. *Nutrition and Cancer* 30: 85–96.

Jacobs DR Jr, Meyer KA, Kushi LH, and Folsom AR (1998a) Whole grain intake may reduce the risk of ischaemic heart disease death in postmenopausal women: the Iowa Women's Health Study. *American Journal of Clinical Nutrition* 68: 248–257.

Jacobs DR Jr, Meyer KA, Kushi LH, and Folsom AR (1999) Is whole grain intake associated with reduced total and cause-specific death rates in older women? The Iowa Women's Health Study. *American Journal of Public Health* 89: 322–329.

Jacobs DR Jr, Meyer HE, and Solvoll K (2001) Reduced mortality among whole grain bread eaters in men and women in the Norwegian County Study. *European Journal of Clinical Nutrition* 55: 137–143.

Lang R and Jebb SA (2003) Who consumes whole grains, and how much? *Proceedings of the Nutrition Society* 62: 123–127.

Lang R, Thane CW, Bolton-Smith C, and Jebb SA (2003) Whole-grain food consumption by British adults from two national dietary surveys. *Public Health Nutrition* 6: 479–484.

Liu S (2002) Dietary carbohydrates, whole grains, and the risk of type 2 diabetes. In: Marquart L, Slavin JL, and Fulcher RG (eds.) *Whole-grain foods in health and disease*, pp. 155–185. Minnesota: American Association of Cereal Chemists, Inc.

Liu S, Manson JE, Stampfer HJ, Hu FB, Giovannucci E, Colditz GA, Manson JE, Hennekens CH, and Willett WC (2000b). A prospective study of whole grain intake and risk of type 2 diabetes mellitus in US women. *American Journal of Public Health* 90: 1409–15.

Liu S, Manson JE, Stampfer MJ, Rexrode KM, Hu FB, Rimm EB, and Willett WC (2000a) Whole grain consumption and risk of ischaemic stroke in women: a prospective study. *Journal of the American Medical Association* 284: 1534–1540.

Liu S, Stampfer HJ, Hu FB, Giovannucci E, Rimm E, Manson JE, Hennekens CH, and Willett WC (1999) Whole grain consumption and risk of coronary heart disease: results from the Nurses' Health Study. *American Journal of Clinical Nutrition* 70: 412–419.

McIntosh GH and Jacobs DR (2002) Cereal-grain foods, fibers and cancer prevention. In: Marquart L, Slavin JL, and Fulcher RG (eds.) *Whole-grain Foods in Health and Disease*, pp. 155–185. Minnesota: American Association of Cereal Chemists, Inc.

McKeown NM, Meigs JB, Liu S, Wilson PWF, and Jacques PF (2002) Whole grain intake is favourably associated with metabolic risk factors for type 2 diabetes and cardiovascular disease in the Framingham Offspring Study. *American Journal of Clinical Nutrition* **76**: 390–398.

Pereira MA, Jacobs DR, Pins JJ, Raatz SK, Gross MD, Slavin JL, and Seaquist ER (2002) Effect of whole grains on insulin sensitivity in overweight hyperinsulinaemic adults. *American Journal of Clinical Nutrition* **75**: 848–855.

Smith AT, Kuznesof S, Richardson DP, and Seal CJ (2003) Behavioural, attitudinal and dietary responses to the consumption of wholegrain foods. *Proceedings of the Nutrition Society* **62**: 1–13.

Z

ZINC

Contents

Deficiency in Developing Countries, Intervention Studies

C Hotz, National Institute of Public Health, Morelos, Mexico

Introduction

Knowledge of the occurrence of zinc deficiency and its importance to human health has increased greatly in recent years. Available evidence indicates that zinc deficiency is an important contributing factor to impaired growth and development, morbidity, and mortality among children in underprivileged settings. Presently, there are few estimates of the prevalence of zinc deficiency in developing countries based on dietary intake or biochemical indices. However, national level estimates of the adequacy of zinc in the food supply and the prevalence of childhood growth stunting can be used to inform on the relative risk of zinc deficiency among countries. National programs to improve zinc status through either supplementation or food fortification are just being initiated.

Recognition of Zinc Deficiency in Developing Countries

The recognition of zinc deficiency as an important contributor to the high rates of morbidity, mortality, and delayed growth and development among children is relatively recent in contrast to the earlier recognition of the importance and widespread occurrence of deficiencies of iodine, vitamin A, and iron. Coordinated efforts to address vitamin A deficiency in less developed countries were formally initiated by the establishment of the International Vitamin A Consultative Group (IVACG) in 1975. In the mid-1980s, similar groups were founded for the control of iodine deficiency disorders (International Council for the Control of Iodine Deficiency Disorders; ICC/IDD) and iron deficiency (International Nutritional Anemias Consultative Group; INACG). It was not until the year 2000 that a similar group emerged, the International Zinc Nutrition Consultative Group (IZiNCG), to promote the control of zinc deficiency in more vulnerable populations.

The detection of zinc deficiency in populations and the recognition of its association with health outcomes have been somewhat more challenging for zinc than for other nutrients, contributing to the delay in efforts to control it. The ability to diagnose zinc deficiency in individuals using biochemical measures is somewhat limited. For example, the concentration of zinc in serum or plasma may not diminish until the depletion of zinc is more advanced, making it less useful for diagnosing mild to moderate zinc deficiency states in individuals. Other possible biochemical indicators of zinc status have not been consistently demonstrated to reflect change in zinc status. These limitations may have subsequently dampened enthusiasm for evaluating zinc status at the population level. Furthermore, the health conditions that are clearly associated with zinc deficiency (e.g., childhood growth stunting, common childhood infections, and mortality; described in further detail below) are general in nature and have multiple causes. This is in contrast to the strong iconic association of iodine deficiency with goiter and cretinism, vitamin A deficiency with eye disorders and blindness, and iron deficiency with easily diagnosable anemia. The nonspecific nature of health outcomes associated with zinc deficiency is in concordance with the role of zinc in a wide variety of biological functions, covering all human physiological systems. Thus, the very nature of zinc metabolism and the ubiquity of zinc in biological functions at the molecular, cellular, and physiological levels has likely contributed to the difficulties and delays in recognizing the important contribution of zinc deficiency to impaired health and development. A brief history of the knowledge of zinc deficiency in developing countries is presented in **Table 1**.

Causes of Zinc Deficiency in Developing Countries

Although the etiology of zinc deficiency in developing countries has not been thoroughly studied, the main contributing factor is believed to be inadequate intake of zinc in bioavailable (i.e., available for absorption across the intestine) forms.

Inadequate Dietary Intake of Zinc

In general, the risk of inadequate intake of dietary zinc within a population may be associated with the nature of the food supply, and its content and relative

Table 1 History of knowledge of zinc deficiency in developing countries

Year	Event or publication
1963	Relationship between zinc deficiency and hypogonadal dwarfism noted in Egypt
1972	The role of zinc deficiency in hypogonadal dwarfism described in Iran
1974	Zinc demonstrated to increase linear growth, weight, and bone age in Iranian pubertal boys
1982	Supplemental zinc demonstrated to increase linear growth in Chinese preschool children
1993	Supplemental zinc during pregnancy demonstrated to increase birth weight and gestational age of infants in India
1996	Supplemental zinc demonstrated to decrease the prevalence of diarrhea and pneumonia among malnourished children in Vietnam
1999	Pooled analysis of randomized, controlled, zinc supplementation trials indicates a significant positive effect of zinc on reducing the incidence of diarrhea and pneumonia
2000	Establishment of the International Zinc Nutrition Consultative Group (IZiNCG)
2001	Mortality reduced by zinc supplementation among low-birth-weight infants in India
	Zinc supplementation recommended as adjunctive therapy for childhood diarrhea
2002	Meta-analysis of randomized, controlled zinc supplementation trials indicates a modest but significant overall improvement in growth

bioavailability of zinc. Animal source foods, in particular shellfish, small whole fish, beef, and organ meats such as liver and kidney, are rich sources of zinc. Furthermore, the zinc contained in animal source foods is more highly bioavailable than from plant source foods; the presence of certain amino acids (e.g., histidine, methioinine), or perhaps other unidentified factors, may facilitate the intestinal absorption of zinc from animal flesh foods. Plant source foods, such as most fruits and vegetables including green leaves, and starchy roots and tubers, have relatively low zinc content. While whole grains and legumes have moderate to high zinc content, these foods also contain large quantities of phytate (phytic acid or myo-inositol hexaphosphate), the most potent identified dietary inhibitor of zinc absorption. The zinc and phytate content, and the phytate:zinc molar ratio of some foods are shown in **Table 2**.

Table 2 The content of zinc and phytate, and the phytate:zinc molar ratio in uncooked foods

Food	Zinc (mg/100 g)	Phytate (mg/100 g)	Phytate:zinc molar ratio
Cereals			
Corn	1.8	800	44
Pasta	0.7	282	40
Rice (milled)	1.1	352	32
Wheat or whole-wheat bread	2.9	845	29
White bread	0.9	30	3
Nuts and legumes			
Lentils/mung beans	1.3	358	27
Peanuts	3.3	1760	53
Peas	2.9	1154	39
Red beans	2.9	1629	56
Roots and tubers			
Cassava	0.3	54	18
Potato	0.3	81	27
Sweet potato	0.5	50	10
Vegetables			
Cabbage	0.1	0	–
Green leaves	0.2	42	21
Onion	0.2	0	–
Tomato	0.1	6	6
Fruits			
Banana	0.2	0	–
Coconut	1.1	324	29
Orange	0.1	0	–
Mango	0.0	20	–
Animal source foods			
Beef	3.0	0	–
Chicken	1.3	0	–
Eggs	1.1	0	–
Fish	0.5	0	–
Milk	0.4	0	–
Pork	1.9	0	–

Plants synthesize phytate, which occurs in highest concentration in seeds and to a lesser extent in vegetative plant parts. Phytate forms chelates with zinc and other minerals; as this compound is largely undigested and is not absorbed, it carries the chelated portion of dietary zinc out of the intestine, thus reducing the amount of zinc available for absorption. The phytate:zinc molar ratio of the diet can be used to estimate the bioavailability of zinc. Populations with a heavy dietary reliance on unrefined cereals or legumes, complemented with only small amounts of zinc-rich animal source foods, will have lower intakes of bioavailable zinc. Although milling cereal grains removes large amounts of phytate, it also removes large amounts of zinc. Thus, among populations with a heavy dietary reliance on refined cereals (e.g., rice) or starchy roots and tubers (e.g., potatoes, cassava) with small amounts of zinc-rich animal foods, the total intake of dietary zinc will be low. In either case, low food intakes due to food insecurity will exacerbate the risk of not meeting daily physiological requirements for absorbed zinc.

Other Causes of Zinc Deficiency

There are a few other commonly occurring conditions in developing country settings that may contribute to zinc deficiency. Diarrhea may not only lead to a reduced absorption of dietary zinc during the episode due to increased intestinal transit time, but may also cause an increase in the loss of body zinc. Under normal physiological conditions, zinc is secreted into the intestine in large quantities together with digestive juices but is largely reabsorbed again; diarrhea may interfere with the reabsorption of this zinc. Given the important role of the intestine in regulating dietary zinc absorption, and the secretion and reabsorption of body zinc during digestion, conditions that affect the health or integrity of the intestine, such as tropical enteropathy, could interfere with the adequate maintenance of zinc balance. The contribution of these conditions to zinc deficiency in developing countries requires investigation.

Prevalence of Zinc Deficiency in Developing Countries: Available Evidence

Relatively little information on population zinc status has been collected at the national or subnational level in developing countries. Thus, only very limited estimates of the prevalence of zinc deficiency are available that are based on the proportion of the population with low concentrations of serum zinc or inadequate dietary zinc intakes. Estimates of the

magnitude of risk of zinc deficiency in a population have therefore been derived from more indirect indicators, such as the:

- adequacy of zinc in the national food supply;
- national prevalence of childhood growth stunting; and
- occurrence of a positive response of health conditions to supplemental zinc as determined by randomized, controlled zinc supplementation trials.

Adequacy of Zinc in the National Food Supply

As described above, the nature of the food supply will provide some information on the likelihood of risk of inadequate dietary zinc within a population. Information compiled by the United Nation's Food and Agriculture Organization has been used to estimate the potential risk of inadequate zinc in the food supply for a large number of countries. This estimate uses country level data on the per capita amounts of 95 different food commodities available for human consumption, and estimates of the zinc content and phytate:zinc molar ratio of these foods, to calculate the per capita amount of bioavailable zinc in the food supply. The per capita amount of bioavailable zinc is compared to the physiological requirement for absorbed zinc weighted for the demographic distribution of the population. The theoretical proportion of the population at risk of inadequate dietary zinc is used to estimate the relative risk of zinc deficiency at the national level. For example, countries with 25% or more of the population at risk of inadequate dietary zinc are considered to be at elevated risk. This information is limited in that it represents the national average situation and cannot identify subnational populations that may be at elevated risk. In the absence of more direct measures of zinc status, such estimates will justify the need to conduct population surveys that measure risk of zinc deficiency more directly.

Estimates of the proportion of the population at risk of inadequate dietary zinc based on food supply data have been calculated for 176 countries; a summary of the tabulations by developing country region is given in **Table 3**, and compared to those from North America. Overall, these estimates suggest that about 20% of the world's population is at risk of inadequate dietary zinc intake.

National Prevalence of Childhood Growth Stunting

Zinc deficiency is a common limiting factor to adequate child growth in developing country settings. A meta-analysis of 25 studies using a randomized, placebo-controlled design, which measured change in linear growth of children following zinc supplementation for at least 2 months, indicated that supplemental

Table 3 Adequacy of dietary zinc in the food supply in major developing country regions, as compared to North America

	Population (millions)	Zinc (mg/caput/day)	Phytate:zinc molar ratio	Zinc from animal source foods (%)	Estimated population at risk of inadequate zinc intake (%)
North America	305	12.5	11	61	10
China	1256	12.4	16	37	14
Latin America and Caribbean	498	10.3	20	42	25
South Asia	1297	10.8	26	11	27
Southeast Asia	504	9.2	24	21	33
Sub-Saharan Africa	581	9.4	26	15	28

Adapted with permission from Food and Nutrition Bulletin (2004) (suppl 2) **25**: S135.
International Zinc Nutrition Consultative Group (Brown KH, Rivera JA, Bhutta Z, Gibson RS, King JC, Ruel M, Sandström B, Wasantwisut E, Hotz C, Lönnerdal B, Lopez de Romaña D, and Peerson J) (2004) Assessment of the risk of zinc deficiency in populations and options for its control. *Food and Nutrition Bulletin* **25**: S91–S202.

zinc had an overall, positive effect on linear growth. This meta-analysis also demonstrated that a low group mean index of child height-for-age (i.e., 1.58 SD below the reference median for height-for-age) predicts an improvement in linear growth in response to supplemental zinc. Therefore, a high prevalence of childhood growth stunting in a population represents an elevated risk of zinc deficiency. The World Health Organization suggests that when the prevalence of children with height-for-age of 2 SD below the reference median is 20% or higher, childhood growth stunting should be considered a problem of public health concern; this prevalence may likewise be indicative of an elevated risk of zinc deficiency. The World Health Organization maintains a global database on the prevalence of low height-for-age at the national and subnational level for a large number of countries.

Occurrence of a Positive Response of Health Conditions to Supplemental Zinc

Suggestive evidence for the widespread occurrence of zinc deficiency in developing regions is derived from the large number of countries from a wide geographical range where positive health changes were observed in response to supplemental zinc. The health conditions that have been positively affected by supplemental zinc, as demonstrated through randomized, controlled, community-based zinc supplementation trials and the locations of these studies are described in detail in the following section.

Consequences of Zinc Deficiency in Developing Countries: Evidence Derived from Zinc Supplementation Trials

In the context of developing country settings, present knowledge on the health consequences of zinc

deficiency has been almost entirely derived from community-based trials of zinc supplementation among populations at possible risk of zinc deficiency. In these trials, individuals in the study population are randomly allocated to receive either a zinc supplement, usually in the form of tablets or syrups, or the same supplement format without zinc (i.e., placebo). The condition under study is then monitored for a given period (typically for 2 months to one year), and the occurrence of or change in the condition is compared between the zinc-supplemented group and the corresponding control group. Given that several other nutritional and environmental factors can influence the health conditions hypothesized to occur with zinc deficiency, such studies have been essential in demonstrating unequivocally the causal role of zinc deficiency in these conditions among human populations. The following section provides an overview of the population groups at elevated risk of zinc deficiency, and the health consequences associated with zinc deficiency, as concluded from these studies.

Groups at Elevated Risk of Zinc Deficiency

In accordance with age and physiological status, some population groups have increased daily physiological requirements for absorbed zinc. The incorporation of zinc in new tissues being synthesized such as occurs during growth and pregnancy or the secretion of zinc in breast milk during lactation require that relatively larger amounts of zinc are absorbed daily. These increased needs for zinc increase the challenge of acquiring sufficient amounts of absorbable zinc from the food supply. Those groups with higher zinc requirements and who are thus at elevated risk of zinc deficiency include:

- infants (particularly those born prematurely);
- young children;

Table 4 Countries from developing regions with documented evidence of improved growth or development in response to supplemental zinc

Region	Country	Population group	Development outcome improved
Eastern Mediterranean	Iran	Pubertal boys	Height, weight, bone age
Latin America and Caribbean	Belize	Preschool children	Height
	Brazil	Low-birth-weight infants	Weight
	Chile	Low-birth-weight infants	Length
		Severely malnourished infants	Length gain
		Preschool children (boys only)	Height
		Preadolescent and adolescent children (boys only)	Height
	Guatemala	Infants (growth stunted)	Length, lean body mass, physical activity
		Preadolescent children	Mid upper arm circumference
	Jamaica	Severely malnourished infants and preschool children	Lean tissue synthesis
South and Southeast Asia	Bangladesh	Infants (low serum zinc concentration)	Weight
		Severely malnourished infants and preschool children	Weight gain
	China	Infants	Length, weight
		Preschool children	Height, weight
		Preadolescent children	Heel-to-knee height[a] Neuropsychological performance
	India	Preschool children	Physical activity level
	Japan	Preadolescent children	Height
	Vietnam	Preschool children (growth stunted)	Height, weight
Sub-Saharan Africa	Ethiopia	Infants (growth-stunted)	Length
	Uganda	Preschool and school-aged children	Mid upper arm circumference

[a]An improvement with supplemental zinc was observed only when administered simultaneously with other micronutrients.

- children recovering from severe malnutrition;
- adolescents; and
- pregnant and lactating women.

At least some evidence exists for the occurrence of zinc deficiency among each of these groups in developing country settings. The elderly may also be at elevated risk of zinc deficiency, due to a decline in adequacy of zinc intakes and possibly a reduction in the absorption of dietary zinc. However, evidence for zinc deficiency among the elderly has thus far only been derived from industrialized countries; elderly populations have not been the subject of study of zinc deficiency in developing countries.

Growth and Development of Children

Many children in developing country settings experience poor growth, in comparison to relatively healthy children from more developed countries. The prevalence of low height-for-age and weight-for-age indices among children under 5 years of age are used as indicators of poor living conditions, to which poor diet, poor environmental and social conditions, and higher exposure to infectious diseases contribute. Similar conditions can result in impaired neurobehavioral development and cognitive function, putting children in developing countries at further disadvantage. Evidence exists for a specific role of zinc in both of these aspects of child development. **Table 4** provides a summary of countries in which improved growth or development in response to supplemental zinc has been clearly demonstrated.

Growth Zinc plays an important role in child growth. Several mechanisms may be involved, including the role of zinc in the transcription and translation of genetic material and, perhaps more importantly, the regulatory role of zinc in the primary endocrine system, which controls growth (i.e., the growth hormone-somatomedin axis). Specifically, zinc status is associated with the concentration of circulating insulin-like growth factor-1, the principal growth factor that controls early childhood growth. Among populations where growth retardation occurs, both height and weight gain have improved following supplemental zinc. Stimulation of linear growth appears to be the primary response, while the increase in body weight likely reflects the synthesis of lean tissue such as bone, cartilage, and muscle associated with linear growth. This is evident because, in general, weight does not increase independently of increased height in response to supplemental zinc.

The magnitude of improvement in linear growth in response to supplemental zinc is, not surprisingly, greater among children experiencing growth retardation (or 'stunting'; >2 SD below the median height-for-age of international reference data). Zinc deficiency has been demonstrated to be an important limiting factor to growth of children across a wide range of geographical settings in developing regions (**Table 4**). It should be noted that not all studies have demonstrated a significant, positive effect of zinc on growth. Possible explanations for this include: the prevalence or severity of growth stunting in the study communities was low; zinc status was adequate; or deficiencies of other growth-limiting nutrients coexisted thus preventing a positive effect of zinc on growth. The latter situation may also explain the observation in some studies of a transient effect of zinc on growth.

Low-birth-weight infants (<2.5 kg) may have additional needs for zinc, presumably to facilitate their rapid postnatal catch-up growth. Some benefits of supplemental zinc to growth have been observed among low-birth-weight infants in the first 6 months of life.

Severely malnourished infants and children have exhibited improved rates of weight gain, height gain, or synthesis of lean tissue when supplemental zinc has been included in their usual rehabilitation treatment regimen. In these recovering children, zinc has been shown to augment the deposition of lean tissue by increasing protein synthesis.

Cognitive function and behavior There are a few possible mechanisms by which zinc may be speculated to affect neurobehavioral function; these include neurotransmission in the synapses or development of the central nervous system via the synthesis of genetic material, proteins, and cell replication. Adequate zinc status appears to be important for certain aspects of neurobehavioral development among infants and children, although these associations are not conclusive. Higher levels of activity, specifically more frequent engagement in walking or playing as opposed to sitting or watching, have been observed among infants in developing country settings in response to supplemental zinc. Nonetheless, other studies have failed to demonstrate an effect of zinc on motor scores as assessed by Bayley Scales or Griffiths' Developmental Assessment and, in one case, a negative effect on the mental development index was observed.

Evidence for improved cognitive function among school-aged children has been derived from studies of urban and rural children in China. In the rural population of children, the positive effect of zinc on cognitive function was dependent on the provision of other supplemental micronutrients, while in the urban group, supplemental zinc had a positive effect that was independent of the provision of other micronutrients. It is possible that some of the inconsistencies in the studies of neurobehavioral development occur due to concurrent deficiencies of other nutrients that also play a role in cognition (e.g., iodine, iron).

Infectious Diseases Among Children

Zinc has many roles in the immune system, contributing both to specific and nonspecific immune functions. Indeed, there is ample information indicating that zinc deficiency makes an important contribution to some of the most common childhood infections that occur in developing countries, as summarized in **Table 5**.

Table 5 Countries from developing regions with documented evidence of a reduced prevalence of infectious disease in response to supplemental zinc for prevention

Region	Country	Population studied	Health condition
Latin America and Caribbean	Mexico	Preschool children	Diarrhea
	Guatemala	Infants	Diarrhea
	Peru	Preschool children	Diarrhea
South and Southeast Asia	India	Infants and preschool children	Diarrhea
	India	Infants and preschool children (recovered from acute diarrhea)	Pneumonia
		Infants (term, small-for-gestational-age)	Mortality
	Vietnam	Infants and preschool children (growth stunted and underweight)	Diarrhea Pneumonia
Sub-Saharan Africa	Burkina Faso	Infants and preschool children	Diarrhea
	Ethiopia	Infants	Diarrhea
Western Pacific	Papua New Guinea	Infants and preschool children	Malaria

Diarrhea Zinc has an important role in both the prevention and treatment of diarrhea, which may be mediated both through functions in immune competence and maintenance of the integrity of the intestine. Studies in various settings indicate that provision of supplemental zinc on a nearly daily basis reduces the incidence of childhood diarrhea by nearly 20%, and reduces the prevalence of diarrhea by about 25%. The magnitude of this decrease is similar to that expected from programs to improve water quality and sanitation. There is no strong evidence to suggest that greater benefits of zinc in diarrhea prevention would occur among children who are growth stunted. Rather, all children living under poor conditions with exposure to diarrheal pathogens may potentially benefit from improved zinc intakes.

Zinc also has therapeutic benefits for recovery from diarrheal infections. Overall, supplemental zinc provided to children during recovery from either acute or persistent diarrhea leads to a reduction in the duration and severity of the episode. It has been recommended that zinc be used in the management of acute diarrhea, in conjunction with oral rehydration therapy. The current recommendation is to provide 10–20 mg of zinc once daily for 10–14 days.

Lower respiratory tract infections Zinc deficiency appears to be associated with an increased incidence of pneumonia. Evidence thus far indicates that supplemental zinc reduces the incidence of pneumonia in children by about 40%.

Malaria Only a few studies to date have considered the possible importance of zinc in protection against malaria. Nonetheless, while it is unlikely that improved zinc status could prevent infection with malarial parasites, it does appear that zinc may reduce the severity of the infection or the symptoms of morbidity associated with the infection. Evidence for this is suggested by a reduction in the number of visits to health facilities due to malaria, but not in the number of cases of malaria as determined during daily surveillance at the child's home, when children in malaria endemic areas were provided with supplemental zinc.

Mortality Given the contribution of zinc deficiency to three of the most common causes of death among children in developing countries (i.e., diarrhea, pneumonia, and malaria) it can be expected that zinc deficiency also contributes substantially to childhood mortality among these populations. Although still limited, available information

does suggest that supplemental zinc leads to sizeable reductions in mortality among vulnerable groups of children. In Bangladesh, evaluation of a program that provided supplemental zinc for 14 days as treatment for diarrhea demonstrated a 68% reduction in mortality among infants and preschool children. Mortality was also reduced by two-thirds following supplemental zinc among low-birth-weight infants in India. A nearly 60% reduction in child mortality was observed among children in Burkina Faso, although this was not statistically significant. Further large-scale studies are required to better quantify the impact of zinc on child mortality.

Pregnancy: Maternal, Fetal and Infant Health

Few firm conclusions can be made as to the consequences of zinc deficiency during pregnancy on maternal, fetal, and infant health. Results from zinc supplementation trials have been inconsistent and therefore difficult to interpret. This may be partly attributed to inadequate study design or failure to consider the zinc status of the women studied. Most earlier studies focused on the evaluation of gestational age and birth weight as primary outcomes. However, zinc deficiency may also manifest itself in more specific qualities of health and development of the fetus and infant, as summarized in **Figure 1**. While there is some evidence from industrialized countries that zinc deficiency contributes to complications during pregnancy, delivery, and postpartum, these outcomes have not been adequately studied in developing countries.

Control of Zinc Deficiency in Developing Countries

Efforts to control zinc deficiency in national programs are only just being initiated. The following information describes the current state of development of zinc nutrition programs, and some direction for the future.

Zinc-Containing Pharmacological Supplements

As exemplified by the results of controlled trials, zinc supplementation is an efficacious (i.e., effective under controlled study conditions) strategy to prevent zinc deficiency. However, the effectiveness of this strategy under realistic conditions will depend on the success of in-country programs to distribute zinc supplements to vulnerable populations and on their use by the intended recipients. At present, few such zinc supplementation programs are in place. It may be more feasible to add zinc to iron

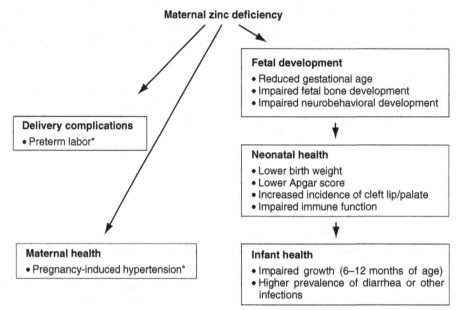

Figure 1 Several consequences of maternal zinc deficiency during pregnancy on maternal health, fetal development, and infant health have been observed in developing and more industrialized countries. These consequences have been confirmed by randomized, placebo-controlled trials of maternal zinc supplementation. Not all of the consequences have been observed in all studies, and the reasons for inconsistent results among studies are not well understood. *Determined from studies in industrialized countries only.

supplements, use of which is widely advocated for the prevention of iron deficiency anemia in young children and women of childbearing age. However, some evidence indicates that when these two minerals are combined, their ability to improve either zinc or iron status diminishes. The competitive interaction between iron and zinc at the level of intestinal absorption or post-absorption may explain this observation. Research is required to determine optimal supplementation schemes for the prevention of iron and zinc deficiencies simultaneously.

Given the recent recommendation for the use of zinc in the management of acute diarrhea and the resultant reduction of childhood mortality observed in one study to date, it is expected that diarrheal treatment programs including supplemental zinc will ensue.

Enrichment (Fortification) of Foods with Zinc

A few countries from developing regions have implemented a policy for the fortification of staple foods with zinc. Mexico established a program whereby wheat and corn (maize) flour producers could voluntarily add zinc to their products (20 mg/kg flour). Indonesia has also implemented a national program for the fortification of wheat flour, which includes addition of zinc. The fortification of condiments, such as fish sauce or seasoning powders in Asia, may serve as an additional vehicle for zinc fortification in the future. Several countries are adding zinc

(and other micronutrients) to foods that are distributed in programs targeted to specific, vulnerable population groups. For example, in Chile and Argentina milk powder for use by young children is fortified with zinc, while in Mexico a milk powder-based supplement with added zinc is directed towards young children as well as pregnant and lactating women. As yet, there is an absence of information on the effectiveness of these programs to improve population zinc status.

Modification of Foods and Diets

Several strategies apart from the use of pharmacological supplements and food fortification have been suggested for the improvement of dietary zinc intake in developing country settings. Cereal crops, such as wheat, corn, and rice, are being bred to contain higher concentrations of zinc in the grain portion. Cereals that have a reduced content of phytate have also been produced but still require further testing of their agricultural viability and effect on improving zinc status when used in the context of a usual diet. Promotion of the production and use of zinc-rich foods through community level education and provision of starter materials could also be used. The efficacy of most of these alternative strategies to improve population zinc status has not yet been tested.

See also: **Anemia**: Iron-Deficiency Anemia.
Supplementation: Dietary Supplements. **Vitamin A**:
Biochemistry and Physiological Role; Deficiency and
Interventions. **Zinc**: Physiology.

Further Reading

Black RE (2003) Zinc deficiency, infectious disease and mortality
in the developing world. *Journal of Nutrition* 133: 1485S–
1489S.
Brown KH, Peerson JM, Rivera J, and Allen LH (2002) Effect of
supplemental zinc on the growth and serum zinc concentrations of prepubertal children: a meta-analysis of randomized
controlled trials. *American Journal of Clinical Nutrition* 75:
1062–1071.
Brown KH and Wuehler SE (2000) *Zinc and Human Health:
Results of Recent Trials and Implications for Program Interventions and Research*. Ottawa: The Micronutrient Initiative/
International Development Research Center.
Brown KH, Wuehler SE, and Peerson JM (2001) The importance
of zinc in human nutrition and estimation of the global prevalence of zinc deficiency. *Food and Nutrition Bulletin* 22:
113–125.
Gibson RS (1994) Zinc nutrition in developing countries. *Nutrition Research Reviews* 7: 151–173.
Gibson RS and Ferguson EL (1998) Nutrition intervention strate-
gies to combat zinc deficiency in developing countries. *Nutri-
tion Research Reviews* 11: 115–131.
International Zinc Nutrition Consultative Group (Brown KH,
Rivera JA, Bhutta Z, Gibson RS, King JC, Ruel M, Sandström
B, Wasantwisut E, Hotz C, Lönnerdal B, Lopez de Romaña D,
and Peerson J) (2004) Assessment of the risk of zinc deficiency
in populations and options for its control. *Food and Nutrition
Bulletin* 25: S91–S202.
Osendarp SJM, West CE, and Black RE on behalf of the Maternal
Zinc Supplementation Study Group (2003) The need for
maternal zinc supplementation in developing countries: an
unresolved issue. *Journal of Nutrition* 133: 817S–827S.
Wood RJ (2000) Assessment of marginal zinc status in humans.
Journal of Nutrition 130: 1350S–1354S.
Zinc Investigators' Collaborative Group (Bhutta ZA, Black RE,
Brown KH, Meeks Gardner J, Gore S, Hidayat A, Khatun F,
Martorell R, Ninh NX, Penny ME, Rosado JL, Roy SK,
Ruel M, Sazawal S, and Shankar A) (1999) Prevention of
diarrhea and pneumonia by zinc supplementation in chil-
dren in developing countries: Pooled analysis of randomized
controlled trials. *Journal of Pediatrics* 135: 689–697.

Physiology

H C Freake, University of Connecticut, Storrs, CT,
USA

Introduction

Zinc is only moderately abundant in nature, ranking
23rd of the elements. Of the trace elements in the
body, it is second only to iron, but, in contrast to
iron, it has a single redox state. Together with its size
and charge characteristics, this has led to its widespread use in proteins of the body. The number of
zinc proteins is unknown but growing, and they
include numerous enzymes and many more nuclear
proteins that regulate gene expression. Further sets of
proteins are responsible for zinc homeostasis. The
binding sites and functions of zinc within some of
these proteins are well understood, but for others
these are less clear. In particular, the links between
the biochemical roles of zinc within proteins and its
physiological functions are often obscure. The range
of physiological functions of zinc is broad and can be
observed in all tissues of the body. In general, zinc is
required for DNA synthesis, cell division and growth,
for protein synthesis and macronutrient metabolism,
and for the development and appropriate function of
most body systems. The lack of an appropriate assessment tool makes it difficult to estimate the prevalence
of zinc deficiency, but undiagnosed marginal zinc
deficiency may be a concern.

The History of Zinc as a Nutrient

The essentiality of zinc for bacterial growth has been
known for almost 150 years. Later, it was shown to be
required by plants and then, in 1934, by rats. In the
succeeding years, the essentiality of zinc was demonstrated for other species. The fact that zinc is used
widely by plants and animals and is therefore reasonably widespread in the food supply led to the position
that human zinc deficiency was unlikely. It was not
until the early 1960s that Prasad and others in Iran
described a syndrome of dwarfism and lack of sexual
development in teenage boys and young adults. The
young Iranian men consumed a diet based on unlea-
vened bread with very little animal protein and also ate
large amounts of clay (geophagia). They were anemic
and responded to treatment with ferrous sulfate
coupled with a more balanced diet including animal
protein. The other symptoms also resolved, but it
seemed unlikely that lack of iron itself was responsible.
Prasad then moved to Egypt, where he encountered a
similar syndrome. His Egyptian patients were not geo-
phagic, but they ate mostly bread and beans and were
infested with *Schistosoma* and hookworm. Zinc deficiency was documented in these individuals, and treatment with zinc was more effective at increasing growth
rates than either iron supplementation or a diet including animal protein. Thus, dietary zinc deficiency was
demonstrated, presumably due to impaired absorption
because of the high fiber and phytate contents of the
diet. While severe zinc deficiency is not a frequent
problem in developed countries, the prevalence of
milder symptoms is unknown. In the USA, mild

symptoms of zinc deficiency have occasionally been reported (see below under Human Zinc Deficiency).

Chemistry of Zinc

The conjunction of the chemical properties of zinc underlies its biological significance. It is a relatively small ion (with an atomic number of 30) and carries a positive charge of two. It attracts electrons as a strong Lewis acid, and this property can be important in its catalytic functions. It has relatively flexible coordination geometry and, while binding its ligands with high affinity, exhibits rapid rates of exchange, which can facilitate chemical reactions and biological processes. All this is coupled with its single redox state, in contrast to the multiple redox states of iron and copper, which eliminates the danger of oxidative damage. While other trace elements may share some of these properties, none share them all. This is what makes zinc so valuable for protein structure and function.

Zinc in Foods

Zinc is associated with proteins in the body and is found associated with proteins in food. Thus, protein-rich foods tend to be good sources (**Table 1**). However, there is great variability, from egg whites, which have almost no zinc, to oysters, at 750 mg kg^{-1}. The physiological function of these high concentrations in oysters is unknown, though the zinc is concentrated in cells thought to serve a phagocytic/host defense function. In addition, the bioavailability of zinc may be quite variable, owing to other food components eaten at the same time.

Table 1 Dietary sources of zinc

Food	Zinc content (mg kg^{-1} raw weight)
Oysters	750
Beef, lean	59
Pork	26
Chicken breast	8
Chicken leg	18
Salmon	4
Egg, whole	11
Egg white	0.3
Milk, whole	4
Cheese, cheddar	31
Wheat, whole flour	29
Wheat, white flour	7
Rice, brown	20
Rice, polished	12
Kidney beans	27
Lentils	36
Potatoes	3
Broccoli	4
Apples	0.4

Grains and legumes may be relatively rich sources, but bioavailability is limited owing to their phytate content. On the other hand, animal proteins appear to enhance zinc absorption.

Control of Zinc Homeostasis

The size and charge characteristics of zinc mandate the use of carriers to traverse biological membranes. Two families of transporters have been described and partially characterized. The ZIP family (ZRT (zinc-regulated transporter)- and IRT (iron-regulated transporter)-related proteins, named after homologous transport proteins in yeast and plants) appears to move zinc into the cytoplasm of the cell, either from outside the cell or from subcellular compartments. The second group of transporters, the CDF (cation diffusion factor) family, is responsible for zinc egress from the cytoplasm. This latter family includes ZnT-1, which has been localized to plasma membranes and functions as a cellular efflux protein, and ZnT-2, which transports zinc into storage vesicles under conditions of high cellular zinc. Collectively, the ZIP and CDF proteins are likely to underlie the homeostatic control of zinc distribution around the body.

Zinc Absorption

The absorption, distribution, and excretion of zinc are shown in **Figure 1**. Overall, about 20–40% of

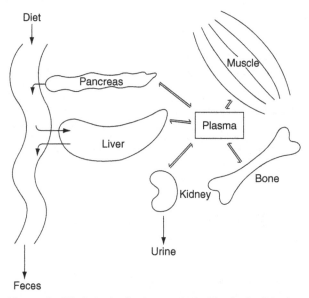

Figure 1 Whole-body zinc homeostasis. Zinc in the intestine comes from the diet and from endogenous secretions. A portion is absorbed, but much is lost in the feces, which are the major route of excretion. Absorbed zinc passes through the liver and then to the general circulation. Zinc is distributed throughout the body, with muscle and bone constituting the largest pools. A minor but controlled amount of zinc is lost in the urine.

consumed zinc is absorbed, depending on the bioavailability within the particular food source. Zinc is absorbed by both saturable and non-saturable processes, with the greatest rates of absorption occurring in the jejunum. Absorption is adjusted to meet needs, being proportionately increased in deficiency states and reduced when intake is high. Zinc status is reflected by the intestinal concentration of the zinc-binding protein metallothionein (MT). MT may trap zinc within the epithelial cells, causing it to be lost in feces as the cells are sloughed off. This may be part of the explanation of how zinc absorption is adjusted to meet needs. Acrodermatitis enteropathica is an autosomal recessive condition of zinc malabsorption, which can lead to severe deficiency. The gene alteration that leads to this condition has recently been identified in *ZIP4*, which encodes one of the zinc transporters. This protein has been localized to the apical membrane of intestinal epithelial cells and, given the severity of the symptoms associated with its inactivation, appears to be necessary for normal zinc absorption. The zinc efflux protein ZnT-1 is found at the basolateral membrane and probably promotes the passage of zinc out of the intestine. Acrodermatitis enteropathica can be treated with large doses of zinc, supporting the existence of paracellular transport at high intake levels. A large amount of zinc is secreted into the gut from the pancreas and intestine (**Figure 1**). Malabsorption syndromes can lead to a failure to reabsorb these endogenous secretions and, hence, to rapid loss of body zinc.

Transport and Distribution

The zinc pool in plasma is relatively small, representing only about 0.1% of total body zinc. It circulates bound to albumin and α-2-macroglobulin, and about 3% is complexed with amino-acids. About fivefold greater amounts of zinc are found in whole blood, with erythrocytes accounting for about 75% of the total. However, about 85% of erythrocyte zinc is complexed within carbonic anhydrase and therefore does not exchange easily. The egress of zinc from the circulation across endothelial cells and into tissues of the body is not well understood. Uptake in association with albumin has been suggested, but members of the ZIP family of transporters are likely to play a role here. The tissue distribution of zinc is relatively uniform. All cells require the mineral, and no cell stores it. The concentration of zinc in the adult human is about $0.5\,\mu\text{mol g}^{-1}$, giving a total body content of about 2 g. More than half is found in skeletal muscle, and about 30% is found in bone. The bone pool appears to be more labile than the muscle pool and has been used as an index of zinc status in experimental animals. The liver represents another labile pool. It receives dietary zinc from the portal circulation and contains about 5% of body zinc.

Excretion

Zinc is lost from the body primarily through the feces (**Figure 1**). Feces contain unabsorbed dietary zinc, zinc contained within intestinal epithelial cells that have been sloughed off, and endogenous zinc secretions into the gut from the pancreas, the gall bladder, and the cells lining the gastrointestinal tract. The endogenous secretions and the extent to which they are reabsorbed can be controlled and constitute an important homeostatic mechanism for regulating zinc status. Zinc losses in urine are relatively minor but do respond to extremes of intake to help maintain homeostasis. Shed skin cells, sweat, hair, menstrual blood, and semen are additional routes of loss.

Zinc Biochemistry

Zinc homeostasis and action involve an intimate association of the mineral with proteins. These proteins include membrane transporters responsible for the absorption of zinc in the gut and its passage into and out of cells and subcellular organelles, transport and delivery proteins (both in the circulation and within cells), sensing proteins that will adjust homeostasis and function according to zinc availability, and a large range of proteins to which zinc is ultimately delivered. Two major classes of these latter proteins are the enzymes and transcription factors. In addition to its association with proteins, zinc within cells is also found associated with membrane lipids and both DNA and RNA. The functions of these pools of zinc are not clear.

Homeostasis

The interaction of zinc with its transporters has not been well characterized, though transmembrane domains have been identified that are thought to be responsible for the transport function. Free concentrations of zinc within the cell appear to be extremely low and may not constitute a sufficient pool for the supply of zinc to its protein ligands. This suggests the existence of delivery proteins, and this role has been suggested for MT, which has been shown to transfer zinc to apoenzymes *in vitro*. MT was originally discovered as a cytoplasmic heavy-metal-binding protein, which was thought to prevent metal toxicity within cells. Additional more significant roles were suggested by the realization that there are multiple MT genes, which have been

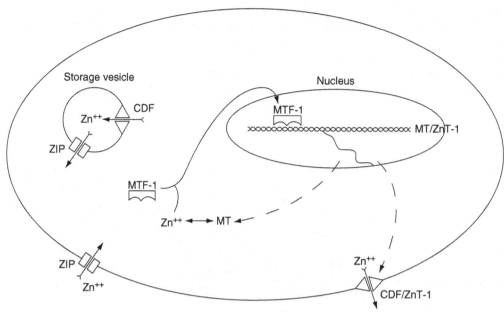

Figure 2 Cellular zinc homeostasis. Zinc is delivered to the cytoplasm from either the extracellular space or vesicles within the cell by members of the ZIP family of transporters. A rise in cellular zinc results in activation and nuclear translocation of MTF-1. In the nucleus, MTF-1 regulates the transcription of a set of target genes, including MT and ZnT-1. MT will bind zinc, and ZnT-1 will transport zinc out across the plasma membrane. MT may govern the delivery of zinc to other proteins within the cell. Other members of the CDF family transport zinc into vesicles.

conserved through evolution. It is a small protein that is unusually rich in cysteine and can bind seven atoms of zinc. MT may influence the subcellular distribution and availability of zinc, since its own distribution varies. For example, the nuclear content of MT varies with the cell cycle. MT expression is regulated not only by heavy metals but also by a range of other signals including glucocorticoids, interleukins, and cyclic adenosine monophosphate. In addition, its zinc-binding activity is influenced by the cellular redox state. For example, an increase in the glutathione disulfide–glutathione ratio results in the release of zinc from MT and thus an increase in its availability for other proteins. However, deletion of individual MT genes in mice has not resulted in major pathologies, questioning the significance of these proteins.

Investigation of the mechanism whereby zinc regulates the expression of MT led to the discovery of the single protein known to act as a zinc sensor within mammalian cells, MTF-1 (metal response element (MRE)-binding transcription factor-1). MTF-1 binds to MREs in the promoter region of MT and other genes and regulates their expression. The ability of MTF-1 to localize to the nucleus and bind to its target genes depends on its zinc content. Thus, an increase in cellular zinc levels results in greater MTF-1 activity and, consequently, increased expression of its target genes. In addition to MT, which will bind more zinc, these include ZnT-1,

which will transport zinc out of the cell. These mechanisms underlying cellular zinc homeostasis are illustrated in **Figure 2**.

Zinc Enzymes

The three-dimensional structures of more than 200 zinc-containing enzymes have now been characterized, and many more enzymes have been identified. All six International Union of Biochemistry classes are represented. Zinc enzymes can be divided into three groups according to the role played by zinc within the protein. In the catalytic group (e.g., carbonic anhydrase), zinc is a direct participant in the catalytic function of the enzyme. The zinc atom is coordinated by three amino-acids from the enzyme and a molecule of water at the active site. In enzymes with structural zinc sites (e.g., protein kinase C), the metal binds four amino-acids within the protein and ensures appropriate folding for bioactivity. Enzymes in which zinc serves a co-catalytic function (e.g., superoxide dismutase) contain two or three zinc atoms, two of which are coordinated by a shared amino-acid residue. Coordination sites are widely spaced on the protein, and the zinc may be used for both structural and catalytic functions. In addition to these three groups, zinc has also been found to serve a bridging function between two separate polypeptides to stabilize a biologically active larger

Table 2 Examples of mammalian zinc-dependent enzymes

Enzyme	Function
RNA polymerase	Transcription and synthesis of mRNA
Carboxypeptidase A	Protein digestion in the intestine
Protein kinase C	Signal transduction
Carbonic anhydrase	Respiration, buffering, and hydration of carbon dioxide
Cytochrome c oxidase	Respiration and electron transport chain
Alcohol dehydrogenase	Ethanol metabolism
Superoxide dismutase	Inactivation of free radicals
Nitric oxide synthase	Signalling and vasodilation
Angiotensin converting enzyme	Blood-pressure regulation and activation of angiotensinogen

complex (e.g., nitric oxide synthase). A selection of zinc enzymes is included in **Table 2**, which helps to illustrate the wide variety of metabolic functions requiring zinc.

Zinc Transcription Factors

There are many zinc enzymes, but there appear to be even more transcription factors that use zinc. These sites have all been identified in the last 20 years and have been less thoroughly investigated than the zinc enzymes. Variable numbers of zinc atoms are each coordinated by four cysteine/histidine residues to stabilize a DNA binding structure. A search of the human genome has revealed over 1000 genes (about 3% of those identified) containing these characteristic zinc finger domains. An important class of zinc finger transcription factors is the steroid/thyroid receptor superfamily, which is responsible for mediating the biological response to a wide range of hormonal and metabolic signals, including retinoic acid and vitamin D. These factors all have nine conserved cysteine residues in the DNA binding region, eight of which are coordinated by two atoms of zinc. Loss of zinc from these sites would interrupt biological function, but it is not clear that this ever happens in a physiological context. Recently, the new array technologies have been used to assess the genome-wide response to changing zinc availability in different tissues, including intestine, liver, and cells of the immune system. The gene products that have been identified as zinc sensitive by these approaches amount to about 5% of the expressed genes within a tissue. They do not necessarily encode zinc proteins themselves but rather proteins whose transcription is altered by zinc. MTF-1 is likely to mediate some but not all of these changes, and other transcription factors whose activity is dependent on zinc may soon be found.

Zinc Physiology

The enormous range of biochemical roles for zinc predicts a large number of physiological functions. The physiological roles of zinc may be further extended to include secondary effects mediated by altered food intake and effects on the functions of other nutrients. While the physiological roles for zinc are well described, it is important to note that the connections between the biochemistry and physiology of zinc remain unclear. Thus, in zinc deficiency the specific zinc-sensitive biochemical step leading to altered physiology is usually unknown. This disconnection will become apparent as the physiological roles of zinc are considered. The broad distribution of zinc through the body at the organ, cellular, and even protein levels suggests that the functions of most systems are dependent upon zinc. Its physiological roles become manifest in cases of deficiency, and that framework will be used to discuss the principal functions here.

Growth

The requirement of zinc for the growth of numerous organisms, ranging from bacteria to humans, is well established. Growth failure is a relatively early consequence of zinc deficiency in experimental animals. Given the lack of a zinc store, in the absence of a sufficient dietary supply zinc will be immediately unavailable for new tissue. Numerous processes seem to contribute to the growth failure. Experiments in animals have shown that zinc deficiency leads to a drop in food intake, though the use of control animals pair-fed an identical amount of a zinc-sufficient diet demonstrates a clear role for a lack of zinc beyond its effects on feeding behavior. The endocrine system is involved with multiple effects of zinc deficiency on the somatotrophic axis, notably a reduction in circulating concentrations of insulin-like growth factor 1 (IGF-1). Again, this appears to be only part of the story since force-feeding a zinc-deficient diet and administering exogenous IGF-1 both fail to correct the growth failure caused by zinc deficiency. Growth of cultured cells is dependent on media zinc. DNA synthesis is interrupted. Production of thymidine kinase mRNA is diminished by the removal of zinc, but again this appears to be only a partial explanation. The IGF-1 signalling pathway within cells also seems to be affected. Zinc is also required for wound healing, presumably owing to related processes.

Immune Function

The immune system appears to be particularly sensitive to zinc deficiency, in comparison with the rest of the body. Lymphopenia and thymic atrophy are observed, and both cell-mediated and antibody-mediated responses are reduced. As with growth, multiple mechanisms appear to be at play. In addition to its generalized effects on DNA synthesis, zinc deficiency appears to induce apoptosis, resulting in a loss of B-cell and T-cell precursors within the bone marrow. Thymulin is a zinc-dependent enzyme that stimulates the development of T cells within the thymus. The production of cytokines by mononuclear cells is also reduced by zinc deficiency. It appears likely that these effects can be of clinical significance. Infections occur more frequently in individuals with acrodermatitis enteropathica, and reduced immune function is accompanied by zinc deficiency in several other conditions, including sickle-cell anemia and various gastrointestinal disorders. In the USA, zinc lozenges have become popular as a treatment for the common cold. Results from controlled trials of this treatment have been variable, but a shortening of cold duration may occur. It would appear reasonable to suppose that treatment effectiveness would depend on initial zinc status, with greater success being seen in individuals with marginal undetected zinc deficiency.

Reproduction

The original description of zinc deficiency in humans included lack of pubertal development. Spermatogenesis is a zinc-dependent process. Seminal fluid is particularly rich in zinc, and the sperm appear to accumulate zinc from this source prior to ejaculation. Zinc is also crucial for normal fetal development, and deficiency leads to abnormalities in humans and animals. Maternal zinc deficiency has been linked with pregnancy-associated morbidity, including pre-term delivery.

Nervous System

The brain is one of the sites that has been shown to be particularly sensitive to zinc deficiency during fetal development, with neural-tube defects and other disorders being found. While this work was performed in animals, a similar relationship appears likely in humans. Zinc is distributed throughout the brain, but greater concentrations are found within the hippocampus. Here, a brain-specific transporter, ZnT-3, concentrates zinc in vesicles within glutamatergic neurones. It is co-secreted with the neurotransmitter and appears to serve as a modulator of neurotransmission. Very high concentrations of zinc ($>100\,\mu M$) are found within the synaptic cleft during this process. In addition, brain injury resulting from ischemia or trauma causes the release of massive amounts of zinc, which is thought to be responsible for the resultant cell death.

Antioxidant Defense System

Although zinc is not itself an antioxidant, there are several ways in which it participates in the antioxidant defense system of the body, with important implications for health. It can bind to thiol groups in proteins, making them less susceptible to oxidation. By displacing redox-reactive metals such as iron and copper from both proteins and lipids it can reduce the metal-induced formation of hydroxyl radicals and thus protect the macromolecules. Its role in inducing MT has already been mentioned, and this protein scavenges hydroxyl radicals. Increased oxidative stress results in the release of zinc from MT, presumably making it more available for other proteins. Copper/zinc superoxide dismutase is an important zinc-containing antioxidant enzyme whose activity is impaired in the deficient state. In general, animal studies have revealed an association between zinc deficiency and increased oxidative stress. The likelihood of increased oxidative stress under conditions of zinc deficiency suggests a potential anticarcinogenic role for this mineral. This connection is further supported by the finding that the tumor suppressor gene p53, which is frequently mutated in human cancers, is a zinc-containing transcription factor whose expression is also dependent on zinc.

Macronutrient Metabolism

Many of the enzymes of intermediary metabolism contain zinc, and deficiency affects all macronutrients. Protein synthesis and DNA and RNA synthesis require zinc. Insulin is secreted from the pancreas and circulates in association with zinc. This secretion is diminished under conditions of zinc deficiency, leading to impaired glucose metabolism. Lipid metabolism is also affected, with zinc deficiency being associated with reductions in circulating high-density lipoproteins.

Human Zinc Deficiency

In addition to dietary inadequacy, there are several routes that lead to zinc deficiency. Acrodermatitis enteropathica, the genetic disorder of zinc malabsorption, has already been mentioned. Other, more generalized, malabsorption syndromes (e.g., coeliac disease) can also lead to zinc deficiency. Deficiency has also resulted from inappropriate intravenous feeding and the use of chelation therapy. Children are likely to be particularly at risk of zinc deficiency, because of its involvement in growth.

Mild

Given the difficulty of assessing marginal impairments in zinc status, the effects of deficiency can often be verified only by a response to treatment. Growth provides a good example of this. Children in Denver, Colorado, who were of low height for their age increased their growth rates in response to zinc supplementation, whereas zinc had no effect in children of normal height. In addition to improved growth, improvements in immune function, taste and smell acuity, and reproductive function have been noted with zinc supplementation.

Severe

Severe human zinc deficiency has been well characterized by the original descriptions in the Middle East and in patients with acrodermatitis enteropathica. The symptoms of mild deficiency are continued and exaggerated. Thus, stunting can be extreme and is accompanied by delayed sexual maturation and impotence. Characteristic skin lesions are found, originating around the mouth and nose but becoming widespread as deficiency develops. Diarrhea is also present. Deficits in taste and smell are accompanied by anorexia and other behavioral changes, including increased irritability and impaired cognitive function. Eye pathologies similar to those seen in vitamin A deficiency are observed.

Zinc Toxicity

Toxicity of zinc from food sources has not been reported and seems unlikely since absorption is homeostatically regulated. Acute gastrointestinal symptoms and headaches have been reported after ingestion of amounts about 10–20-fold higher than the recommended intakes. Chronic ingestion of these large amounts has been shown to impair immune response and lipoprotein metabolism. However, the key danger of excessive zinc intake is reduced copper status. This is probably due to a zinc-induced blockage of copper absorption and in fact is clinically useful in individuals with Wilson's disease, a condition of copper toxicity. In the USA, an upper limit of $40 \, \text{mg day}^{-1}$ has been set for adults, because of the threat to copper status. The popularity of zinc lozenges for treatment of the common cold could lead to this intake being exceeded. Thus, the use of these treatments should be of limited duration.

Assessment

The prevalence of marginal zinc deficiency in human populations is unknown because of the lack of a good means of assessing zinc status. Measurement of plasma zinc is straightforward, but it does not serve as a reliable indicator of zinc status. Plasma zinc is a quantitatively minor pool that can be easily influenced by minor shifts in tissue zinc. Plasma concentrations do not fall with decreasing dietary intake, except at very low intakes. Plasma zinc can also be affected by factors unrelated to zinc status (e.g., time of day, stress, and infection). Cellular components of blood can be assayed, but erythrocyte concentrations of zinc are maintained in deficient states and variable results have been found with leucocytes. Hair zinc concentrations may reflect available zinc but will also depend on the rate of hair growth.

Several different zinc-dependent enzymes have been investigated as potential markers of zinc status, but none have proved reliable. MT in blood cells has been suggested as a useful indicator of zinc status, assayed at either the protein or the mRNA level. MT expression is likely to be regulated by factors other than zinc and therefore may lack the specificity required of a good indicator. The gene-array approaches that have recently been used to determine the global effects of zinc deficiency within a tissue would appear to offer hope for the identification of an appropriate functional marker of zinc status.

Recommended Intakes

In the absence of a reliable index of zinc status, both the US Food and Nutrition Board and the Food and Agriculture Organization (FAO)/World Health Organization (WHO) Expert Committee used the factorial approach to estimate human zinc requirements. As shown in **Table 3**, the FAO/WHO give three sets of recommendations, depending on the zinc bioavailability of the diet. The US Food and Nutrition Board figures fall between those given for moderate- and low-availability diets. Both groups also set upper limits for intake, based largely on the risk of impairing copper status. These values are similar (40 mg for the US Food and Nutrition Board, 45 mg for FAO/WHO, for adults).

Table 3 Recommended intakes of zinc

Age group		US–Canadian recommended dietary allowance	FAO/WHO reference nutrient intake Bioavailability		
			High	Moderate	Low
Children (1–3 years old)		3	2.4	4.1	8.3
Adolescents (14–18 years old)	Female	9	4.3	7.2	14.4
	Male	11	5.1	8.6	17.1
Adults (>19 years old)	Female	8	3.0	4.9	9.8
	Male	11	4.2	7.0	14.0
Pregnant women	Third trimester	11	6.0	10.0	20.0
Lactating women	0–3 months	12	5.8	9.5	19.0

See also: **Antioxidants**: Diet and Antioxidant Defense; Observational Studies; Intervention Studies. **Copper**.

Further Reading

Andrews GK (2001) Cellular zinc sensors: MTF-1 regulation of gene expression. *Biometals* **14**: 223–237.

Cousins RJ, Blanchard RK, Moore JB *et al.* (2003) Regulation of zinc metabolism and genomic outcomes. *Journal of Nutrition* **133**(5S-1): 1521S–1526S.

FAO/WHO (2002) *Human Vitamin and Mineral Requirements*. Report of a joint FAO/WHO expert consultation, Bangkok, Thailand, pp. 257–270. Rome: Food and Nutrition Division of the Food and Agriculture Organization.

Gaither LA and Eide DJ (2001) Eukaryotic zinc transporters and their regulation. *Biometals* **14**: 251–270.

Institute of Medicine (2001) Dietary reference intakes for vitamin A, vitamin K, arsenic, boron, chromium, copper, iodine, iron, manganese, molybdenum, nickel, silicon, vanadium and zinc. pp. 442–501. Washington, DC: National Academy Press.

MacDonald RS (2000) The role of zinc in growth and cell proliferation. *Journal of Nutrition* **130**(5S): 1500S–1508S.

Maret W (2001) Zinc biochemistry, physiology, and homeostasis – recent insights and current trends. *Biometals* **14**: 187–190.

Mills CF (ed.) (1989) *Zinc in Human Biology*. London: Springer-Verlag.

Prasad AS (1991) Discovery of human zinc deficiency and studies in an experimental human model. *American Journal of Clinical Nutrition* **53**: 403–412.

Vallee BL and Falchuk KH (1993) The biochemical basis of zinc physiology. *Physiological Reviews* **73**: 79–118.

INDEX

Printed in the United States
By Bookmasters